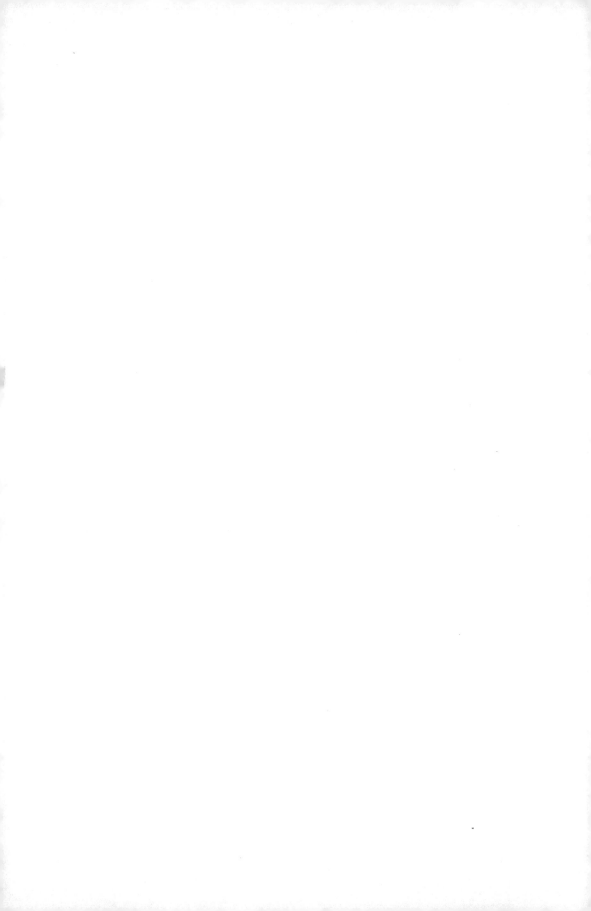

Hereditary Tumors

Edited by
Heike Allgayer, Helga Rehder
and Simone Fulda

Related Titles

R. A. Meyers (Ed.)

Cancer

From Mechanisms to Therapeutic
Approaches

2007
ISBN: 978-3-527-31768-4

K.-M., Debatin, S. Fulda (Eds.)

**Apoptosis and Cancer
Therapy**

From Cutting-edge Science to Novel
Therapeutic Concepts

2006
ISBN: 978-3-527-31237-5

H. zur Hausen

**Infections Causing Human
Cancer**

2006
ISBN: 978-3-527-31056-2

M. S. A. Tuffaha

**Phenotypic and Genotypic
Diagnosis of Malignancies**

An Immunohistochemical and
Molecular Approach

2008
ISBN: 978-3-527-31881-0

C. S. S. R. Kumar (Ed.)

**Nanomaterials for Cancer
Diagnosis**

2007
ISBN: 978-3-527-31387-7

C. S. S. R. Kumar (Ed.)

**Nanomaterials for Cancer
Therapy**

2006
ISBN: 978-3-527-31386-0

Hereditary Tumors

From Genes to Clinical Consequences

Edited by
Heike Allgayer, Helga Rehder,
and Simone Fulda

WILEY-BLACKWELL

WILEY-VCH Verlag GmbH & Co. KGaA

The Editors

Prof. Dr. Heike Allgayer, PhD
University of Heidelberg
and DKFZ (German Cancer Research Center)
Heidelberg
Medical Faculty Mannheim
Theodor-Kutzer-Ufer 1–3
68167 Mannheim
Germany

Prof. Dr. Helga Rehder
Medical University Vienna
Department of Medical Genetics
Währinger Strasse 10
1090 Wien
Austria

Prof. Dr. Simone Fulda
Ulm University Children's Hospital
Eythstrasse 24
89075 Ulm
Germany

Library of Congress Card No.: applied for

British Library Cataloguing-in-Publication Data
A catalogue record for this book is available from the British Library.

Bibliographic information published by the Deutsche Nationalbibliothek
The Deutsche Nationalbibliothek lists this publication in the Deutsche Nationalbibliografie; detailed bibliographic data are available on the Internet at http://dnb.d-nb.de.

© 2009 WILEY-VCH Verlag GmbH & Co. KGaA, Weinheim

Typesetting SNP Best-set Typesetter Ltd., Hong Kong
Printing Strauss GmbH, Mörlenbach
Binding Litges & Dopf GmbH, Heppenheim

Printed in the Federal Republic of Germany
Printed on acid-free paper

ISBN: 978-3-527-32028-8

Foreword

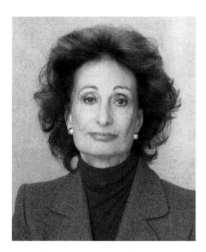 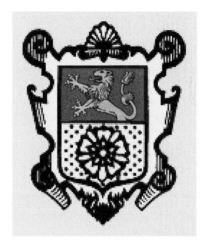

This book will be published in the fourteenth year of the IzS Foundation – a great pleasure for me!

The beginnings of the Foundation in the early 1990s were really not that easy. One group of people maintained that if women are to be supported, then they should be the unemployed, the sick, or mothers with children. If those to be supported must be academic women, then at least they should be the ones with problems, for whatever reason. Another group asserted that an award can only be given to someone dedicated to gender equality, women's rights, or similar issues.

In my opinion, support is already available for the aforementioned groups – perhaps not enough, but, after all, there is a large social network. Officials charged with ensuring women's rights are certainly necessary to implement existing laws but, I think, they are not essential. Hopefully, the need for these officials will soon disappear – because who among us wants to be a "token woman"?

What is really important is to permit women to employ their intellectual potential positively, so that they receive encouragement and support on their often

Hereditary Tumors: From Genes to Clinical Consequences
Edited by Heike Allgayer, Helga Rehder and Simone Fulda
Copyright © 2009 WILEY-VCH Verlag GmbH & Co. KGaA, Weinheim
ISBN: 978-3-527-32028-8

thorny path – support in terms of saying "you are great, don't be deterred, and stay on your course!".

I would like to repeat three statements I once gave as the Founder of the IzS Foundation:

- We support the intellectual elite of women, so that they do stay at their work and don't go back to the kitchen for ever.
- A person who supports the intellectual elite also supports others – indirectly, but perhaps more efficiently.
- We support the status of women not via a bottom-up approach, but by raising standards.

These are the reasons why the IzS scientific awards were created. They certainly are a financial stimulus, but it is much more important to publicly highlight these excellent scientific women!

In order to achieve these aims and ensure their effective endurance, we stimulate an efficient, interdisciplinary network among the recipients. For this reason, the IzS Foundation has initiated the IzS Fellowship to include all our award recipients, with the central aim that they support and coach one another.

This includes, but is not restricted to, informal regular e-mail and telephone contacts, meetings on the occasion of the annual award ceremony organized by the Foundation Board, and additional seminars about important career issues. For example, the last Fellowship seminar was held on "Contact with the Media."

At present, the members of the Fellowship are ten recipients of the Medical Research Award, two co-opted members, and two honorary members. The ten Award recipients are Babette Simon (Full Professor and Vice President, Marburg University, Germany), Barbara Rehermann (Full Professor, NIH, Frederick, USA), Rita Schmutzler (Full Professor, University of Cologne, Germany), Claudia Frank (Associate Professor, now in own practice), Simone Fulda (Full Professor, University of Ulm, Germany), Heike Allgayer (Full Professor, University and German Cancer Research Center Heidelberg, Germany), Carola Berking (Associate Professor, Ludwig Maximilians University Munich, Germany), Silke Anders (Medical Research Associate and Guest Scientist, University of Luebeck and Bernstein Center for Computational Neuroscience, Berlin, Germany), Rohini Kuner (Full Professor, University of Heidelberg, Germany), and Henriette Löffler-Stastka (Full Professor, University of Vienna, Austria). Further members of the Fellowship are Isabel Mundry (composer, Full Professor), Shi-Yeon Sung (musical conductor), Natalie Clein, Kaori Yamagami, and Eun Sung Hong (cellists), as the winners of the Music/Culture Award. With increasing interactions between all Fellows, we find striking similarities in career mechanisms and obstacles. In 2008, Dr Rafaela Hillerbrand (University of Oxford, UK) also joined the Fellowship as the first basic scientist to win the new IzS Basic Research and Informatics Award.

Two awards for promoting human rights have been given:

- In 2002 to "Forward Germany" e.V., working against female gender mutilation in Germany,
- In 2007 to Seyran Ates, German–Turkish lawyer, living in Berlin, for her work to improve the situation of Muslim women in Germany.

We are on the way!

I congratulate the IzS Fellows who created this book on the increasingly important topic of Hereditary Tumors, collaborating with a significant majority of female authors as experts in the respective fields – but certainly equally acknowledging the expertise of their male colleagues and authors. I thank all of them sincerely, above all Heike Allgayer for this outstanding work!

Let us go forward together to improve the status of women!

Dr med. Ingrid Gräfin zu Solms-Wildenfels
Founder and Donor, the Ingrid zu Solms-(IzS)-Foundation
A foundation dedicated to the support of the female intellectual
elite in science, culture, and to ensuring human rights

Frankfurt, Germany, January 14, 2008

Preface

Due to recent rapid advances in genomics, there has been an enormous progress over the last years in our understanding of hereditary and familial tumors and cancer syndromes. It is now well appreciated that hereditary conditions, such as germline mutations or polymorphisms, may have an important impact on tumorigenesis and tumor progression in humans. Also, the genetic composition may substantially impinge on the individual response to cancer therapy. However, we were surprised to learn that no comprehensive book so far compiles these tremendous achievements into an overall and state-of the art picture of hereditary and familial tumors. In response to this demand, the objective of this book is to give the latest and updated overview on the existing knowledge on hereditary aspects of human cancers, to elucidate their molecular mechanisms, to discuss the diagnostic potential of genetic changes, and to summarize cutting-edge developments in disease management and treatment of hereditary tumors and cancer syndromes.

The structure of the book provides a first general section outlining essential mechanisms relevant for tumorigenesis, progression and metastasis, and specific molecular events contributing to hereditary tumor diseases. In a second section, overviews on the syndromal types of hereditary tumors are given, followed by a specific section in which hereditary tumor conditions are discussed for specific organs and sites. Finally, a last section provides general thoughts, trends and examples for genetic counseling, psycho-oncology, and molecular targeted therapy. By providing a framework on how our knowledge on genetic causes of hereditary tumors can be translated into clinical application, we believe that the book will be of interest to a broad readership, including geneticists, oncologists, pathologists, molecular and cell biologists, and those working in pharmaceutical and biotechnological industries.

Frankfurt/Main, Mannheim/Heidelberg,
Ulm, Vienna, October 2008

Heike Allgayer, Simone Fulda,
Helga Rehder, and the Fellowship
of the Ingrid zu Solms-Foundation

Hereditary Tumors: From Genes to Clinical Consequences
Edited by Heike Allgayer, Helga Rehder and Simone Fulda
Copyright © 2009 WILEY-VCH Verlag GmbH & Co. KGaA, Weinheim
ISBN: 978-3-527-32028-8

Contents

List of Contributors

Heike Allgayer*
University of Heidelberg
and DKFZ (German Cancer
Research Center) Heidelberg
Medical Faculty Mannheim
Chair of Experimental Surgery
Theodor-Kutzer-Ufer 1–3
68167 Mannheim
Germany

Carola Berking*
Ludwig-Maximilians-Universität
München
Klinik und Poliklinik für
Dermatologie und Allergologie
Frauenlobstrasse 9–11
80337 München
Germany

Anja Katrin Bosserhoff
University of Regensburg
Institute of Pathology
Molecular Pathology
Franz-Josef-Strauss-Allee 11
93053 Regensburg
Germany

Krystyna H. Chrzanowska
The Children's Memorial Health
Institute
Department of Medical Genetics
Al. Dzieci Polskich 20
04-736 Warsaw
Poland

Sarah Danson
University of Sheffield
Academic Department of Clinical
Oncology
Cancer Research Centre
Weston Park Hospital
Whitham Road
Sheffield, S10 2SJ
United Kingdom

Maria Debiec-Rychter
Catholic University of Leuven
Center for Human Genetics
Herestraat 49
3000 Leuven
Belgium

Martin Digweed
Charité-Universitätsmedizin Berlin
Institut für Humangenetik
Augustenburger Platz 1
13353 Berlin
Germany

*indicates a fellow and awardee of the Ingrid zu Solms-Foundation.

Hereditary Tumors: From Genes to Clinical Consequences
Edited by Heike Allgayer, Helga Rehder and Simone Fulda
Copyright © 2009 WILEY-VCH Verlag GmbH & Co. KGaA, Weinheim
ISBN: 978-3-527-32028-8

Helen Dimaras
The Division of Hematology/
Oncology
The Hospital for Sick Children
Room 7260
555 University Ave
Toronto, Ontario M5G 1X8
Canada

Steffen Emmert
Georg-August-University of
Göttingen
Department of Dermatology
and Venerology
von-Siebold-Strasse 3
37075 Göttingen
Germany

Christa Fonatsch
Medical University Vienna
Department of Medical Genetics
Währinger Strasse 10
1090 Vienna
Austria

Waltraut Friedl
University of Bonn
Institute of Human Genetics
Wilhelmstrasse 31
53111 Bonn
Germany

Simone Fulda*
Ulm University
Children's Hospital
Eythstrasse 24
89075 Ulm
Germany

Dorothea Gadzicki
Hannover Medical School
Institute of Cell and Molecular
Pathology
Carl-Neuberg-Strasse 1
30625 Hannover
Germany

Brenda L. Gallie
University of Toronto
University Health Network
Department of Applied Molecular
Oncology
Princess Margaret Hospital/Ontario
Cancer Institute
610 University Avenue
Toronto, Ontario M5G 2M9
Canada

Gabriele Gillessen-Kaesbach
Universitätsklinikum
Schleswig-Holstein
Institut für Humangenetik Lübeck
Ratzeburger Allee 160
23538 Lübeck
Germany

Nils Habbe
Philipps-Universität Marburg
Universitätsklinikum Gießen
und Marburg
Baldingerstrasse
35033 Marburg
Germany

Nicoline Hoogerbrugge
Radboud University Nijmegen
Medical Centre
849 Human Genetics
Postbox 9101
6500 HB Nijmegen
The Netherlands

Hildegard Kehrer-Sawatzki
University of Ulm
Institute of Human Genetics
Albert-Einstein-Allee 11
89081 Ulm
Germany

Gisela Keller
Technische Universität München
Institut für Pathologie
Trogerstrasse 18
81675 München
Germany

Marion Kiechle
Technical University of Munich
Clinic for Gynecology and
Obstetrics
Klinikum Rechts der Isar
Ismaningerstrasse 22
81675 Munich
Germany

Eric Legius
Catholic University of Leuven
Centre for Human Genetics
Herestraat 49
3000 Leuven
Belgium

Christine Marosi
Medizinische Universität Wien
Allgemeines Krankenhaus
Klinische Abteilung für
Onkologie
Währinger Gürtel 18–20
1090 Vienna
Austria

Gabriela Möslein
St. Josefs Hospital Bochum-Linden
(Helios)
Department of Visceral Surgery
Coloproctology
Axtstrasse 35
44879 Bochum
Germany

Mechthild Neises
Medical School Hannover
Pychosomatic Gynecology
Clinic Psychosomatic and
Psychotherapy
Carl-Neuberg-Strasse 1
30625 Hannover
Germany

Sabine J. Presser
Charité Campus Virchow-Klinikum
Klinik für Allgemein-, Viszeral- und
Transplantationschirurgie
Augustenburger Platz 1
13353 Berlin
Germany

Helga Rehder*
Medical University Vienna
Department of Medical Genetics
Währinger Strasse 10
1090 Vienna
Austria

Brigitte Royer-Pokora
Heinrich-Heine-University
Institute for Human Genetics
and Anthropology
Moorenstrasse 5
40225 Düsseldorf
Germany

Brigitte Schlegelberger
Hannover Medical School
Institute of Cell and Molecular
Pathology
Carl-Neuberg-Strasse 1
30625 Hannover
Germany

Rita Katharina Schmutzler*
University Hospital Cologne
Center for Hereditary Breast and
Ovarian Cancer
Department of Obstetrics and
Gynecology
Kerpener Strasse 34
50931 Cologne
Germany

Eva Seemanova
Charles University Hospital
Department of Clinical Genetics
Vúvalu 84
15018 Praha
Czechia

Babette Simon*
Philipps-Universität Marburg
Universitätsklinikum Gießen
und Marburg
Baldingerstrasse
35033 Marburg
Germany

Karl Sperling
Charité-Universitätsmedizin
Berlin
Institut für Humangenetik
Augustenburger Platz 1
13353 Berlin
Germany

Liesbeth Spruijt
Radboud University Nijmegen Medical
Centre
849 Human Genetics
Postbox 9101
6500 HB Nijmegen
The Netherlands

Ortrud K. Steinlein*
Ludwig Maximilians University
of Munich
University Hospital
Institute of Human Genetics
Goethestrasse 29
80336 Munich
Germany

M Dawn Teare
University of Sheffield
Mathematical Modelling and
Genetic Epidemiology
The Medical School
Beech Hill Road
Sheffield, S10 2RX
United Kingdom

Holger Vogelsang
Klinikum Garmisch-Partenkirchen
Abteilung für Allgemein-, Viszeral-,
Thorax-, Gefäss- und endokrine
Chirurgie
Auenstrasse 6
82467 Garmisch-Partenkirchen
Germany

Stefanie Vogt
University of Bonn
Institute of Human Genetics
Wilhelmstrasse 31
53111 Bonn
Germany

Raphaela Waidelich
University of Munich
Department of Urology
Marchioninistrasse 15
81377 Munich
Germany

Eva Wardelmann
Universitätsklinikum Bonn
Institut für Pathologie
Sigmund-Freud-Strasse 25
53127 Bonn
Germany

Theresia Weber
University Hospital Ulm
Department of Surgery
Steinhoevelstrasse 9
89075 Ulm
Germany

Katharina Wimmer
Medical University Vienna
Department of Medical Genetics
Währinger Straße 10
1090 Vienna
Austria

Penella Woll
University of Sheffield
Academic Department of
Clinical Oncology
Cancer Research Centre
Weston Park Hospital
Whitham Road
Sheffield, S10 2SJ
United Kingdom

Barbara Wollenberg
Universitätsklinikum
Schleswig-Holstein
Campus Lübeck
Klinik für Hals-Nasen-Ohren-
Heilkunde
Ratzeburger Allee 160
23538 Lübeck
Germany

Part I
Hereditary Tumors – General Aspects

1
General Insights Into Tumor Invasion, Progression, and Metastasis

Heike Allgayer

Summary

Invasion, progression, and metastasis are the hallmarks of malignant tumors, regardless of potentially hereditary compounds. Therefore, this introductory chapter will give a general overview of the major steps of the metastatic cascade, outline major phenomena contributing to metastasis, and introduce major molecules promoting these processes. Finally, current preliminary knowledge on potentially hereditary aspects of these molecules will be briefly discussed. However, this particular aspect is in desperate need of extensive further investigation.

1.1
The Metastatic Cascade

One of the hallmarks of malignant tumors, as opposed to benign tumors or physiological processes such as embryogenesis and wound healing, is an uncontrolled destruction of surrounding tissue (invasion), and the formation of destructive metastases. Tumor recurrence and metastasis are certainly the major limiting issues as to life expectancy of patients with malignant tumors, and certainly they represent the most pressing problem to any clinician treating cancer patients. Therefore, a description of the major steps of the metastatic cascade and major molecular events promoting metastasis are included in the general introduction of the present book.

The metastatic cascade occurs via five decisive major steps:
1. Local invasion
2. Intravasation
3. Dissemination
4. Extravasation, and finally
5. Establishment of distant metastasis (Figure 1.1)

The initial step of *local invasion* involves several molecular processes such as the loss in cell–cell adhesion and also cell–matrix adhesion, which often is accompa-

Hereditary Tumors: From Genes to Clinical Consequences
Edited by Heike Allgayer, Helga Rehder and Simone Fulda
Copyright © 2009 WILEY-VCH Verlag GmbH & Co. KGaA, Weinheim
ISBN: 978-3-527-32028-8

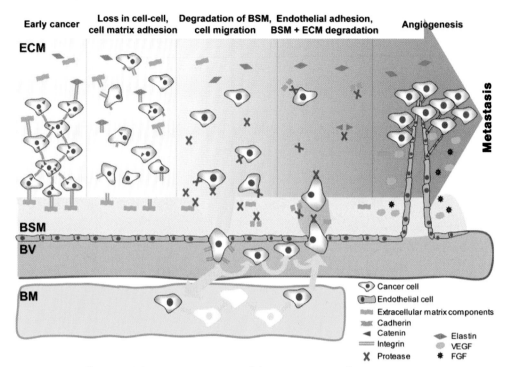

Figure 1.1 Schematic representation of the metastatic cascade. ECM, extracellular matrix; BSM, basement membrane; BV, blood vessel; BM, bone marrow. (Figure cited from [1]).

nied by a downregulation of diverse adhesion molecules, an enhanced migratory potential of cancer cells, and an efficient and uncontrolled local destruction of components of the surrounding extracellular matrix such as proteoglycans, collagen IV, vitronectin, or laminin.

The second step of *intravasation* reflects the ability of tumor cells to invade lymph and especially blood vessels. This again is characterized by the ability of the tumor cells to specifically destroy components of the basement membrane of vessels, such as collagen IV or laminin, and to transmigrate through basement membranes and endothelial layers.

The ability of tumor cells to enter lymphatic or blood vessels is the prerequisite for the third step of metastasis, which is the systemic *dissemination* of tumor cells throughout the body. Increasing evidence suggests that, even in early stages of solid tumors, disseminated tumor cells can be found in lymph nodes as well as the bone marrow of cancer patients, both compartments potentially acting as a filter for spreading tumor cells (Figure 1.2) [2–5]. Disseminated tumor cells in lymph nodes and bone marrow have been detected in patients with various malignant diseases, such as breast, gastric, colon, and lung cancers [6–20]. How-

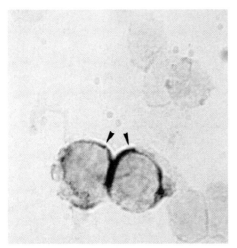

Figure 1.2 Disseminated tumor cells in the bone marrow of a patient with gastric cancer. Tumor cells have been detected with immunocytochemistry, using cytokeratin 18 as a marker (red). Arrows indicate an additional staining (black) for the invasion-related molecule u-PAR (see text). (Figure cited from [1]).

ever, since their prognostic relevance is still controversial, there is ongoing debate about the biological relevance of these cells. Increasing evidence suggests that certain phenotypic markers such as erb-B2, u-PAR, molecules of immune response, or proliferation markers, as well as long-term development of these cells over time after curative tumor resection of solid tumors, might indicate tumor cells critical for the development of a minimal residual disease component that might give rise to later tumor recurrences [5, 7, 21–23]. However, debate is still ongoing.

After systemic dissemination, the fourth step within the metastatic cascade is the *extravasation* of the tumor cell at the metastatic target site, which again involves transmigration through the endothelium as well as successful destruction of the basement membrane.

The fifth and final step, which is the *establishment of distant metastasis* at the target site, is probably the most complicated and involves several different molecular processes which need to interact successfully for metastasis establishment. Again, tumor cells need to destroy components of the extracellular matrix, be able to migrate at the metastatic site, and especially to divide, proliferate, and stimulate the generation of novel tumor vasculature providing them with nutrients and oxygen (neoangiogenesis). Therefore, a successful and complicated interaction between molecules of adhesion, migration, proteolysis and invasion, angiogenesis, cell growth, and proliferation is necessary to establish metastasis.

An additional important phenomenon to be discussed in the context of the metastatic cascade is the phenomenon of "dormancy". It has often been observed in tumor patients that tumor recurrence and metastasis do not occur immediately, but can occur even several years after curative resection of the primary tumor. There is increasing evidence that tumor cells can be kept in a quiescent state, most likely corresponding to a G0/G1-arrest, which enables tumor cells to survive in the body for several years. After being reactivated, these dormant cells might give rise to tumor recurrence and metastasis, even many years after curative tumor resection. The phenomenon of dormancy and especially the molecular and micro-environmental conditions inducing, or releasing cells from dormancy, are the subject of intense current investigations by several research groups [1].

In summary, the metastatic cascade consists of five major steps, which are brought about by the complex interplay between many different molecules. Still, however, the major molecules driving the metastatic cascade can be summarized as a few major molecular groups: (i) molecules of adhesion/migration; (ii) molecules of invasion, which in mainly represented by proteases; and (iii) molecules promoting angiogenesis, growth, and proliferation. Major molecules of these classes will be discussed below. However, it should be emphasized that one of the major hallmarks of successful metastasis in general is *interaction*.

First, there is intensive interaction between the different molecular groups involved in metastasis at the molecular level. For example, it is well-known that growth factor receptors or certain factors of angiogenesis, such as the VEGF/VEGF-R-family, via specific signaling cascades and transcription factors, can induce the expression of genes relevant for promoting tumor-associated proteolysis, migration, or invasion. On the other hand, as will be discussed below, certain invasion-related molecules are able to initiate signaling cascades, which again promote proliferation or angiogenesis, or can even provide molecular switches between tumor cell proliferation and dormancy (see Section 1.2.2.4). Furthermore, it is well-known that major signaling molecules such as K-Ras or c-Src, often found activated in tumors and especially in tumor metastasis, can induce the expression of several molecular classes related to metastasis, such as genes promoting proliferation, migration, and invasion [1].

Second, there is increasing evidence that invasion and metastasis most efficiently rely on complex interactions between tumor cells and surrounding stromal cells such as tumor-associated macrophages, endothelia, or fibroblasts [24–27]. Several studies indicate that, for example, receptors for tumor cell growth, angiogenesis, or invasion are being overexpressed by cancer cells, whereas the stimulating ligands, such as EGF, VEGFs, or u-PA are being recruited from the surrounding stroma. Therefore, cancer cell metastasis is an interactive process between different classes of molecules, cancer cells and their environment, and especially cancer cells and surrounding benign stromal cell types. This certainly is one of the explanations why, despite of the dangerous nature of processes leading towards metastasis, fortunately the process of metastasis is highly inefficient, and only a minority of primary tumor cells will finally succeed in establishing metastasis [28].

1.2
Key Molecules Promoting Metastasis

This chapter will briefly discuss major molecules and molecular classes contributing to metastasis. Since tumor-associated proteases and especially the u-PA-system have been shown to be major players in most steps of the metastatic cascade, there will be an emphasis on these. In general, we encourage the reader to consult specialist reviews and articles, to widen their knowledge on specific molecules.

1.2.1
Adhesion and Migration

The phenomena of adhesion and migration represent a complex interplay between components of the cytoskeleton, especially the actin cytoskeleton, molecules of cell–cell-adhesion, molecules of cell–matrix adhesion, specific subcellular molecular aggregations, such as focal adhesion contacts or desmosomes, and specific signaling cascades interacting with, or initiating them. For a complete overview of mechanisms of cell migration and adhesion, the reader should consult additional literature and specialized books, since a complete description of all molecules and phenomena in this context would exceed a single chapter. In the context of cancer and metastasis, however, a few molecules should be highlighted. Regarding cell–cell-adhesion, it has been shown that especially cadherins (in particular E-cadherin) are often downregulated in cancers, thus enhancing migration of tumor cells and supporting the transition of the epithelial tumor cell to a mesenchymal type (epithelial mesenchymal transition, EMT). Cadherins are transmembrane molecules that interact transcellularly with intracellular catenins, providing interactions with signaling molecules regulating, for example, the rearrangement of actin fibers, which contribute to major mechanisms of cell motility such as lamellipodia, fibropodia, or membrane ruffling. In this context, the adenomatous polyposis coli protein (APC), to be discussed later in the context of hereditary colorectal cancer, has been described as forming a complex with β-catenin in its wildtype form, inducing degradation of β-catenin. Major signaling molecules regulating actin rearrangement are Rho, Rac, and Cdc42, in addition to PI3K (phosphoinositide 3-kinase) [29, 30]. It has been shown that these signaling molecules are often activated in cancer, thus supporting phenomena related to cytoskeletal rearrangement, adhesion, and migration.

One of the major molecular classes of cell–matrix adhesion molecules highly relevant to cancer progression and metastasis is the class of integrins. Integrins are transmembraneous adhesion molecules presenting as heterodimers, consisting of one α-chain and one β-chain each. Currently, there are 16 known α- and 8 β-chains. Extracellular ligands for integrins are molecules of the extracellular matrix, such as vitronectin or laminin, whereas intracellular ligands, such as talin, enable connections to the actin cytoskeleton. Furthermore, integrins have been shown to activate signaling molecules, such as focal adhesion kinase (FAK), Src,

Ras, or mitogen-activated protein kinases (MAPK). Therefore, integrins are important adhesion molecules providing a link between the extracellular matrix and the cytoskeleton, at the same time promoting phenomena such as cytoskeletal reorganization, migration, but also cell proliferation and cell survival. It has been shown that integrins cluster in focal adhesion contacts, this again enhancing the expression of genes related to progression (e.g. EGF, FGF), apoptosis, the cell cycle, invasion, and angiogenesis (e.g. VEGFs). Certain integrins have been suggested to be related to cancer cells, or especially to endothelia found in tumor vessels (e.g. alpha-5beta1, alphavbeta3, alphavbeta5). Therefore, novel compounds targeting certain integrins potentially are attractive candidates for novel cancer therapeutics [31, 32].

1.2.2
Tumor-Associated Proteolysis and Invasion

As stated above, most of the specific steps of the metastatic cascade involve the degradation of extracellular matrix components, such as type IV collagen, laminin, vitronectin, proteoglycans, and others. This proteolytic degradation necessary for local invasion, intravasation, extravasation, and establishment of distant metastasis is accomplished by a series of tumor-associated proteases [33] which, by their proteolytic capacities, enable several different steps of the metastatic cascade (Figure 1.1) [34]. According to the catalytically active site of these proteases, they are classified into serine, aspartic, cysteine, threonine, and metalloproteinases (MMPs) [33]. The proteases are either secreted by the tumor cells, or by cells in the surrounding stromal compartment recruited by the tumor cells. These enzymes do not differ from the enzymes which are involved in several tissue remodeling processes such as wound healing, fibrinolysis, inflammation, embryogenesis, and angiogenesis [35–38]. In fact, the quantity rather than the quality of their expression contributes to the invasive phenotype of malignant cells [39].

One of the major molecular systems shown to be decisive for invasion and metastasis in many different cancer types is the urokinase- or u-PA-system. The u-PA-system consists of urokinase-type plasminogen activator (u-PA), the glyco-lipid-anchored receptor (u-PAR), the two serpin inhibitors plasminogen activator inhibitor-1 (PAI-1) and plasminogen activator inhibitor-2 (PAI-2), and nexin 1, which up to now has not been shown to play a major role.

1.2.2.1 u-PA
One of the best characterized "tumor-associated proteases" is the u-PA, which has been implicated in the invasive phenotype of tumor cells. u-PA is a serine protease with a molecular mass of 55 kDa. It is an important component in the fibrinolytic system converting plasminogen to an active enzyme, plasmin. Enhanced activity of plasmin promotes the degradation of extracellular matrix components including fibrin, fibronectin (FN), proteoglycans and, as the main molecules in basement membranes, laminin and collagen IV, in part by activating MMP-2/9 [38, 40, 41]. u-PA is produced as an inactive single-chain protein secreted from cells of the urogenital system, leukocytes, fibroblasts, and also tumor cells including breast, colon, ovary, gastric, cervix, endometrium, bladder, kidney, and brain tumor

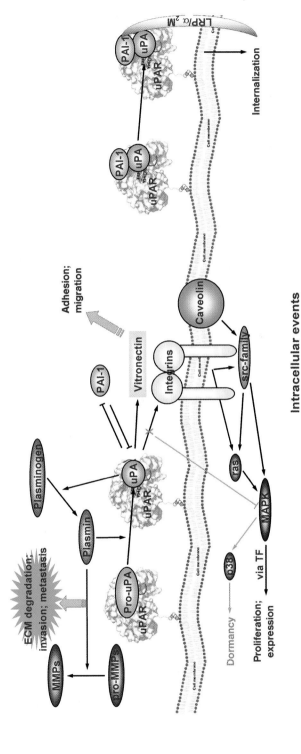

Figure 1.3 Functional properties of the urokinase receptor (u-PAR). The drawing of the molecular structure of u-PAR has been adapted from the crystal structure recently published [47]. (Figure cited from [63]).

tissues [38]. It is proteolytically activated either in the extracellular space or bound to the urokinase-receptor (u-PAR) [41, 42]. u-PA consists of two disulfide bridge-linked polypeptide chains, a C-terminal serine proteinase domain, and an N-terminal A-chain. It is released from the cells in the single-chain form (pro-u-PA). Plasmin can catalyze the conversion of pro-u-PA to the active two-chain-form u-PA, preferentially at the u-PA-receptor.

1.2.2.2 u-PAR

The 55–60 kDa heavily glycosylated, disulfide-linked cell surface receptor (u-PAR) binds both single-chain pro-u-PA and active two-chain u-PA [43, 44]. Binding of the A-chain of the active two-chain form of u-PA allows activation of ubiquitously available plasminogen and initiation of the proteolytic cascade by the catalytic B-chain [45]. The u-PAR consists of three similar repeats of approximately 90 residues each, the last of which is anchored to the cell membrane via glycosyl-phosphatidylinositol [46]. This GPI-anchor is hypothesized to enable high intra-membrane mobility [44, 46]. Furthermore, the u-PAR is glycosylated at N-residues of glucosamine and sialic acid within the binding site, thereby regulating its affinity (KD of 0.1–1.0 nM) for u-PA [46]. Receptor-bound u-PA, as compared to the fluid phase enzyme, activates plasminogen more efficiently, this being reflected by a 40-fold decrease in km of urokinase for its substrate [46]. Recently, the crystal structure of a soluble form of human u-PAR was reported. Based on the crystal structure of the u-PAR-peptide complex, a model of the human u-PA–u-PAR complex was constructed, revealing for the first time how the modular structure of u-PAR may guide u-PA-focused proteolysis at the cell surface, and control cell adhesion, migration, and invasion [47].

1.2.2.3 Plasminogen Activator Inhibitors

The two best known inhibitors for u-PA in the context of cancer are the glycoproteins plasminogen activator inhibitor-1 and -2 (PAI-1 and PAI-2, respectively), belonging to the gene family of serine protease inhibitors called serpins [48–50]. In the context of cancer, especially PAI-1 forms a complex with two-chain u-PA [51], and it has also been shown to form a reversible complex with single-chain u-PA [52]. Receptor-bound u-PA is inactivated by PAI-1 (-2), the trimeric complex u-PAR/u-PA/PAI is internalized into the cell together with a-2-macroglobulin receptor and its ligand [53–56], free u-PAR is recycled to the cell surface, and binding and activation of a second u-PA-molecule to the receptor can occur.

1.2.2.4 Evidence for Diverse Functions of the u-PAR System Relevant for Cancers

It has been shown that the u-PAR is colocalized with integrins and acts as a core-ceptor for vitronectin [57–59]. Furthermore, the u-PAR can be found localized at cellular focal contacts, lamellipodia, and caveolae, and has been shown to induce the phosphorylation of FAK, cytoskeletal proteins, and Src-family members [57, 60–62]. A switch between considerably different signaling cascades brought about by u-PAR-associated interaction can promote opposing phenomena, such as proliferation and dormancy (see below this section). A schematic illustration of the most important functions and interactions of u-PAR is given in Figure 1.3.

Numerous studies have shown an overexpression of the u-PAR gene in diverse human malignant tumors in contrast to the corresponding normal tissue and/or surrounding stromal cells [63–67] and suggested u-PAR as a characteristic of the invasive or even the malignant phenotype [68–70]. Much experimental evidence has convincingly shown that an overexpression of the u-PAR in diverse *in-vitro* and *in-vivo* models enhances local invasion, but also intravasation as specifically shown in an elegant chicken embryo model [71–77].

Regarding clinical studies in patient tissues, Pyke and coworkers postulated an *in-vivo* paracrine interaction between tumor and surrounding stromal cells, the former overexpressing u-PAR, the latter secreting u-PA and PAIs [65].

Moreover, prospective studies on diverse cancers involving large patient numbers have demonstrated a correlation of high u-PAR (and/or u-PA/PAI-1) expression with short survival times and advanced tumor stages. Thus, the u-PAR and/or u-PA/PAI-1 have already been shown to be significant prognostic risk factors in many cancers, including breast [78, 79], lung [80], colon [81, 82], esophageal, and gastric cancer [83, 84], and some of these studies reported an independent impact on survival probability in multivariate analysis, this recently being confirmed in an independent patient series in our own studies [84]. First studies already implicated the clinical use of the u-PA-system as a diagnostic tool to take more precise therapeutic decisions. For example, a large-scale study by Harbeck and her group addressed the issue of the predictive impact of u-PA/PAI-1 in 3424 primary breast cancer patients with regard to adjuvant chemo- and/or endocrine therapy. In this study, u-PA and PAI-1 levels in primary tumor tissue provided clear information on relapse risk and treatment response, supporting the notion that the u-PA-system will help to tailor adjuvant therapy concepts in breast cancer [85]. Moreover, in our own studies, we showed that the u-PAR might be one of the phenotyptic characteristics for the metastatically relevant phenotype of disseminated tumor cells found in the bone marrow of gastric cancer patients (Figure 1.2), since we found evidence for a quantitative increase of bone marrow-derived tumor cells harboring the u-PAR, in the follow-up of curatively resected gastric cancer patients [22]. Moreover, an expression of the u-PAR on disseminated tumor cells in the bone marrow was an independent prognostic marker for survival [23].

From the observation that disseminated tumor cells can be detected in the bone marrow of patients for many years after curative tumor surgery, it can be speculated that some of these cells are dormant. First evidence that u-PAR can play a role in tumor cell dormancy came from studies showing that a u-PAR-antisense strategy in a human squamous carcinoma cell line, resulting in a significant reduction of u-PAR gene expression, induced tumor cell dormancy. Moreover, permanent dormancy could be achieved by prolonged u-PAR-suppression [73]. Kook and coauthors investigated control cells with high u-PAR protein amounts, producing large tumors within four weeks on the chorioallantoic membrane (CAM) model, whereas u-PAR-downregulated cell clones did not recover their malignant potential, even after 10 weeks on the CAM. In nude mice, downregulation of u-PAR-gene expression in Hep3-cells using antisense technology was sufficient to induce enhanced tumor dormancy with a rapid G_0/G_1 arrest *in vivo* [86].

These data clearly indicated that dormancy could be induced by suppressing u-PAR gene expression. Previous results with immunocolocalization, resonance energy transfer, and functional studies had suggested integrin receptor families as potential interaction partners of u-PAR [58, 59]. These results were confirmed by co-immuno-precipitation of integrin α5β1 with u-PAR in the Hep3 cell model. Moreover, FN, a class of high-molecular-weight adhesive glycoproteins playing a prominent role in mediating ECM-function, is closely associated with the α5 subunit of the integrin α5β1-receptor [87]. Functional association between u-PAR, α5β1 integrins, and FN in tumorigenic cells is necessary for their optimal adhesion to FN, and for transducing the FN-dependent activation of extracellular regulated kinase (ERK) [88]. Exciting studies of Aguirre-Ghiso showed that the interaction between u-PAR and integrins apparently can provide a switch between tumor cell proliferation and dormancy, since there is an activation of the MAP-kinase pathway when u-PAR interacts with integrins, leading to proliferation. However, when the u-PAR interaction with integrins is interrupted, the P38 pathway is activated, and the tumor cell can go into dormancy [88]. Reconsidering the phenomena we described in the first part of this chapter on disseminated tumor cells in bone marrow, we consider u-PAR to be a very likely candidate to provide a switch between proliferating and dormant tumor cells in this compartment, especially since the bone marrow is known to be rich in FN [87].

Many recent studies show that u-PAR can be regulated by many different growth factors and also factors of angiogenesis, such as epidemial growth factor (EGF), basic fibroblast growth factor (FGF), vascular endothelial growth factor (VEGF), transforming growth factor β type 1 (TGF β1), protein kinase C and A, (PKC, PKA) the MAPK-, and the JNK-pathway [89–95]. Our own novel study showed that u-PAR-expression and invasion can be downregulated by tumor-suppressor Pdcd4 [96]. This underlines the functional interactions between genes related to invasion and proteolysis and factors of proliferation and angiogenesis. Furthermore, the recent discovery of microRNAs as a completely new way to regulate eukaryotic gene expression increasingly gives exciting insight into particular micro-RNAs (miRs) to be associated with carcinogenesis or tumor progression, since some miRs have been found to be overexpressed or downregulated in many tumors as opposed to corresponding normal tissues, suggesting that particular miRs can act as oncogenes ("onco-miRs"), or tumor suppressor genes. miRs regulate the expression of target genes by binding to specific target sites within the 3′UTR of mRNAs, leading to a post-transcriptional negative regulation of the target, potentially in some cases also affecting mRNA stability (for review see [97, 98]). Initial functional studies have identified first targets associated with cancer progression for miRs. For example, miR-15 and miR-16 have been shown to negatively regulate Bcl-2, an antiapoptotic molecule, and first reports suggest that a deletion of these two miRs promotes leukemogenesis and lymphomagenesis (see Chapter 23 on leukemias). Others reported that the microRNA let-7 negatively regulates Ras-oncogenes [98]. In our own study, we recently gave first evidence that miR-21 negatively regulates the tumor suppressor Pdcd4, which had been seen to down-regulate u-PAR (see paragraph above), and that it can promote local invasion, *in vivo* intravasation, and the formation of distant metastasis in cultured colorectal cancer [99]. Therefore, it is to be expected that this and potentially further miRs yet to be discovered will be additional important regulators of the metastatic cascade, and of essential invasion-related molecules.

Finally, many studies in the past have characterized the transcriptional regulation of the u-PAR gene as well as activating signaling cascades. Among them are oncogene-like transcription factors such as AP-1, and again important signaling molecules such as Src and K-Ras, which often are activated during cancer progression and metastasis. Recently, in our own translational studies we characterized novel high-risk groups of cancer patients by transcriptional and signaling-related activators of u-PAR within patient groups judged to be uncritical by clinical staging parameters [100]. These and other translational and clinical studies show that a detailed knowledge of regulatory pathways of genes related to invasion and metastasis can be applied clinically, to more precisely identify patients that are high risk for developing tumor recurrence and metastasis.

In addition to the u-PAR system, many other tumor-associated proteolytic factors have been extensively described that promote local invasion, and also intravasation and metastasis. In particular, some important players in invasion and metastasis can be found within the group of matrix metalloproteinases (MT-MMPs). An aspect of them has already been mentioned in the context of the u-PA system. Up to now, 28 MT-MMPs have been described, and their number is potentially still increasing. Probably the most important representatives relevant for the metastatic cascade are MMP-1 (collagenase-1), which has been shown to be overexpressed in different solid cancer types, and MMP-2 and MMP-9, representing the 72-kDa and 92-kDa isoform of collagenase-IV. Both isoforms are essential for invading basement membranes of vessels. Comparable to mechanisms described for the u-PAR-system, MT-MMTs interact with specific inhibitors (tissue inhibitors of metalloproteinases, TIMPs), and also with membrane-bound metalloproteinases (MT-MMPs). Six membrane-bound MT-MMPs have been described to date, and recent studies suggest that, similar to the u-PA-system, they do not only promote invasion and metastasis, but also additional phenomena important for progression and metastasis, such as the epithelial–mesenchymal transition (EMT). Via regulation of E-cadherin, MT-MMP-1 has recently been shown to interrupt cell–cell adhesion [101–103]. In summary, the large group of MT-MMTs, comparable to principles described for the u-PAR-system, represent a complex interplay between proteases, specific inhibitors (TIMPs), and membrane-bound molecules, which in concerted action do not only promote invasion and metastasis, but also additional phenomena, such as adhesion, migration, or epithelial–mesenchymal transition.

1.2.3
Factors for Tumor Growth and Angiogenesis

As already stated, for the establishment of a distant metastasis many different aspects such as the destruction of surrounding tissue, local invasion, cell division,

proliferation, a :. However,
neoangiogenesi or the successful establish e. Steps of
neoangiogenesis

1. The secretion ...giogeneic factors, such as, especially, VEGF via tumor or also endothelial cells.

2. The degradation of local basement membranes and migration through basement membranes by endothelial cells, followed by the formation of first capillary sprouts.

3. Endothelial proliferation and branching of the capillary sprouts, which is accompanied by the initiation of blood circulation through the new vessels.

4. The formation of anastomoses between new capillaries, the maturation of vessels, and the formation of novel basement membranes.

There are exciting studies suggesting that molecules expressed by neoangioge-netic vessels in tumor tissue differ from the molecular equipment found in normal vessels (e.g. intregrin $\alpha v \beta 3$) [104, 105] and that tumor- or organ-specific targeting can be achieved by techniques considering such molecular differences. These encouraging observations need to be followed in further studies.

Proangiogenetic factors especially involved in angiogenesis of tumor metasta-sis are, for example, the family of VEGF/VEGF-receptors (see detailed reviews [106, 107]), angiopoietins (ANG), such as ANG-1 and ANG-2 (together with espe-cially the receptor TIE-2), FGF, PDGF, TGF-β, and potentially also PAI-1 out of the u-PA-system. Exciting current research is exploring the potentially differen-tial roles of members of the human ANG-family in angiogenesis, but also other phenomena, such as mitogenesis, inflammation, or vascular extravasation. Cur-rently, the human ANG-family is described as a family of the ligands ANG-1, ANG-2, and ANG-4, their cognate TIE-2-receptor, and a closely related orphan receptor, TIE-1. Studies with knockout and transgenic mice suggest the impor-tant role of ANGs in both vascular angiogenesis and lymphogenesis. Currently, a pivotal role in the interaction between endothelial and perivascular cells is assigned to ANG-1. For ANG-2, proangiogenic, but also antiangiogenic activities, in part as an interplay with VEGF or FGF, have been proposed. In addition, especially ANG-2 has been associated with aggressive tumor growth, which might be linked to TIE-2-receptor activation. Since expression of the TIE-2-receptor has increasingly been characterized in tumor cells, and an interaction of ANGs with $\alpha 5 \beta 1$- and $\alpha v \beta 5$-integrins has been described recently, it is assumed that the ANGs promote additional tumor-associated phenomena such as tumor growth and development, over and above angiogenesis. This includes paracrine and autocrine molecular mechanisms in tumor cells involving TIE-2. Therefore, the ANG family, in parallel to already known major molecules such as VEGFs, are of increasing interest for novel targeting approaches in the context of angiogenesis [108].

It is well established that factors such as VEGF/VEGF-R, a family of ligands and tyrosine kinase receptors, can stimulate numerous essential signaling pathways, such as the Ras/MAP-kinase pathway, FAK, PI3-kinase/Akt, PKC, NOS, SHC, and others, which promote the expression of genes relevant for tumor cell proliferation, cell survival, migration, and cytoskeletal rearrangement. These phenomena again promote angiogenesis as well as the establishment and outgrowth of metastasis. The secretion of factors such as VEGF can be stimulated by, for example, hypoxia, which is known to be a condition often found in the center of tumors and especially metastases, hypoxia inducible factors (HIFs) and, again by essential signaling pathways relevant for tumor progression and metastasis such as Src, Ras, or others. Thus, many molecular mechanisms of angiogenesis, proliferation, antiapoptosis, migration, cytoskeletal remodeling, and invasion are networking together to achieve a successful metastatic cascade. For a more detailed description of molecular factors and pathways promoting angiogenesis, the reader should consider essential reviews in this field [106–108].

As mentioned above, many of these and further molecules and pathways are also essential pathways to stimulate tumor cell proliferation and growth. In particular, among the tyrosine kinase receptors there are, for example, EGF/EGF-R, which have been shown to be overexpressed in many solid cancers, c-erb-B2, and potentially other members of the EGF-receptor family, VEGF/VEGF-R [107], c-Kit, and others; among the signaling cascades, the major players promoting proliferation such as Src, Ras, MAP-kinases, FAK, PI3-kinase/Akt, PKC, and others have already been mentioned. The most interesting aspect of most of these molecules is that many of them already represent targets for novel molecular therapeutic concepts, which already have entered first clinical trials with promising results. This is specifically true for EGF-R, as a target in colorectal and lung cancer, c-erb-B2 as a target in breast cancer, c-Kit as a target in GIST-tumors (see Chapters 18 and 27 and VEGF, Src, Ras, and PI3-kinase as targets in different solid cancers. For a more detailed description of novel molecular targeted therapy, please refer to Chapter 30 at the end of this book.

Besides the aforementioned molecules, also molecules promoting migration, invasion, and intravasation, such as integrins, MMPs, and the u-PAR-system, are currently being investigated as targets for second-generation targeting strategies. Overall, the increasing potential of targeting many different molecules promoting different aspects of the metastatic cascade is certainly an exciting and highly promising current development, supporting the hope that the most limiting and lethal characteristic of malignant tumors, the metastatic cascade, can soon be blocked or at least slowed, enhancing the potential for survival and quality of life for cancer patients.

1.3
Potential Hereditary Aspects of Molecules Promoting Metastasis

Certainly, in the context of this book on hereditary cancers, it is a pressing question as to whether molecules promoting the metastatic cascade as described above are prone to hereditary genetic changes. Out of the adhesion molecules, most evidence for hereditary components has been suggested for the E-cadherin/β-catenin/APC/Wnt-pathway. A number of studies have already reported on DNA-variations within the E-cadherin gene in some cancers, and especially in hereditary gastric cancer. Here, diverse germline mutations within the human E-cadherin (CDH1)-gene have been reported [109–111]. The first study on DNA-variations within this gene has been published recently for prostate cancer [112]. Polymorphisms in gastric cancer have been described especially for E-cadherin and also the APC gene [113], as well as in patients with double gastric and colorectal adenocarcinomas. In the latter, changes of expression of β-catenin have also been reported [114]. However, some studies suggest that, for example, mutations of β-catenin and APC-genes cannot only be found in hereditary colorectal or gastric cancer, but also in some "sporadic" cancers, which do not meet the classical clinical criteria for hereditary cancer diagnosis [114, 115]. These findings raise the interesting question as to what extent a differentiation between hereditary cancers and "sporadic" cancers can be made in individual cases. A detailed discussion on hereditary gastric and colorectal cancers as well as the E-cadherin/β-catenin/APC-pathway will be given in specific chapters on hereditary gastric and colorectal cancer in this book. Furthermore, β-catenin mutations have been reported to coincide with *WT1*-mutations in patients with Wilms tumor (see Chapter 14).

Concerning further molecules described above in the context of migration and adhesion, little is known about potential hereditary genetic variations or mutations in, for example, integrins, Rho, Rac, and Cdc42. Single mutations in the Rho/Rac/Cdc42-cascade have been described; however, it is not clear as to whether such mutations can be genetically inherited.

Concerning tumor-associated proteases, no systematic studies have been conducted so far as to potential genetic variations within promoters or structural genes of these molecules decisive for invasion and metastasis. Such further studies are desperately needed. There are single reports about polymorphisms in MMPs that might increase the risk of lung cancer (see Chapter 10). For microRNAs, first studies have suggested that the deletion of particular miRs, such as miR-15 and miR-16, occur via chromosomal deletion, especially in leukemias (see Chapter 23).

Concerning molecules of cell growth, proliferation, and angiogenesis, no convincing reports have suggested hereditary changes within the genes for EGF-R, the ANGs, or VEGF-Rs. There have been few reports on genetic alterations for c-erb-B2 in patients with BRCA1- or BRCA2-mutation carriers, which are associated with hereditary breast cancer [116]. Single reports implicate MET receptor mutations in hereditary papillary renal cell carcinomas (see Chapter 15). Still, there needs to be more studies on potential functional interrelations between these observations. Regarding essential signaling cascades promoting tumor proliferation, progression, and metastasis, single studies suggested c-Src kinase activation to be related to development of early diffuse gastric cancer in which a hereditary component is implicated [117], and one study suggested Src-inhibition as an antiproliferative treatment for medullary thyroid cancer, which is one component of MEN-type 2 [118]. For discussions on hereditary MEN-type 2, see Chapter 9. Regarding activating mutations of K-ras, some studies suggest that they might rather occur in non-hereditary colorectal cancers, and might not be related to microsatellite instability [119, 120]. This is interesting, especially since a recent study suggested a decreased likelihood of metastasis in patients with microsatellite-instable cancers. Still, more and larger studies need to clarify relationships between activating mutations of prominent signaling molecules such as K-ras, and conditions such as microsatellite instability often found in hereditary cancer types, e.g. on hereditary colon cancer (see Chapters 3 and 20).

In summary, there need to be many more studies in the future, investigating the important question of potentially hereditary components modifying expression and/or activation of crucial molecules promoting the metastatic cascade. Such studies will lead to further refinements on how to treat metastases in cancer patients, and in particular patients with inherited cancer types.

Acknowledgments

The author was supported by the Alfried Krupp von Bohlen und Halbach Foundation, Essen, the Wilhelm Sander Foundation, Munich, the Auguste Schädel Dantscher Foundation, Garmisch, the Dr. Heller Bühler-Foundation Heidelberg, the B. Braun Foundation, Melsungen, the Hector Stiftung Foundation, Weinheim, and the Dr Ingrid zu Solms Foundation, Frankfurt/M, Germany. Furthermore, the author received funding for translational studies on compounds from the Merck and Novartis companies, Europe. The author wishes to thank all of her mentors and supporters, as well as all members of her departments at Mannheim Medical Faculty, University of Heidelberg, and the German Cancer Research Center, Heidelberg, Germany.

References

1 Laufs, S., Schumacher, J. and Allgayer, H. (2006) Urokinase-receptor (u-PAR): an essential player in multiple games of cancer. *Cell Cycle*, **5** (16), 1–12.

2 Cote, R.J., Beattie, E.J., Chaiwun, B., Shi, S.R., Harvey, J., Chen, S.C., Sherrod, A.E., Groshen, S. and Taylor, C.R. (1995) Detection of occult bone marrow micrometastases in patients with operable lung carcinoma. *Annals of Surgery*, **222**, 415–23.

3 Ellis, G., Ferguson, M., Yamanaka, E., Livingston, R.B. and Gown, A.M. (1989) Monoclonal antibodies for detection of occult carcinoma cells in bone marrow of breast cancer patients. *Cancer*, **63**, 2509–14.

4 Braun, S. and Pantel, K. (1996) Biological characteristics of micrometastatic carcinoma cells in bone marrow. *Current Topics in Microbiology and Immunology*, **213** (Pt 1), 163–77.

5 Braun, S. and Naume, B. (2005) Circulating and disseminated tumor cells. *Journal of Clinical Oncology*, **23**, 1623–6.

6 Lindemann, F., Schlimok, G., Dirschedl, P., Witte, J. and Riethmuller, G. (1992) Prognostic significance of micrometastatic tumour cells in bone marrow of colorectal cancer patients. *Lancet*, **340**, 685–9.

7 Pantel, K. and Brakenhoff, R.H. (2004) Dissecting the metastatic cascade. *Nature Reviews Cancer*, **4**, 448–56.

8 Pantel, K. and Woelfle, U. (2005) Detection and molecular characterisation of disseminated tumour cells: implications for anti-cancer therapy. *Biochimica et Biophysica Acta*, **1756**, 53–64.

9 Cote, R.J., Rosen, P.P., Lesser, M.L., Old, L.J. and Osborne, M.P. (1991) Prediction of early relapse in patients with operable breast cancer by detection of occult bone marrow micrometastases. *Journal of Clinical Oncology*, **9**, 1749–56.

10 Osborne, M.P. and Rosen, P.P. (1994) Detection and management of bone marrow micrometastases in breast cancer. *Oncology (Williston. Park)*, **8**, 25–31.

11 Pantel, K., Schlimok, G., Angstwurm, M., Weckermann, D., Schmaus, W., Gath, H., Passlick, B., Izbicki, J.R. and Riethmuller, G. (1994) Methodological analysis of immunocytochemical screening for disseminated epithelial tumor cells in bone marrow. *Journal of Hematotherapy*, **3**, 165–73.

12 Riesenberg, R., Oberneder, R., Kriegmair, M., Epp, M., Bitzer, U., Hofstetter, A., Braun, S., Riethmuller, G. and Pantel, K. (1993) Immuno-cytochemical double staining of cytokeratin and prostate specific antigen in individual prostatic tumour cells. *Histochemistry*, **99**, 61–6.

13 Moss, T.J., Reynolds, C.P., Sather, H.N., Romansky, S.G., Hammond, G.D. and Seeger, R.C. (1991) Prognostic value of immunocytologic detection of bone marrow metastases in neuroblastoma. *The New England Journal of Medicine*, **324**, 219–26.

14 Mansi, J.L., Easton, D., Berger, U., Gazet, J.C., Ford, H.T., Dearnaley, D. and Coombes, R.C. (1991) Bone marrow micrometastases in primary breast cancer: prognostic significance after 6 years' follow-up. *European Journal of Cancer*, **27**, 1552–5.

15 Jauch, K.W., Heiss, M.M., Gruetzner, U., Funke, I., Pantel, K., Babic, R., Eissner, H.J., Riethmueller, G. and Schildberg, F.W. (1996) Prognostic significance of bone marrow micrometastases in patients with gastric cancer. *Journal of Clinical Oncology*, **14**, 1810–17.

16 Soeth, E., Roder, C., Juhl, H., Kruger, U., Kremer, B. and Kalthoff, H. (1996) The detection of disseminated tumor cells in bone marrow from colorectal-cancer patients by a cytokeratin-20-specific nested reverse-transcriptase-polymerase-chain reaction is related to the stage of disease. *International Journal of Cancer*, **69**, 278–82.

17 Zippelius, A. and Pantel, K. (2000) RT-PCR-based detection of occult disseminated tumor cells in peripheral blood and bone marrow of patients with solid tumors. An overview. *Annals of the New York Academy of Sciences*, **906**, 110–23.

18 Izbicki, J.R., Hosch, S.B., Pichlmeier, U., Rehders, A., Busch, C., Niendorf, A., Passlick, B., Broelsch, C.E. and Pantel, K. (1997) Prognostic value of immuno-histochemically identifiable tumor cells in lymph nodes of patients with completely resected esophageal cancer. *The New England Journal of Medicine*, **337**, 1188–94.

19 Funke, I. and Schraut, W. (1998) Meta-analyses of studies on bone marrow micrometastases: an independent prognostic impact remains to be sub-stantiated. *Journal of Clinical Oncology*, **16**, 557–66.

20 Janni, W., Hepp, F., Rjosk, D., Kentenich, C., Strobl, B., Schindlbeck, C., Hantschmann, P., Sommer, H., Pantel, K. and Braun, S. (2001) The fate and prognostic value of occult metastatic cells in the bone marrow of patients with breast carcinoma between primary treatment and recurrence. *Cancer*, **92**, 46–53.

21 Reimers, N., Zafrakas, K., Assmann, V., Egen, C., Riethdorf, L., Riethdorf, S., Berger, J., Ebel, S., Janicke, F., Sauter, G. and Pantel, K. (2004) Expression of extracellular matrix metalloproteases inducer on micrometastatic and primary mammary carcinoma cells. *Clinical Cancer Research*, **10**, 3422–8.

22 Heiss, M.M., Allgayer, H., Gruetzner, K.U., Funke, I., Babic, R., Jauch, K.W. and Schildberg, F.W. (1995) Individual development and uPA-receptor-expression of disseminated tumour cells in bone marrow: a reference to early systemic disease in solid cancer. *Nature Medicine*, **1** (10), 1035–9.

23 Heiss, M.M., Simon, E.H., Beyer, B.C.M., Grützner, K.U., Tarabichi, A., Babic, R., Schildberg, F.W. and Allgayer, H. (2002) Minimal residual disease in gastric cancer: first evidence of an independent prognostic relevance of urokinase receptor gene expression by disseminated tumor cells in a large series of patients. *Journal of Clinical Oncology*, **20** (8), 2005–16.

24 Pyke, C., Kristensen, P., Ralfkiaer, E., Eriksen, J. and Dano, K. (1991) The plasminogen activation system in human colon cancer: messenger RNA for the inhibitor PAI-1 is located in endothelial cells in the tumor stroma. *Cancer Research*, **51**, 4067–71.

25 Nikitenko, L. and Boshoff, C. (2006) Endothelial cells in cancer. *Handbook of Experimental Pharmacology*, **176** (Pt 2), 307–34.

26 Ji, R.C. (2006) Lymphatic endothelial cells, lymphangiogenesis, and extra-cellular matrix. *Lymphatic Research and Biology*, **4** (2), 83–100.

27 Pawelek, J., Chakraborty, A., Lazova, R., Yilmaz, Y., Cooper, D., Brash, D. and Handerson, T. (2006) Co-opting macrophage traits in cancer progression: a consequence of tumor cell fusion? *Contributions to Microbiology*, **13**, 1338–55.

28 Townson, J.L. and Chambers, A.F. (2006) Dormancy of solitary metastatic cells. *Cell Cycle*, **5** (16), 1755–0.

29 Barber, M.A. and Welch, H.C. (2006) PI3K and RAC signalling in leukocyte and cancer cell migration. *Bulletin du Cancer*, **93** (1), E44–52.

30 Reynolds, A.B. and Rocznia-Ferguson, A. (2004) Emerging roles for p120-catenin in cell adhesion and cancer. *Oncogene*, **23** (48), 7947–56.

31 Jin, H. and Varner, J. (2004) Integrins: roles in cancer development and as treatment targets. *British Journal of Cancer*, **90** (3), 561–5.

32 Scatena, M. and Giachelli, C. (2002) The alpha(v)beta3 integrin, NF-kappaB, osteoprotegerin endothelial cell survival pathway. Potential role in angiogenesis. *Trends in Cardiovascular Medicine*, **12** (2), 83–8.

33 Schmitt M.J.F.G.H. (1992) Tumor-associated proteases. *Fibrinolysis* **6**, 3–26.

34 Dvorak, H.F. (1986) Tumors: wounds that do not heal. Similarities between tumor stroma generation and wound healing. *The New England Journal of Medicine*, **315**, 1650–9.

35 Blasi, F. (1988) Surface receptors for urokinase plasminogen activator. *Fibrinolysis*, **2**, 73–84.

36 Dano, K., Andreasen, P.A., Grondahl-Hansen, J., Kristensen, P., Nielsen, L.S. and Skriver, L. (1985) Plasminogen activators, tissue degradation, and cancer. *Advances in Cancer Research*, **44**, 139–266.

37 Liotta, L.A., Steeg, P.S. and Stetler-Stevenson, W.G. (1991) Cancer metastasis and angiogenesis: an imbalance of positive and negative regulation. *Cell*, **64**, 327–36.

38 Andreasen, P.A., Egelund, R. and Petersen, H.H. (2000) The plasminogen activation system in tumor growth, invasion, and metastasis. *Cellular and Molecular Life Sciences*, **57**, 25–40.

39 Ludwig, T. (2005) Local proteolytic activity in tumor cell invasion and metastasis. *Bioessays*, **27**, 1181–91.

40 Duffy, M.J. (1992) The role of proteolytic enzymes in cancer invasion and metastasis. *Clinical and Experimental Metastasis*, **10**, 145–55.

41 Gunzler, W.A., Steffens, G.J., Otting, F., Kim, S.M., Frankus, E. and Flohe, L. (1982) The primary structure of high molecular mass urokinase from human urine. The complete amino acid sequence of the A chain. *Hoppe-Seyler's Zeitschrift fur Physiologische Chemie*, **363**, 1155–65.

42 Vassalli, J.D., Dayer, J.M., Wohlwend, A. and Belin, D. (1984) Concomitant secretion of prourokinase and of a plasminogen activator-specific inhibitor by cultured human monocytes-macrophages. *The Journal of Experimental Medicine*, **159**, 1653–68.

43 Cubellis, M.V., Nolli, M.L., Cassani, G. and Blasi, F. (1986) Binding of single-chain prourokinase to the urokinase receptor of human U937 cells. *The Journal of Biological Chemistry*, **261**, 15819–22.

44 Stoppelli, M.P., Tacchetti, C., Cubellis, M.V., Corti, A., Hearing, V.J., Cassani, G., Appella, E. and Blasi, F. (1986) Autocrine saturation of pro-urokinase receptors on human A431 cells. *Cell*, **45**, 675–84.

45 Stoppelli, M.P., Corti, A., Soffientini, A., Cassani, G., Blasi, F. and Assoian, R.K. (1985) Differentiation-enhanced binding of the amino-terminal fragment of human urokinase plasminogen activator to a specific receptor on U937 monocytes. *Proceedings of the National Academy of Sciences of the United States of America*, **82**, 4939–43.

46 Ploug, M., Gardsvoll, H., Jorgensen, T.J., Lonborg, H.L. and Dano, K. (2002) Structural analysis of the interaction between urokinase-type plasminogen activator and its receptor: a potential target for anti-invasive cancer therapy. *Biochemical Society Transactions*, **30**, 177–83.

47 Llinas, P., Le Du, M.H., Gardsvoll, H., Dano, K., Ploug, M., Gilquin, B., Stura, E.A. and Menez, A. (2005) Crystal structure of the human urokinase plasminogen activator receptor bound to an antagonist peptide. *The EMBO Journal*, **24**, 1655–63.

48 Ny, T., Sawdey, M., Lawrence, D., Millan, J.L. and Loskutoff, D.J. (1986) Cloning and sequence of a cDNA coding for the human beta-migrating endothelial-cell-type plasminogen activator inhibitor. *Proceedings of the National Academy of Sciences*

of the United States of America, **83**, 6776–80.

49 Antalis, T.M., Clark, M.A., Barnes, T., Lehrbach, P.R., Devine, P.L., Schevzov, G., Goss, N.H., Stephens, R.W. and Tolstoshev, P. (1988) Cloning and expression of a cDNA coding for a human monocyte-derived plasminogen activator inhibitor. *Proceedings of the National Academy of Sciences of the United States of America*, **85**, 985–9.

50 Ye, R.D., Ahern, S.M., Le Beau, M.M., Lebo, R.V. and Sadler, J.E. (1989) Structure of the gene for human plasminogen activator inhibitor-2. The nearest mammalian homologue of chicken ovalbumin. *The Journal of Biological Chemistry*, **264**, 5495–502.

51 Andreasen, P.A., Nielsen, L.S., Kristensen, P., Grondahl-Hansen, J., Skriver, L. and Dano, K. (1986) Plasminogen activator inhibitor from human fibrosarcoma cells binds urokinase-type plasminogen activator, but not its proenzyme. *The Journal of Biological Chemistry*, **261**, 7644–51.

52 Manchanda, N. and Schwartz, B.S. (1995) Interaction of single-chain urokinase and plasminogen activator inhibitor type 1. *The Journal of Biological Chemistry*, **270**, 20032–35.

53 Olson, D., Pollanen, J., Hoyer-Hansen, G., Ronne, E., Sakaguchi, K., Wun, T.C., Appella, E., Dano, K. and Blasi, F. (1992) Internalization of the urokinase-plasminogen activator inhibitor type-1 complex is mediated by the urokinase receptor. *The Journal of Biological Chemistry*, **267**, 9129–33.

54 Cubellis, M.V., Wun, T.C. and Blasi, F. (1990) Receptor-mediated internalization and degradation of urokinase is caused by its specific inhibitor PAI-1. *The EMBO Journal*, **9**, 1079–85.

55 Conese, M., Olson, D. and Blasi, F. (1994) Protease nexin-1-urokinase complexes are internalized and degraded through a mechanism that requires both urokinase receptor and alpha 2-macroglobulin receptor. *The Journal of Biological Chemistry*, **269**, 17886–92.

56 Andreasen, P.A., Kjoller, L., Christensen, L. and Duffy, M.J. (1997) The urokinase-type plasminogen activator system in cancer metastasis: a review. *International Journal of Cancer*, **72**, 1–22.

57 May, A.E., Kanse, S.M., Lund, L.R., Gisler, R.H., Imhof, B.A. and Preissner, K.T. (1998) Urokinase receptor (CD87) regulates leukocyte recruitment via beta 2 integrins in vivo. *The Journal of Experimental Medicine*, **188**, 1029–37.

58 Xue, W., Mizukami, I., Todd, R.F. III and Petty, H.R. (1997) Urokinase-type plasminogen activator receptors associate with beta1 and beta3 integrins of fibrosarcoma cells: dependence on extracellular matrix components. *Cancer Research*, **57**, 1682–9.

59 Wei, Y., Lukashev, M., Simon, D.I., Bodary, S.C., Rosenberg, S., Doyle, M.V. and Chapman, H.A. (1996) Regulation of integrin function by the urokinase receptor. *Science*, **273**, 1551–5.

60 Tang, H., Kerins, D.M., Hao, Q., Inagami, T. and Vaughan, D.E. (1998) The urokinase-type plasminogen activator receptor mediates tyrosine phosphorylation of focal adhesion proteins and activation of mitogen-activated protein kinase in cultured endothelial cells. *The Journal of Biological Chemistry*, **273**, 18268–72.

61 Stahl, A. and Mueller, B.M. (1995) The urokinase-type plasminogen activator receptor, a GPI-linked protein, is localized in caveolae. *The Journal of Cell Biology*, **129**, 335–44.

62 Pollanen, J., Hedman, K., Nielsen, L.S., Dano, K. and Vaheri, A. (1988) Ultrastructural localization of plasma membrane-associated urokinase-type plasminogen activator at focal contacts. *The Journal of Cell Biology*, **106**, 87–95.

63 Allgayer, H. (2006) Molecular regulation of an invasion-related molecule–options for tumour staging and clinical strategies. *European Journal of Cancer*, **42**, 811–19.

64 Sier, C.F., Verspaget, H.W., Griffioen, G., Ganesh, S., Vloedgraven, H.J. and Lamers, C.B. (1993) Plasminogen activators in normal tissue and carcinomas of the human oesophagus and stomach. *Gut*, **34**, 80–5.

65 Pyke, C., Kristensen, P., Ralfkiaer, E., Eriksen, J. and Dano, K. (1991) The plasminogen activation system in human colon cancer: messenger RNA for the inhibitor PAI-1 is located in endothelial cells in the tumor stroma. *Cancer Research*, **51**, 4067–71.

66 Romer, J., Pyke, C., Lund, L.R., Eriksen, J., Kristensen, P., Ronne, E., Hoyer-Hansen, G., Dano, K. and Brunner, N. (1994) Expression of uPA and its receptor by both neoplastic and stromal cells during xenograft invasion. *International Journal of Cancer*, **57**, 553–60.

67 Morita, S., Sato, A., Hayakawa, H., Ihara, H., Urano, T., Takada, Y. and Takada, A. (1998) Cancer cells overexpress mRNA of urokinase-type plasminogen activator, its receptor and inhibitors in human non-small-cell lung cancer tissue: analysis by Northern blotting and *in situ* hybridization. *International Journal of Cancer*, **78**, 286–92.

68 Wang, H., Skibber, J., Juarez, J. and Boyd, D. (1994) Transcriptional activation of the urokinase receptor gene in invasive colon cancer. *International Journal of Cancer*, **58**, 650–7.

69 Bianchi, E., Cohen, R.L., Thor, A.T., Todd, R.F. III, Mizukami, I.F., Lawrence, D.A., Ljung, B.M., Shuman, M.A. and Smith, H.S. (1994) The urokinase receptor is expressed in invasive breast cancer but not in normal breast tissue. *Cancer Research*, **54**, 861–6.

70 Hollas, W., Blasi, F. and Boyd, D. (1991) Role of the urokinase receptor in facilitating extracellular matrix invasion by cultured colon cancer. *Cancer Research*, **51**, 3690–5.

71 Kariko, K., Kuo, A., Boyd, D., Okada, S.S., Cines, D.B. and Barnathan, E.S. (1993) Overexpression of urokinase receptor increases matrix invasion without altering cell migration in a human osteosarcoma cell line. *Cancer Research*, **53**, 3109–17.

72 Ossowski, L. (1988) *In vivo* invasion of modified chorioallantoic membrane by tumor cells: the role of cell surface-bound

urokinase. *The Journal of Cell Biology*, **107**, 2437–45.

73 Kook, Y.H., Adamski, J., Zelent, A. and Ossowski, L. (1994) The effect of antisense inhibition of urokinase receptor in human squamous cell carcinoma on malignancy. *The EMBO Journal*, **13**, 3983–91.

74 Quattrone, A., Fibbi, G., Anichini, E., Pucci, M., Zamperini, A., Capaccioli, S. and Del Rosso, M. (1995) Reversion of the invasive phenotype of transformed human fibroblasts by anti-messenger oligonucleotide inhibition of urokinase receptor gene expression. *Cancer Research*, **55**, 90–5.

75 Mohanam, S., Sawaya, R., McCutcheon, I., Ali-Osman, F., Boyd, D. and Rao, J.S. (1993) Modulation of *in vitro* invasion of human glioblastoma cells by urokinase-type plasminogen activator receptor antibody. *Cancer Research*, **53**, 4143–7.

76 Liu, G., Shuman, M.A. and Cohen, R.L. (1995) Co-expression of urokinase, urokinase receptor and PAI-1 is necessary for optimum invasiveness of cultured lung cancer cells. *International Journal of Cancer*, **60**, 501–6.

77 Kim, J., Yu, W., Kovalski, K. and Ossowski, L. (1998) Requirement for specific proteases in cancer cell intravasation as revealed by a novel semiquantitative PCR-based assay. *Cell*, **94**, 353–62.

78 Janicke, F., Schmitt, M., Pache, L., Ulm, K., Harbeck, N., Hofler, H. and Graeff, H. (1993) Urokinase (uPA) and its inhibitor PAI-1 are strong and independent prognostic factors in node-negative breast cancer. *Breast Cancer Research and Treatment*, **24**, 195–208.

79 Duffy, M.J., Reilly, D., O'Sullivan, C., O'Higgins, N., Fennelly, J.J. and Andreasen, P. (1990) Urokinase-plasminogen activator, a new and independent prognostic marker in breast cancer. *Cancer Research*, **50**, 6827–9.

80 Pedersen, H., Grondahl-Hansen, J., Francis, D., Osterlind, K., Hansen, H.H. Dano, K. and Brunner, N. (1994) Urokinase and plasminogen activator inhibitor type 1 in pulmonary

adenocarcinoma. *Cancer Research*, **54**, 120–3.

81 Mulcahy, H.E., Duffy, M.J., Gibbons, D., McCarthy, P., Parfrey, N.A., O'Donoghue, D.P. and Sheahan, K. (1994) Urokinase-type plasminogen activator and outcome in Dukes' B colorectal cancer. *Lancet*, **344**, 583–4.

82 Ganesh, S., Sier, C.F., Heerding, M.M., Griffioen, G., Lamers, C.B. and Verspaget, H.W. (1994) Urokinase receptor and colorectal cancer survival. *Lancet*, **344**, 401–2.

83 Nekarda, H., Schlegel, P., Schmitt, M., Stark, M., Mueller, J.D., Fink, U. and Siewert, J.R. (1998) Strong prognostic impact of tumor-associated urokinase-type plasminogen activator in completely resected adenocarcinoma of the esophagus. *Clinical Cancer Research*, **4**, 1755–63.

84 Beyer, B.C., Heiss, M.M., Simon, E.H., Gruetzner, K.U., Babic, R., Jauch, K.W., Schildberg, F.W. and Allgayer, H. (2006) Urokinase system expression in gastric carcinoma: prognostic impact in an independent patient series and first evidence of predictive value in preoperative biopsy and intestinal metaplasia specimens. *Cancer*, **106**, 1026–35.

85 Harbeck, N., Kates, R.E., Look, M.P., Meijer-Van Gelder, M.E., Klijn, J.G., Kruger, A., Kiechle, M., Janicke, F., Schmitt, M. and Foekens, J.A. (2002) Enhanced benefit from adjuvant chemotherapy in breast cancer patients classified high-risk according to urokinase-type plasminogen activator (uPA) and plasminogen activator inhibitor type 1 (n = 3424). *Cancer Research*, **62**, 4617–22.

86 Yu, W., Kim, J. and Ossowski, L. (1997) Reduction in surface urokinase receptor forces malignant cells into a protracted state of dormancy. *The Journal of Cell Biology*, **137**, 767–77.

87 Pankov, R. and Yamada, K.M. (2002) Fibronectin at a glance. *Journal of Cell Science*, **115**, 3861–3.

88 Aguirre-Ghiso, J.A., Kovalski, K. and Ossowski, L. (1999) Tumor dormancy induced by downregulation of urokinase receptor in human carcinoma involves integrin and MAPK signaling. *The Journal of Cell Biology*, **147**, 89–104.

89 Lengyel, E., Wang, H., Stepp, E., Juarez, J., Wang, Y., Doe, W., Pfarr, C.M. and Boyd, D. (1996) Requirement of an upstream AP-1 motif for the constitutive and phorbol ester-inducible expression of the urokinase-type plasminogen activator receptor gene. *The Journal of Biological Chemistry*, **271**, 23176–84.

90 Gum, R., Juarez, J., Allgayer, H., Mazar, A., Wang, Y. and Boyd, D. (1998) Stimulation of urokinase-type plasminogen activator receptor expression by PMA requires JNK1-dependent and -independent signaling modules. *Oncogene*, **17**, 213–25.

91 Lund, L.R., Ellis, V., Ronne, E., Pyke, C. and Dano, K. (1995) Transcriptional and post-transcriptional regulation of the receptor for urokinase-type plasminogen activator by cytokines and tumour promoters in the human lung carcinoma cell line A549. *The Biochemical Journal*, **310** (Pt 1), 345–52.

92 Boyd, D. (1989) Examination of the effects of epidermal growth factor on the production of urokinase and the expression of the plasminogen activator receptor in a human colon cancer cell line. *Cancer Research*, **49**, 2427–32.

93 Mandriota, S.J., Seghezzi, G., Vassalli, J.D., Ferrara, N., Wasi, S., Mazzieri, R., Mignatti, P. and Pepper, M.S. (1995) Vascular endothelial growth factor increases urokinase receptor expression in vascular endothelial cells. *The Journal of Biological Chemistry*, **270**, 9709–16.

94 Li, C., Liu, J.N. and Gurewich, V. (1995) Urokinase-type plasminogen activator-induced monocyte adhesion requires a carboxyl-terminal lysine and cAMP-dependent signal transduction. *The Journal of Biological Chemistry*, **270**, 30282–5.

95 Lengyel, E., Wang, H., Gum, R., Simon, C., Wang, Y. and Boyd, D. (1997) Elevated urokinase-type plasminogen

activator receptor expression in a colon cancer cell line is due to a constitutively activated extracellular signal-regulated kinase-1-dependent signaling cascade. *Oncogene*, **14**, 2563–73.

96 Leupold, J.H., Yang, H-S, Colburn, N.H., Boyd, D.D., Lengyel, E.R., Post, S. and Allgayer, H. (2007) Tumor suppressor Pdcd4 inhibits invasion and regulates urokinase-receptor (uPAR) gene expression via Sp-transcription factors. *Oncogene*, **26** (31), 4550–62.

97 Hammond, S.C.M. (2006) MicroRNAsas oncogenes. *Current Opinion in Genetics and Development*, **16**, 4–9.

98 Esquela-Kerscher, A. and Slack, F.J. (2006) Oncomirs–microRNAs with a role in cancer. *Nature Reviews*, **6**, 259–69.

99 Asangani, I.A., Rasheed, S.A.K., Nikolova, D.A., Leupold, J.H., Colburn, N.H., Post, S. and Allgayer, H. (2007) MicroRNA-21 (miR-21) post-transcriptionally downregulates tumor suppressor Pdcd4 and stimulates invasion, intravasation and metastasis in colorectal cancer. *Oncogene*, 1–9.

100 Maurer, G.D., Leupold, J.H., Schewe, D.M., Biller, T., Kates, R.E., Hornung, H.-M., Lau-Werner, U., Post, S. and Allgayer, H. (2007) First analysis of specific transcriptional regulators as predictors of independent prognostic relevance in resected colorectal cancer. *Clinical Cancer Research*, **13** (4), 1123–32.

101 Zucker, S. and Cao, J. (2006) Molecular mechanisms of matrix metalloproteinase (MT-MMP) induction of cancer cell migration and metastasis. *European Journal of Cancer*, **4** (6 Suppl), 7–8.

102 Cao, J., Chiarelli, C., Kozarekar, P. *et al.* (2005) Membrane type 1-matrix metalloproteinase promotes human prostrate cancer invasion and metastasis. *Thrombosis and Haemostasis*, **93** (4), 770–8.

103 Wolf, D.A., Zhou, C. and Wee, S. (2003) The COP9 signalosome: an assembly and maintenance platform for cullin ubiquitin ligases?. *Nature Cell Biology*, **5** (12), 1029–33.

104 Arap, W., Paqualini, R. and Ruoslahti, E. (1998) Cancer treatment by targeted drug

delivery to tumor vasculature in a mouse model. *Science,* **279** (5349), 323–4.

105 Rajotte, D., Arap, W., Hagedorn, M., Koivunen, E., Pasqualini, R. and Ruoslahti, E. (1998) Molecular heterogeneity of the vascular endothelium revealed by in vivo phage display. *The Journal of Clinical Investigation,* **102** (2), 430–7.

106 Folkman, J. (2006) Angiogenesis. *Annual Review of Medicine,* **57**, 1–18.

107 Folkman, J. (2007) Angiogenesis: an organizing principle for drug discovery? *Nature Reviews Drug Discovery* **6** (4), 273–86.

108 Shim, W.S.N., Ho, I.A.W. and Wong, P.E.H. (2007) Angiopoietin: a TIE(d) balance in tumor angiogenesis. *Molecular Cancer Research,* **5** (7), 655–65.

109 Norton, J.A., Ham, C.M., Van Dam, J. *et al.* (2007) CDH1 truncating mutations in the E-cadherin gene: an indication for total gastrectomy to treat hereditary diffuse gastric cancer. *Annals of Surgery,* **245** (6), 873–6.

110 More, H., Humar, B., Weber, W. *et al.* (2007) Identification of seven novel germline mutations in the human E-cadherin (CDH1) gene. *Human Mutation,* **28** (2), 2003.

111 Bacani, J.T., Soares, M., Zwingerman, R. *et al.* (2006) CDH1/E-cadherin germline mutations in early-onset gastric cancer. *Journal of Medical Genetics,* **43** (11), 867–72.

112 Cybulski, C., Wokolorczyk, D., Jakubowska, D. *et al.* (2007) DNA variation in MSR1, RNASEL and E-cadherin genes in prostate cancer in Poland. *Urologia Internationalis,* **79** (1), 44–9.

113 Wu, M.S., Chen, C.J. and Lin, J.T. (2003) Genetic alterations and polymorphisms in gastric cancer. *Journal of the Formosan Medical Association,* **102** (7), 447–58.

114 Kim, J.C., Koo, K.H., Kim, H.C. *et al.* (2004) Geno- and pheno-typic characterization in ten patients with double-primary gastric and colorectal adenocarcinomas. *International Journal of Colorectal Disease,* **19** (6), 561–8.

115 Miyaki, M., Iijima, T., Kimura, J. *et al.* (1999) Frequent mutation of beta-catenin and APC genes in primary colorectal tumors from patients with hereditary nonpolyposis colorectal cancer. *Cancer Research,* **59** (18), 4506–9.

116 Adem, C., Soderberg, C.L., Hafner, K. *et al.* (2004) ERBB2, TBX2, RPS6KB1, and MYC alterations in breast tissues of BRCA1 and BRCA1 mutation carriers. *Genes Chromosomes Cancer,* **41** (1), 1–11.

117 Humar, B., Fukuzawa, R., Blair, V. *et al.* (2007) Destabilized adhesion in the gastric proliferative zone and c-Src kinase activation mark the development of early diffuse gastric cancer. *Cancer Research,* **67** (6), 2480–9.

118 Liu, Z., Falola, J., Zhu, X. *et al.* (2004) Antiproliferative effects of Src inhibition on medullary thyroid cancer. *The Journal of Clinical Endocrinology and Metabolism,* **89** (7), 3503–9.

119 Malesci, A., Laghi, L., Bianchi, P. *et al.* (2007) Reduced likelihood of metastases in patients with microsatellite-unstable colorectal cancer. *Clinical Cancer Research,* **13** (13), 3831–9.

120 Söreide, K., Janssen, E.A., Siland, H., Körner, H. and Baak, J.P. (2006) Microsatellite instability in colorectal cancer. *The British Journal of Surgery,* **93** (4), 395–406.

2
The Genetic Background of Hereditary Tumor Diseases

Ortrud K. Steinlein

Summary

High penetrance mutations in several tumor predisposition genes have been identified that contribute to different hereditary cancer syndromes. Many of these mutations follow an autosomal dominant mode of inheritance, thus predisposition carriers are often found in subsequent generations. For several tumor predisposition genes, the basic mechanisms they play in cancer pathogenesis are well understood, however, several questions remain. Extensive research is still needed to uncover the molecular basis of phenomena such as reduced penetrance, cell-type specificity, and variability of associated clinical features.

2.1
Introduction

During the last few decades, an increasing number of well-defined cancer predisposition syndromes have been described (Table 2.1). Recognition and correct clinical diagnosis of these syndromes requires a basic understanding of the clinical course, the syndrome-specific spectrum of tumor types, and the respective mode of inheritance. Research has already gained considerable insight into the molecular mechanisms underlying different hereditary tumor predispositions. However, our knowledge today is far from complete. Several questions still have not been answered satisfactorily, including how and when an inherited predisposition gives rise to tumor development, and why these tumors are often cell-type specific. Early models, such as Knudson's "two hit" hypothesis, have now been proven experimentally to be sound, but these models are able to explain only a small part of the genetic mechanisms underlying cancer predisposition syndromes [1–3]. These genetic mechanisms are far more diverse and complex, according to the large number and various functions of tumor predisposition genes involved in the different syndromes.

Hereditary Tumors: From Genes to Clinical Consequences
Edited by Heike Allgayer, Helga Rehder and Simone Fulda
Copyright © 2009 WILEY-VCH Verlag GmbH & Co. KGaA, Weinheim
ISBN: 978-3-527-32028-8

Table 2.1 Selected cancer predisposition syndromes.

Inheritance	Syndrome	Gene	Chromosome
Autosomal dominant			
	Familial breast cancer	*BRCA1*	17q21
		BRCA2	13q12
	Multiple endocrine neoplasia type 1	*MEN1*	11q13
	Multiple endocrine neoplasia type 2	*RET*	10q11
	Familial retinoblastoma	*RB1*	13q14
	Familial polyposis	*APC*	5q21
	MutYH-associated polyposis	*MutYH*	1p34.3-1p32.1
	Hereditary nonpolyposis colorectal cancer	*MSH2*	2p16
		MLH1	3p21
		Others	
	Familial Wilms tumor	*WT1*	11p13
	Neurofibromatosis type 1	*NF1*	17q11
	Neurofibromatosis type 2	*NF2*	22q12
	Von Hippel Lindau disease	*VHL*	3p25
	Gorlin syndrome	*PTCH*	9q22
	Hereditary diffuse gastric cancer	*CDHE*	16q22.1
	Li Fraumeni syndrome	*TP53*	17q13
Autosomal recessive			
	Xeroderma pigmentosum	*XPA-XPG*	At least 8 loci
		XPV	
	Fanconi anemia	*FANCA-FANCD1* [*FANCD1(=BRCA1)*]) *FANCD2* *FANCE-FANCG* *FANCJ* *FANCL-FANCN*	Multiple complementation groups
	Bloom syndrome	*BLM*	15q26

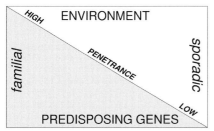

Figure 2.1 Gene penetrance in cancer. Highly penetrant germline mutations (left part) can cause cancer with little or no environmental influences. Low penetrance mutations (middle) increase the risk of certain malignancies but require the interaction with environmental predisposing factors. The right part of the model represents malignancies that are caused by a combination of somatic mutations and environmental influences, without a preexisting inherited predisposition.

2.2
Sporadic Versus Hereditary Tumors

Malignancies are traditionally divided into sporadic and familial (or hereditary) cases. This distinction is mostly based on clinical and anamnestic data, since genetic tests are available only for a small number of cases. However, a classification based on clinical data has several pitfalls. The absence of a family history of cancer in an apparently sporadic case can be misleading, as the true familial nature of the disorder might be masked by small family size or insufficient family data. Also, familial occurrence of malignancies does not necessarily imply a genetic origin, as it includes families in which multiple affected individuals occurred by chance, as well as those in which low-risk predisposition genes are segregating, as well as families with high-risk genetic predispositions [4, 5]. From a genetic point of view the great majority (~95%) of malignancies belong to the large group of multifactorial disorders, in which inherited and acquired (or somatic) low-penetrance genetic predisposition factors interact with various environmental factors [6]. Only a small portion of malignancies are due to monogenic inheritance, with high recurrence risks in relatives [7] (Figure 2.1). Overall, the portion of monogenic malignancies can be roughly estimated to be about 5%. The ratio of monogenic versus multifactorial cases not only varies between different tumor types, but for some tumor types it also depends on the ethnic and/or regional background of the patient sample [8, 9]. In the affected families it is not the tumor itself that is inherited, but the predisposition to develop this tumor.

2.2.1
Sporadic Malignancies Are More Common

The identification of families at risk for hereditary tumor predispositions is rarely a straightforward process. One of the difficulties is that the genotype not always equals the phenotype [10, 11]. The impact a certain genotype has on the observable physical condition of an individual (or a cell) depends on various factors, including the mode of inheritance, the penetrance of the gene mutation, and the average age of manifestation. These variables have to be taken into consideration in families with suspected or proven hereditary tumor predispositions. The clinical phenotype presents one of the greatest challenges regarding the correct identification of high-risk constellations, for example the differentiation between high-risk family members and those with only low risks. Most malignancies observed in hereditary tumor predispositions also occur sporadically in the general population [12]. Thus, the type of malignancy observed rarely allows us to distinguish between monogenic and multifactorial forms. Hints pointing to a tumor of sporadic rather than monogenic origin might be a malignancy type that is not typical for any of the known hereditary tumor predispositions, and/or a tumor that is known to commonly have a strong environmental background (e.g. carcinogens, radiation exposure). For most malignancies, such a distinction based mainly on the tumor type and patients' history is not feasible. This can be best demonstrated for breast or colorectal cancer. Both types of cancer have a high frequency in the general population and are in most cases sporadic. Multiple affected members in the same family do not necessarily indicate a monogenic form of these malignancies, and even in families with an autosomal dominant mode of inheritance, affected family members with sporadic forms of the malignancy might be present.

2.2.2
Red Flags for Hereditary Tumors

"Red flags" indicating that one of the rare monogenic tumor predispositions might be present are a young age at onset, multiple tumors in the same patient, and the presence of the same or related malignancies in close relatives. For several hereditary tumor predispositions, such red flags have been used to formulate guidelines that are helpful in identifying families at risk. An example are the Amsterdam criteria for colorectal cancer that require at least three relatives with this type of cancer, one or more diagnosed under the age of 50 years, before a clinical diagnosis of an hereditary predisposition for colorectal cancer should be made [13]. In some disorders, specific laboratory tests are helpful in recognizing the rare monogenic forms. Tumors in hereditary nonpolyposis colorectal cancer (HNPCC) are frequently showing microsatellite instability caused by the predisposing mutations in genes coding for mismatch repair (MMR) proteins [14]. In sporadic colorectal tumors, microsatellite instability is only present in about 15% of cases. In breast cancer, one of the main problems in identifying high-risk families is caused by the fact that this tumor type is a common disorder that affects 1 in 10 women (life-time risk). Thus, multiple affected members in the same family are not an unusual finding, and such apparently familial cases of breast cancer are more often due to chance than to monogenic inheritance, especially if these malignancies mostly occurred in women over 50 years of age. On the other hand, the dominant inheritance patterns of hereditary breast cancer predispositions are often masked in families by reduced penetrance (not all mutation carriers develop cancer) and the variability of the age of onset (mutation carriers are healthy at the time of ascertainment, but might develop cancer later in life) [15]. Small family sizes are another factor that can make it difficult to recognize high-risk families, because of the low number of affected individuals per generation in such families. Once a sufficient likelihood for a hereditary tumor predisposition is established and high-risk individuals are identified, the possibilities of symptomatic and presymptomatic (predictive) testing can be explored.

2.3
Inheritance Patterns in Hereditary Tumor Predispositions

2.3.1
Autosomal Dominant Inheritance

Nearly all of the known types of inheritance patterns are found in the different hereditary tumor predispositions, but the autosomal dominant mode of inheritance is the most commonly observed one (Figures 2.1 and 2.2A). Usually, in autosomal dominant inheritance, only one copy of a mutated gene needs to be passed to the next generation to cause the associated phenotype in the offspring. As in many other autosomal dominant disorders, in hereditary tumor predispositions it is not a clinical phenotype that is inherited, but rather a predisposition that might, or might not, lead to clinical symptoms, in this case a certain kind of tumor or malignancy. The children of predisposition carriers have a 50% chance of inheriting the predisposing parental allele, irrespective of their sex. Predisposition carriers are usually heterozygous for the disease allele; homozygous individuals that inherited such alleles from both parents have been rarely reported for autosomal dominant disorders. This could be due to the low frequency of such alleles in the population that renders it unlikely that both parents (if unrelated) are heterozygotes. Another explanation could be that homozygosity for certain predisposition alleles might cause a more severe or even lethal phenotype [16]. In most tumor predispositions with an autosomal dominant mode of inheritance, the average age

(A)   (B)

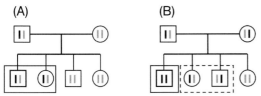

Figure 2.2 Inheritance models. Segregation patterns in dominant (A) and recessively (B) inherited tumor predisposition alleles. Black bars, mutated allele; solid box, affected individual; hatched box, healthy carriers of the predisposition allele.

of onset and life expectance does not interfere with reproduction. This means that the rate of *de novo* mutations is low in these disorders, otherwise the number of affected individuals would increase with each generation. Such a balance between *de novo* mutation rates and reproductive fitness is well-known for different genetic conditions.

2.3.2
Autosomal Recessive Inheritance

Disorders that usually cause death before reproduction are characterized by either high rates of autosomal dominant *de novo* mutations or, more often, by recessive inheritance (Figure 2.2B). Thus it is not surprising that many hereditary cancer predispositions in children follow the latter inheritance pattern. In autosomal recessive inheritance, both alleles of the tumor predisposition gene carry a mutation, because both (usually healthy) parents need to pass on a mutated allele to establish the predisposition in the next generation. The parents of an affected individual are usually healthy, heterozygote carriers of the mutation. In general, homozygotes for recessive disorders are rarely found in subsequent generations. Such a phenomenon, called "pseudo-dominance", is mostly known from inbred populations, or populations from geographical regions where certain recessive mutations reached high frequency because they help to protect heterozygote carriers against certain environmental risks (heterozygote advantage). Children of two heterozygote parents have a 25% chance of inheriting both parental alleles and therefore the predisposition. Their chance of being heterozygote carriers like their parents is 50%, while a 25% chance exists that such a child only inherits the two wildtype alleles. Examples of tumor predisposition syndromes with an autosomal recessive mode of inheritance are Ataxia telangiectasia, Bloom syndrome, and Xeroderma pigmentosum [17–19]. Ataxia telangiectasia is a multisystem disorder caused by mutations in the *ATM* gene on chromosome 11. The *ATM* gene is involved in cell cycle arrest following DNA damage, and seems to be required for the activation of the breast cancer-causing gene *BRCA1*. Thus it is not surprising that, in addition to its role in Ataxia telangiectasia, *ATM* mutations if present in a heterozygous state are able to confer an at least moderately increased risk for breast cancer [20]. This example demonstrates that at least for some mutations, no clear-cut boundaries between recessive and dominant inheritance exist.

2.4
Genotype–Phenotype Relations in Hereditary Tumor Predispositions

A phenomenon often encountered in genetic traits is reduced penetrance. This term describes the fraction of mutation carriers that manifest the specific phenotype. In hereditary tumor predispositions, penetrances vary widely, and even within the same syndrome there are differences in penetrance between the tumor types typically found in affected families. For example, the penetrance rates for breast cancer in female *BRCA1* mutation carriers are 65% (cumulative risk by age 70 years), while ovarian cancer has a much lower penetrance rate in these individuals (39%). The corresponding estimates for *BRCA2* mutation carriers are even lower; meta analyses demonstrated penetrance rates of 45% and 11%, respectively [15, 21]. Even within the same gene, the penetrance rates are not identical for different mutations. This is demonstrated by I1307K, a low penetrance mutation/polymorphism in the *APC* gene. It is found mainly in Ashkenazi Jews (with a heterozygote frequency of 5% to 7%). This amino acid exchange appears to be associated with a relative risk of colorectal cancer of between 1.5 and 2.2, while "classical" or high-penetrance APC gene mutations confer a considerably higher risk for this type of cancer [22]. In many dominant disorders, the condition shows different degrees of manifestation, clinically observed as different degrees of severity or affectedness. An example is neurofibromatosis, in which some mutation carriers show the full-blown picture with numerous cutaneous neurofibromas, subcutaneous plexiform neurofibromas, café-au-lait spots, psychomotor retardation, and increased malignancy rates, while others—even in the same family—may show only a few café-au-lait spots. The phenomenon is referred to by either variable expression or incomplete penetrance [23].

2.4.1
Mechanisms Underlying Genotype–Phenotype Relations

The mechanisms underlying reduced penetrance or variable expression have so far only been analyzed in detail in a few model disorders. One of these is retinoblastoma, in which one out of ten individuals carrying an *RB1* mutation will not develop the tumor [24, 25]. According to the "two-hit" hypothesis of Knudson (see Section 2.5.1), reduced penetrance has to be expected because the development of a retinoblastoma depends on the chance occurrence of the second mutation. However, such stochastic effects are not able to fully explain the phenomena of variable expression. Of equal importance is the nature of the predisposing mutation. Most of the known *RB1* mutations are truncating, for example, nonsense or frameshift mutations that are located in internal exons. These classes of mutations are usually associated with bilateral retinoblastoma, without showing much genotype-phenotype variation. It is likely that transcripts with premature stop codons trigger nonsense-mediated decay so that only the transcripts of the normal *RB1* allele remain.

Another class of mutations causes aberrant splicing. Many of these so-called splice site mutations cause out-of-frame transcripts with premature termination codons too. However, in some of them the effect of the mutation on the respective splice site is "leaky", meaning a fraction of the normal transcript is still spliced from the mutated preRNA [26]. In these patients, the dosage of the normal transcript is higher than in patients with truncating mutations, explaining why these mutations tend to be associated with a milder phenotype (e.g. unilateral retinoblastoma). Such a milder phenotype is also often observed in patients carrying mutations in the *RB1* gene promoter [25, 27]. Mutations in regulating sequence motives such as promoters often decrease gene activity but do not shut it down completely.

Another mechanism that is able to rescue at least part of the *RB1* function includes the use of alternative translation start points. For example, an *RB1* mutation has been described that comprises a 23-basepair duplication in the first exon, producing a premature chain termination in exon 2. Such a mutation can usually be expected to completely abolish gene function and produce a severe clinical phenotype. However, expression studies showed that alternative in-frame translation start sites are used to generate truncated *RB1* products. Clinically, this mutation resulted in low-penetrance retinoblastomas, indicating that at least a partial rescue of *RB1* function had occurred [28].

2.5
From Predisposition to Cancer – Is One Gene Enough?

Since first published in 1971, Knudson's two-hit hypothesis has provided an illustrative model for the understanding of tumor pathogenesis. Alfred Knudson suggested that mutations in both alleles of a tumor suppressor gene are needed before a tumor starts to form [1]. The main difference between sporadic malignancies and familial tumor syndromes is that in the latter the patients are already born with the first mutation in all their cells. This germline mutation might inactivate one allele of a certain tumor suppressor gene, but tumorigenesis does not start before the second allele is knocked out by another, somatic mutation. In sporadic tumors, both alleles need to be inactivated by somatic mutations hitting the same cell, thus two independently occurring mutational events are required. Such a somatic-two-hit-scenario has a much lower probability than the occurrence of a second hit in one of numerous cells of an individual already carrying a germline mutation. These differences in probability are one of the main reasons why sporadic tumors usually occur at a later age than their familial counterparts [1].

2.5.1
Experimental Evidence for the Two-Hit Hypothesis

Experimental support for Knudson's two-hit hypothesis has been first found in studies of sporadic and hereditary retinoblastoma, in which mutations in both alleles of the tumor suppressor gene *RB1* are found [29]. In hereditary retinoblastoma the family members at risk are already born with an inactivating mutation on one of their *RB1* alleles. The second hit is a somatic mutation that in many cases involves the partial or complete loss of the second *RB1* allele in a certain cell. If polymorphic genetic markers are part of the deletion this second mutation can be observed as a loss of heterozygosity (LOH) [24, 30]. Such a LOH has been demonstrated not only to be a key event in hereditary tumor syndromes such as retinoblastoma, Wilms tumor, or Li Fraumeni syndrome, but is also found in up to 50% of chromosomes in sporadic tumors [30–32]. The systematic search for LOH has been repeatedly used to successfully locate formerly unknown genes involved in tumor formation or progression in the genome. Examples include the identification of the *RET* oncogene in multiple endocrine neoplasia, as well as the *NF2* gene in neurofibromatosis type 2 [33–35].

2.5.2
"Multi Hit" and Recruitment Hypotheses

More recent studies suggested that the two-hit mechanism may not be universal but that other, more complicated mechanisms might exist [36]. Alternative mechanisms of tumorigenesis have been found in hereditary tumors as well as in sporadic malignancies with their more complex etiology. One of these models was introduced by Vogelstein who described a multi-step process in which clonal expansion of cells that have accumulated three to seven mutations occur [37]. Each subsequent mutation provides a selective advantage to the progeny cells, first with respect to proliferation and, in later stages, to escape apoptosis or other growth control mechanisms. Evidence for this multi-step model of tumorigenesis is again found in studies of retinoblastoma where LOH can be detected only in about 60% of both hereditary and non-hereditary cases. Furthermore, many retinoblastomas show additional genomic mutations in chromosomal regions other than the *RB1* region [38, 39]. These findings strongly suggest that the loss of both copies of *RB1* is not sufficient to cause retinoblastoma, but that the malignant transformation requires additional mutational events. Gallie *et al.* therefore introduced the "multi-hit" model in which the loss of the two *RB1* alleles can lead to benign retinoma, but another mutational event affecting one of the apoptosis pathways is required for progression to malignant retinoblastoma [40]. Another hypothesis of tumor formation is based on the observation that some tumors do not always show evidence of clonality. Examples are subependymal giant cell astrocytomas in tuberous sclerosis, or neurofibromas in neurofibromatosis type 1 [41, 42]. The recruitment hypothesis postulates that after the second hit the cells that are now endangered by a complete loss of function recruit surrounding haploinsufficient cells for their own rescue [3]. The recruited cells become part of the forming tumor and mask the clonality of the original clonal cell formation. These examples demonstrate that pathogenesis in inherited tumor syndromes, as well as in sporadic malignancies, is a heterogeneous process in which different possible pathways exist. Knudson's two-hit hypothesis has played an important role in our understanding of the pathobiological processes underlying tumorigenesis, but it provides just one (albeit important) of the many existing pieces of the puzzle.

2.6
The Phenomena of Cell-Type Specificity

In most hereditary tumor syndromes only one particular cell type commonly develops the malignancy, although the inherited germline mutation is present in all cells of the body. Other tumor predispositions are characterized by a main lesion but also include an increased risk for malignancies in one or a few additional, often unrelated cell types. Furthermore, some genes are known that can be associated with different, family-specific predisposition syndromes. Different authors have speculated about the mechanisms underlying those observations, but so far the experimental data supporting the various hypotheses are scarce [43].

2.6.1
Colocalization of Additional Mechanisms

The simplest explanation for the tissue-restricted tumor phenotype demonstrated by most disorders would be a cell-type specific expression of the predisposing gene. However, the genes associated with inherited tumor predispositions are mostly not known to show tissue specific expression patterns, but are often active in many if not all parts of the body. A more feasible model would be that different cell types may have different tumor suppressor mechanisms, and that a syndrome-specific cell type suppressor mechanism colocalizes with the cancer predisposition gene in the genome [44]. In its most simplified form, such a tumor suppressor mechanism could consist of the regulation of a cell-type specific growth-promoting gene or a gene involved in genetic stability. The genomic element coding for the suppressor mechanism could be localized in an intron of the predisposing gene, overlap it, or be in the flanking regions. Such a suppressor mechanism could take different forms, such as a regulatory genomic element (e.g. regulatory genes, transcription factors, microRNA) or an insulator element that normally prevents the flow of transcriptional activity to neighboring genes [43, 45]. A tumor would then arise if one allele of the cell-type specific suppressor mechanism is co-mutated by the second-hit mutation that also knocks out the remaining intact allele of the predisposition gene. Such a co-mutation could be caused, for example, by a small subcytogenetic deletion, a mutation type commonly found as a second hit mutation in different hereditary tumors [30]. The co-mutation of the suppressor mechanism would have a pro-proliferative effect that would only be active in cells of a certain type, ensuring the cell-type or organ specificity of the respective hereditary tumor predisposition. Co-mutations in other cell types would have no tumorigenic effects, since the proposed suppressor mechanism is not engaged in these cells.

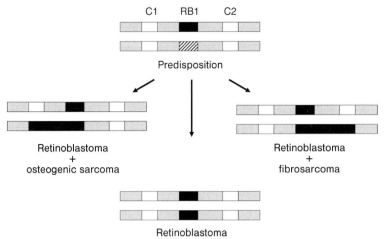

Figure 2.3 Retinoblastoma and associated malignancies. Model of two cell-type specific regulatory elements explaining the occurrence of different, less common malignancies in addition to the main tumor type. *RB1*, retinoblastoma gene; C1, C2, cell-type specific regulatory elements; small black boxes, *RB1* gene mutation; large black boxes, second hit mutation; shaded small box, normal *RB1* allele.

2.6.2
The Involvement of More Than One Cell Type

A slightly modified version of the model discussed above could apply to hereditary tumor syndromes that predispose to malignancies in more than one cell type [43, 46]. An example of such a predisposition is (again) inherited retinoblastoma in which the most common lesion is retinoma and retinoblastoma, with occasional manifestations of osteogenic sarcomas and (possible) fibrosarcomas. These latter tumor types could be explained by the existence of two or more cell-type specific tumor suppressor mechanisms within or in close proximity to the predisposing *RB1* gene (Figure 2.3). Additional examples of hereditary tumor syndromes to which this extended model of cell-type specificity could apply are familial adenomatous polyposis coli (FAP), and von Hippel–Lindau syndrome. In FAP, the basic phenotype is of multiple polyps of the colon. Some FAP families with germline *APC* mutations develop additional symptoms, such as brain tumors (Turcot's syndrome), or soft tissue tumors (Gardner syndrome) [47]. Patients with von Hippel–Lindau syndrome are at risk of phaeochromocytomas, renal tumors, and different vascular tumor types [48]. It is possible that different forms of cell-type specific tumor suppressor mechanisms (e.g. cell cycle regulators, apoptosis control mechanisms, or DNA integrity control mechanisms) are linked to the respective predisposing genes in these syndromes.

2.6.3
Cell-Type Specificity in Recessive Inheritance

Most hereditary tumor syndromes follow an autosomal dominant mode of inheritance; however, examples such as Xeroderma pigmentosum mentioned above show autosomal recessive inheritance [49]. In these syndromes, the predisposition already requires the inheritance of two mutated alleles, thus additional "hits" in other genes are needed to start tumorigenesis. One possibility would be that this additional hit targets a cell-type specific tumor suppressor mechanism. Such a simplified model would not even require that the suppressor mechanism is closely linked to, or even on the same chromosome, as the recessively inherited predisposition gene.

2.7
Conclusions and Future Directions

Inherited tumor predispositions still represent a challenge for genetics and oncology. The relationship between a given mutation and the clinically observed phenotype is often anything but straightforward, making it difficult to analyze the complex mechanisms of tumor pathogenesis. The effect of high-penetrance mutations in tumor predisposition genes is often modulated by various, mostly unknown factors such as low-penetrance susceptibility genes, somatic mutations, and environmental influences. Nevertheless, inherited tumor predispositions represent only one end of a continuum that includes the complete spectrum from familial to sporadic cases of cancer. Low penetrance mutations or modifier genes account for much of the low-level genetic predisposition, underlying the more common sporadic cases of cancer. Identifying such modifier genes, and understanding the mechanisms they participate in, presents a great challenge for cancer research, but will be of great importance for the future development of new preventive and therapeutic strategies.

References

1 Knudson, A.G. (1971) Mutation and cancer: statistical study of retinoblastoma. *Proceedings of the National Academy of Sciences of The United States of America*, **68**, 820–3.

2 Santarosa, M. and Ashworth, A. (2004) Haploinsufficiency for tumour suppressor genes: when you don't need to go all the way. *Biochimica et Biophysica Acta*, **1654**, 105–22.

3 Tucker, T. and Friedman, J.M. (2002) Pathogenesis of hereditary tumors: beyond the "two-hit" hypothesis. *Clinical Genetics*, **62**, 345–57.

4 Bishop, J.N., Harland, M. and Bishop, D.T. (2006) The genetics of melanoma. *British Journal of Hospital Medicine (London)*, **67**, 299–304.

5 Rostagno, P., Gioanni, J., Garino, E., Vallino, P., Namer, M. and Frenay, M.

(2003) A mutation analysis of the BRCA1 gene in 140 families from southeast France with a history of breast and/or ovarian cancer. *Journal of Human Genetics*, **48**, 362–6.

6 Korpershoek, E., Van Nederveen, F.H., Dannenberg, H., Petri, B.J., Komminoth, P., Perren, A., Lenders, J.W., Verhofstad, A.A., De Herder, W.W., De Krijger, R.R. and Dinjens, W.N. (2006) Genetic analyses of apparently sporadic pheochromocytomas: the Rotterdam experience. *Annals of the New York Academy of Sciences*, **1073**, 138–48.

7 Cunningham, J.M., Kim, C.Y., Christensen, E.R., Tester, D.J., Parc, Y., Burgart, L.J., Halling, K.C., McDonnell, S.K., Schaid, D.J., Walsh Vockley, C., Kubly, V., Nelson, H., Michels, V.V. and Thibodeau, S.N. (2001) The frequency of hereditary defective mismatch repair in a prospective series of unselected colorectal carcinomas. *American Journal of Human Genetics*, **69**, 780–90.

8 Struewing, J.P., Hartge, P., Wacholder, S., Baker, S.M., Berlin, M., McAdams, M., Timmerman, M.M., Brody, L.C. and Tucker, M.A. (1997) The risk of cancer associated with specific mutations of BRCA1 and BRCA2 among Ashkenazi Jews. *The New England Journal of Medicine*, **336**, 1401–8.

9 Fodor, F.H., Weston, A., Bleiweiss, I.J., McCurdy, L.D., Walsh, M.M., Tartter, P.I., Brower, S.T. and Eng, C.M. (1998) Frequency and carrier risk associated with common BRCA1 and BRCA2 mutations in Ashkenazi Jewish breast cancer patients. *American Journal of Human Genetics*, **63**, 45–51.

10 Turner, J.J., Leotlela, P.D., Pannett, A.A., Forbes, S.A., Bassett, J.H., Harding, B., Christie, P.T., Bowen-Jones, D., Ellard, S., Hattersley, A., Jackson, C.E., Pope, R., Quarrell, O.W., Trembath, R. and Thakker, R.V. (2002) Frequent occurrence of an intron 4 mutation in multiple endocrine neoplasia type 1. *The Journal of Clinical Endocrinology and Metabolism*, **87**, 2688–93.

11 Hohenstein, P. and Fodde, R. (2003) Of mice and (wo)men: genotype-phenotype correlations in BRCA1.

Human Molecular Genetics, **12** (Spec No 2), R271–7.

12 Boyd, J., Sonoda, Y., Federici, M.G., Bogomolniy, F., Rhei, E., Maresco, D.L., Saigo, P.E., Almadrones, L.A., Barakat, R.R., Brown, C.L., Chi, D.S., Curtin, J.P., Poynor, E.A. and Hoskins, W.J. (2000) Clinicopathologic features of BRCA-linked and sporadic ovarian cancer. *The Journal of the American Medical Association*, **283**, 2260–5.

13 Park, J.G., Vasen, H.F., Park, K.J., Peltomaki, P., Ponz de Leon, M., Rodriguez-Bigas, M.A., Lubinski, J., Beck, N.E., Bisgaard, M.L., Miyaki, M., Wijnen, J.T., Baba, S. and Lynch, H.T. (1999) Suspected hereditary nonpolyposis colorectal cancer: International Collaborative Group on Hereditary Non-Polyposis Colorectal Cancer (ICG-HNPCC) criteria and results of genetic diagnosis. *Diseases of the Colon and Rectum*, **42**, 710–15.

14 Boland, C.R., Thibodeau, S.N., Hamilton, S.R., Sidransky, D., Eshleman, J.R., Burt, R.W., Meltzer, S.J., Rodriguez-Bigas, M.A., Fodde, R., Ranzani, G.N. and Srivastava, S. (1998) A National Cancer Institute Workshop on Microsatellite Instability for cancer detection and familial predisposition: development of international criteria for the determination of microsatellite instability in colorectal cancer. *Cancer Research*, **58**, 5248–57.

15 Antoniou, A., Pharoah, P.D., Narod, S., Risch, H.A., Eyfjord, J.E., Hopper, J.L., Loman, N., Olsson, H., Johannsson, O., Borg, A., Pasini, B., Radice, P., Manoukian, S., Eccles, D.M., Tang, N., Olah, E., Anton-Culver, H., Warner, E., Lubinski, J., Gronwald, J., Gorski, B., Tulinius, H., Thorlacius, S., Eerola, H., Nevanlinna, H., Syrjäkoski, K., Kallioniemi, O.P., Thompson, D., Evans, C., Peto, J., Lalloo, F., Evans, D.G. and Easton, D.F. (2003) Average risks of breast and ovarian cancer associated with BRCA1 or BRCA2 mutations detected in case Series unselected for family history: a combined analysis of 22 studies. *American Journal of Human Genetics*, **72**, 1117–30.

16 Rousseau, F., Bonaventure, J., Legeai-Mallet, L., Pelet, A., Rozet, J.M.,

Maroteaux, P., Le Merrer, M. and Munnich, A. (1994) Mutations in the gene encoding fibroblast growth factor receptor-3 in achondroplasia. *Nature,* **371**, 252–4.

17 Chaganti, R.S., Schonberg, S. and German, J. (1974) A manyfold increase in sister chromatid exchanges in Bloom's syndrome lymphocytes. *Proceedings of the National Academy of Sciences of the United States of America,* **71**, 4508–12.

18 Flejter, W.L., McDaniel, L.D., Johns, D., Friedberg, E.C. and Schultz, R.A. (1992) Correction of xeroderma pigmentosum complementation group D mutant cell phenotypes by chromosome and gene transfer: involvement of the human ERCC2 DNA repair gene. *Proceedings of the National Academy of Sciences of the United States of America,* **89**, 261–5.

19 Savitsky, K., Bar-Shira, A., Gilad, S., Rotman, G., Ziv, Y., Vanagaite, L., Tagle, D.A., Smith, S., Uziel, T., Sfez, S., Ashkenazi, M., Pecker, I., Frydman, M., Harnik, R., Patanjali, S.R., Simmons, A., Clines, G.A., Sartiel, A., Gatti, R.A., Chessa, L., Sanal, O., Lavin, M.F., Jaspers, N.G., Taylor, A.M., Arlett, C.F., Miki, T., Weissman, S.M., Lovett, M., Collins, F.S. and Shiloh, Y. (1995) A single ataxia telangiectasia gene with a product similar to PI-3 kinase. *Science,* **268**, 1749–53.

20 Renwick, A., Thompson, D., Seal, S., Kelly, P., Chagtai, T., Ahmed, M., North, B., Jayatilake, H., Barfoot, R., Spanova, K., McGuffog, L., Evans, D.G. and Eccles, D., Breast Cancer Susceptibility Collaboration (UK), Easton, D.F., Stratton, M.R. and Rahman, N. (2006) ATM mutations that cause ataxia-telangiectasia are breast cancer susceptibility alleles. *Nature Genetics,* **38**, 873–5.

21 King, M.C., Marks, J.H. and Mandell, J.B. (2003) Breast and ovarian cancer risks due to inherited mutations in BRCA1 and BRCA2. *Science,* **302**, 643–6.

22 Locker, G.Y. and Lynch, H.T. (2004) Genetic factors and colorectal cancer in Ashkenazi Jews. *Familial Cancer,* **3**, 215–21.

23 Easton, D.F., Ponder, M.A., Huson, S.M. and Ponder, B.A. (1993) An analysis of variation in expression of neurofibromatosis (NF) type 1 (NF1): evidence for modifying genes. *American Journal of Human Genetics,* **53**, 305–13.

24 Scheffer, H., te Meerman, G.J., Kruize, Y.C., van den Berg, A.H., Penninga, D.P., Tan, K.E., der Kinderen, D.J. and Buys, C.H. (1989) Linkage analysis of families with hereditary retinoblastoma: nonpenetrance of mutation, revealed by combined use of markers within and flanking the RB1 gene. *American Journal of Human Genetics,* **45**, 252–60.

25 Sakai, T., Ohtani, N., McGee, T.L., Robbins, P.D. and Dryja, T.P. (1991) Oncogenic germ-line mutations in Sp1 and ATF sites in the human retinoblastoma gene. *Nature,* **353**, 83–6.

26 Benn, D.E., Croxson, M.S., Tucker, K., Bambach, C.P., Richardson, A.L., Delbridge, L., Pullan, P.T., Hammond, J., Marsh, D.J. and Robinson, B.G. (2003) Novel succinate dehydrogenase subunit B (SDHB) mutations in familial phaeochromocytomas and paragangliomas, but an absence of somatic SDHB mutations in sporadic phaeochromocytomas. *Oncogene,* **22**, 1358–64.

27 Otterson, G.A., Chen, W., Coxon, A.B., Khleif, S.N. and Kaye, F.J. (1997) Incomplete penetrance of familial retinoblastoma linked to germ-line mutations that result in partial loss of RB function. *Proceedings of the National Academy of Sciences of the United States of America,* **94**, 12036–40.

28 Sánchez-Sánchez, F., Ramírez-Castillejo, C., Weekes, D.B., Beneyto, M., Prieto, F., Nájera, C. and Mittnacht, S. (2007) Attenuation of disease phenotype through alternative translation initiation in low-penetrance retinoblastoma. *Human Mutation,* **28**, 159–67.

29 Cavenee, W.K., Dryja, T.P., Phillips, R.A., Benedict, W.F., Godbout, R., Gallie, B.L., Murphree, A.L., Strong, L.C. and White, R.L. (1983) Expression of recessive alleles by chromosomal mechanisms in retinoblastoma. *Nature,* **305**, 779–84.

30 Hagstrom, S.A. and Dryja, T.P. (1999) Mitotic recombination map of 13cen-13q14 derived from an investigation of loss of heterozygosity in retinoblastomas.

Proceedings of the National Academy of Sciences of the United States of America, **96**, 2952–7.

31 Fearon, E.R., Vogelstein, B. and Feinberg, A.P. (1984) Somatic deletion and duplication of genes on chromosome 11 in Wilms' tumours. *Nature*, **309**, 176–8.

32 Varley, J.M., Thorncroft, M., McGown, G., Appleby, J., Kelsey, A.M., Tricker, K.J., Evans, D.G. and Birch, J.M. (1997) A detailed study of loss of heterozygosity on chromosome 17 in tumours from Li-Fraumeni patients carrying a mutation to the TP53 gene. *Oncogene*, **14**, 865–71.

33 Mulligan, L.M., Kwok, J.B., Healey, C.S., Elsdon, M.J., Eng, C., Gardner, E., Love, D.R., Mole, S.E., Moore, J.K. and Papi, L. (1993) Germ-line mutations of the RET proto-oncogene in multiple endocrine neoplasia type 2A. *Nature*, **363**, 458–60.

34 Seizinger, B.R., Martuza, R.L. and Gusella, J.F. (1986) Loss of genes on chromosome 22 in tumorigenesis of human acoustic neuroma. *Nature*, **322**, 644–547.

35 Watson, C.J., Gaunt, L., Evans, G., Patel, K., Harris, R. and Strachan, T. (1993) A disease-associated germline deletion maps the type 2 neurofibromatosis (NF2) gene between the Ewing sarcoma region and the leukaemia inhibitory factor locus. *Human Molecular Genetics*, **2**, 701–4.

36 Paige, A.J. (2003) Redefining tumour suppressor genes: exceptions to the two-hit hypothesis. *Cellular and Molecular Life Sciences*, **60**, 2147–63.

37 Vogelstein, B. and Kinzler, K.W. (1993) The multistep nature of cancer. *Trends in Genetics*, **9**, 138–41.

38 Potluri, V.R., Helson, L., Ellsworth, R.M., Reid, T. and Gilbert, F. (1986) Chromosomal abnormalities in human retinoblastoma. A review. *Cancer*, **58**, 663–71.

39 Squire, J., Gallie, B.L. and Phillips, R.A. (1985) A detailed analysis of chromosomal changes in heritable and non-heritable retinoblastoma. *Human Genetics*, **70**, 291–301.

40 Gallie, B.L., Campbell, C., Devlin, H., Duckett, A. and Squire, J.A. (1999) Developmental basis of retinal-specific induction of cancer by RB mutation. *Cancer Research*, **7** (59 Suppl), 1731s–5.

41 Fialkow, P.J., Sagebiel, R.W., Gartler, S.M. and Rimoin, D.L. (1971) Multiple cell origin of hereditary neurofibromas. *The New England Journal of Medicine*, **284**, 298–300.

42 Däschner, K., Assum, G., Eisenbarth, I., Krone, W., Hoffmeyer, S., Wortmann, S., Heymer, B. and Kehrer-Sawatzki, H. (1997) Clonal origin of tumor cells in a plexiform neurofibroma with LOH in NF1 intron 38 and in dermal neurofibromas without LOH of the NF1 gene. *Biochemical and Biophysical Research Communications*, **234**, 346–50.

43 Bignold, L.P. (2004) The cell-type-specificity of inherited predispositions to tumours: review and hypothesis. *Cancer Letters*, **216**, 127–46.

44 Godbout, R., Dryja, T.P., Squire, J., Gallie, B.L. and Phillips, R.A. (1983) Somatic inactivation of genes on chromosome 13 is a common event in retinoblastoma. *Nature*, **304**, 451–3.

45 Geyer, P.K. and Clark, I. (2002) Protecting against promiscuity: the regulatory role of insulators. *Cellular and Molecular Life Sciences*, **59**, 2112–27.

46 Bignold, L.P. (2003) Initiation of genetic instability and tumour formation: a review and hypothesis of a nongenotoxic mechanism. *Cellular and Molecular Life Sciences*, **60**, 1107–17.

47 Foulkes, W.D. (1995) A tale of four syndromes: familial adenomatous polyposis, Gardner syndrome, attenuated APC and Turcot syndrome. *Monthly Journal of the Association of Physicians*, **88**, 853–63.

48 Lonser, R.R., Glenn, G.M., Walther, M., Chew, E.Y., Libutti, S.K., Linehan, W.M. and Oldfield, E.H. (2003) von Hippel-Lindau disease. *Lancet*, **361**, 2059–67.

49 Cleaver, J.E. (1968) Defective repair replication of DNA in xeroderma pigmentosum. *Nature*, **218**, 652–6.

Part II
Syndromal Types of Hereditary Tumors

3
Family Cancer Syndromes

Helga Rehder

Summary

Familial cancer syndromes are defined by an inherited predisposition to a syndrome specific pattern of different tumor types and sites, aggregating within families, to earlier onset of tumor development and to the occurrence of multiple primary tumors in affected individuals. The different tumors of a familial cancer syndrome share common causative genes and molecular pathways. A first mutation always represents a predisposing germline mutation that was either inherited, or arose from a new mutation in a parental germ cell. Local tumor manifestation requires at least one additional somatic "second hit" mutation. Since Knudson's "two hit hypothesis", a model to explain multifocal primary tumors in hereditary retinoblastoma, a great number of family cancer syndromes have been recognized. This chapter does not claim completeness but rather aims to summarize and emphasize those conditions for which predisposing genes have been identified and respective tests can be offered. Since this chapter provides a comprehensive overview and synopsis on cancer family syndromes, some contents might be overlapping with previous, organ-specific chapters. The reader is advised to refer to these chapters for additional information on particular hereditary cancer conditions. Malformation syndromes, presenting with an increased tumor risk (Chapter 4 on Genetic Dysmorphic Syndromes), and hereditary solitary cancers are not the subject of this comprehensive chapter. The reader is also advised to refer to organ specific chapters for additional information on particular hereditary cancer conditions.

3.1
Introduction

A cancer family syndrome was first described by Warthin, 1913 [1], who over a 30-year period studied a family with a clustering of endometrial and gastric cancers. When, 53 years later, Lynch and coworkers published on their two families that, in addition to endometrial and gastric cancers, presented with an even wider range of different tumors and with family members affected by

Hereditary Tumors: From Genes to Clinical Consequences
Edited by Heike Allgayer, Helga Rehder and Simone Fulda
Copyright © 2009 WILEY-VCH Verlag GmbH & Co. KGaA, Weinheim
ISBN: 978-3-527-32028-8

multiple primary neoplasias, the term "cancer family syndrome" was coined, but it was clearly restricted to the "Lynch cancer family syndrome" [2]. In 1969, a second syndromal tumor disorder was described by Li and Fraumeni [3], characterized by a familial aggregation of childhood soft tissue sarcomas, early onset breast cancer, and other neoplasms. By analogy with the "cancer family syndrome", it was designated as "sarcoma family syndrome". For other cancer syndromes that were recognized in subsequent years, the term cancer family syndrome was no more disposable. The terms "hereditary cancer predisposition syndromes", "inherited cancer susceptibility syndromes", "familial or hereditary cancer syndromes", or "family cancer syndromes" are now widely used [4–6]. However, none of these latter terms focuses on the fact that, besides familial aggregation, the many different tumors within a "cancer family", that belong to a "family of tumors", are related by their common genetic origin and common molecular pathways.

Hereditary cancer syndromes are clinically characterized by a genetic predisposition:

- For a distinctive pattern of different, site and type specific tumors that aggregate within families,
- For an earlier onset of tumor development, and
- For the tendency of a gene carrier to develop multiple primary tumors.

In the majority of cases, and as in hereditary solitary cancers, the heterozygous germline mutation needs additional hits to develop a tumor. Somatic second hits refer to loss of heterozygosity (LOH) by loss of the normal wildtype allele and reduction to hemi- or homozygosity for the mutated allele, to acquired mutations in other interacting genes, to regulatory inactivation, and to alteration in gene methylation, affecting the grade of gene activity.

Hundreds of genes and proteins, essential to regulate normal cell division and apoptosis, and also DNA replication and repair, can undergo mutations and thus be responsible for susceptibility to the differing hereditary cancer syndromes and subsequent uncontrolled cancerous growth. Predominant molecular mechanisms are transformation of a proto-oncogene into an oncogene by a "gain of function" mutation, inactivation of a tumor suppressor gene, and inactivation of a mismatch repair (MMR) gene by "loss of function" mutations.

Penetrance of mutations predisposing to family cancer syndromes is usually high. Since most of these mutations are autosomal dominant, the risk of a member of a cancer family being a gene carrier and to develop one or more tumors is close to 50%. Aggressive tumor screening programs and invasive prophylactic measures are components of preventive oncology. They require thorough risk assessments and predictive gene tests, by clinicians, geneticists, and psychologists, after profound information and counseling of those at risk.

Table 3.1 covers most familial cancer syndromes for which responsible gene mutations have been identified. Further information on clinical and genetic aspects and on available gene tests can be found on the websites http://facd.uicc.org/, www.ncbi.nlm.nih.gov/entrez?db=omim and www.genetests.org.

Table 3.1 Family cancer syndromes – in alphabetical order.

CFS	Syndrome specific tumors/ features	Associated tumors	Trait	Incidence	Genes involved	Gene loca lization	OMIM No.	References
Ataxia-telangiectasia	Leukemia, usually of T-cell origin Lymphoma, usually of B-cell origin	Breast/ovarian/gastric/ pancreatic cancers – in adults	AR	~1:100000– 1:300000 p	*ATM*	11q22.3	#208900 *251260	[6]
Bannayan-Ruvalcaba-Riley syndrome (BRRS) (Bannayan Zonana/ Riley-Smith/ Ruvalcaba-Myhre-Smith syndrome; PTEN hamartoma tumor syndrome – allelic to Cowden syndrome)	Intestinal hamartomas with angiomatous, lipomatous and lymphangiomatous components Skin tumors • lipomas • haemangiomas (in the presence of macrocephaly)	Meningioma Follicular cell tumor of thyroid	AD	Not known	*PTEN*	10q23.31	#153480 *601728	[7, 8]
Birt-Hogg-Dubé syndrome	Cutaneous hamartomas • fibrofolliculomas • trichodiscomas • acrochordons Lung cysts and pneumothorax	Renal tumors • chromophobe carcinomas (cc) • oncocytomas or hybrids with cc • clear cell and papillary cancer Parathyroid adenomas Thyroid adenomas/ carcinomas Parotid oncocytomas Angiolipomas	AD	~6% of FRT	*FLCN*	17p11.2	#135150 *607273	[9, 10]

Table 3.1 *Continued*

CFS	Syndrome specific tumors/ features	Associated tumors	Trait	Incidence	Genes involved	Gene loca lization	OMIM No.	References
Bloom's syndrome	Immunodeficiency Erythematous skin lesions (sun-sensitive) Small body size Diabetes mellitus Chronic pulmonary disease	Leukemia/ lymphoma Multiple cancers – early onset • GI-/respiratory tract • breast/hepatocellular cancers • urogenital tract incl. Wilms tumor • and others	AR	~300 pc	RecQL3	15q26.1	#210900 *604610	[11, 12]
Breast/ovarian cancer type 1	Breast cancer Ovarian cancer	Papillary serous carcinoma of peritoneum Prostate cancer Colon cancer	AD	1:500–1000 carrier rate	BRCA1	17q21	+113705	[13]
Breast/ovarian cancer type 2	Breast cancer (including males) Ovarian cancer	Prostate cancer Pancreatic/colon cancer Other gastrointestinal cancers Leukemias Melanomas	AD	1:50–700 carrier rate	BRCA2	13q12.3	+600185	[13]

Syndrome	Clinical features		Inheritance	Gene	Locus	OMIM	Ref.
Carney syndrome (complex) (Carney complex type 1 (CNC1)* Carney complex type 2 (CNC2)** NAME syndrome LAMB syndrome)	Myxomas • atrial/ventricular of the heart • eyelid • subcutaneous • myxoid uterine leiomyoma • myxoid neurofibroma Pigmented skin lesions (spotty) • nevi, ephelides, blue nevi • centrofacial / mucosal lentigines • red hair, hirsuitism Endocrine hyperactivity • thyroid, adrenal, pituitary Hyper-/dysplasia/ Cushing disease/ Acromegaly	Sertoli cell tumor (large cell, calcified) Leydig cell tumor Adrenal/pituitary adenoma Mammary ductal fibroadenoma Schwannoma (e.g. melanotic) Thyroid cancer Phaeochromocytoma	AD >200 pc	PRKAR1A (CNC1) CNC2	17q23-q24 2p16 (amplifications/ deletions of CNC2 region)	#160980 *188830 %605244	[14, 15]
Carney complex variant (questionable CS)	see: CARNEY syndrome plus distal arthrogryposis (trismus-pseudocamptodaktyly)	see: CARNEY syndrome	–	MYH8	17p13.1	#160980 %608837	[14, 15]

Table 3.1 *Continued*

CFS	Syndrome specific tumors/ features	Trait	Incidence	Genes involved	Gene loca lization	OMIM No.	References
Costello syndrome (faciocutaneoskeletal syndrome)	Papillomata • perioral • nasal • anal Sqamous acanthomas of skin (skin and heart anomalies)	AD	~250 pc	*HRAS*	11p15.5	#218040 *190020	[16]
Cowden syndrome (PTEN harmatoma-tumor syndrome – allelic with BRRS)	Mucocutaneous lesions: • facial trichilemmomas • papillomatous papules • acral keratosis • subcutaneous lipomas Intest. hamarto-matous polyps Breast lesions incl. fibroadenoma Thyroid lesions incl. adenoma Macrocephaly	AD	1:200 000 p	*PTEN*	10q23.31	#158350 *601728	[8, 17]

Associated tumors (Costello syndrome): Epithelioma, Bladder cancer, Rhabdomyosarcoma, Ganglioneuroblastoma, Vestibular schwannoma

Associated tumors (Cowden syndrome): Breast cancer (30–50%), Endometrial cancer (10%), Ovarian and uterine cancer, Thyroid cancer (3–10%), Colon and bladder cancer, Meningioma

Syndrome	Cancer	Extracolonic tumors	Inheritance	Frequency	Gene	Location	OMIM	References
Familial adenomatous polyposis (FAP)	Colorectal adenomatous polyps Precancerous polyps Colorectal cancer	Extracolonic tumors • upper GI-tract • osteoma/desmoids • childhood hepatoblastoma • adrenal corticoid tumors • thyroid/bile duct cancers	AD	~1:35000p	APC	5q21-q22	+175100	[18, 19]
Gardner syndrome (Familial adnomatous polyposis, FAP)	see: FAP		AD	See: FAP	APC	5q21-q22	+175100	[20]
Gorlin syndrome (nevoid basal cell carcinoma syndrome) (basal cell nevus syndrome)	Basal cell cancers Palmar and plantar pits Odontogenic keratocysts Calcification of the falx cerebri	Childhood medulloblastoma (5%) Ovarian fibromas Cardiac fibromas/ rhabdomyomas Meningioma/ mesenchymoma/ lymphoma/fibrosarcoma	AD	1:40000p	PTCH	9q22.3	#109400 *601309	[9, 21, 22]
Hereditary diffuse gastric cancer (CHDGC+LBC with lobular breast cancer)	Diffuse gastric cancer Lobular breast cancer	Endometrial cancer Ovarian cancer	AD	Not known	CDH1	16q22.1	+192090	[128]

Table 3.1 *Continued*

CFS	Syndrome specific tumors/ features	Associated tumors	Trait	Incidence	Genes involved	Gene loca lization	OMIM No.	References
Hyperparathyreoidism-jaw tumor syndrome (HRPT2)	Parathyroid adenoma/carcinoma Ossifying fibromas of the jaw	Renal tumors • cortical adenoma/ hamartoma • Wilms tumor – late onset • papillary/clear cell carcinoma Pancreatic adenocarcinoma Testicular germ cell tumor Hurthle cell thyroid adenoma	AD	Not known	HRPT2	1q25-q31	#145001 *607393	[23, 24]
Juvenile polyposis syndrome	Hamartomatous juvenile polyps in • small intestine and stomach • colorectum	Colorectal cancer	AD	1:16000– 100000 p	BMPR1A SMAD4	10q22.3 18q21.1	#174900 *601299 *600993	[17, 25]
LAMB syndrome (lentigines, atrial myxoma, mucocutaneous myxoma, blue nevi)	see: CARNEY syndrome			–				

Li–Fraumeni 1 syndrome (LFS1) • Sarcoma family syndrome of Li and Fraumeni • SBLA syndrome (**s**arcoma, **b**reast and **b**rain tumors, **l**eukemia, **l**aryngeal and **l**ung cancer, **a**drenal cortical carcinoma)	Sarcomas: • soft tissue sarcoma (fibro-/lipo-/leiomyosarcoma) • osteosarcoma • childhood rhabdomyosarcoma Breast cancer (premenopausal) Brain tumor • medulloblastoma • glioblastoma/glioma • choroid plexus carcinoma Acute leukemia Lung adenocarcinoma Adrenal cortical carcinoma	Gastric/colorectal cancer Ovarian cancer Melanoma Laryngeal carcinoma Lymphoma Gonadal germ cell tumor Endometrial cancer Thyroid/pancreatic cancer Prostate cancer Cervical cancer Wilms tumor Malignant phyllodes breast tumor	AD	~400 pc	*TP53*	17p13.1	#151623 %191170	[26, 27]
Li–Fraumeni 2 syndrome (LFS2)	see: LFS1	see: LFS1	AD	See: LFS1	*CHEK2*	2q12.1	#609265 %604373	[28]
Li–Fraumeni 3 syndrome (LFS3)	see: LFS1	see: LFS1	AD	See: LFS1			#151623 %609266	[29]
Li–Fraumeni-like syndrome (LFL) • not strictly confirming the definition of LFS	see: LFS1	see: LFS1	AD	See: LFS1	*TP53* *CHEK2* *BRCA2*	17p13.1 2q12.1 13q12.3	#151623 %191170 %604373 %600185	[30]

Table 3.1 *Continued*

CFS	Syndrome specific tumors/features	Associated tumors	Trait	Incidence	Genes involved	Gene localization	OMIM No.	References
Lynch syndrome (II) • (Lynch) cancer family syndrome • HNPCC – hereditary nonpolyposis colorectal cancer – with extracolonic tumors	Adenocarcinomas of the colon, mostly proximal and multiple Adenomas of the colon, mostly dyplastic and multiple Endometrial carcinoma	Gastric adenocarcinoma Ovarian cancer Hepatobiliary tract cancers Transitional cancer of ureter/renal pelvis Small bowel cancers Brain-/CNS tumors Duodenal and jejunal cancer Skin tumors	AD	1–3% CC 1–1.5% EC	MLH1	3p21.3	#114400 *120436	[31, 32]
Melanoma-astrocytoma syndrome	Malignant melanoma (multiple) Atypical nevi	Neural system tumors • astrocytoma • medulloblastoma • glioblastoma multiforme • ependymoma/ meningioma • glioma/neurofibroma • acoustic neurilemmoma	AD	Single families	CDKN2A CDKN2B (contiguous 9p21deletiom)	9p21	#155755 *600160	[33, 34]
Melanoma-pancreatic cancer syndrome (Familial atypical multiple mole melanoma-pancreatic cancer syndrome, FAMMMPC)	Malignant melanoma (multiple) Multiple atypical (precursor) nevi	Pancreatic cancer Breast cancer Squamous cell carcinoma	AD	12% of PC	CDKN2A/p16	9p21	#606719 *600160	[35–37]

MEN1 syndrome (Multiple endocrine neoplasias type 1) (Werner syndrome)	Endocrine tumors of the • parathyroids • anterior pituitary • GEP-tract-	Facial angiofibromas Collagenomas Lipomas Mengiomas/ependymomas Leiomyomas	AD	1:30000 p	*MEN1*	11q13	+131100	[38, 39]
MEN2A syndrome (Sipple syndrome)	Medullary thyroid carcinoma Cutanous lichen amyloidosis Hirschsprung disease	Phaeochromocytoma Parathyroid adenoma	AD	MEN2A+2B 1:30000 p	*RET*	10q11.2	#171400	[40]
MEN2B syndrome (Wagenmann–Froboese syndrome) (Mucosal neuroma syndrome)	Medullary thyroid carcinoma Mucosal neuromas Dysmorphic features	Phaeochromocytoma Ganglioneuroma (gastrointestinal)	AD	MEN2A+2B 1:30000 p	*RET*	10q11.2	#162300	[40]
Muir–Torre syndrome (MTS)	Sebaceous gland tumours: • sebaceous adenomas • sebaceous epitheliomas • sebaceous carcinoma (24–30%) • keratoacanthoma with sebaceous differentiation	Visceral malignancies: • gastrointestinal cancers (61%) (colorectal 50%) • genitourinary cancers (24%) (endometrial 15%)	AD	not known	*MSH2, MLH1* deletion	2p22–p21 3p21.3	#158320 *609309 *120436	[41]

Table 3.1 *Continued*

CFS	Syndrome specific tumors/features	Associated tumors	Trait	Incidence	Genes involved	Gene localization	OMIM No.	References
NAME syndrome (nevi, atrial myxoma, mucinosis of skin, endocrine overactivity)	see: Carney syndrome	see: Carney syndrome		–				
Neurofibromatosis 1 (NF1) (von Recklinghausen disease)	Neurofibromas • dermal • subdermal • spinal • visceral • neurofibrosarcoma Pigmentary changes • café au lait spots/ freckling • Lisch nodules Scoliosis	Cranial tumours • optic glioma • pilocytic astrocytoma • menigioma/ ependymoma • hypothalamic tumor Fibro-/ Neurofibrosarcoma Malignant periph. Schwannoma Rhabdomyosarcoma Phaeochromocytoma Parathyroid adenoma Duodenal carcinoid tumor Pilocytic astrocytoma Non-lymphocytic leukaemia	AD	1:2500–3000i	NF1	17q11.2	+162200	[42, 43]
Neurofibromatosis 2 (NF2)	Vestibular schwannoma uni- and bilateral)	Cutaneous schwannoma Meningioma Glioma Neurofibroma Ependymoma/ astrocytoma (rare)	AD	1:25 000i	NF2	22q12.2	#101000 *607379	[44]

Syndrome	Clinical features	Tumors		Inheritance	Incidence	Gene	Location	OMIM	Ref.
Nijmegen breakage syndrome	Short stature Progressive microcephaly Recurrent respiratory infections	B-cell Lymphoma Glioma Medulloblastoma Rhabdomyosarcoma		AR	Not known	NBN	8q21	#251260 602667	[17, 45]
Peutz–Jeghers syndrome (PJS) (Hamartomatous intestinal polyposis, polyps-and-spots syndrome)	Hamartomatous polyps • small intestine (64%) • colon (53%) and rectum (32%) • stomach (49%) • biliary tract • nasal and bronchial • bladder, ureteral and renal pelvis Mucocutaneous pigmentation (95%) • lips and buccal mucosa • hands (palms), arms, feet and legs	Any type of cancer (81%), e.g. • gastrointestinal (66%) incl. pancreas • breast (32%) and ovary • adenoma malignum of cervix • lung, thyroid Benign, hormone producing sex-cord tumors of ovary/testis		AD	1:25 00–1:280 000 p	STK11	19p13.3	#175200 *602216	
Retinoblastoma	Retinoblastoma • unilateral • bilateral (~40%)	Osteosarcoma/ Ewing sarcoma Soft tissue sarcomas Melanoma Pineoblastoma Lung cancer/Bladder cancer Leukemia/lymphoma		AD	1:28 000 i	RB1	13q14.1–13q14.2	+180200	[46]

Table 3.1 *Continued*

CFS	Syndrome specific tumors/features	Associated tumors	Trait	Incidence	Genes involved	Gene localization	OMIM No.	References
Reed syndrome (Hereditary leiomyomatosis and renal cell cancer, LRCC)	Cutaneous • leiomyomas • leiomyosarcoma (rare) Uterine • leiomyomas/fibroids • leiomyosarcoma (rare)	Renal cancer • papillary type 2 • tubulo-papillary • collectin tubules Leydig cell tumour of testis	AD	Not known	*FH*	1q42.1	#605839 *136850	[47, 48]
Rhabdoid predisposition syndrome	Atyp. teratoid/rhabdoid tumors of • kidney • brain	Other brain tumours • PNET • medulloblastoma/schwannoma • anaplastic ependymoma • chorioid plexus carcinoma • meningioma/pinealoblastoma • Ewing-/rhabdomyo-sarcoma	AD	Not known	*SNF5/ INI1*	22q11 deletion/duplication	#609322 *601607	[49–51]

Disease	Clinical features	Inheritance	Frequency	Gene	Locus	OMIM	Ref.
Rothmund–Thomson syndrome (Poikiloderma atrophicans and cataract)	Poikiloderma • erythema on face and limbs (rash) • reticular hyper- and hypopigmentation (chronic phase) • teleangiectases & punctate atrophy / Sparse hair / hyperkeratosis / Dysmorphic features / cataract / Skeletal & dental anomalies / Osteogenic sarcoma / Basal cell carcinoma / Squamous cell carcinoma (skin) / Leukemia / Hodgkin lymphoma (after therapy)	AR	~300 pc	*RECQL4~*	8q24.3	#268400 *603780	[52, 53]
Tuberous sclerosis complex (Morbus Bourneville-Pringle)	Skin lesions: • facial angiofibromas • hypomelanotic macules • shagreen patches / fibrous plaques / Brain hamartomas: • glial nodules / (sub)cortical tubers • astrocytomas / ependymomas / Renal angio-myolipomas / Cardiac rhabdo-myomas / Pulmonary lymphangiomatosis / Malignant angiomyolipoma / Renal cell carcinoma / Hamartomatous rectal polyps / Hamartomas in liver/spleen / Renal/bone cysts / Subungual/sublingual fibromas / Retinal achromic patches / Cerebral radial migration lines	AD	1:6000 p	*TSC1* *TSC2*	9q34 16p13.3	#191100 *605284 *191092	[54, 55]

Table 3.1 Continued

CFS	Syndrome specific tumors/features	Associated tumors	Trait	Incidence	Genes involved	Gene localization	OMIM No.	References
Turcot syndrome (Mismatch repair cancer indrome) (Brain tumor-polyposis indrome)	Brain tumours • medulloblastoma (APC complex) • glioblastoma (MMR defect) • astrocytoma/ependymoma Colonic tumors • colorectal polyps (APC complex) • colorectal adenomas (MMR defect) • colorectal cancer	Sebaceous cysts Café au lait spots Basal cell carcinoma Papillary thyroid carcinoma Leukemia	AD	Not known	APC MHL1 MSH2 PMS2 MSH6	5q21-q22 3p21.3 2p22-p21 7p22 2p16	#276300 *120436 *609309 +600259 +600678	[56, 57]
von Hippel–Lindau syndrome (VHL)	Haemangioblastomas • retinal • cerebellar • spinal • pancreatic Renal cell carcinoma Phaeochromocytoma Pancreatic tumors	Haemangiomas • pulmonary • hepatic • renal • adrenal Paraganglioma Tumors of epididymis • papillary cystadenoma(bilateral) • hypernephroid tumor/cysts	AD	~1:50000p	VHL	11q13 3p26-p25	#193300 *608537 *168461	[58–60]

	Premature aging / tumors	Inheritance	Incidence/prevalence	Gene	Locus	MIM number	References
Werner syndrome (Progeria of the adult)	Premature aging • atrophic skin/ skin ulcers • pigmentary alterations • soft tissue calcifications • graying of hair/ balding • osteoporosis • diabetes mellitus • arteriosclerosis/ myocard. infarct • hypogonadism/ early menopause — Soft tissue sarcomas Osteosarcomas Acral lentiginous melanoma Meningioma Thyroid carcinoma	AR	1:20– 40000 I (Japan) 1:200000 I (USA)	WRN	8p12p11.2	#277700 *604611	[61–63]
Xeroderma pigmentosum	Skin photosensitivity freckle like lesions poikiloderma/ skin atrophy teleangiektasia/ keratoses angioma/ keratoacanthoma photophobia — Early onset skin cancer • basal cell carcinoma • squamous cell carcinoma • malignant melanoma Tongue cancer	AR	1:1000000– 1:100000 p	XPA XPB XPC XPD XPE XPF XPG XPV	9q22.3 2q21 3p25 19q13.2-.3 11p12-p11 16p13.3-.1 13q33 6p21–p12	#278700 #610651 +278720 #278730 #278740 #278760 #278780 #278750	[64, 65]

MIM number prefixes: # = phenotype description, molecular basis known; * = gene with known sequence; + = gene with known sequence and phenotype; % = mendelian phenotype and locus, molecular basis unknown; AD = autosomal dominant; AR = autosomal recessive; CC = colon cancer; EC = endometrial cancer; FRT = familial renal tumours; GI = gastrointestinal; i = incidence; p = prevalence; pc = published cases; PC = pancreatic cancer; PNET = primitive neuroectodermal tumors.

The reader is also advised to refer to organ-specific chapters for additional information on particular hereditary cancer conditions.

3.2
Hereditary Non-Polyposis Colon Cancer Syndromes (HNPCC)

Lynch syndrome, or Lynch syndrome II, refers to hereditary non-polyposis colorectal cancer type 2 (HNPCC2), a cancer family syndrome that, in addition to increased occurrence of site specific, mostly proximal multiple primary adenomas and adenocarcinomas of the colon characteristic for HNPCC1 (or familial colon cancer), show a distinct pattern of extracolonic tumors [66]. These include endometrial carcinoma and also gastric, ovarian, hepatobiliary, proximal urinary, and small intestinal cancers, and brain tumors. For clinical diagnosis of HNPCC2, the Amsterdam criteria, defined for HNPCC1, had been modified to Amsterdam criteria II [31]:

- At least three relatives with an HNPCC-related cancer, one of whom is a first-degree relative of the other two;
- At least two successive affected generations;
- At least one of the HNPCC-related cancers diagnosed before the age of 50 years; and
- Exclusion of familial adnomatous polyposis (FAP).

However, since the Amsterdam criteria were too restrictive, giving a diagnostic sensitivity and specificity for HNPCC of only 60 and 70%, respectively, less stringent Bethesda guidelines have been created and then modified for persons whose colonic tumors should be tested for microsatellite instability (MSI) to recognize possible carriers of HNPCC-specific mismatch repair gene (MMR) mutations. This distinctly raised the sensitivity but lowered the specificity [67]. In addition, immunohistochemistry of tumor tissues were recommended using antibodies against MMR proteins [68].

Lynch syndrome (HNPCC2) as HNPCC1 and also variant and atypical HNPCC, are due to mutations in MMR genes. Their proteins are responsible for repairing nucleotide mismatches, insertions, or deletions, mistakes that were made during DNA replication. Heterozygous MMR mutations, as may be found in the germline of HNPCC family members, do not interfere with MMR. Although inherited in a dominant manner, they function in a recessive manner at the cellular level, requiring reduction to homozygosity. Homozygous MMR mutations, resulting from somatic LOH, lead to cells lacking MMR, to an accumulation of mutations causing MSI, and to malignant transformation. Several MMR genes have been associated with HNPCC:

MLH1 (homolog of MutL of *E. coli* 1) was identified as a human MMR gene [32]. Over 200 different mutations have been reported so far. *MLH1* mutations are predominantly found in HNPCC2 and in HNPCC variants, including Muir–Torre and Turcot syndromes. Mhl1 protein coordinates the binding of other proteins involved in MMR, including helicases, single-stranded-DNA binding-protein, proliferating cell nuclear antigen, and DNA polymerases [69].

MSH2 (homolog of MutS *E. coli* 2) was found to carry mutations in HNPCC [70]. It accounts for 50% of HNPCC1 mutations, and also for cases of HNPCC variant Muir–Torre and Turcot syndromes. Almost 200 *MSH2* mutations have been recognized. Msh2 protein functions by forming a heterodimer with *MSH3* or *MSH6* proteins that, as a clamp, slides along the DNA to identify mismatches [71].

MSH6 mutations account for some families with atypical HNPCC, displaying a high frequency of hyper- and dysplastic lesions and carcinomas of the endometrium (73% in female carriers as compared to about 30% in *MSH2* and *MLH1* carriers) [72]. Over 30 different mutations have been identified.

PMS2 (postmeiotic segregation increase 2) mutations are found in the Turcot MMR cancer syndrome, and rarely in HNPCC1/2 families. They cause defective protein–protein interaction with other MMR proteins.

In addition, *PMS1*-, *TGFBR2*-, and *MLH3* mutations of questionable significance have been found in a very few HNPCC families.

The life-time risk of HNPCC gene carriers to develop a colon cancer is 69% (vs. 5.5% in the general population), the mean age of onset being 61 years [73]. About two-thirds of colon cancers occur in the right colon. Life-time risk for endometrium cancer is 20–60% (vs. 2.7%), followed by a risk for gastric cancer of 11–19% (vs. <1%), ovarian cancer of 9–12% (vs. 1.6%), hepatobiliary cancer of 4–5% (vs. <1%), small bowel cancer of 1–4% (vs. <1%), and brain tumors of 1–3% (vs. <1%) (American Cancer Society Surveillance Research, 2002).

Muir–Torre syndrome represents a Lynch syndrome variant. It combines HNPCC2-related low-grade gastrointestinal, urogenital, and gynaecologic malignancies with skin lesions such as sebaceous epitheliomas, adenomas and carcinomas, keratoacanthomas, and basal cell carcinomas. Sixty-one percent of the patients develop early proximal colon cancer, and 22% of female patients develop endometrial cancer. In the majority of cases, the internal malignancies precede the sebaceous tumors [74]. *MSH2* gene mutations account for 93% of the Muir–Torre syndromes, and only a few are due to mutations in the *MHL1* gene, this being in contrast to HNPCC, with an almost equal distribution of *MSH2* and *MHL1* mutations [41, 75].

The *"mismatch repair cancer syndrome"* corresponds to the "MMR-associated type of *Turcot* syndrome", and is another HNPCC2 variant. It is characterized by childhood brain tumors, mainly glioblastomas in association with colorectal adenomas that may become malignant, and has also been named "brain tumor-polyposis syndrome type 1" (BPT1). Other features, such as early onset leukemia and skin lesions comprising sebaceous cysts, café au lait spots, and basal cell carcinoma, were added later [56, 57]. MMR gene mutations were found mainly in the *PMS2* gene, but also in the *MHL1*, *MSH2*, and *MSH6* genes.

3.3
APC-Associated Polyposis Syndromes

Familial adenomatous polyposis (FAP) may now be considered a colon cancer pre-disposition syndrome [18]. In the classical form defined earlier, FAP was restricted to the occurrence of myriads of partly precancerous adenomatous polyps[1] (see also Fig. 16.1) of the colon developing at the age of 7 to 36 years, and of colorectal cancer with the mean age of diagnosis of 40 years. In the presence of variable extracolonic manifestations occurring in approximately 20% of FAP individuals, and including polyps in the gastric fundus and duodenum and associated tumors outside the gastrointestinal tract, the condition was regarded as "APC-associated polyposis" and classified as Gardner or Turcot syndrome, or as attenuated FAP. Meanwhile, the terms FAP and Gardner syndrome are used synonymously because of the overlap of phenotypes, the multiple identical mutations, and the occurrence in sibships. FAP and APC-associated conditions are caused by mutation in the *APC* (adenomatous polyposis of the colon) gene. Its protein acts as a tumor suppressor after binding to other proteins, antagonizing the signaling pathway of the oncogene *WNT1*. Through regulation of ß-catenin, it maintains normal apoptosis and decreases cell proliferation. Loss of the APC protein thus contributes to cancer progression [19]. More than 800 germline mutations have been found, almost always causing truncation of the APC protein. The APC protein is functionally active only as a homeodimer. Binding of a truncated to a normal APC molecule causes inactivation of the functioning APC protein. Binding depends on the length of the truncated molecule. Distal mutations, leaving long truncated molecules that are capable of binding and thus inactivation, result in a more aggressive disease, while proximal mutations leaving short truncated protein molecules that are unable to bind, cause mild disease manifestations [76]. Furthermore, the phaeno-typic expression of FAP is related to the localization of the mutation within the APC gene, for example, osteomas and desmoid tumors are correlated with a truncating mutation between codon 1403 and 1578 [77].

Gardner syndrome and FAP are synonymous terms. In the past, Gardner syndrome was regarded as a distinct clinical entity characterized by the association of colonic adenomatous polyposis and colon cancer with extracolonic tumors, such as of the upper gastrointestinal tract (80–90%), childhood hepatoblastoma (1%), osteoma commonly found in the jaw and skull (80%), soft tissue tumors, especially desmoid tumors (12–38%), and, rarely, other associated cancers. The latter included adrenal cortical carcinoma, papillary carcinoma of the thyroid, and bile duct cancer. Dental anomalies and congenital hypertrophy of the retinal pigment epithelium (CHRPE) are frequent (80%) and may be used for FAP screening. The Gardner phenotype, representing a severe manifestation of FAP, is correlated to mutations within a specific region of the APC gene [20].

Turcot syndrome families are APC-associated in two-thirds of cases by carrying an *APC* gene mutation, and are classified as "brain tumor-polyposis syndrome

---

1) According to the WHO classification adenomatous polyps are no more designated as polyps but as adenomas. The term polyp is now restricted to hamartomatous polyps.

type 2" (BPT2). BPT2 differs from the aforementioned "BPT1–MMR repair cancer syndrome" by an increased risk of medulloblastoma-type brain tumors and colorectal polyposis, as compared to the malignant gliomas and predominant colorectal adenomas in BPT1 [78].

Attenuated AFP (AAPC) defines a milder "APC-associated condition" with fewer polyps, late onset colonic carcinoma, presence of upper gastrointestinal tumors, but rare CHRPE lesions and desmoid tumors. AAPC is caused by very proximal or very distal truncating *APC* mutations (before codon 157 of after codon 1464) [79].

3.4
Hamartomatous Tumor Syndromes

In *Peutz–Jeghers syndrome* (PJS), characteristic hamartomatous polyps[2)] are most common in the small intestine (64%), but may also involve the colon (53%), stomach (49%), and rectum (32%), and rarely the upper and lower respiratory tract, the ureter, and bladder. They can cause death by bleeding and intussusception. In 95% of the patients, hamartomatous polyposis is accompanied by mucocutaneous hyperpigmentation causing dark blue spots, especially on palms, plantar areas, lips, and buccal mucosa that fade after puberty. Malignant transformation of the small intestinal polyps is rare, but the risk of developing any kind of cancer is increased about four-fold with a cumulative risk of 85% by the age of 70 years [45]. Cancers observed in PJS involved the gastrointestinal tract and the pancreas, and also the lung and breast. Rarely, testicular and ovarian sex cord tumors with annular tubules (SCTAT), and especially aggressive "adenoma malignum of the cervix uteri" have been described. Clinical diagnosis of Peutz-Jeghers syndrome is based on the histological verification of a hamartomatous polyp displaying characteristic arborized patterns of smooth muscle proliferation and epithelial displacement, appearing as pseudocarcinomatous invasion (see also Fig. 16.1). In the absence of this verification, two of the three criteria "positive family history, mucocutaneous hyperpigmentations, and/or polyposis coli", have to be present [17]. The gene responsible for Peutz-Jeghers syndrome is *STK11* (previously *LKB1X1*). It codes for serine/threonine protein kinase 11 that is involved in apoptosis through p53 pathways in epithelial cells, in the regulation of cellular proliferation by affecting G1 cell cycle arrest, in cell polarity, and in the inhibition of AMP-activated protein kinase and mTOR pathways [80, 81]. Most STK11 mutations result in protein truncation, leading to an earlier onset of the disease than missense mutations, deletions, and splice site variants [82].

Cowden syndrome (CS) is one of the "PTEN hamartomatous tumor syndromes" that are caused by a germline mutation of the tumor suppressor gene *PTEN*. CS encounters benign lesions, mostly hamartomatous in nature, of the skin and mucous membranes, breast, thyroid, uterus, and gastrointestinal tract, and

---

2) Hamartoma is defined as a tumourlike non-neoplastic condition arising from local differentiated tissues by simple tissue growth and not by mono- or polyclonal cell proliferation resulting in true tumors.

also fibromas and lipomas. Mucocutaneous lesions, occurring in 99% of the patients, include facial trichilemmomas/epitheliomas, papillomatous papules, acral keratosis, and oesophageal acanthosis, while intestinal hamartomatous or hyperplastic polyps are observed in only 30% of the patients [17, 83]. Together with cerebellar dysplastic gangliocytoma (Lhermitte-Duclos disease, see also Fig. 5.1), leading to seizures, skin lesions are considered pathognomonic for CS. About 40% of individuals with CS are macrocephalic, and there is a high risk of cancer, the life-time risk for breast cancer amounting to 50%, and that of thyroid and endometrial cancer to about 10%. These features represent major diagnostic criteria. A high risk for breast cancer also accounts for males. Cancers of the skin and genitourinary tract, especially melanoma and renal cell carcinomas, and also other benign tumors and tumor-like lesions including intestinal polyps, are considered minor diagnostic criteria. An increased risk for colorectal cancers, progressing from gastrointestinal hamartomas, is under discussion [84]. Diagnosis of CS requires at least six mucocutaneous lesions or two major criteria, or one major and three minor criteria or four minor criteria [83].

PTEN gene mutations are responsible for Cowden and other *PTEN* hamartomatous tumor syndromes. *PTEN* encodes an almost ubiquitously expressed dual specificity phosphatase, a major lipid phosphatase that downregulates the PI3K/ Akt pathway to cause G1 arrest (by nuclear PTEN) and apoptosis (by cytoplasmatic PTEN) [85]. More than 150, mostly unique missense and nonsense mutations, deletions, and insertions are listed, 76% resulting in truncation, lack, or dysfunction of the protein. There is a clustering of mutations in exon 5. *PTEN* mutations are identified in 85% of the CS and 65% of the BRRS (Bannayan–Riley–Ruvalcaba syndrome) cases. In about 10% of individuals with CS, mutations in the *PTEN* promoter have been found, while 10% of individuals with BRRS have a large deletion [86].

Bannayan–Riley–Ruvalcaba syndrome (BRRS) is allelic to CS. Besides overlapping mucocutaneous features, it shows a slightly different phenotype with high birth weight and length (>97th percentile), decelerated postnatal growth, macrocephaly, and gross motor delay as a more constant feature, mental retardation in about 50% of the cases, multiple lipomas, haemangiomas and gastrointestinal hamartomatous polyps, and, in males, pigmented macules on the glans penis. A number of dysmorphic features and Hashimoto thyroiditis have also been described [7]. Neoplasias mainly comprise meningiomas and thyroid follicular cell tumors. It is not yet clear whether BRRS patients have the same cancer risk as individuals with CS. Since CS and BRRS were found as different phenotypes within the same families, and a genotype/phenotype failed to detect a correlation with either CS or BRRS, Lachlan and coworkers [8] concluded that they represent one condition with variable expression and age-related penetrance.

In *Proteus and Proteus-like syndromes*, characterized by asymmetric hamartomatous overgrowth of multiple tissues, leading to lipomas, lymph- and haemangiomas, connective tissue and epidermal nevi, and to hyperostoses, somatic, and germline *PTEN* mutations have been found [87]. Tumors are rare but have been reported as ovarian cystadenomas, testicular tumors, tumors of the central nervous system, including meningioma, and parotoid monomorphic adenomas [88, 89]. A somatic mosaic hypothesis was put forward [90] to explain the local aspect of overgrowth.

Juvenile polyposis syndrome (JPS) is another hamartomatous polyposis syndrome. It presents with characteristic "juvenile type hamartomatous polyps" in the stomach, small intestine, and colorectum, which are distinct from the "Peutz-Jeghers type hamartomatous polyps" by demonstrating mucous filled dilated glands, a smooth surface with normal epithelium, dense stroma, an absence of smooth muscle proliferation, and frequent inflammatory infiltration (see also Fig. 16.1). Hamartomatous juvenile polyps can develop at any age, but are mostly diagnosed under the age of 20 years and in the generalized form not before the age of 6 years. Diagnosis of JPS requires more than five juvenile polyps in the colorectum or multiple polyps throughout the gastrointestinal tract, or any number of polyps in a positive family history [17]. There is an increased risk for gastrointestinal, mainly colorectal, cancer with a cumulative life-time risk of 55% [91]. Four genes have been associated with JPS:

BMPR1A, encodes a type 1 receptor of the bone morphogenetic proteins. The BMP pathway leads to the phosphorylation of SMAD4 and downregulates cell proliferation, especially proliferation of cells of the gastrointestinal tract [92]. *BMPR1A* nonsense, missense, frameshift, and splice site mutations account for 21% of the JPS cases.

SMAD4 encodes a protein that functions as a mediator of the TGF-beta signaling pathway. It mediates growth inhibitory signals from the cell surface to the nucleus. Most mutations are unique and account for 18% of the JPS cases [92]. *BMPR1A* and *SMAD4* mutations have a more prominent phenotype of JPS.

ENG is a member of the beta-TGF superfamily, such as *BMPR1A* and *SMAD4*. *ENG* mutations have been shown to cause hereditary hemorrhagic teleangiectasia (HHT1): Their significance for JPS, with or without associated HHT1, is still under discussion [25].

PTEN germline mutations had been described earlier in JPS. After clinical re-examination, the cases are now considered to correspond to CS or BRRS. However, Delatte and coworkers [93] presented nine cases displaying severe early onset juvenile polyposis in the presence of a large more than one MB germline deletion in 10q23.2–q23.4. Since the deletion encompasses the *BMPR1A* and the *PTEN* locus, they suggested this contiguous gene deletion, causing hemizygosity for both genes, to be the etiologic basis for the subset of JP termed "juvenile polyposis of infancy".

3.5
Familial Endocrine Tumor Syndromes

The *multiple endocrine neoplasias type 1* (MEN1) represent an example of familial endocrine tumor syndromes, predisposing to over 20 different benign endocrine and non-endocrine tumors. Clinical diagnosis request the presence of two of three endocrine hormonal active tumors of the parathyroids, causing hypercalcemia, the anterior pituitary (mainly prolactinomas), or of the gastro-entero-pancreatic (GEP) tract. GEP tumors include gastrinoma, leading to Zollinger–Ellison syndrome, pancreatic insulinoma or glucagonoma, causing hypo- and hyperglycaemia, respectively, and VIPoma, secreting a vasoactive intestinal peptide and causing watery diarrhea, hypokalemia, and achlohydria (WDHA) [38]. Thymic and bronchial carcinoids are non-hormone secreting as are the majority of adrenocortical tumors (20–40%). Among the nonendocrine tumors, angiofibromas (88%), collagenomas (72%), lipomas (34%), meningiomas (8%), ependymoma (1%), and leiomyomas have been described and claimed to be helpful in diagnosis of cases prior to the appearance of a hormone secreting tumor [39]. Although malignancies are not a feature of classical MEN1, gastrinomas may include a malignant, metastasizing component, as may thymic carcinoids by demonstrating aggressive growth.

MEN1 is caused by **MEN1** gene mutations. *MEN1* encodes menin, a multifunctional nuclear protein that is thought to be involved in the regulation of DNA replication and repair and in transcription. Over 400 different mutations have been described. Most of these are nonsense mutations and deletions and lead to protein truncation. Premature centromere division and hypersensitivity to alkylating agents has been demonstrated in individuals with a heterozygous *MEN1* mutation. LOH has been shown to occur in tumor tissues [94].

Hyperparathyroidism-Jaw tumor syndrome (HPT-JT) is a rare familial condition in which parathyroid adenomas are associated with a predisposition for ossifying fibromas of the jaw and various renal lesions. The latter may include renal cysts and hamartomas, and also renal mesoblastic nephroblastoma (late onset Wilms tumor), papillary, and clear cell renal carcinoma (Figure 3.1) [23]. Parathyroid carcinoma, pancreas adenocarcinoma, testicular mixed germ cell tumor, and Hurthle cell thyroid adenoma have also been described. Germline mutations have been found in the **HRPT2** gene, a putative tumor suppressor gene. The encoded protein has been named parafibromin [24]. LOH has been demonstrated in malignant tumors, but not in all parathyroid adenomas, suggesting alternative mechanisms for tumorigenesis of parathyroid tumors in HPT-JP patients [23].

The **multiple endocrine neoplasias type 2** (MEN2) comprise the subtypes MEN2A (60–90%), MEN2B (5%), and FMTC (5–35%). They all are familial disorders that share an almost 100% risk for early onset medullary thyroid carcinoma. But only in MEN2A and MEN2B, is there a predisposition for additional tumors, mainly for potentially malignant pheochromocytoma (50%). In MEN2A, parathyroid adenomas are observed in 20–30% of the cases that are rather uncommon in MEN2B. MEN2B individuals show a 40% rate of gastrointestinal ganglioneuromas and also prominent mucosal neuromas of the tongue, palate, and lips. The gene responsible for FMTC, MEN2A, and MEN2b is the **RET** gene, a protooncogene. It encodes a transmembrane tyrosine kinase receptor. The protein plays a role in cell growth and cell differentiation. "Ligand dependent" dimerization of the RET receptor protein after binding to the glial cell derived nerve growth factor GDNF or to NTN, and also to GDNF or NTN receptor proteins, results in autophosphorylation of intracellular RET tyrosine kinase domains that function as docking sites for intracellular signaling proteins, and allow downstream activation of the mitogen-

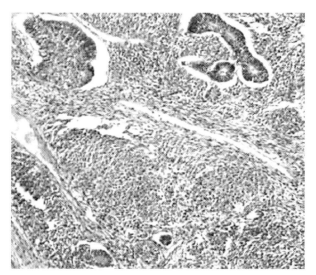

Figure 3.1 Nephroblastoma (Wilms tumor): Embryonal neoplasm, derived from nephrogenic blastemal cells, trying to imitate renal differentiation with stromal, blastemalm and tubular elements; see *"Li–Fraumeni syndrome"* (HE, ×2.5).

activated protein kinase signaling cascade [40]. Mutations in the cystein-rich extracellular and transmembrane domains of RET enable "ligand independent" RET-dimerization and permanent activation of signaling pathways. They are responsible for most FMTC and MEN2A cases. The classical codon 918 point mutations, responsible for 95% of the MEN2B, lies within the catalytic core of the intracellular tyrosine kinase domain, and allows autophosphorylation and thus permanent activation "without dimerization" of the RET receptors. In contrast to the "gain of function" mutations in MEN 2, mutations that cause Hirschsprung disease (HSCR) are "loss of function" mutations [95]. For families in which MEN 2A and HSCR cosegregate, models to explain how the same mutation can cause gain of function and loss of function have been proposed [96].

The **Carney complex** (CNC1 and CNC2) is characterized by endocrine tumors or overactivity in the setting of myxomas, schwannomas, and spotty mucocutaneous pigmentations, the latter comprising multiple lentigines on the face, lips, conjunctiva, vaginal and penile mucosa, and also (epitheloid) blue nevi. Myxomas have been observed in approximately 70% of patients as subcutaneous myxomas at mucosal-ephithelial junctions, preferably at inner eyelid borders, as cardiac, usually multiple pedunculated myxomas of endocardial origin that may be associated by a heart malformation, as myxomatosis of the breast, and rarely as osteochondro-myxoma of the bone (Figure 3.2). A frequent endocrine tumor-like lesion is the primary pigmented (micro) nodular adrenocortical disease (PPNAD) occurring in 25% of CNC individuals, and leading to cortisol overproduction and Cushing syndrome. Seventy-five percent of CNC individuals present with thyroid adenomas, 10% with growth hormone producing pituitary adenomas causing acromegaly, and 10% with psammomatous melanotic schwannomas that involve the gastroin-

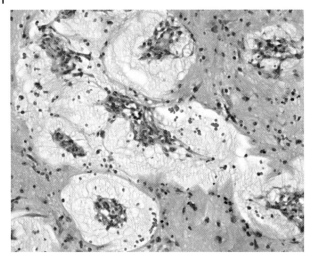

Figure 3.2 Cardiac (atrial) myxoma: Tumor cells characterized by abundant eosinophilic cytoplasm and indistinct cell borders, also forming complex ring structures around blood vessels embedded in a myxoid matrix; see *"Carney complex"* (HE, ×20) (R. Moll, Marburg).

testinal tract and the skin, and metastasize in about 10% of the cases [97]. Ductal adenomas or intraductal papillomas of the breast may also occur. Fifty percent of male patients present with testicular tumors, mostly bilateral "large-cell calcifying Sertoli cell tumors" that, when hormone producing, lead to precocious puberty. Malignancies are uncommon, but thyroid carcinomas have been described, suggesting that the thyroid pathology in CNC ranges from follicular hyperplasia and/or cystic changes to carcinoma [14]. A condition called the CNC variant, associated with additional distal arthrogryposis and shows mutations in the MYH8 gene, is now considered a distinct disorder [98]. Two gene loci have been related to CNC, but only one responsible (*CNC1*) gene has as yet been identified.

PRKARIA1A, a tumor suppressor gene, encodes the R1α regulatory subunit of cAMP-dependent protein kinase A (PKA) that is an important effector molecule in many endocrine signaling pathways. Almost all pathologic mutations result in the truncation of the protein. They account for 65% of CNC cases [15]. Complete inactivation of PRKAR1A at the tissue level follows degradation of the mRNA (NMD), or LOH.

3.6
Familial Cancer Associated Genodermatoses

Nevoid basal cell carcinoma (Gorlin) syndrome (NBCCS) was delineated by Gorlin and Goltz [9, 21]. Major features include multiple (up to hundreds) basal cell carcinomas or one BCC before the age of 30 years (85%), multiple palmar or plantar pits (80%), odontogenic keratocysts (75%), bilamellar calcification of the falx cerebri (65%), and tentorium cerebelli (20%), and a first degree relative with NBCCS. Minor features comprise relative macrocephaly with an occipito-frontal circumference (OFC) of more than 97th percentile (50%), a coarse face (54%) with hypertelorism (40%), frontal bossing (27%) and cleft lip and palate (5%), epidermal cysts and facial milia (50%), bridged sella (68%), splayed or fused ribs and vertebrae, kyphoscoliosis, and pectus deformities, short fourth metacarpal, and also ovarian calcifications and fibromas (25%), lymphomesenteric cysts, and cardiac fibromas or rhabdomyomas (2%). Meningioma, hepatic mesenchymoma, lymphoma, and fibrosarcoma have also been reported. Five percent of affected children develop medulloblastoma and other primitive neuroectodermal tumors (PNET). Clinical diagnosis of NBCCS requires the presence of two major, or one major and two minor criteria. Some authors claim that palmar and plantar pits are pathognomonic [99, 100]. Seventy percent to 80% of NBCCS cases are familial. New dominant mutations seem to be correlated with increased paternal age. Individuals with NBCCS are susceptible to X-irradiation. The gene associated with NBCCS is **PTCH1**, the human homolog to the drosophila *patched* gene, encodes a 12-pass transmembrane protein that represses the signaling activity of the membrane-bound proto-oncogene smoothed (SMOH). It also functions as a receptor for the sonic hedgehog (SHH) signaling protein. When PTCH1 is bound to SHH, SMOH is freed from suppression for downstream signaling. Thus, *PTCH1* exhibits tumor suppressor function, mutations activating the proto-oncogene *SMOH*. Activating mutations in *SMOH* have only been found in sporadic basal cell carcinomas [101]. *PTCH1*-mutations, including "in frame" and mostly "out of frame" deletions, insertions, duplications, and also missense mutations, are detected in over 50% of affected individuals [22]. In the presence of a germline mutation, tumor development requires LOH through a second somatic mutation of the wildtype allele. LOH may be triggered by UV or irradiation, as has been shown by the occurrence of thousands of basal cell carcinomas after radiotherapy of a childhood medulloblastoma [9]. 9q interstitial deletions, when covering the *PTCH1* locus, may lead to NBCCS with additional features [102].

The **Melanoma-pancreatic cancer syndrome** (see also Chapters 20 and 24 on pancreatic cancer and melanoma), also known as familial atypical multiple mole melanoma-pancreatic cancer syndrome (FAMMM-PC), is a subset of familial atypical multiple mole melanoma (FAMMM) [36]. It shares common features with the Melanoma-astrocytoma syndrome, namely the restriction to two tumor sites, the skin tumor always being a melanoma, the presence of numerous atypical nevi of more than 5 mm in diameter, and the causative involvement of the tumor suppressor gene **CDKN2A** that is mutated in 20% of the FAMMM families. *CDKN2A* encodes a cyclin-dependent kinase inhibitor p16 and the p53 activator p14^{ARF}, the latter by an alternative and independent exon 1ß spliced to exon 2 of the *CDKN2A* gene. Both proteins are cell cycle regulators, p16 producing G1 cell cycle arrest by inhibiting phosphorylation of the retinoblastoma (Rb) protein, and p14^{ARF} acting at the p53 and Rb pathways by preventing binding of the proto-oncogene MDM2 to p53 and Rb, thus arresting both G1 and G2 phases of cell division [35]. *CDKN2A* mutations have been identified in FAMMM-PC families. No significant differences in the types and locations of mutations were found between melanoma prone families with and without pancreas carcinoma [103]. However, an increased risk of developing pancreas cancer was associated with the *p16-Leiden* mutation, a 19bp deletion of exon 2 of the *CDKN2A* gene [104]. Twelve percent of the pancreatic cancer families and 60% of FAMMM families present with p16 mutations.

The **Melanoma-astrocytoma syndrome** is another rare subset of FAMMM. It is characterized by the dual predisposition to melanoma, including atypical melanocytic nevi and neural system tumors, most commonly astrocytomas. Other associated neural tumors have been described as medulloblastoma, glioblastoma multiforme, ependy-moma, glioma, meningioma, neurofibroma, and acoustic neurilemmoma [33]. Mutations have been described as large deletions of the chromosomal band 9p21, containing the *CDNK2A* and *CDNK2B* genes, and encoding p16 and p15 and also p14^{ARF} by differential splicing. It was suggested that either loss of p14^{ARF} function, or disruption of p16 expression, was the critical abnormality, rather than the contiguous loss of *CDKN2A* and *CDKN2B* genes [34].

The **Birt–Hogg–Dubé syndrome** (BHD) is defined by the triad of adult onset fibro-folliculomas, trichodiscomas, and acrochordons (skin tags), representing hamartomas that show up as whitish perfollicular skin papules predominantly on the face, neck, and trunk [9]. The cutaneous lesions were found to be associated with emphysema-like multifocal lung cysts and spontaneous pneumothorax in 89% of affected individuals, and with renal tumors in 15%. Other less frequent findings were parathyroid adenomas, parotid oncocytomas, thyroid multinodular adenomas, medullary carcinoma, angiolipoma, and flecked chorioretinopathy, while previous reports on an association with colonic polyps and carcinomas were not confirmed [100]. Renal tumors most commonly present as hybrid oncocytoma and chromophobe renal cell carcinomas (50%), chromophobe (34%) and clear cell type carcinomas (9%), oncocytomas (5%), and papillary carcinomas (2%) [105]. The gene responsible for BHD syndrome is the **FLCN** gene. It encodes folliculin, widely expressed in different tissues, including skin and skin appendages, type1 pneumocytes, distal renal nephrons, and secretory cells. It functions as a tumor suppressor gene. *FLCN* mutations were found in 84% of BHD patients. The majority of mutations cause protein truncation [10].

Rothmund Thomson syndrome is an autosomal-recessive tumor associated geno-dermatosis starting with erythema, swelling, and blistering of the face, limbs, and buttocks between the age of three to six months, later changing to a chronic phase with reticulated hypo- and hyperpigmentations, teleangiectases, and punctuate atrophy of the skin – a condition named poikiloderma. Scalp hair, including eyebrows and eyelashes is sparse. Juvenile cataracts (6%), skeletal and dental anomalies, and dysmorphic features may occur. Affected individuals carry a risk of early osteosarcoma (32%) and skin cancer (5%) [52]. Haematologic disorders may include leukemia. Non-Hodgkin lymphoma has been observed following cytostatic therapy of osteosarcoma, and a higher risk for secondary malignancies has been suggested. The syndrome is due to mutation of the **RECQL4** gene, a member of the RecQ helicases family that promotes unwinding of the DNA helix. However, *RECQL4* encodes an ATP dependent DNA helicase Q4 that does not demonstrate helicase activity, but rather is involved in the initiation of DNA replication [53]. In 70% of patients with the clinical diagnosis of Rothmund-Thomson syndrome, different truncating *RECQL4* mutations were found, and it was stated that only truncating mutations are associated with a risk of osteosarcoma. Few cases not affected by osteosarcoma demonstrated missense mutations of unclear functional significance [52]. The finding of cell lines with trisomy 8 in lymphocytes of RTS patients was interpreted as acquired somatic mosaicism, indicating instability of lymphocyte chromosomes [106].

Werner syndrome is a rare autosomal recessive "adult progeroid syndrome", more commonly reported in Japan. It is featured by signs of premature aging, chromosomal instability, and increased cancer incidence. Cardinal signs, starting in the twenties, are atrophy and pigmentary alterations, especially of the facial skin, premature graying and thinning of hair and balding, scleroderma-like skin changes in the limbs, ulcers and soft tissue calcifications, bilateral cataracts, type 2 diabetes mellitus, hypogonadism, and osteoporosis. Early arteriosclerosis may lead to myocardial infarcts. Malignancies occur in about 10% of the patients with a ratio of mesenchymal to epithelial tumors of 1:1 as compared to a ratio of 1:10 in the normal aging population. Predominant tumors are soft tissue sarcoma and osteosarcoma, leukemia, benign and malignant meningioma, acral lentiginous melanoma, and thyroid cancer [61]. In about 90% of cases, Werner syndrome results from a mutation in the **WRN** gene, which encodes a member of the RecQ family (see Rothmund Thomson and Bloom's syndrome), possessing helicase and exonuclease activities. The WRN protein can unwind and digest aberrant DNA structures. It also regulates processes of DNA recombination and repair and is thus important for maintenance of genome stability. A great number of different mutations have been identified that result in stop codons, frame shift, or exon skipping. Twenty percent to 25% of WRN mutations correspond to a 1336C>T transition. In the Japanese population, a founder mutation IVS 25–1G > C has been found in 60% of the mutant alleles [62, 107]. In tumor cells of Werner syndrome patients, it was demonstrated that *WRN* function was abrogated by transcriptional silencing associated with CpG island-promotor hypermethylation [63].

Tuberous sclerosis complex (TSC) refers to a hereditary tumor syndrome that presents with hamartomas in child- and adulthood, involving many different organs. TSC shows a predominance of almost 100%. About two-thirds of the cases represent new mutations. Characteristic skin lesions occur in more than 90% of the patients. They include hypomelanotic macules, facial angiofibromas (previously termed adenoma sebaceum), shagreen patches, and fibrous facial plaques. Other major features are brain hamartomas (70%) such as subependymal glial nodules, cortical/subcortical tubers, and also giant cell astrocytomas (<14%) or ependymomas (see also Fig. 5.6). Furthermore, cardiac rhabdomyomas (48–68%)

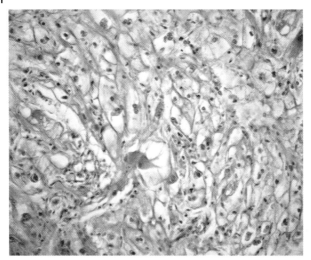

Figure 3.3 Rhabdomyoma of the heart: Hamartoma consisting of enlarged, vacuolated, and clearly demarcated tumor cells and occasional spider cells with radial cytoplasmic extensions. Occasional cross striation can be demonstrated immunhistochemically; see *"Tuberous sclerosis"* (HE, ×20).

that are mostly congenital and may regress and disappear, renal angiomyolipomas (75%) that are more common in affected children and females and pulmonary lymphangiomyomatosis, found almost exclusively in women, are observed (Figs. 3.3 and 3.4) [54, 55]. Hamartomatous rectal polyps, hamartomas in liver and spleen, multiple renal and bone cysts, pits in the dental enamel, subungual and sublingual fibromas, retinal achromic patches, and cerebral white matter radial migration lines are considered minor features. Renal cell carcinoma and malignant angiomyolipoma have also been described [108, 109]. Many children with TSC show behavioral and cognitive impairment and seizures. The reported association of TSC with polycystic kidneys result from microdeletions in chromosome region 16p13.3, with a loss of both contiguous genes *TSC2* and *PKD1*, the latter being responsible for autosomal dominant polycystic kidney disease [110]. Two genes were shown to be capable each of causing TSC:

TSC1 encodes a protein called hamartin and **TSC2** encodes a protein called tuberin. Hamartin and tuberin form a heterodimer, and in concert regulate cell growth and proliferation via the inhibition of the mTOR pathway. Deficiency in tuberin and hamartin cause activation of cell proliferation and increase in cell size, thus leading to hamartomas and to giant cell formation, as seen in brain tumors and cardiac rhabdomyomas [111]. The TSC1-TSC2 complex is also thought to be involved in the regulation of mesenchymal differentiation, since cells from all components of the angiomyolipomas and lymphangiomyomatosis were shown to have identical somatic second hit mutations, suggesting derivation from a common progenitor [54]. Furthermore, focal cell adhesion seems to be deficient in *TSC1*

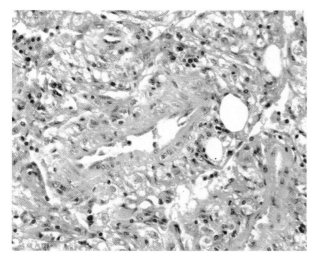

Figure 3.4 Angiomyolipoma of the kidney: Mesenchymal neoplasm showing disordered arrangement of various mature tissues at a site, where these tissues normally do not reside (choristoma). They comprise thick-walled blood vessels, smooth muscle cells, and fat cells; see *"Tuberous sclerosis"* (HE, ×20) (R. Moll, Marburg).

and *TSC2* mutations. This gave rise to the hypothesis of an increased migratory potential of TSC cells, allowing "benign metastasis" of hamartoma cells from the kidneys into the lungs [112]. About 30% of the familial and about 15% of the simplex cases are TSC1 mutations, and about 50% of the familial and about 70% of the simplex cases are TSC2 mutations. About 20% are thought to be due to somatic mosaicism. More than 300 TSC1 and more than 800 TSC2 allele variants have been identified, showing missense mutations and large deletions more common in TSC2, and nonsense and small deletions more common in TSC1 [113]. TSC1 mutations coincide with a milder phenotype concerning the risk for renal malignancy, cognitive, and behavioral disorders [113].

Muir-Torre, Cowden, Bannayan-Riley-Ruvalkaba, Gardner, and Carney syndromes represent other typical cancer associated genodermatoses. They are dealt with under the subheadings "familial (non-)polyposis-" and "endocrine tumor syndromes" of this chapter.

3.7
Familial Renal Cancer Syndromes

Van Hippel–Lindau syndrome (VHL) predisposes to multiple cysts, for example, in the kidney (76%), pancreas (30–70%), and epididymis, and to a variety of benign and malignant tumors. Retinal angiomas (70%) may be the initial tumor lesion

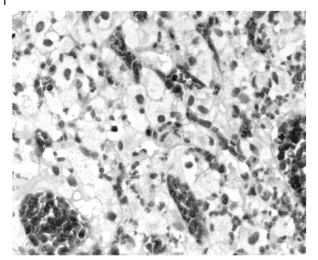

Figure 3.5 Cerebellar haemangioblastoma: Disease specific neoplasm displaying proliferated capillaries with characteristic foamy tumor cells in between; see *"van Hippel–Lindau disease"* (HE, × 40) (A. Pagenstecher, Marburg).

diagnosed at about 25 years of age. They are histologically identical to the disease specific cerebellar and spinal haemangioblastomas (55–59%) (see also Fig. 3.5). In addition, epididymal cystadenomas (25–60%), renal clear cell carcinomas (24–28%), phaeochromocytomas (7–19%), and pancreatic tumors (rare) occur, the latter comprising haemangioblastoma, neuroendo-crine tumors, insulinoma, and carcinoma. Cystadenomas have also been observed in females in the broad ligament. Pulmonary haemangioblastomas, thoracic paraganglioma, and endolymphatic sac tumors (10%) of the membranous labyrinth, causing hearing loss, have been described [59, 60, 114, 115]. VHL shows intrafamilial variability. About 20% of the cases are due to new mutations. Penetrance reaches almost 100% by the age of 65 years. With respect to the likelihood of developing phaeochromocytoma or renal cell carcinoma, four subtypes had been delineated:

- VHL1 = low risk of phaeochromocytoma,
- VHL2A = high risk of phaeochromocytoma, low risk of renal cell carcinoma,
- VHL2B = high risk of phaeochromocytoma, high risk of renal cell carcinoma,
- VHL2C = risk for phaeochromocytoma only [116].

VHL is due to mutation of the **VHL** gene, encoding the multifunctional tumor suppressor protein pVHL. pVHL is involved in transcriptional regulation, posttranscriptional gene expression, protein folding, extracellular matrix formation, and ubiquitinylation [58]. Its best known function so far is the oxygen dependent regulation of the hypoxia inducible factor HIF-1α, and its approximate 60 target genes, many of them coding for growth factors such as VEGF, PDGF, TGF, and EPO [59]. Over 300 germline mutations have been described, including deletions, frameshift, nonsense, missense, and splice site mutations, codon 167 being a hot spot. With respect to the genotype/phenotype correlation, it has been shown that VHL1 is associated with mutations that cause protein loss or disturbance of protein folding by an up-regulation of HIF-1α. VHL2A and VHL2B show missense mutations and up-regulation of HIF-1α, and additional microtubuli destabilization in VHL2A. The VHL2C phenotype is due to missense mutations that maintain the function of HIF-1α degradation, but cause limited binding to fibronectin. LOH has been shown in benign tumors and cysts. For malignant transformation, additional mutations in modifier genes are needed [59].

Hereditary leiomyomatosis and renal cell cancer (Reed) syndrome (HLRCC) is defined by single or multiple painful cutaneous leiomyomas (76%) and/or a single renal cell cancer (62%) [47, 48]. Affected women always show leiomyomata/fibroids of the uterus that may be large and numerous. The leiomyomas rarely become malignant leiomyosarcomas. Leydig cell tumors have also been described, as have some single other tumors such as breast and prostate cancer. However, the latter are not related to the disorder. The renal tumor tends to be aggressive and displays a unique histological and cytologic pattern, corresponding to a type 2 papillary, tubulo-papillary, or a collecting duct renal carcinoma. Mean age of diagnosis is 10 to 47 years. The disorder is due to mutation of the *FH* gene encoding fumarate hydratase, an enzyme responsible for the transformation of fumarate to L-malate in the tricarbocylic acid cycle. It was demonstrated that FH inhibition, together with elevated intracellular fumarate, coincides with HIF upregulation (see von Hippel-Lindau), this leading to the stimulation of numerous growth factor target genes, and thus supporting the role of FH as tumor suppressor [117]. Most mutations in HLRCC are missense mutations. LOH has been shown in tumor tissues [48].

Rhabdoid tumor predisposition syndrome is a rare condition characterized by highly malignant atypical teratoid/rhabdoid tumors (AT/RT) (see also Fig. 5.4). Typically, they present with eccentric vesicular nuclei, prominent nucleoli, distinct nuclear membranes, and globular cytoplasmic inclusions, and develop in children younger than 2 years of age. They were first described in the kidneys and mistaken for sarcomatous variants of Wilms tumors (Fig. 3.6). Extrarenal primary manifestations of AT/RT were shown to occur in the posterior fossa, and/or the subtentorial compartment of the brain, occasionally in the pineal and cervical region, often diagnosed as medulloblastoma, anaplastic ependymoma, chorioid plexus carcinomas, schwannomas, meningiomas, sPNET, pinealoblastoma, rhabdomyosarcoma, or Ewing sarcoma [118–120]. A CNS malignancy is found in 13.5% of cases with a renal rhabdoid tumor [121]. The responsible gene for the AT/RT predisposition was found in a frequently deleted chromosomal region 22q11.2 and was identified as the *SNF5/INI1* tumor suppressor gene. Its product forms part of the SW1/SNF chromatin remodeling complex, thought to be responsible for ploidy control. Tumor associated *SNF5/INI1* mutations exacerbate poly-and aneuploidization by abrogating chromosome segregation [122]. Most germline mutations, leading to truncation or protein loss by duplications and/or large deletions, are due to new mutations [49, 50]. However, familial cases, demonstrating incomplete penetrance

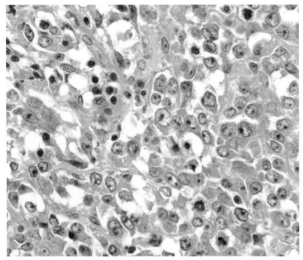

Figure 3.6 Rhabdoid tumor of the kidney: Characteristic
monomorphic pattern of non-cohesive blastemal cells with
eccentric vesicular nuclei, prominent nucleoli, distinct nuclear
membranes and occasional pale cytoplasmic inclusions;
see *"Rhabdoid tumour disposition syndrome"* (HE, ×20)
(R. Moll, Marburg).

via non penetrant males, have been described [51]. LOH with loss of the wildtype
allele is needed for tumor development. It is not clear whether reported brain
tumor types represent misdiagnosed rhabdoid tumors [51], or whether *SNF5/INI1*
mutations can cause other primitive neuroectodermal tumors without a rhabdoid
phenotype [119].

3.8
Sarcoma Family Syndrome

Li–Fraumeni syndrome (LFS) features a *sarcoma family syndrome*, first described
in 1969. It contrasts the *cancer family* and *hereditary cancer syndromes* by a wider
range of tumors, originating in tissues derived from the ecto- or entodermal germ
layer, and also by a predisposition to sarcomas that arise in tissues of mesodermal
origin. LFS shows a tendency towards an unusually early onset of tumor development, especially in families with a germline *TP53* mutation [26]. This also explains
the occurrence of typical childhood tumors, such as embryonal rhabdomyosarcoma, medullo-, neuro-, glio-, and nephroblastoma (Wilms tumor) (Fig. 3.1).
The observed tumor types and sites of LFS are listed in Table 3.1, the six classical
tumors being breast cancer ($25.8\%^{TP53+}/24.6\%^{TP53-}$), soft tissue sarcoma ($19.7\%^{TP53+}/$
$17.8\%^{TP53-}$), osteosarcoma ($14.9\%^{TP53+}/13.7\%^{TP53-}$), brain tumor ($13.2\%^{TP53+}/$
$2.7\%^{TP53-}$), leukemia and lymphoma ($5.3\%^{TP53+}/6.8\%^{TP53-}$), and adrenocortical
carcinoma ($3\%^{TP53+}/0\%^{TP53-}$) [26]. Classic LFS is defined by

- a proband with a sarcoma before the age of 45 years,
- a first-degree relative with any cancer before the age of 45 years, and
- an additional first- or second-degree relative in the same lineage with any cancer before the age of 45 years, or
- a sarcoma at any age [3].

Tumor conditions, suggesting LFS, but not strictly conforming to this definition, are designated as Li–Fraumeni-like syndrome (LFL) [123, 124]. LFS and LFL are genetically heterogenous.

A heterozygous germline *TP53* mutation underlies about 80% of LFS – and 20% of LFL families [26]. Tumor development is associated with LOH, denoting somatic loss of the normal wildtype allele. *TP53* codes for the tumor suppressor protein p53, a cellular gatekeeper for growth and division. It determines whether cells undergo a delay of cell cycle progression for purposes of DNA repair or programmed cell death (apoptosis), by stimulating the production of p21 that interacts with the cell division-stimulating protein cdk2. P53 mutations cause an inability to set off the appropriate chain of events when presented with damaged DNA, and thus promotes the development of a wide spectrum of tumor types [125]. More than 200 distinct germline *TP53* mutations have been described, the vast majority occurring in exons 5 to 8. Most mutations represent missense mutations, but also duplications, inversions, large deletions, and splice site mutations have been observed.

A heterozygous germline mutation of **CHEK2** (checkpoint kinase 2), another tumor suppressor gene, has been detected in a subset of *TP53* negative LFS- and LFL families, leading to the delineation of a Li–Fraumeni syndrome type 2 (LFS2) [28]. *CHEK2* encodes the serine/threonine-protein kinase chk2 that mediates the phosphorylation of p53 at Ser^{22}, which is essential for the stabilization of p53 after DNA damage. After LOH, *CHEK2* mutations fail to activate p53 after DNA damage, or lead to gross instability of the chk2 protein. Chk2 also binds and regulates BRCA1 [27, 126].

A Li–Fraumeni syndrome type 3 (LFS3) was defined after mapping of a third LFS predisposition locus to human chromosome 1q23 [29]. Recently, mutations in the **BRCA2** gene have been associated with Li–Fraumeni-like syndrome [30].

LFS is a highly penetrant tumor syndrome, with an overall life-time cancer risk calculated at 85% [127]. Fifty-six percent of tumors in LFS families occur prior to the age of 30 years, and in LFL families 44% were diagnosed before the age of 30 years [27]. Frameshift *TP53* mutations confer a higher cancer risk than certain missense mutations.

References

1 Warthin, A.S. (1913) Heredity with reference to carcinoma. *Archives of Internal Medicine*, **12**, 546–55.
2 Lynch, H.T., Smyrk, T.C., Watson, P., Lanspa, S.J., Lynch, J.F., Lynch, P.M., Cavalieri, R.J. and Boland, C.R. (1993) Genetics, natural history, tumor spectrum, and pathology of hereditary nonpolyposis colorectal cancer: an updated review. *Gastroenterology*, **104**, 1535–49.

3 Li, F.P. and Fraumeni, J.F. (1969) Soft tissue sarcomas, breast cancer, and other neoplasms. A family syndrome? *Annals of Internal Medicine*, **71**, 747–52.

4 Garber, J.E. and Offit, K. (2005) Hereditary cancer predisposition syndromes. Review. *Journal of Clinical Oncology*, **23** (2), 276–92.

5 Field, M., Shanley, S. and Kirk, J. (2007) Inherited cancer susceptibility syndromes in paediatric practice. Review. *Journal of Paediatrics and Child Health*, **43**, 219–29.

6 Hecht, F. (2007) Familial cancer syndromes catalog with comments. *Cytogenetic and Genome Research*, **118**, 222–8.

7 Marsh, D.J., Kum, J.B., Lunetta, K.L., Benett, M.J., Gorlin, R.J., Ahmed, S.F., Bodurtha, J., Crowe, C., Curtis, M.A., Dasouki, M., Dunn, T., Feit, H. *et al.* (1999) PTEN mutation spectrum and genotype-phenotype correlations in Bannayan-Riley-Ruvalcaba syndrome suggest a single entity with Cowden syndrome. *Human Molecular Genetics*, **8**, 1461–72.

8 Lachlan, K.L., Lucassen, A.M., Bunyan, D. and Temple, I.K. (2007) Cowden syndrome and Bannayan-Riley-Ruvalcaba syndrome represent one condition with variable expression and age-related penetrance: results of a clinical study of PTEN mutation carriers. *Journal of Medical Genetics*, **44**, 579–85.

9 Burgdorf, W.H.C. (2006) Cancer-associated genodermatoses: a personal history. *Experimental Dermatology*, **15**, 653–66.

10 Schmidt, L.S., Nickerson, M.L., Warren, M.B., Glenn, G.M., Toro, J.R., Merino, M.J., Turner, M.L., Choyke, P.L., Sharma, N., Peterson, J., Morrison, P., Maher, E.R., Walther, M.M., Zbar, B. and Linehan, W.M. (2005) Germline BHD-mutation spectrum and phenotype analysis of a large cohort of families with Birt-Hogg-Dubé syndrome. *American Journal of Human Genetics*, **76**, 1023–33.

11 German, J. (1997) Bloom's syndrome. XX. The first 100 cancers. *Cancer Genetics and Cytogenetics*, **93**, 100–6.

12 Stavropoulos, D.J., Bradshaw, P.S., Li, X., Pasic, I., Truong, K., Ikura, M., Ungrin, M. and Meyn, M.S. (2002) The Bloom syndrome helicase BLM interacts with TRF2 in ALT cells and promotes telomeric DNA synthesis. *Human Molecular Genetics*, **11**, 3135–44.

13 Malone, K.E., Daling, J.R., Doody, D.R., Hsu, L., Bernstein, L., Coates, R.J., Marchbanks, P.A., Simon, M.S., McDonald, J.A., Norman, S.A., Strom, B.L., Burkman, R.T., Ursin, G., Deapen, D., Weiss, L.K., Folger, S., Madeoy, J.J., Friedrichsen, D.M., Suter, N.M., Humphrey, M.C., Spirtas, R. and Ostrander, E.A. (2006) Prevalence and predictors of BRCA1 and BRCA2 mutations in a population-based study of breast cancer in white and black American women ages 35 to 64 years. *Cancer Research*, **66**, 8297–308.

14 Stratakis, C.A., Kirschner, L.S. and Carney, J.A. (2001) Clinical and molecular features of the Carney complex: diagnostic criteria and recommendations for patient evaluation. *The Journal of Clinical Endocrinology and Metabolism*, **86**, 4041–6.

15 Veugelers, M., Bressan, M., McDermott, D.A., Weremowicz, S., Morton, C.C., Mabry, C.C., Lefaivre, J.F., Zunamon, A., Destree, A., Chaudron, J.M. and Basson, C.T. (2004) Mutation of perinatal myosin heavy chain associated with a Carney complex variant. *The New England Journal of Medicine*, **351**, 460–9.

16 White, S.M., Graham, J.M., Kerr, B., Gripp, K., Weksberg, R., Cytrynbaum, C., Reeder, J.L., Stewart, F.J., Edwards, M., Wilson, M. and Bankier, A. (2005) The adult phenotype in Costello syndrome. *American Journal of Medical Genetics*, **136A**, 128–35.

17 Zbuk, K.M. and Eng, C. (2007) Hamartomatous polyposis syndromes. Review. *Nature Clinical Practice Gastroenterology and Hepatology*, **4** (9), 492–502.

18 Vasen, H.F., Moeslein, G., Alonso, A., Aretz, S., Bernstein, I., Bertario, L., Blanco, I., Bulow, S., Burn, J., Capella, G., Colas, C., Engel, C., Frayling, I., Friedl, W., Hes, F., Hodgson, S., Jarvinen, H., Mecklin, J.P., Moller, P.,

Myrhoj, T., Nagengast, F.M., Parc, Y., Phillips, R. and Clark, S., Ponz de Leon, M., Renkonen-Sinisalo, L., Sampson, J., Stormrken, A., Tejpar, S., Thomas, H. and Wijnen, J. (2008) Guidelines for the clinical management of familial adenomatous polyposis (FAP). *Gut*, **57(5)**, 704–13.

19 Hanson, C.A. and Miller, J.R. (2005) Non-traditional roles for the adenomatous polyposis coli (APC) tumor suppressor protein. *Gene*, **361**, 1–12.

20 Davies, D.R., Armstrong, J.G., Thakker, N., Horner, K., Guy, S.P., Clancy, T., Sloan, P., Blair, V., Dodd, C., Warness, T.W., Harris, R. and Evans, D.G.R. (1995) Severe Gardner syndrome in families with mutations restricted to a specific region of the APC gene. *American Journal of Human Genetics*, **57**, 1151–8.

21 Gorlin, R.J. (2004) Nevoid basal cell carcinoma (Gorlin) syndrome. *Genetics in Medicine*, **6**, 530–9.

22 Klein, R.D., Dykas, D.J. and Bale, A.E. (2005) Clinical testing for the nevoid basal cell carcinoma syndrome in a DNA diagnostic laboratory. *Genetics in Medicine*, **7**, 611–19.

23 Haven, C.J., Wong, F.K., Van Dam, E.W.C.M., van der Luijt, R., van Asperen, C., Jansen, J., Rosenberg, C., De Wit, M., Roijers, J., Hoppener, J., Lips, C.J., Larsson, C., The, B.T. and Morreau, H. (2000) A genotypic and histopathological study of a large Dutch kindred with hyperparathyroidism-jaw tumor syndrome. *The Journal of Clinical Endocrinology and Metabolism*, **85**, 1449–54.

24 Carpten, J.D., Robbins, C.M., Villablanca, A., Forsberg, L., Presciuttini, S., Larsson, C. and Hobbs, M.R. (2002) HRPT2, encoding parafibromin, is mutated in hyperpara-thyroidism-jaw tumour syndrome. *Nature Genetics*, **32**, 676–80.

25 Howe, J.R., Haidle, J.L., Lal, G., Bair, J., Song, C., Pechman, B., Chinnathambi, S. and Lynch, H.T. (2007) ENG mutations in *MADH4/BMPR1A* mutation negative patients with juvenile polyposis. *Clinical Genetics*, **71**, 91–2.

26 Varley, J.M., Evans, D.G.R. and Birch, J.M. (1997) Li-Fraumeni syndrome: a molecular and clinical review. *British Journal of Cancer*, **76**, 1–14.

27 Olivier, M., Goldgar, D.E., Sodha, N., Ohgaki, H., Kleihues, P., Hainaut, P. and Eeles, R.A. (2003) Li-Fraumeni and related syndromes: correlation between tumour type, family structure, and TP53 genotype. *Cancer Research*, **63**, 6643–50.

28 Bell, D.W., Varley, J.M., Szadlo, T.E., Kang, D.H., Wahrer, D.C., Shannon, K. E., Lubratovich, M., Verselis, S.J., Isselbacher, K.J., Fraumeni, J.F., Birch, J. M., Li, F.P., Garber, J.E. and Haber, D.A. (1999) Heterozygous germ line hCHK2 mutations in Li-Fraumeni syndrome. *Science*, **286**, 2528–31.

29 Bachinski, L.L., Olufemi, S.-E., Zhou, X., Wu, C.-C., Yip, L., Shete, S., Lozano, G., Amos, C.I., Strong, L.C. and Krahe, R. (2005) Genetic Mapping of a third Li-Fraumeni syndrome predisposition locus to human chromosome 1q23. *Cancer Research*, **65**, 427–31.

30 Evans, D.G., Wu, C.L. and Birch, J.M. (2008) *BRCA2*: a cause of Li-Fraumeni-like syndrome. *Journal of Medical Genetics*, **45**, 62–3.

31 Lenz, H.J. (2005) First Amsterdam, then Bethesda, now Melbourne? *Journal of Clinical Oncology*, **23**, 6445–9.

32 Papadopoulos, N., Nicolaides, N.C., Wei, Y.F., Ruben, S.M., Carter, K.C., Rosen, C.A., Haseltine, W.A., Fleischmann, R. D., Fraser, C.M. and Adams, M.D. (1994) Mutation of a mutL homolog in hereditary colon cancer. *Science*, **263**, 1625–9.

33 Azizi, E., Friedman, J., Pavlotsky, F., Iscovich, J., Bornstein, A., Shafir, R., Trau, H., Brenner, H. and Nass, D. (1995) Familial cutaneous malignant melanoma and tumors of the nervous system. A hereditary cancer syndrome. *Cancer*, **76**, 1571–8.

34 Randerson-Moor, J.A., Harland, M., Williams, S., Cuthbert-Heavens, D., Sheridan, E., Aveyard, J., Sibley, K., Whitaker, L., Knowles, M., Bishop, J.N. and Bishop, D.T. (2001) A germline deletion of p14 [ARF] but not *CDKN2A* in a melanoma-neural system tumour

syndrome family. *Human Molecular Genetics*, **10**, 55–62.

35 Bartsch, D.K., Sina-Frey, M., Lang, S., Wild, A., Gerdes, B., Barth, P., Kress, R., Grützmann, R., Colombo-Benkmann, M., Ziegler, A., Hahn, S.A., Rothmund, M. and Rieder, H. (2002) CDKN2A germline mutations in familial pancreatic cancer. *Annals of Surgery*, **6**, 730–7.

36 Lynch, H.T., Brand, R.E., Hogg, D., Deters, C.A., Fusaro, R.M., Lynch, J.F., Liu, L., Knezetic, J., Lassam, N.J., Goggins, M. and Kern, C. (2002) Phenotypic variation in eight extended CDKN2A germline mutation familial atypical multiple mole melanoma-pancreatic carcinoma-prone families: the familial atypical multiple mole melanoma-pancreatic carcinoma syndrome. *Cancer*, **94**, 84–96.

37 Lynch, H.T., Fusaro, R.M., Lynch, J.F. and Brand, R. (2008) Pancreatic cancer and the FAMMM syndrome. *Familial Cancer*, **7(1)**, 103–12.

38 Asgharian, B., Turner, M.L., Gibril, F., Entsuah, L.K., Serrano, J. and Jensen, R.T. (2004) Cutaneous tumors in patients with multiple endocrine neoplasm type 1 (MEN1) and gastrinomas: prospective study of frequency and development of criteria with high sensitivity and specificity MEN1. *The Journal of Clinical Endocrinology and Metabolism*, **89**, 5328–36.

39 Kloeppel, G., Perren, A. and Heitz, P.U. (2004) The gastroenteropancreatic neuroendocrine cell system and its tumors: the WHO classification. *Annals of the New York Academy of Sciences*, **1014**, 13–27.

40 Santoro, M., Melillo, R.M., Carlomagno, F., Vecchio, G. and Fusco, A. (2004) Mini review: RET: normal and abnormal functions. *Endocrinology*, **145**, 5448–51.

41 Yanaba, K., Nakagawa, H., Takeda, Y., Koyama, N. and Sugano, K. (2008) Muir-Torre syndrome caused by partial duplication of MSH2 gene by Alu-mediated nonhomologous recombination. *The British Journal of Dermatology*, **158**, 150–6.

42 DeBella, K., Szudek, J. and Friedman, J.M. (2000) Use of the national institutes of health criteria for diagnosis of neurofibromatosis 1 in children. *Pediatrics*, **105**, 608–14.

43 Wimmer, K., Roca, X., Beiglbock, H., Callens, T., Etzler, J., Rao, A.R., Krainer, A.R., Fonatsch, C. and Messiaen, L. (2007) Extensive in silico analysis of NF1 splicing defects. *Human Mutation*, **28**, 599–612.

44 Baser, M.E., Friedman, J.M., Walace, A.J., Ramsden, R.T., Joe, H. and Evans, D.G. (2002) Evaluation of clinical diagnostic criteria for neurofibromatosis 2. *Neurology*, **59**, 1759–65.

45 Hearle, N., Schumacher, V., Menko, F.H., Olschwang, S., Boardman, L.A., Gille, J.J.P., Keller, J.J., Westerman, A.M., Scott, R.J., Lim, W., Trimbath, J.D., Giardiello, F.M., Gruber, S.B., Offerhaus, G.J.A., de Rooij, F.W.M., Wilson, J.H.P., Hansmann, A., Möslein, G., Royer-Pokora, B., Vogel, T., Phillips, R.K.S., Spigelman, A.D. and Houlston, R.S. (2006) Frequency and spectrum of cancers in the Peutz-Jeghers syndrome. *Clinical Cancer Research*, **12**, 3209–15.

46 Lohmann, D.R. and Gallie, B.L. (2004) Retinoblastoma: revisiting the model prototype of inherited cancer. *American Journal of Medical Genetics*, **129**, 23–8.

47 Alam, N.A., Barclay, E., Rowan, A.J., Tyrer, J.P., Calonje, E., Manek, S., Kelsell, D., Leigh, I., Olpin, S. and Tomlinson, J.P.M. (2005) Clinical features of multiple cutaneous and uterine leiomyomatosis. *Archives of Dermatology*, **141**, 199–206.

48 Wei, M.H., Toure, O., Glenn, G.M., Pithukpakorn, M., Neckers, L., Stolle, C., Choyke, P., Grubb, R., Middelton, L., Turner, M.L., Walther, M.M., Merino, M.J., Zbar, B., Linehan, W.M. and Toro, J.R. (2006) Novel mutations in FH and expansion of the spectrum of phenotypes expressed in families with hereditary leiomyomatosis and renal cell cancer. *Journal of Medical Genetics*, **43**, 18–27.

49 Sévenet, N., Sheridan, E., Amram, D., Schneider, P., Handgretinger, R. and Delattre, O. (1999) Constitutional mutations of the hSNF5/INI1 gene predispose to a variety of cancers.

American Journal of Human Genetics, **65**, 1342–8.

50 Wieser, R., Fritz, B., Ullmann, R., Müller, J., Galhuber, M., Storlazzi, C.T., Ramaswamy, A., Christiansen, H., Shimizu, N., and Rehder, H. (2005) Novel Rearrangement of chromosome band 22q11.2 causing 22q11 micro-deletion syndrome-like phenotype and rhabdoid tumor of the kidney. *Human Mutation*, **26**, 1–6.

51 Ammerlaan, A.C., Ararou, A., Houben, M.P.W.A., Baas, F., Tijssen, C.C., Teepen, J.L.J.M., Wesseling, P. and Hulsebos, T.J.M. (2008) Long-term survival and transmission of INI1-mutation via nonpenetrant males in a family with rhabdoid tumour predisposition syndrome. *British Journal of Cancer*, **98**, 474–9.

52 Wang, L.L., Gannavarapu, A., Kozinetz, C.A., Levy, M.L., Lewis, R.A., Chintagumpala, M.M., Ruiz-Maldanado, R., Contreras-Ruiz, J., Cunniff, C., Erickson, R.P., Lev, D., Rogers, M., Zackai, E.H. and Plon, S.E. (2003) Association between osteosarcoma and deleterious mutations in the RECQL4 gene in Rothmund-Thomson syndrome. *Journal of National Cancer Institute*, **95**, 669–74.

53 Sangrithi, M.N., Bernal, J.A., Madine, M., Phipott, A., Lee, J., Dunphy, W.G. and Ventikaraman, A.R. (2005) Initiation of DNA replication requires the RECQL4 protein mutated in Rothmund-Thomson syndrome. *Cell*, **121**, 887–98.

54 Crino, P.B., Nathanson, K.L. and Henske, E.P. (2006) The tuberous sclerosis complex. Review. *The New England Journal of Medicine*, **355**, 1345–56.

55 Jozwiak, J., Jozwiak, S. and Wöodarski, P. (2008) Possible mechanisms of disease development in tuberous sclerosis. *The Lancet Oncology*, **9**, 73–9.

56 Ostergaard, J.R., Sunde, L. and Okkels, H. (2005) Neurofibromatosis von Recklinghausen type I phenotype and early onset of cancers in siblings compound heterozygous for mutations in MSH6. *American Journal of Medical Genetics*, **139A**, 96–105.

57 Auclair, J., Leroux, D., Desseigne, F., Lasset, C., Saurin, J.C., Joly, M.O., Pinson, S., Xu, X.L., Montmain, G., Ruano, E., Navarro, C., Puisieux, A. and Wang, Q. (2007) Novel biallelic mutations in MSH6 and PMS2 genes: gene conversion as a likely cause of PMS2 gene inactivation. *Human Mutation*, **28**, 1084–90.

58 Kaelin, W.G. Jr (2002) Molecular basis of the VHL hereditary cancer syndrome. *Nature Reviews Cancer*, **2**, 673–82.

59 Decker, H.J. (2006) Von Hippel-Lindau syndrome. *Medgen*, **18**, 355–61.

60 Huang, J.S., Huang, C.J., Chen, S.K., Chien, C.C., Chen, C.W. and Lin, C.M. (2007) Associations between VHL genotype and clinical phenotype in familial von Hippel-Lindau disease. *European Journal of Clinical Investigationy*, **37**, 492–500.

61 Goto, M., Miller, R.W., Ishikawa, Y. and Sugano, H. (1996) Excess of rare cancers in Werner syndrome (adult progeria). *Cancer Epidemiology, Biomarkers and Prevention*, **5**, 239–46.

62 Huang, S., Lee, L., Hanson, N.B., Lenaerts, C., Hoehn, H., Poot, M., Rubin, C.D., Chen, D.F., Yang, C.C., Juch, H., Dorn, T., Spiegel, R., Oral, E.A., Abid, M., Battisti, C., Lucci-Cordisco, C., Neri, G., Steed, E.H., Kidd, A., Isley, W., Showalter, D., Vittone, J.L., Konstantinow, A., Ring, J., Meyer, P., Wnger, S.L., von Herbay, A., Wollina, U., Schuelke, M., Huizenga, C.R., Leistritz, D.F., Martin, G.M., Mian, I.S. and Oshima, J. (2006) The spectrum of WRN mutations in Werner syndrome patients. *Human Mutation*, **27**, 558–67.

63 Agrelo, R., Cheng, W.-H., Setien, F., Ropero, S., Espada, J., Fraga, M.F., Herranz, M., Paz, M.F., Sanchez-Cespedes, M., Artiga, M.J., Guerrero, D., Castells, A., von Kobbe, C., Bohr, V.A. and Esteller, M. (2006) Epigenetic inactivation of the premature aging Werner syndrome gene in human cancer. *PNAS*, **103**, 8822–7.

64 Bootsma, D., Kraemer, K.H., Cleaver, J.E. and Hoeijmakers, J.H.J. (revised 2002) Nucleotide excision repair syndromes: xeroderma pigmentosum, Cockayne syndrome, and trichiodystrophy, in *The*

Metabolic and Molecular Bases of Inherited Disease (OMMBID) (eds C.R. Scriver, A.L. Beaudet, W.S. Sly, D. Valle and B. Vogelstein), McGraw-Hill, New York, Chap. 28, www.ommbid.com

65 Blankenburg, S., Konig, I.R., Moessner, R., Laspe, P., Thomas, K.M., Krueger, U., Khan, S.G., Westphal, G., Berking, C., Volkenandt, M., Reich, K., Neumann, C., Ziegler, A., Kraemer, K. H. and Emmerts, S. (2005) Assessment of 3 xeroderma pigmentosum group C gene polymorphisms and risk of cutaneous melanoma: a case-control study. *Carcinogenesis*, **26**, 1085–90.

66 Boland, C.R. and Troncale, F.J. (1984) Familial colonic cancer without antecedent polyposis. *Annals of Internal Medicine*, **100**, 700–1.

67 Lipton, L.R., Johnson, V., Cummings, C., Fisher, S., Risby, P., Eftekhar Sadat, A.T., Cranston, T., Izatt, L., Sasieni, P., Hodgson, S.V., Thomas, H.J.W. and Tomlinson, I.P.M. (2004) Refining the Amsterdam criteria and Bethesda guidelines: testing algorithms for the prediction of mismatch repair mutation status in the familial cancer clinic. *Journal of Clinical Oncology*, **24**, 4934–43.

68 Southey, M.C., Jenkins, M.A., Mead, L., Whitty, J., Trivett, M., Tesoriero, A.A., Smith, L.D., Jennings, K., Grubb, G., Royce, S.G., Walsh, M.D., Barker, M.A., Young, J.P., Jass, J.R., St John, D.J., Macrae, F.A., Giles, G.G. and Hopper, J.L. (2005) Use of molecular tumor characteristics to prioritize mismatch repair gene testing in early-onset colorectal cancer. *Journal of Clinical Oncology*, **23**, 6524–32.

69 Peltomäki, P. (2003) Role of DNA mismatch repair defects in the pathogenesis of human cancer. *Journal of Clinical Oncology*, **21**, 1174–9.

70 Leach, F.S., Nicolaides, N.C., Papadopoulos, N., Liu, B., Jen, J., Parsons, R., Peltomäki, P., Sistonen, P., Aaltonen, L.A., Nyström-Lahti, M. *et al.* (1993) Mutations of a mutS homolog in hereditary nonpolyposis colorectal cancer. *Cell*, **75**, 1215–25.

71 Fishel, R., Lescoe, M.K., Rao, M.R., Copeland, N.G., Jenkins, N.A., Garber, J., Kane, M. and Kolodner, R. (1993) The human mutator gene homolog MSH2 and its association with hereditary nonpolyposis colon cancer. *Cell*, **75**, 1027–38.

72 Wijnen, J., de Leeuw, W., Vasen, H., van der Klift, H., Moller, P., Stormorken, A., Meijers-Heijboer, H., Lindhout, D., Menko, F., Vossen, S., Moslein, G., Tops, G., Brocker Vriends, A., Wu, Y., Hofstra, R., Sijmons, R., Cornelisse, C., Morreau, H. and Fodde, R. (1999) Familial endometrial cancer in female carriers of MSH6 germline mutations. *Nature Genetics*, **23**, 142–4.

73 Hampel, H., Stephens, J.A., Pukkala, E., Sankila, R., Aaltonen, L.A., Mecklin, J.P. and de la Chapelle, A. (2005) Cancer Risk in hereditary nonpolyposis colorectal cancer syndrome: later age of onset. *Gastroenterology*, **129**, 415–21.

74 Akhtar, S., Oza, K.K., Khan, S.A. and Wright, J. (1999) Muir-Torre syndrome: case report of a patient with concurrent jejunal and ureteral cancer and a review of the literature. *Journal of the American Academy of Dermatology*, **41**, 707–9.

75 Mangold, E., Pagenstecher, C., Leister, M., Mathiak, M., Rutten, A., Friedl, W., Propping, P., Ruzicka, T. and Kruse, R. (2004) A genotype-phenotype correlation in HNPCC: strong predominance of msh2 mutations in 41 patients with Muir-Torre syndrome. *Journal of Medical Genetics*, **41**, 567–72.

76 Su, L.K., Vogelstein, B. and Kinzler, K.W. (1993) Association of the APC tumor suppressor protein with catenins. *Science*, **262**, 1734–7.

77 Caspari, R., Olschwang, S., Friedl, W., Mandl, M., Böker, T., Augustin, A., Kadmon, M., Möslein, G., Thomas, G. *et al.* (1995) Familial adenomatous polyposis: desmoid tumors and lack of ophthalmic lesions (CHRPE) associated with APC mutations beyond codon 1444. *Human Molecular Genetics*, **4**, 337–40.

78 Hamilton, S.R., Liu, B., Parson, R.E., Papadopoulos, N., Jen, J., Powell, S.M., Krush, A.J., Berk, T., Cohen, Z., Tetu, B. *et al.* (1995) The molecular basis of Turcot's syndrome. *The New England Journal of Medicine*, **332**, 839–47.

79 Knudson, A.L., Bisgaard, M.L. and Bulow, S. (2003) Attenuated familial adenomatous polyposis (AFAP). A review of the literature. *Familial Cancer*, **2**, 43–55.

80 Forcet, C., Etienne-Manneville, S., Gaude, H., Fournier, L., Debilly, S., Salmi, M., Baas, A., Olschwang, S., Clevers, H. and Billaud, M. (2005) Functional analysis of Peutz-Jeghers mutations reveals that the LKB C-terminal region exerts a crucial role in regulating both the AMPK pathway and the cell polarity. *Human Molecular Genetics*, **14**, 1283–92.

81 Alessi, D.R., Sakamoto, K. and Bayascas, J.R. (2006) LKB1-dependent signalling pathways. *Annual Review of Biochemistry*, **75**, 137–63.

82 Amos, C.I., Keitheri-Cheteri, M.B., Sabripour, M., Wei, C., McGarrity, T.J. Seldin, M.F., Nations, L., Lynch, P.M., Fidder, H., Friedman, E. and Frazier, M.L. (2004) Genotype-phenotype correlations in Peutz-Jeghers syndrome. *Journal of Medical Genetics*, **41**, 327–33.

83 Eng, C. (2000) Will the real Cowden syndrome please stand up: revised diagnostic criteria. *Journal of Medical Genetics*, **37**, 828–30.

84 Bosserhoff, A.K., Grussendorf-Conen, E.I., Rübben, A., Rudnik-Schöneborn, S., Zerres, K., Buettner, R. and Merkeblach-Bruse, S. (2006) Multiple colon carcinomas in a patient with Cowden syndrome. *International Journal of Molecular Medicine*, **18**, 643–7.

85 Chung, J.H. and Eng, C. (2005) Nuclear-cytoplasmic partitioning of phosphatase and tensin homologue deleted on chromosome 10 (PTEN) differentially regulates the cell cycle and apoptosis. *Cancer Research*, **65**, 8096–100.

86 Zhou, X.P., Ivanovich, J., Matloff, E., Patterson, A., Pierpont, M.E., Russo, D., Nassif, N.T., Eng, C., Waite, K.A., Pilarski, R., Hampel, H., Fernandez, M.J., Bos, C., Dasouki, M., Felman, G. L. and Greenberg, L.A. (2003) Germline PTEN promoter mutations and deletions in Cowden/Bannayan-Riley-Ruvalcaba syndrome result in aberrant PTEN protein and dysregulation of the phophoinositol-3-kinase/Akt pathway. *American Journal of Human Genetics*, **73**, 404–11.

87 Smith, J.M., Kirk, E.P.E., Theodoso-poulos, G., Marshall, G.M., Walker J., Rogers, M., Field, M., Brereton, J.J. and Marsh, D.J. (2002) Germline mutation of the tumour suppressor *PTEN* in Proteus syndrome. *Journal of Medical Genetics*, **39**, 937–40.

88 Cohen, M.M. Jr (1999) Overgrowth syndromes: an update. *Advances in Pediatrics*, **46**, 441–91.

89 Gilbert-Barness, E., Cohen, M.M. and Opitz, J.M. (2000) Multiple meningiomas, craniofacial hyperostosis and retinal abnormalities in Proteus syndrome. *American Journal of Medical Genetics*, **93**, 234–40.

90 Happle, R., Steijlen, P.M., Theile, U., Karitzky, D., Tinschert, S., Albrecht-Nebe, H. and Kuster, W. (1997) Patchy dermal hypoplasia as a characteristic feature of Proteus syndrome. *Archives of Dermatology*, **133**, 77–80.

91 Howe, J.R., Roth, S., Ringold, J.C., Summers, R.W., Järwinen, H.J., Sistonen, P., Tomlinson, I.P., Houlston, R.S., Bevan, S., Mitros, F.A., Stone, E.M. and Aaltonen, L.A. (1998) Mutations in the SMAD4/DPC4 gene in juvenile polyposis. *Science*, **280**, 1086–8.

92 Howe, J.R., Sayed, M.G., Ahmed, A.F., Ringold, J., Larsen-Haidle, J., Merg, A., Mitros, F.A., Vaccaro, C.A., Petersen, G.M., Giardiello, F.M., Tinley, S.T., Aaltonen, L.A. and Lynch, H.T. (2004) The prevalence of MADH4 and BMPR1A mutations in juvenile polyposis and absence of *BMPR2, BMPR1B* and *ACVR1* mutations. *Journal of Medical Genetics*, **41**, 484–91.

93 Delatte, C., Sanlaville, D., Mougenot, J.F., Vermeesch, J.R., Houdayer, C., de Blois, M.C., Genevieve, D., Goulet, O., Fryns, J.P., Jaubert, F., Vekemans, M., Lyonnet, S., Romana, S., Eng, C. and Stoppa-Lyonnet, D. (2006) Contiguous gene deletion within chromosome arm 10q is associated with juvenile polyposis of infancy, reflecting cooperation between the *BMPR1A* and *PTEN* tumor-suppressor genes. *American Journal of Human Genetics*, **78**, 1066–74.

94 Agarwal, S.K., Lee Burns, A., Sukhodolets, K.E., Kennedy, P.A., Obungu, V.H., Hickman, A.B., Mullendore, M.E., Whitten, I., Skarulis, M.C., Simonds, W.F., Mateo, C., Crabtree, J.S., Scacheri, P.C., Ji, Y., Novotny, E.A., Garrett-Beal, L., Ward, J.M., Libutti, S.K., Richard Alexander, H., Cerrato, A., Parisi, M.J., Santa Anna, A.S., Oliver, B., Chandrasekharappa, S.C., Collins, F.S., Spiegel, A.M. and Marx, S.J. (2004) Molecular pathology of the MEN1 gene. *Annals of the New York Academy of Sciences*, **1014**, 189–98.

95 Manie, S., Santoro, M., Fusco, A. and Billaud, M. (2001) The RET receptor: function in development and dysfunction in congenital malformation. *Trends in Genetics*, **17**, 580–9.

96 Takahashi, M., Asai, N., Iwashita, T., Murakami, H. and Ito, S. (1999) Molecular mechanisms of development of multiple endocrine neoplasia 2 by RET mutations. *Journal of Internal Medicine*, **243**, 509–13.

97 Carney, J.A. (1995) Carney complex: the complex of myxomas, spotty pigmentation, endocrine overactivity, and schwannomas. *Seminars in Dermatology*, **14**, 90–8.

98 Stratakis, C.A., Bertherat, J. and Carney, J.A. (2004) Mutation of perinatal myosin heavy chain (Letter). *The New England Journal of Medicine*, **351**, 2556 only.

99 Kimonis, V.E., Goldstein, A.M., Pastakia, B., Yang, M.L., Kase, R., DiGiovanna, J.J., Bale, A.E. and Bale, S. J. (1997) Clinical manifestations in 105 persons with nevoid basal cell carcinoma syndrome. *American Journal of Medical Genetics*, **69**, 299–308.

100 Somoano, B., Niendorf, K.B. and Tsao, H. (2005) Hereditary cancer syndromes of the skin. *Clinics in Dermatology*, **23**, 85–106.

101 Cohen M.M. Jr (2003) The hedgehog signaling network. *American Journal of Medical Genetics*, **123A**, 5–28.

102 Midro, A.T., Panasiuk, B., Tümer, Z., Stankiewicz, P., Silahtaroglu, A., Lupski, J.R., Zemanova, Z., Stasiewicz-Jarocka, B., Hubert, E., Tarasów, E.,

Famulski, W., Zadrozna-Tolwinska, B., Wasilewska, E., Kirchhoff, M., Kalscheuer, V., Michalova, K. and Tommerup, N. (2004) Interstitial deletion 9q22.32-q33.2 associated with additional familial translocation t(9;17)(q34.11;p11.2) in a patient with Gorlin-Goltz syndrome and features of nail-patella syndrome. *American Journal of Medical Genetics*, **124A**, 179–91.

103 Goldstein, A.M. (2004) Familial melanoma, pancreatic cancer and germline CDKN2A mutations. *Human Mutation*, **23**, 630.

104 Vasen, H.F.A., Gruis, N.A., Frants, R.R., van der Velden, P.A., Hille, E.T.M. and Bergman, W. (2000) Risk of developing pancreatic cancer in families with familial atypical multiple mole melanoma associated with a specific 19 deletion of p16(p16-Leiden). *International Journal of Cancer*, **87**, 809–11.

105 Pavlovich, C.P., Walther, M.M., Eyler, R.A., Hewitt, S.M., Zbar, B., Linehan, W. M. and Merino, M.J. (2002) Renal tumors in the Birt-Hogg-Dubé syndrome. *The American journal of Surgical Pathology*, **26**, 1542–52.

106 Lindor, N.M., Devries, E.M., Michels, V.V., Schad, C.R., Jalal, S.M., Donnovan, K.M., Smithson, W.A., Kvols, L.K., Thibodeau, S.N. and Dewald, G.W. (1996) Rothmund-Thomson syndrome in siblings: evidence for acquired in vivo mosaicism. *Clinical Genetics*, **49**, 124–9.

107 Satoh, M., Imai, M., Sugimoto, M., Goto, M. and Furuichi, Y. (1999) Prevalence of Werner's syndrome heterozygotes in Japan. *Lancet*, **353**, 1766.

108 Cook, J.A., Oliver, K., Mueller, R.F. and Sampson, J. (1996) A cross sectional study of trenal involvement in tuberous sclerosis. *Journal of Medical Genetics*, **33**, 448–84.

109 Patel, U., Simpson, E., Kingswood, J.C. and Saggar-Malik, A.K. (2005) Tuberous sclerosis complex: analysis of growth rates aids differentiation of renal cell carcinoma from atypical or minimal-fat-containing angiomyolipoma. *Clinical Radiology*, **60**, 665–73.

110 Brook-Carter, P.T., Peral, B., Ward, C.J., Thompson, P., Hughes, J., Maheshwar,

M.M., Nellist, M., Gamble, V., Harris, P.C. and Sampson, J.R. (1994) Deletion of TSC2 and PKD1 genes associated with severe infantile polycystic kidney disease – a contiguous gene syndrome. *Nature Genetics*, **8**, 328–32.

111 Roux, P.P., Ballif, B.A., Anjum, R., Gygi, S.P. and Blenis, J. (2004) Tumor-promoting phorbol esters and activated Ras inactivate the tuberous sclerosis tumor suppressor com-plex via p90 ribosomal S6 kinase. *Proceedings of the National Academy of Sciences of the United States of America*, **101**, 13489–94.

112 Karbowniczek, M., Astrinidis, A., Balsara, B.R. *et al.* (2003) Recurrent lymphangio-myomatosis after transplantation: genetic analyses reveal a metastatic mechanism. *American Journal of Respiratory and Critical care Medicine*, **167**, 967–82.

113 Sancak, O., Nellist, M., Goedbloed, M., Elfferich, P., Wouters, C., Maat-Kievit, A., Zonnenberg, B., Verhoef, S., Halley, D. and van den Ouweland, A. (2005) Mutational analysis of the TSC1 and TSC2 genes in a diagnostic setting: genotype-phenotype correlations and comparison of diagnostic DNA techniques in tuberous sclerosis complex. *European Journal of Human Genetics*, **13**, 731–41.

114 Gläsker, S. (2005) Central nervous system manifestations in VHL: genetic, pathology and clinical phenotypic features. *Familial Cancer*, **4**, 37–42.

115 Wong, W.T., Agrón, E., Coleman, H.R., Reed, G.F., Csaky, K., Peterson, J., Glenn, G., Linehan, M., Albert, P. and Chew, E.Y. (2007) Genotype-phenotype correlation in von Hippel-Lindau disease with retinal angiomatosis. *Archives of Ophthalmology*, **125**, 239–45.

116 Zbar, B., Kishida, T., Chen, F., Schmidt, L., Maher, E.R., Richards, F.M., Crossey, P.A., Webster, A.R., Affara, N.A., Ferguson-Smith, M.A., Brauch, H., Glavac, D., Neumann, H.P., Tisherman, S., Mulvihill, J.J., Gross, D.J., Shuin, T., Whaley, J., Seizinger, B., Kley, N., Olschwang, S., Boisson, C., Richard, S., Lips, C.H., Lerman, M. *et al.* (1996) Germline mutations in the Von Hippel-Lindau disease (VJL)

gene in families from North America, Europe, and Japan. *Human Mutation*, **8**, 348–57.

117 Isaacs, J.S., Jung, Y.J., Mole, D.R., Lee, S., Torres-Cabala, C., Chung, Y.L., Merino, M., Trepel, J., Zbar, B., Toro, J., Ratcliffe, P.J., Linehan, W.M. and Neckers, L. (2005) HIF over-expression correlates with biallelic loss of fumarate hydratase in renal cancer: novel role of fumarate in regulation of HIF stability. *Cancer Cell*, **8**, 143–53.

118 Burger, P.C., Yu, I.-T., Tihan, T., Friedman, H.S., Strother, D.R., Kepner, J.L., Duffner, P.K. and Kun, L.E. and Perlman, E.J. (1998) Atypical teratoid/rhabdoid tumor of the central nervous system: a highly malignant tumor of infancy and childhood frequently mistaken for medulloblastoma: a pediatric oncology group study. *The American journal of Surgical Pathology*, **22**, 1083–92.

119 Haberler, C., Laggner, U., Slavc, I., Czech, T., Ambros, I.M., Ambros, P.F., Budka, H. and Hainfellner, J.A. (2006) Immunhistochemical analysis of INI1 protein in malignant pediatric CNS tumors: lack of INI1 in atypical teratoid/rhabdoid tumors and in a fraction of primitive neuroectodermal tumors without rhabdoid phenotype. *The American journal of Surgical Pathology*, **30**, 1462–8.

120 Hulsebos, T.J.M., Plomp, A.S., Wolterman, R.A., Robanus-Maandag, E.X., Baas, F. and Wesseling, P. (2007) Germline mutation of INI1/SMARCB1 in familial schwannomatosis. *American Journal of Human Genetics*, **80**, 805–10.

121 Weeks, D.A., Beckwith, J.B., Mierau, G.W. and Luckey, D.W. (1989) Rhabdoid tumor of kidney: a report of 111 cases from the National Wilms' Tumor Study Pathology Center. *The American journal of Surgical Pathology*, **13**, 439–58.

122 Vries, R.G.J., Bezrookove, V., Zuijderduijn, L.M.P., Kia, S.K., Howeling, A., Oruetxebarria, I., Raap, A.K. and Verrijzer, C.P. (2005) Cancer-associated mutations in chromatin remodeler hSNF5 promote chromosomal instability by compromising the mitotic checkpoint. *Genes and Development*, **19**, 665–70.

123 Birch, J.M., Hartley, A.L., Tricker, K.J., Prosser, J., Condie, A., Kelsey, A.M., Harris, M., Jones, P.H., Binchy, A., Crowther, D. *et al.* (1994) Prevalence and diversity of constitutional mutations in the p53 gene among 21 Li-Fraumeni families. *Cancer Research*, **54**, 1298–304.

124 Eeles, R.A. (1995) Germline mutations in the TP53 gene. *Cancer Surveys*, **25**, 1001–124.

125 Levine, A.J. (1997) p53, the cellular gatekeeper for growth and division. *Cell*, **88**, 323–31.

126 Lee, S.B., Kim, S.H., Bell, D.W., Wahrer, D.C.R., Schiripo, T.A., Jorczak, M.M., Sgroi, D.C., Garber, J.E., Li, F.P., Nichols, K.E., Varley, J.M., Godwin, A. K., Shannon, K.M. and Harlow, E. Haber, D.A. (2001) Destabilization of CHK2 by a missense mutation associated with Li-Fraumeni syndrome. *Cancer Research*, **61**, 8062–7.

127 Le Bihan, C., Moutou, C., Brugieres, L., Feunteun, J. and Bonaiti-Pellie, C. (1995) ARCAD: a method for estimating age-dependent disease risk associated with mutation carrier status from family data. *Genetic Epidemiology*, **12**, 13–25.

128 Schrader, K.A., Masciari, S., Boyd, N., Wiyrick, S., Kaurah, P., Senz, J., Burke, W., Lynch, H.T., Garber, J.E. and Huntsman, D.G. (2008) Hereditary diffuse gastric cancer: association with lobular breast cancer. *Familial Cancer* **7**, 73–82.

4
Genetic Dysmorphic Syndromes Leading to Tumorigenesis

Gabriele Gillessen-Kaesbach

Summary

In 1957, a three times higher incidence of leukemia in children with Down's syndrome was described [1]. The association of Wilms tumor in children with Beckwith–Wiedemann syndrome is now well established. Ataxia-teleangiectasia, Fanconi syndrome, Nijmegen breakage syndrome, and Bloom syndrome are further examples resulting from mutations in genes contributing to genome stability with a predisposition to develop cancer. During recent years, a growing number of dysmorphic syndromes are known to be associated with tumorigenesis (Proteus syndrome, Noonan syndrome, Costello syndrome, Sotos syndrome, etc.).

Genetic, as well as environmental factors, play a role in the development of cancer. Common pathways are suspected to be involved in tumorigenesis and the etiology of congenital anomalies. In several studies it has been shown that patients with congenital anomalies have an increased risk of malignancies, in comparison to control children. The first study establishing the incidence and spectrum of clinical genetic syndromes concurring with malignancies in children was published by Merks *et al.* [2]. They found 7.5% of patients with cancer had a suspected genetic syndrome. This number is considerably higher than the prevalence of syndromes in the general population. It is of note that a high number of syndromes associated with tumors were first detected in this study. This means that clinically well defined syndromes in children with cancer are often overlooked by standard pediatric care. Therefore, it is recommended that every child with cancer should be examined by a clinical geneticist or pediatrician trained in dysmorphology.

4.1
Overgrowth Syndromes

Overgrowth syndromes are characterized by height and weight measurements 2–3 standard deviations above the mean for age and sex. The relationship between

Hereditary Tumors: From Genes to Clinical Consequences
Edited by Heike Allgayer, Helga Rehder and Simone Fulda
Copyright © 2009 WILEY-VCH Verlag GmbH & Co. KGaA, Weinheim
ISBN: 978-3-527-32028-8

malignancies and overgrowth syndromes has been extensively described [3, 4]. Frequently seen are kidney and liver tumors, as well as neuroblastoma, osteosarcoma, and leukemia.

4.1.1
Beckwith–Wiedemann Syndrome (BWS)

Macrosomia, macroglossia, and omphalocele are the diagnostically important clinical signs characterizing Beckwith–Wiedemann syndrome (BWS). Hemihyperplasia may affect segmental regions of the body or selected organs. Patients with BWS display a rather recognizable facial phenotype including prominent eyes, midline facial nevus flammeus, macroglossia, anterior earlobe creases, and posterior helical pits. Most patients with BWS have birth measurements above the 97th percentile for gestational age [5]. However, it is noteworthy that increased growth parameters normalize with puberty, resulting in adult heights between the 50th and 90th centiles [5, 6]. Mental development may be delayed in cases with duplication of 11p15, or due to undetected episodes of hypoglycemia present in about 30–50% of infants with BWS [6]. Visceromegaly of the liver, spleen, pancreas, kidneys, and adrenal glands are further features in this condition.

The genetic mechanisms in BWS, in which genetic imprinting, somatic mosaicism, and multiple genes are involved, are complex and have recently been reviewed [7, 8]. The phenotypic variability and risk for malignancy are related to the underlying genetic etiology [9].

The condition has been localized to the chromosomal region 11p15. BWS is most often sporadic (85%), whereas cytogenetic aberrations (translocations, inversions, or duplications) involving 11p15 are present in only 1% of patients with BWS [10]. However, cytogenetic testing is necessary in order to interpret the results of molecular analysis, and for evaluation of the risk for recurrence. Autosomal dominant inheritance with preferential maternal transmission has been documented in about 10–15% of cases. Due to a high phenotypic variability even within families, a careful examination of the pedigree is recommended.

BWS results from the abnormal expression of imprinted genes on 11p15. Alterations in two clusters (DMR1 and DMR2) of imprinted genes lead to changes of expression of genes responsible for BWS. Domain 1 (DMR1), which is located on the telomeric end of the imprinted gene cluster in 11p15, contains the genes insulin-like growth factor 2 (*IGF2*, paternally expressed), and *H19* (maternally expressed). About 25% of patients show loss of imprinting (LOI) of *IGF2*, resulting in expression of both parental alleles. A second domain, DMR2, which is centromeric to DMR1, contains several imprinted genes including: *KCNQ1, KCNQ1OT1(LIT1) CDKN1C, PHLDA*, and *SLC22A18. LIT1* is paternally expressed, whereas *KCNQ1*and *CDKN1C* are maternally expressed. Hypomethylation of DMR2 and LOI of *LIT1* are present in about 50% of the patients with sporadic BWS. In the remaining cases, paternal uniparental disomy (UPD) of 11p15 (20%), mutations of *CDKN1C* (5–10%), chromosomal rearrangements (duplications, inversions, and translocations) (1%), or other epigenetic alterations are present [8]. In some patients the molecular etiology cannot be resolved.

Patients with BWS have an increased risk (5–10%) of developing embryonal tumors, especially between the first 5–8 years [6, 11–13]. This risk is influenced by several factors such as the presence of hemihyperplasia, nephromegaly, and molecular etiology. The most common tumors are Wilms tumor and hepatoblastoma, but also rhabdomyosarcoma, adrenocortical carcinoma, and neuroblastoma can occur [11, 14]. Patients with LOI of *LIT1* have a risk of 1–5% of malignancy, whereas the risk in patients with LOI of *H19* is much higher (35–45%). Paternal UPD11p15 is associated with a risk of 25–30% of developing a tumor. In patients with a normal methylation pattern there seems to be a risk of 10–15% for malignancies [13]. Although the spectrum of tumors varies with the underlying molecular defect, Wilms tumor is the most frequent embryonal tumor, especially in patients with paternal uniparental disomy 11p15 and *H19* hypermethylation, whereas patients with a loss of methylation in DMR2 are more susceptible to developing rhabdomyosarcoma, hepatoblastoma, and, less frequently, gonadoblastoma, neuroblastoma, or adrenocortical carcinoma [14].

Regular surveillance for tumors in children with BWS independent from the molecular etiology is recommended [15–17]. At the time of diagnosis, an MRI of the abdomen should be performed [18], followed by quarterly abdominal ultrasounds and serum AFP testing of alphafetoprotein (AFP) [19].

4.1.2
Isolated Hemihyperplasia (IHH)

Isolated hemihyperplasia (IHH) is an abnormality of cell proliferation leading to asymmetric overgrowth of one or more regions of the body. Hemihyperplasia can occur as one part of different overgrowth syndromes or in isolation. In addition, IHH is often found in cytogenetic anomalies, especially mosaicism. Molecular studies revealing methylation defects of the *LIT1* (hypomethylation) and *H19* (hypermethylation) genes on chromosome 11p give evidence that epigenetic changes can result in a phenotype different from BWS [20, 21].

In patients with IHH, there is an increased risk (~6%) of embryonal cancers in childhood, particularly Wilms tumor [22–24]. Most common are adrenal cortical carcinoma and hepatoblastoma, but also pheochromocytoma, testicular carcinoma, undifferentiated sarcoma, and leiomyosarcoma can occur. Patients with isolated hemihypertrophy due to uniparental disomy at 11p15 seem to have a high tumor risk [25].

Most of the tumors occur in the abdomen, which makes it reasonable to recommend regular abdominal ultrasound and physical examination, serum (AFP and beta human chorionic gonadotropin), and urine screening (vanillymandelic acid, homovanillic acid, and catecholamines) every 3 months up to an age of 7 years [4].

4.1.3
Proteus Syndrome (PS)

Proteus syndrome (PS) is characterized by asymmetric overgrowth of different parts of the body [26–28]. Frequently found are lipomas, epidermal nevi, vascular and lymphatic malformations, and cranial hyperostoses. There seems to exist a facial phenotype comprising dolichocephaly, long face, low nasal bridge, and anteverted nares. Diagnostic guidelines have been developed by Biesecker [29, 30]. Zhou *et al.* [31] reported a boy with congenital hemihypertrophy, epidermal nevi, macrocephaly, lipomas, arteriovenous malformations, and normal intellect. A clinical diagnosis of Proteus-like syndrome was suggested. Mutational analysis of the DNA from peripheral blood revealed heterozygosity for a single base transversion, resulting in a nonsense mutation R335X leading to a premature stop, whereas analysis of DNA from a nevus, lipoma, and arteriovenous mass was found to carry an additional second hit R130X mutation on the allele opposite the germline mutation R335X. These mutations have been reported in patients with Cowden and Bannayan–Zonana syndromes. It has been speculated that the second hit, R130X, occurred early in embryonic development, and may even represent germline mosaicism. Thus, as to whether *PTEN* may play a role in patients with Proteus or Proteus like-syndrome with implications for cancer development is still unclear.

In PS, most malignancies occur under the age of 20 years, and often unusual types of tumors have been described such as ovarian (cystadenoma of the ovary), testicular (adenocarcinoma), meningeal and parotid neoplasms [27, 32, 33]. Multiple tumors can occur in the same patient. MRI screening of the brain (every two years), physical examination, and abdominal ultrasound (once a year) are recommended.

4.1.4
Sotos Syndrome (SS)

Sotos syndrome (SS) is an autosomal dominant disorder characterized by hypotonia, accelerated growth, macrodolichocephaly, receding anterior hairline, sparse hair, frontal bossing, ocular hypertelorism, and a prominent chin. Most patients show delayed development and behavioral problems [34]. Mild dilation of the cerebral ventricles, non-specific EEG changes, and seizures have been observed. Bone age is often accelerated, but decreases after the age of 5 years. Height is usually above the 97th centile. It is important to note that both height and head circumference are within the upper normal range in 10% of the individuals, indicating that overgrowth is not obligatory for the diagnosis of SS.

In 2002, the causative gene *NSD1* localized in 5q35 was identified in patients with SS [35]. The results indicate that haploinsufficiency of *NSD1* is the major cause of SS. Microdeletions are frequent in the Japanese population (52%), but seem to be rare in Caucasians (6–10%) [36, 37].

An increased risk (2–3%) for tumors was described [38–40]. Most tumors occurred after the age of 5 years. The most frequent tumor types are leukemia and lymphoma with a preponderance in males [41]. In contrast to other overgrowth syndromes, embryonal tumors are not the most common. More than 20 different tumors have been described in patients with SS, among them Wilms tumor, lymphomas, neuroblastoma, acute leukemia, hepatocarcinoma, blastoma of the lung, small cell carcinoma of the lung, yolk sac tumor of the testis, epidermoid carcinoma of the vagina, and diffuse gastric carcinoma [4]. It is of note that a variety of benign tumors (osteochondroma of the bone, sacrococcygeal teratoma, ganglioglioma, fibroma of the heart and ovary) have been reported. Due to the huge spectrum of malignancies, it is difficult to define a specific screening protocol. Generally, a physical examination, abdominal ultrasound, as well as serum and urine screening, should be performed every four months.

4.1.5
Weaver Syndrome (WS)

Patients with Weaver syndrome (WS) are usually macrosomic at birth. The face is characterized by a broad forehead, large ears, hypertelorism, micrognathia (but with a pointed, dimpled chin), and a long philtrum. Flaring of the metaphyses of the long bones and significantly advanced bone age in infants are helpful in establishing the clinical diagnosis. Most patients show developmental delay [42]. Multiple reports give evidence that WS is an autosomal dominant condition. There is ongoing debate as to whether SS and WS are representatives of locus or allelic heterogeneity [43]. The facial appearance bears somewhat similar features, but experienced dysmorphologists strongly believe they are distinct. The underlying defect is still unknown. *NSD1* mutations have been found in some rare patients; however, the diagnosis of WS was not convincing [37, 38, 44].

The risk for malignancies in patients with WS seems to be low. There are two reports of neuroblastoma [45, 46], one patient with a sacrococcygeal teratoma [47] and one with an ovarian endodermal sinus tumor [48]. Screening (physical examination, abdominal ultrasound, serum screening, and urine analysis) are recommended once a year.

4.1.6
Simpson–Golabi–Behmel Syndrome (SGBS)

Simpson–Golabi–Behmel syndrome (SGBS) is an X-linked condition characterized by pre- and postnatal overgrowth, coarse face, macroglossia, organomegaly, congenital heart defects, and variable mental retardation [49–51]. There is considerable overlap with BWS. About 100 patients with SGBS have been reported to date [52].

Mutations in the glypican 3 gene *(CPC3)* (point mutations and deletions) at Xq26 have been identified by [53]. The reported frequency for tumors is 10%. All tumors are intra-abdominal (Wilms tumor, hepatoblastoma, adrenal neuroblastoma, gonadoblastoma, hepatocellular carcinoma) [4, 54]. Tumor screening should include abdominal ultrasound, urine analysis, and biochemical testing for embryonal tumors.

4.1.7
Bannayan–Riley–Ruvalcaba Syndrome (BRRS)

Bannayan–Riley–Ruvalcaba syndrome (BRRS) is characterized by high birth measurements, macrocephaly, intestinal polyposis, developmental delay, lipomas, and pigmented spots on the penis [55–57]. The three independent descriptions were recognized to be a single entity and renamed by Cohen in 1990 [58]. Mutations in the *PTEN* gene have been identified in patients with BRRS [59], as well as in patients with Cowden syndrome [60]. In 1999, Marsh *et al.* [61] suggested that the spectrum of disorders be referred to as PTEN hamartoma tumor syndrome (PHTS). *PTEN* is a tumor suppressor gene localized at 10q23.21 and plays an important role in malignancy. In BRRS mostly benign tumors such lipomas, angiolipomas, and hamartoma are observed [28]. Up to now, malignant tumors (thyroid carcinoma, breast cancer, ganglioneuroma) were only reported in three patients [28, 62].

4.2
Syndromes with Mutations in the Mitogen-Activated Protein Kinase (MAPK)-RAS Pathway

Noonan syndrome (NS) is an autosomal dominant condition characterized by specific dysmorphic facial features, congenital heart disease, and short stature. Cardio-facio-cutaneous (CFC) and Costello (CS) syndromes are two autosomal dominant disorders showing overlapping features to NS. These three conditions are members of the MAPK-RAS pathway, which transduces a large variety of cellular responses, including cellular growth, differentiation, inflammation, and apoptosis. Clinically, it is often difficult to make an accurate diagnosis, especially in neonates and young children. Given the fact that there are different risks of neoplasia in these conditions, it is important to provide a molecular diagnosis, especially in making management decisions.

4.2.1
Noonan Syndrome (NS)

Noonan syndrome (NS), first described in 1963 [63], is a common autosomal dominant dysmorphic syndrome characterized by short stature, hypertelorism, a downward eye slant, and low-set posteriorly rotated ears. Other features include short stature, short neck with webbing or redundancy of skin, cardiac anomalies, epicanthic folds, deafness, mild intellectual and motor delay, and a bleeding diathesis [64]. There is great variability in expression, and especially the facial phenotype becomes less pronounced with age [65]. Pulmonary stenosis is the most frequent cardiac defect in NS and hypertrophic cardiomyopathy is present in about 20% of patients, which has an estimated incidence of 1 in 1000 to 2500 live births [66]. In about 50% of patients with a clinical diagnosis of NS, gain-of-function mutations in the *PTPN11* gene (12q24.1) have been identified [67]. The *PTPN11* gene encodes the non-receptor-type protein tyrosine phosphatase SHP-2 [67]. In 1969, Gorlin *et al.* [68] described the LEOPARD syndrome (LS) which is an acronym for the following features: multiple **L**entigines, **E**lectrocardiographic conduction abnormalities, **O**cular hypertelorism, **P**ulmonic stenosis, **A**bnormal genitalia, **R**etardation of growth, and sensorineural **D**eafness. LS shares a variety of clinical features with Noonan syndrome. Digilio *et al.* [69] identified *PTPN11* mutations in 8 of 10 (80%) infants with LS, indicating that these two disorders are allelic. Subsequently, Pandit *et al.* [70] demonstrated that, in addition, gain of function mutations in the *RAF1* gene, which encodes a serine-threonine kinase that activates *MEK1* and *MEK2*, are responsible for a subgroup of patients with LS and NS showing hypertrophic cardiomyopathy.

De novo germline mutations of the *KRAS* gene have also been disclosed in individuals with NS, but account for less than 5% of cases [71]. In about 17–20% of patients with NS, gain-of-function mutations in the *SOS1* gene [72, 73] have been identified. The *SOS1* gene encodes a RAS-specific guanine nucleotide exchange factor.

Children with NS have an increased incidence of juvenile myelomonocytic leukemia (JMML), myelodysplastic syndrome (MDS), and acute myeloid leukemia (AML) [74, 75]. However, the clinical course is much milder than in the isolated forms. Tartaglia *et al.* [76] show that patients with NS and JMML have germline gain of function mutations in *PTPN11*, whereas somatic mutations in this gene account for about 34% of non-syndromic JMML, and for a small percentage of patients with non-syndromic MDS and AML. It is of note that patients with NS with JMML mainly harbor the 218-C mutation in *PTPN11*, which is a rare mutation in isolated NS, highlighting that specific mutated alleles indicate a risk for JMML. In 2006, Tartaglia *et al.* [77] proposed a model that splits NS- and leukemia-associated *PTPN11* mutations in two major classes of activating lesions with differential perturbing effects on development and hematopoiesis. These results documented a strict correlation between the identity of the lesion and disease, and demonstrated that NS-causative mutations have less potency for promoting SHP2 gain of function, than do leukemia-associated ones.

4.2.2
Cardio-Facio-Cutaneous Syndrome (CFC)

Cardio-facio-cutaneous (CFC) syndrome is characterized by a distinctive facial appearance, heart defects, cutaneous abnormalities, and mental retardation. Postnatal feeding problems can be severe. The heart defects include pulmonic stenosis, atrial septal defect, and hypertrophic cardiomyopathy. Some patients have ectodermal abnormalities such as sparse, curly and friable hair, hyperkeratotic skin lesions, or a generalized ichthyosis-like condition. Typical facial characteristics include high forehead with bitemporal constriction, hypoplastic supraorbital ridges, down slanting palpebral fissures, a depressed nasal bridge, and posteriorly angulated ears with prominent helices. There is a considerable phenotypic overlap of CFC syndrome with Noonan and Costello syndromes [78]. Recently germline missense mutations in *KRAS* (5%), *BRAF* (75–80%), and *MEK1/MEK2* (10–15%) [79, 80] have been identified in patients with CFC syndrome, whereas somatic mutations in these genes are present in various tumors. There seems to a very low incidence of neoplasms in CFC syndrome. To date, only two patients are reported to have an acute lymphatic leukaemia [81, 82]. As to whether this association is coincidental or causal is unknown at the moment.

4.2.3
Costello Syndrome (CS)

Costello syndrome (CS) is a rare multiple congenital anomaly syndrome, associated in all cases with a characteristic coarse face with full lips and a large mouth, curly or sparse hair, short stature, severe feeding problems, and failure to thrive. Other features include cardiac anomalies, soft skin with deep palmar and plantar creases, and mental retardation. Facial papillomata, particularly nasolabial, often develop in later childhood [83]. In 2005, Aoki *et al.* [84] were able to demonstrate that heterozygous *de novo* germline mutations in *HRAS*, a member of the MAPK-RAS pathway, are causative for CS. Patients with CS have a predisposition to develop benign or malignant neoplasia. The most common malignancies in CS are embryonal rhabdomyosarcoma, transitional cell carcinoma, and neuroblastoma. About a quarter of the reported patients with CS developed a malignancy, including rhabdomyosarcoma, neuroblastoma, ganglioneuroblastoma, bladder carcinoma, acoustic neuroma, and epitheliomata. The incidence of solid tumors is similar to that in BWS. Most frequently, rhabdomyosarcoma, originated from the abdomen, pelvis, or urogenital areas occur [85].

Regular tumor screening is recommended: ultrasound examination of the abdomen and pelvis every 3 to 6 months until the age of 8 to 10 years looking for rhabdomyosarcoma and abdominal neuroblastoma, urine catecholamine metabolite analysis every 6 to 12 months until age 5 years for neuroblastoma, and urine analysis for hematuria annually, for bladder carcinoma after age 10 years.

4.2.4
Noonan-Neurofibromatosis Syndrome (NFNS)

Neurofibromatosis type 1 (NF) and Noonan syndrome (NS) are two distinctive conditions (see Chapter 6 on neurofibromatosis). In 1985, Allanson and colleagues [86] described patients with features of both, neurofibromatosis type 1 and NS (café-au lait spots, pulmonic stenosis, short stature, and pectus anomalies). Subsequently, further reports of this association have been described [87]. There was an ongoing debate whether NFNS is a variant of NF1 or NS, whether there is a chance association, or whether they are two distinct disorders. Mutations in the *NF1* gene have been reported in patients with the NFNS phenotype [88]. Interestingly, DeLuca *et al.* [89] were able to identify a mutation in the *NF1* gene in 16/17 patients with a NFNS phenotype, indicating that *NF1* mutations represent the major molecular event underlying NFNS. None of these patients carried a mutation in the *PTPN11* gene. A mutation in the *NF1* gene and the *PTPN11* gene has been described in only one patient with NFNS [90], a finding which was not supported in other studies. The identification of specific NF1 alleles recurring in NFNS, together with evidence that these alleles cosegregate with the condition in families, as well as the presence of a specific mutational spectrum, suggests that NFNS is a phenotypic variant of NF1. From a molecular point of view, the clinical overlap between NF1 and NS is evident because the gene products of *NF1* (neurofibrin) and *PTPN11* (SHP-2) run in a common pathway. Mutations in the *PTPN11* gene usually show a gain of function resulting in excessive SHP-2 activity, whereas mutations in the *NF1* gene generally result in haploinsuffiency of neurofibrin through a loss of function. Neurofibrin and SHP-2 show antagonistic function on RAS-mediated transduction cascades, which modulate cell response to several growth-factor and cytokine receptors [91]. Consistent with these findings, patients with NF1 and NS are predisposed to develop similar hematologic malignancies [91, 92]. However, until now there are only a few reports describing an association of malignancy and NFNS. Klopfenstein *et al.* [93] reported two unrelated boys with NFNS who developed acute lymphoblastic leukemia. Oguzkan *et al.* [94] described a patient with the NFNS phenotype with rhabdomyosarcoma of the bladder. Molecular analysis revealed a deletion in the *NF1* gene.

4.3
Miscellaneous Dysmorphic Syndromes Leading to Tumorigenesis

There are a number of further dysmorphic syndromes associated with cancer. However, some of these conditions are very rarely reported and, in others, the frequency of tumours is only documented in a single case report, therefore, in the following only more common syndromes with an increased frequency of malignancies are described.

4.3.1
Gorlin Syndrome (Nevoid Basal Cell Carcinoma Syndrome, NBCCS)

Patients with NBCCS have characteristic dysmorphic facial features such as macrocephaly, frontal and temporo-parietal bossing, and prominent supraorbital ridges. In 50%, relative macrocephaly is present. The jaw is prognathic, the nasal root is broad, and there may be telecanthus or even true hypertelorism. In addition, numerous basal cell cancers (BCC) and epidermal cysts of the skin, odontogenic keratocysts of the jaws, as well as palmar and plantar pits are present. There are a number of radiological signs, such as bifid, fused, or partially missing ribs which occur in about 60% of cases. Kyphoscoliosis occurs in 30–40% and spina bifida occulta in about 60%. Short metacarpals, pre- or postaxial polydactyly, syndactyly of the second and third fingers, and Sprengel deformity are also seen but less frequently. The multiple nevoid basal cell carcinomas appear after puberty, especially on the face and neck, but also on the trunk and other parts of the body. Various neoplasms or hamartoma can occur [95, 96]. Kimonis *et al.* [97] introduced major criteria and minor criteria which can be used in making the diagnosis of Gorlin syndrome by the presence of two major, or one major and two minor criteria.

Major criteria are:

1. More than two BCCs or one under the age of 20 years;
2. Odontogenic keratocysts;
3. Three or more palmar pits;
4. Bilamellar calcification of falx cerebri;
5. Bifid, fused, or splayed ribs;
6. First-degree relative with NBCCS.

Minor criteria consist of:

1. Macrocephaly adjusted for height;
2. Frontal bossing, cleft lip/palate, hypertelorism;
3. Sprengel deformity, syndactyly of digits;
4. Bridging of sella turcica, hemivertebrae, flame-shaped radiolucencies;
5. Ovarian fibroma;
6. Medulloblastoma.

Gorlin and Goltz [96] suggested autosomal dominant inheritance with complete penetrance and variable expressivity. New mutations are present in about 35–50%. The gene has been mapped to 9q22.3 [98, 99]. Mutations in the *PTC* gene (*PTCH*), a human homolog of the Drosophila "patched" gene was identified as being the causative gene for NBCCS [100, 101]. The *PTC* gene, which plays a role in the hedgehog signaling pathway [102], is also mutated in non-syndromic forms of basal cell carcinomas. Mutations are detected in 60–85%. There is no obvious genotype-phenotype correlation [103]. About 5% of children with NBCCS develop medulloblastoma (now often called primitive neuroectodermal tumor, PNET). Peak incidence is 2 years of age [104]. This tumor tends to be of desmoplastic histology [105] and to have a favorable prognosis. In children with medulloblastoma, NBCCS should be excluded. Awareness of the risk of medulloblastoma in the first years of life is important, and may justify developmental assessment and physical examination every six months. Patients with NBCCS are abnormally sensitive to radiotherapeutic doses of ionizing radiation, and several patients treated this way have developed an unusually large number of basal cell tumors in the irradiated area a short time after exposure [106]. Therefore, frequent neuro-imaging should be avoided because of risks associated with radiation. No other tumors occur at a frequency that warrants special surveillance.

4.3.2
Rubinstein-Taybi Syndrome (RSTS)

Rubinstein–Taybi syndrome (RSTS) is an autosomal dominant condition characterized by distinctive facial features, microcephaly, broad and often angulated thumbs and big toes, short stature, and moderate to severe mental retardation [107]. The characteristic craniofacial features are highly arched eyebrows, down slanting palpebral fissures, broad nasal bridge, the columella extending below the nares, highly arched palate, and mild micrognathia. The presence of talon cusps at the permanent incisors can be of diagnostic help. Prenatal growth is often normal, but height, weight, and head circumference percentiles rapidly drop in the first few months of life. Obesity may occur in childhood or adolescence. IQ scores range from 25 to 79. Average IQ is between 36 and 51. Other variable findings are colobomata, cataracts, congenital heart defects, renal abnormalities, and cryptorchidism [108]. Patients with a cytogenetic aberration in 16p13.3 [109–111] helped to identify the *CBP*-gene (CREB binding protein) as the major causative gene for RSTS [112]. Microdeletions of the *CBP* gene are only found in about 10%, whereas a mutation is present in 30–50% of the patients with RSTS [113, 114]. The fact that *CBP* has a homolog *EP300* located in 22q13.2 initiated a search in *EP300* for mutations in patients with RSTS. Until now, mutations have only been described in 3% of patients [115]. Molecular confirmation of the clinical diagnosis is only possible in about half of the patients suspected of having RSTS.

In 1995, Miller and Rubinstein [116] noted that patients with RSTS have an increased risk of tumor formation. Among more than 700 patients, 17 had malignant tumors and 19 had benign tumors. Twelve of these tumors were located in the nervous system, including oligodendroglioma, medulloblastoma, neuroblastoma, and meningioma. Other tumor types included rhabdomyosarcoma and leukemias, among others. The authors suggested that about 5% of patients with RSTS develop neoplasms, which is similar to the frequency of malignancy in neurofibromatosis type 1. Petrij *et al.* [112] suggested that the risk of cancer, as well as the formation of keloids, may be explained by the role proposed for *CBP* in cAMP-regulated cell immortalization. It is of note that *CBP* and *EP300* participate in various tumor-suppressor pathways, and somatic mutations of these genes occur in a number of malignancies [117, 118]. Therefore, regular clinical surveillance is recommended in order to early recognize developing malignancies.

4.3.3
Rothmund–Thomson Syndrome (RTS)

Rothmund–Thomson syndrome (RTS) is an autosomal recessive condition characterized by infantile poikiloderma, sparse hair, small stature, skeletal and dental abnormalities, cataracts, and hypogonadism. The skin is typically normal at birth. Poikiloderma starts in infancy, usually between age 3 to 6 months, as erythema on the cheeks and face (acute phase), and spreads to involve the extensor surfaces of the extremities. The trunk and abdomen are usually spared, the buttocks may be involved. Gradually, the rash changes into a more chronic phase with hyper- and hypopigmentation, telangiectasias, and areas of punctate atrophy. These changes, described as poikiloderma, persist throughout life [119–121].

Skeletal abnormalities include dysplasias, absent or malformed bones (such as absent radii), osteopenia, and delayed bone formation. Kitao *et al.* [122] identified mutations in the helicase gene *RECQL4* located in 8q24.3. In RTS, an increased frequency of malignancies, especially osteosarcomas, has been reported. The overall prevalence of cancers in adults with RTS syndrome is unknown. Osteosarcoma is the most commonly reported malignancy [123, 124]. In addition, an increased risk for skin cancers such as basal cell carcinoma and squamous cell carcinoma is known [125, 126]. It is important to note that secondary malignancies (Hodgkin- and non-Hodgkin lymphomata) have been observed [121]. On the other hand, it has been recommended that in patients with osteosarcoma and skin changes, RTS should be excluded [127]. Skeletal radiographs of the long bones by age 5 years should be obligatory for all patients with RTS [121].

References

1 Krivit, W. and Good, R.A. (1957) Simultaneous occurrence of mongolism and leukemia; report of a nationwide survey. *American Journal of Diseases of Children*, **94**, 289–93.

2 Merks, J.H., Caron, H.N. and Hennekam, R.C. (2005) High incidence of malformation syndromes in a series of 1073 children with cancer. *American Journal of Medical Genetics Part A*, **34**, 132–43.

3 Cohen, M.M. Jr (1989) A comprehensive and critical assessment of overgrowth and overgrowth syndromes, in advances, in *Human Genetics*, Vol. 18 (eds H. Harris and K. Hirschhorn), Plenum Press, New York, pp. 373–76.

4 Lapunzina, P. (2005) Risk of tumorigenesis in overgrowth syndromes: a comprehensive review. *American Journal of Medical Genetics Part C*, **137**, 53–71.

5 Weng, E.Y., Moeschler, J.B. and Graham J.M. Jr (1995) Longitudinal observations on 15 children with Wiedemann–Beckwith syndrome.

American Journal of Medical Genetics, **56**, 366–73.

6 Pettenati, M.J., Haines, J.L., Higgins, R.R., Wappner, R.S., Palmer, C.G. and Weaver, D.D. (1986) Wiedemann–Beckwith syndrome: presentation of clinical and cytogenetic data on 22 new cases and review of literature. *Human Genetics*, **74**, 143–54.

7 Weksberg, R., Smith, A.C., Squire, J. and Sadowski, P. (2003) Beckwith–Wiedemann syndrome. *Molecular Genetics*, **12** (Spec No 1), R61–8.

8 Weksberg, R., Shuman, C. and Smith, A.C. (2005) Beckwith–Wiedemann syndrome. *American Journal of Medical Genetics Part C*, **137**, 12–23.

9 Cooper, W.N., Luharia, A., Evans, G.A., Raza, H., Haire, A.C., Grundy, R., Bowdin, S.C. and Riccio, A. *et al.* (2005) Molecular subtypes and phenotypic expression of Beckwith–Wiedemann syndrome. *European Journal of Human Genetics*, **13**, 1025–13.

10 Slavotinek, A., Gaunt, L. and Donnai, D. (1997) Paternally inherited duplications of 11p15.5 and Beckwith–Wiedemann

syndrome. *Journal of Medical Genetics*, **34**, 819–26.

11 Bliek, J., Gicquel, C., Gaston, V., Le Bouc, Y. and Mannens, M. (2004) Epigenotyping as a tool for the prediction of tumor risk and tumor type in patients with Beckwith–Wiedemann syndrome (BWS). *Journal of Pediatrics*, **145**, 796–9.

12 Sotelo-Avila, C.M. and Gooch, W.M. III (1976) Neoplasms associated with the Beckwith–Wiedemann syndrome. *Perspectives in Pediatric Pathology*, **3**, 255–72.

13 Rump, P., Zeegers, M.P. and van Essen, A.J. (2005) Tumor risk in Beckwith–Wiedemann syndrome: a review and meta-analysis. *American Journal of Medical Genetics Part A*, **136A**, 95–104.

14 Weksberg, R., Nishikawa, J., Caluseriu, O., Fei, Y.L., Shuman, C., Wei, C., Steele, L., Cameron, J. *et al.* (2001) Tumor development in the Beckwith–Wiedemann syndrome is associated with a variety of constitutional molecular 11p15 alterations including imprinting defects of KCNQ1OT1. *Human Molecular Genetics*, **10**, 2989–3000.

15 Craft, A.W., Parker, L., Stiller, C. and Cole, M. (1995) Screening for Wilms tumor in patients with aniridia, Beckwith syndrome, or hemihypertrophy. *Medical and Pediatric Oncology*, **24**, 231–4.

16 De Baun, M.R., Siegel, M.J. and Choyke, P.L. (1998) Nephromegaly in infancy and early childhood: a risk factor for Wilms tumor in Beckwith–Wiedemann syndrome. *Journal of Pediatrics*, **132**, 401–4.

17 Choyke, P.L., Siegel, M.J., Craft, A.W., Green, D.M. and DeBaun, M.R. (1999) Screening for Wilms tumor in children with Beckwith–Wiedemann syndrome or idiopathic hemihypertrophy. *Medical and Pediatric Oncology*, **32**, 196–200.

18 Clericuzio, C.L., DÁngio, G.J., Duncan, M., Green, D.M. and Knudson A.G. Jr (1993) Summary and recommendations of the workshop held at the first international conference on molecular and clinical genetics of childhood renal tumors, Albuquerque, New Mexico,

May 14–16. *Medical and Pediatric Oncology*, **21**, 233–6.

19 Everman, D.B., Shuman, C., Dzolganowski, B., O'riordan, M.A., Weksberg, R., Robin, N.H. (2000) Serum alpha-fetoprotein levels in Beckwith–Wiedemann syndrome. *Journal of Pediatrics*, **137**, 123–7.

20 West, P.M., Love, D.R., Stapleton, P. and Winship, I.M. (2003) Paternal uniparental disomy in monozygotic twins discordant for hemihypertrophy. *Journal of Medical Genetics*, **40**, 223–6.

21 Martin, R.A., Grange, D.K., Zehnbauer, B. and DeBaun, M.R. (2005) LIT1 and H19 methylation defects in isolated hemihyperplasia. *American Journal of Medical Genetics*, **134**, 129–31.

22 Hoyme, H.E., Seaver, L.H., Jones, K.L., Procopio, F., Crooks, W. and Feingold, M. (1998) Isolated hemihyperplasia (hemihypertrophy): report of a prospective multicenter study of the incidence of neoplasia and review. *American Journal of Medical Genetics*, **79**, 274–8.

23 Fraurmeni, J.F. Jr, Geiser, C.F. and Manning, M.D. (1967) Wilms tumor and congenital hemihypertrophy: report of five new cases and review of literature. *Pediatrics*, **40**, 886–99.

24 Niemitz, E.L., Feinberg, A.P., Brandenburg, S.A., Grundy, P.E. and DeBaun, M.R. (2005) Children with idiopathic hemihypertrophy and Beckwith–Wiedemann syndrome have different constitutional epigenotypes associated with Wilms tumor. *American Journal of Human Genetics*, **77**, 887–91.

25 Shuman, C., Smith, A.C., Steele, L., Ray, P.N., Clericuzio, C., Zackai, E., Parisi, M.A. Meadows, A. *et al.* (2006) Constitutional UPD for chromosome 11p15 in individuals with isolated hemihyperplasia is associated with high tumor risk and occurs following assisted reproductive technologies. *American Journal of Medical Genetics*, **140A**, 1497–503.

26 Wiedemann, H.R., Burgio, G.R., Aldenhoff, P., Kunze, J., Kaufmann, H.J. and Schirg, E. (1983) The Proteus syndrome: partial gigantism of the hands and/or feet, nevi, hemihypertrophy, subcutaneous tumors, macrocephaly or

other skull anomalies and possible accelerated growth and visceral affections. *European Journal of Pediatrics*, **140**, 5–12.

27 Cohen, M.M. Jr (1993) Proteus syndrome: clinical evidence for somatic mosaicism and selective review. *American Journal of Medical Genetics*, **47**, 645–52.

28 Cohen, M.M. Jr, Neri, G. and Weksberg, R. (2002) *Overgrowth Syndromes*, Oxford University Press, New York.

29 Biesecker, L.G., Happle, R., Mulliken, J.B., Weksberg, R., Graham, J.M. Jr, Viljoen, D.L. and Cohen, M.M. Jr (1999) Proteus syndrome: diagnostic criteria, differential diagnosis, and patient evaluation. *American Journal of Medical Genetics*, **84**, 389–95.

30 Biesecker, L.G. (2001) The multifaceted challenges of Proteus syndrome. *The Journal of the American Medical Association*, **285**, 2240–3.

31 Zhou, X.P., Marsh, D.J., Hampel, H., Mulliken, J.B., Gimm, O. and Eng, C. (2000) Germline and germline mosaic PTEN mutations associated with a Proteus-like syndrome of hemihypertrophy, lower limb asymmetry, arteriovenous malformations and lipomatosis. *Human Molecular Genetics*, **9**, 765–8.

32 Gordon, P.L., Wilroy, R.S., Lasater, O.E. and Cohen, M.M. Jr (1995) Neoplasms in Proteus syndrome. *American Journal of Medical Genetics*, **57**, 74–8.

33 Gilbert-Barness, E., Cohen, M.M. Jr and Opitz, J.M. (2000) Multiple meningiomas, craniofacial hyperostosis and retinal abnormalities in Proteus syndrome. *American Journal of Medical Genetics*, **93**, 234–40.

34 Cole, T.R.P. and Hughes, H.E. (1994) Sotos syndrome: a study of the diagnostic criteria and natural history. *Journal of Medical Genetics*, **31**, 20–32.

35 Kurotaki, N., Imaizumi, K., Harada, N., Masuno, M., Kondoh, T., Nagai, T., Ohashi, H., Naritomi, K. *et al.* (2002) Haploinsufficiency of NSD1 causes Sotos syndrome. *Nature Genetics*, **30**, 365–6.

36 Turkmen, S., Gillessen-Kaesbach, G., Meinecke, P., Albrecht, B., Neumann, L.M., Hesse, V., Palanduz, S., Balg, S. *et al.* (2003) Mutations in NSD1 are responsible for Sotos syndrome, but are not a frequent finding in other overgrowth phenotypes. *European Journal of Human Genetics*, **11**, 858–65.

37 Tatton-Brown, K., Douglas, J., Coleman, K., Baujat, G., Cole, T.R.P., Das, S., Horn, D., Hughes, H.E. *et al.* (2005) Genotype-phenotype associations in Sotos syndrome: an analysis of 266 individuals with NSD1 aberrations. *American Journal of Human Genetics*, **77**, 193–204.

38 Maldonado, V., Gaynon, P.S. and Poznanski, A.K. (1984) Cerebral gigantism associated with Wilms tumor. *American Journal of Diseases of Children*, **138**, 486–8.

39 Nance, M.A., Neglia, J.P., Talwar, D. and Berry, S.A. (1990) Neuroblastoma in a patient with Sotos syndrome. *Journal of Medical Genetics*, **27**, 130–2.

40 Hersh, J.H., Cole, T.R., Bloom, A.S., Bertolone, S.J., Hughes, H.E. (1992) Risk of malignancy in Sotos syndrome. *Journal of Pediatrics*, **120**, 572–4.

41 Martinez-Glez, V. and Lapunzina, P. (2007) Sotos syndrome is associated with leukemia/lymphoma. *American Journal of Medical Genetics*, **143A**, 1244–5.

42 Cole, T.R.P., Dennis, N.R. and Hughes, H.E. (1992) Weaver syndrome. *Journal of Medical Genetics*, **29**, 332–7.

43 Opitz, J.M., Weaver, D.W. and Reynolds J.F. Jr (1998) The syndromes of Sotos and Weaver: reports and review. *American Journal of Medical Genetics*, **79**, 294–304.

44 Douglas, J., Hanks, S., Temple, I.K., Davies, S., Murray, A., Upadhyaya, M., Tomkins, S., Hughes, H.E. *et al.* (2003) NSD1 mutations are the major cause of Sotos syndrome and occur in some cases of Weaver syndrome but are rare in other overgrowth phenotypes. *American Journal of Human Genetics*, **72**, 132–43.

45 Muhonen, M.G. and Menezes, A.H. (1990) Weaver syndrome and instability of the upper cervical spine. *Journal of Pediatrics*, **116**, 596–9.

46 Huffman, C., McCandless, D., Jasty, R., Matloub, J., Robinson, H.B., Weaver, D.D. and Cohen M.M. Jr (2001) Weaver

syndrome with neuroblastoma and cardiovascular anomalies. *American Journal of Medical Genetics*, **99**, 252–5.

47 Kelly, T.E., Alford, B.A. and Abel, M. (2000) Cervical spine anomalies and tumors in Weaver syndrome. *American Journal of Medical Genetics*, **95**, 492–5.

48 Derry, C., Temple, I.K. and Venkat-Raman, K. (2001) A probable case of familial Weaver syndrome associated with neoplasia. *Journal of Medical Genetics*, **36**, 725–8.

49 Simpson, J.L., Landey, S., New, M. and German, J. (1975) A previously unrecognized X-linked syndrome of dysmorphia. *Birth Defects Original Article Series*, **XI** (2), 18–24.

50 Golabi, M. and Rosen, L. (1984) A new X-linked mental retardation-overgrowth syndrome. *American Journal of Medical Genetics*, **17**, 345–58.

51 Behmel, A., Plochl, E. and Rosenkranz, W. (1984) A new X-linked dysplasia gigantism syndrome: identical with the Simpson dysplasia syndrome? *Human Genetics*, **67**, 409–13.

52 Lin, A.E., Ner, G., Hughes-Benzie, R. and Weksberg, R. (1999) Cardiac anomalies in the Simpson–Golabi–Behmel syndrome. *American Journal of Medical Genetics*, **83**, 378–81.

53 Pilia, G., Hughes-Benzie, R.M. and MacKenzie, A. (1996) Mutations in GPC3, a glypican gene, cause the Simpson–Golabi–Behmel overgrowth syndrome. *Nature Genetics*, **12**, 241–7.

54 Li, M., Shuman, C., Fei, Y., Cutiongco, E., Bender, H.A. and Stevens, C. (2001) GPC3 mutation analysis in a spectrum of patients with overgrowth expands the phenotype of Simpson–Golabi–Behmel syndrome. *American Journal of Medical Genetics*, **102**, 161–8.

55 Bannayan, G.A. (1971) Lipomatosis, angiomatosis, and macrencephalia: a previously undescribed congenital syndrome. *Archives of Pathology*, **92**, 1–5.

56 Riley, H.D. Jr and Smith, W.R. (1960) Macrocephaly, pseudopapilledema and multiple hemangiomata: a previously undescribed heredofamilial syndrome. *Pediatrics*, **26**, 293–300.

57 Ruvalcaba, R.H.A., Myhre, S. and Smith, D.W. (1980) Sotos syndrome with intestinal polyposis and pigmentary changes of the genitalia. *Clinical Genetics*, **18**, 413–16.

58 Cohen M.M. Jr (1990) Bannayan–Riley–Ruvalcaba syndrome: renaming three formerly recognized syndromes as one etiologic entity. *American Journal of Medical Genetics*, **35**, 291.

59 Celebi, J.T., Tsou, H.C., Chen, F.F., Zhang, H., Ping, X.L., Lebwohl, M.G., Kezis, J. and Peacocke, M. (1996) Phenotypic findings of Cowden syndrome and Bannayan–Zonana syndrome in a family associated with a single germline mutation in PTEN. *Journal of Medical Genetics*, **36**, 360–4.

60 Marsh, D.J., Dahia, P.L.M., Zheng, Z., Liaw, D., Parsons, R., Gorlin, R.J. and Eng, C. (1997) Germline mutations in PTEN are present in Bannayan–Zonana syndrome. *Nature Genetics*, **16**, 333–4.

61 Marsh, D.J., Kum, J.B., Lunetta, K.L., Bennett, M.J., Gorlin, R.J., Ahmed, S.F., Bodurtha, J., Crowe, C. *et al.* (1999) PTEN mutation spectrum and genotype-phenotype correlations in Bannayan–Riley–Ruvalcaba syndrome suggest a single entity with Cowden syndrome. *Human Molecular Genetics*, **8**, 1461–72.

62 Haggitt, R.C. and Reid, B.J. (1986) Hereditary gastrointestinal polyposis syndromes. *The American journal of Surgical Pathology*, **10**, 871–87.

63 Noonan, J.A. and Ehmke, D.A. (1963) Associated non cardiac malformations in children with congenital heart disease. *Journal of Pediatrics*, **63**, 468–70.

64 Allanson, J.E. (1987) Noonan syndrome. *Journal of Medical Genetics*, **24**, 9–13.

65 Allanson, J.E., Hall, J.G., Hughes, H.E., Preus, M. and Witt, R.D. (1985) Noonan syndrome: the changing phenotype. *American Journal of Medical Genetics*, **21**, 507–14.

66 Allanson, J.E. (2007) Noonan syndrome. *American Journal of Medical Genetics Part C*, 274–9.

67 Tartaglia, M., Mehler, E.L., Goldberg, R., Zampino, G., Brunner, H.G., Kremer, H., van der Burgt, I., Crosby, A.H. *et al.* (2001) Mutations in PTPN11, encoding the protein tyrosine phosphatase SHP-2, cause Noonan syndrome. *Nature Genetics*, **29**, 465–8.

68 Gorlin, R.J., Anderson, R.C. and Blaw, M.E. (1969) Multiple lentigines syndrome: complex comprising multiple lentigines, electrocardiographic conduction abnormalities, ocular hypertelorism, pulmonary stenosis, abnormalities of genitalia, retardation of growth, sensorineural deafness, and autosomal dominant hereditary pattern. *American Journal of Diseases of Children*, **117**, 652–62.

69 Digilio, M.C., Conti, E., Sarkozy, A., Mingarelli, R., Dottorini, T., Marino, B., Pizzuti, A. and Dallapiccola, B. (2002) Grouping of multiple-lentigines/ LEOPARD and Noonan syndromes on the PTPN11 gene. *American Journal of Human Genetics*, **71**, 389–94.

70 Pandit, B., Sarkozy, A., Pennacchio, L.A., Carta, C., Oishi, K., Martinelli, S., Pogna, E.A., Schackwitz, W. *et al.* (2007) Gain-of-function RAF1 mutations cause Noonan and LEOPARD syndromes with hypertrophic cardiomyopathy. *Nature Genetics*, **39** (8), 1007–12.

71 Schubbert, S., Zenker, M., Rowe, S.L., Boll, S., Klein, C., Bollag, G., van der Burgt, I., Musante, L. *et al.* (2006) Germline KRAS mutations cause Noonan syndrome. *Nature Genetics*, **38**, 331–6.

72 Roberts, A.E., Araki, T., Swanson, K.D.S., Montgomery, K.T., Schiripo, T.A., Joshi, V.A., Li, L., Yassin, Y. *et al.* (2007) Germline gain-of-function mutations in SOS1 cause Noonan syndrome. *Nature Genetics*, **39**, 70–4.

73 Tartaglia, M., Pennacchio, L.A., Zhao, C., Yadav, K.K., Fodale, V., Sarkozy, A., Pandit, B., Oishi, K. *et al.* (2007) Gain-of-function SOS1 mutations cause a distinctive form of Noonan syndrome. *Nature Genetics*, **39**, 75–9.

74 Bader-Meunier, B., Tchernia, G., Mielot, F., Fontaine, J.L., Thomas, C., Lyonnet, S., Lavergne, J.M. and Dommergues, J.P. (1997) Occurrence of myeloproliferative disorder in patients with Noonan syndrome. *Journal of Pediatrics*, **130**, 885–9.

75 Choong, K., Freedmann, M.H., Chitayat, D., Kelly, E.N., Taylor, G. and Zipursky, A. (1999) Juvenile myelomonocytic leukemia and Noonan syndrome. *Journal of Pediatric Hematology and Oncology*, **21**, 523–7.

76 Tartaglia, M., Niemeyer, C.M., Fragale, A., Song, X., Buechner, J., Jung, A., Hahlen, K., Hasle, H. *et al.* (2003) Somatic mutations in PTPN11 in juvenile myelomonocytic leukemia, myelody-splastic syndromes and acute myeloid leukaemia. *Nature Genetics*, **34**, 148–50.

77 Tartaglia, M., Martinelli, S., Stella, L., Bocchinfuso, G., Flex, E., Corddedu, V. Zampino, G., van der Burgt, I. *et al.* (2006) Diversity and functional consequences of germline and somatic PTPN11 mutations in human disease. *American Journal of Human Genetics*, **78**, 279–90.

78 Roberts, A., Allanson, J., Jadico, S.K., Kavamura, M.I., Noonan, J., Opitz, J.M. and Young, T. (2006) The cardiofaciocutaneous syndrome. *Journal of Medical Genetics*, **43**, 833–42.

79 Niihori, T., Aoki, Y., Narumi, Y., Neri, G., Cave, H., Verloes, A., Okamoto, N., Hennekam, R.C.M. *et al.* (2006) Germline KRAS and BRAF mutations in cardio-facio-cutaneous syndrome. *Nature Genetics*, **38**, 294–6.

80 Rodriguez-Viciana, P., Tetsu, O., Tidyman, W.E., Estep, A.L., Conger, B.A., Santa Cruz, M., McCormick, F. and Rauen, K.A. (2006) Germline mutations in genes within the MAPK pathway cause cardio-facio-cutaneous syndrome. *Science*, **311**, 1287–90.

81 Van Den Berg, H. and Hennekam, R.C.M. (1999) Acute lymphoblastic leukaemia in a patient with cardio-faciocutaneous syndrome. *Journal of Medical Genetics*, **36**, 799–800.

82 Makita, Y., Narumi, Y., Yoshida, M., Niihori, T., Kure, S., Fujieda, K., Matsubara, Y. and Aoki, Y. (2007) Leukemia in cardio-facio-cutaneous (CFC) syndrome: a patient with a germline mutation in BRAF proto-oncogene. *Journal of Pediatric Hematology and Oncology*, **29**, 287–90.

83 Kerr, B., Delrue, M.A., Sigaudy, S., Perveen, R., Marche, M., Burgelin, I., Stef, M., Tang, B. *et al.* (2006) Genotype-phenotype correlation in Costello syndrome: HRAS mutation analysis in 43 cases. *Journal of Medical Genetics*, **43**, 401–5.

84 Aoki, Y., Niihori, T., Kawame, H., Kurosawa, K., Ohashi, H., Tanaka, Y., Filocamo, M., Kato, K. *et al.* (2005) Germline mutations in HRAS proto-oncogene cause Costello syndrome. *Nature Genetics*, **37**, 1038–40.

85 Gripp, K.W. (2005) Tumor predisposition in Costello syndrome. *American Journal of Medical Genetics Part C*, **137**, 72–7.

86 Allanson, J.E., Hall, J.G. and Van Allen, M.I. (1985) Noonan phenotype associated with neurofibromatosis. *American Journal of Medical Genetics*, **21**, 457–62.

87 Bahuau, M., Houdayer, C., Assouline, B., Blanchet-Bardon, C., Le Merrer, M., Lyonnet, S., Giraud, S., Recan, D. *et al.* (1998) Novel recurrent nonsense mutation causing neurofibromatosis type 1 (NF1) in a family segregating both NF1 and Noonan syndrome. *American Journal of Medical Genetics*, **75**, 265–72.

88 Baralle, D., Mattocks, C., Kalidas, K., Elmslie, F., Whittaker, J., Lees, M., Ragge, N., Patton, M.A. *et al.* (2003) Different mutations in the NF1 gene are associated with neurofibromatosis-Noonan syndrome (NFNS). *American Journal of Medical Genetics*, **119A**, 1–8.

89 De Luca, A., Bottillo, I., Sarkozy, A., Carta, C., Neri, C., Bellacchio, E., Schirinzi, A., Conti, E. *et al.* (2005) NF1 gene mutations represent the major molecular event underlying neurofibromatosis-Noonan syndrome. *American Journal of Human Genetics*, **77**, 1092–101.

90 Bertola, D.R., Pereira, A.C., Passetti, F., de Oliveira, P.S., Messiaen, L., Gelb, B.D., Kim, C.A. and Krieger, J.E. (2005) Neurofibromatosis-Noonan syndrome: molecular evidence of the concurrence of both disorders in a patient. *American Journal of Medical Genetics*, **136A**, 242–5.

91 Tartaglia, M., Niemeyer, C.M., Shannon, K.M. and Loh, M.L. (2004) 2004) SHP-2 and myeloid malignancies. *Current Opinion in Hematology*, **11** (1), 44–50. Review.

92 Stevenson, D.A., Viskochil, D.H., Rope, A.F. and Carey, J.C. (2006) Clinical and molecular aspects of an informative family with neurofibromatosis type 1 and Noonan phenotype. *Clinical Genetics*, **69**, 246–53.

93 Klopfenstein, K.J., Sommer, A. and Ruymann, F.B. (1999) Neurofibromatosis-Noonan syndrome and acute lympho-blastic leukemia: a report of two cases. *Journal of Pediatric Hematology and Oncology*, **21**, 158–60.

94 Oguzkan, S., Terzi, Y.K., Guler, E., Derbent, M., Agras, P.I., Saatci, U. and Ayter, S. (2006) Two neurofibro-matosis type 1 cases associated with rhabdomyosarcoma of the bladder, one with a large deletion in the NF1 gene. *Cancer Genetics and Cytogenetics*, **164**, 159–63.

95 Gorlin, R.J. (1987) Nevoid basal-cell carcinoma syndrome. *Medicine*, **66**, 98–113.

96 Gorlin, R.J. and Goltz, R.W. (1960) Multiple nevoid basal-cell epithelioma, jaw cysts and bifid rib: a syndrome. *The New England Journal of Medicine*, **262**, 908–12.

97 Kimonis, V.E., Goldstein, A.M., Pastakia, B., Yang, M.L., Kase, R., DiGiovanna, J.J., Bale, A.E. and Bale, S.J. (1997) Clinical manifestations in 105 persons with nevoid basal cell carcinoma syndrome. *American Journal of Medical Genetics*, **69**, 299–308.

98 Farndon, P.A., Del Mastro, R.G., Evans, D.G.R. and Kilpatrick, M.W. (1992) Location of gene for Gorlin syndrome. *Lancet*, **339**, 581–2.

99 Reis, A., Kuster, W., Linss, G., Gebel, E., Hamm, H., Fuhrmann, W., Wolff, G., Groth, W. *et al.* (1992) Localisation of gene for the naevoid basal-cell carcinoma syndrome. *Lancet*, **339**, 617.

100 Johnson, R.L., Rothman, A.L., Xie, J., Goodrich, L.V., Bare, J.W., Bonifas, J.M., Quinn, E.H., Myers, R.M., Cox, D. R., Epstein, E.H. Jr and Scott, M.P. (1996) Human homolog of patched, a candidate gene for the basal cell nevus syndrome. *Science*, **272**, 1668–71.

101 Hahn, H., Gillies, S., Negus, K., Smyth, I., Pressman, C., Leffell, D.J., Gerrard, B., Goldstein, A.M. *et al.* (1996) Mutations of

the human homolog of drosophila patched in the nevoid basal cell carcinoma syndrome. *Cell*, **85**, 841–52.

102 Stone, D.M., Phillips, H., Noll, M., Hooper, J.E., de Sauvage, F., Rosenthal, A., Hynes, M., Armanini, M. *et al.* (1996) The tumour-suppressor gene patched encodes a candidate receptor for sonic hedgehog. *Nature*, **384**, 129–34.

103 Wicking, C., Shanley, S., Smyth, I., Gillies, S., Negus, K., Graham, S., Suthers, G., Haites, N. *et al.* (1997) Most germline mutations in the nevoid basal cell carcinoma syndrome lead to a premature termination of the PATCHED protein, and no genotype-phenotype correlations are evident. *American Journal of Human Genetics*, **60**, 21–6.

104 Cowan, R., Hoban, P., Kelsey, A., Birch, J.M., Gattamaneni, R. and Evans, D.G. (1997) The gene for the naevoid basal cell carcinoma syndrome acts as a tumour-suppressor gene in medulloblastoma. *British Journal of Cancer*, **76**, 141–5.

105 Amlashi, S.F., Riffaud, L., Brassier, G. and Morandi, X. (2003) Nevoid basal cell carcinoma syndrome: relation with desmoplastic medulloblastoma in infancy. A population-based study and review of the literature. *Cancer*, **98**, 618–24.

106 Featherstone, T., Taylor, A.M.R. and Harnden, D.G. (1983) Studies on the radiosensitivity of cells from patients with basal cell naevus syndrome. *American Journal of Human Genetics*, **35**, 58–66.

107 Rubinstein, J.H. and Taybi, H. (1963) Broad thumbs and toes and facial abnormalities. *American Journal of Diseases of Children*, **105**, 588–608.

108 Hennekam, R.C.M. (2006) Rubinstein–Taybi syndrome. *European Journal of Human Genetics*, **14**, 981–5.

109 Imaizumi, K. and Kuroki, Y. (1991) Rubinstein–Taybi syndrome with *de novo* reciprocal translocation t(2;16) (p13.3;p13.3). *American Journal of Medical Genetics*, **38**, 636–9.

110 Tommerup, N., van der Hagen, C.B. and Heiberg, A. (1992) Tentative assignment of a locus for Rubinstein–Taybi syndrome to 16p13.3 by a *de novo* reciprocal translocation, t(7;16) (q34;p13.3). *American Journal of Medical Genetics*, **44**, 237–41.

111 Lacombe, D., Saura, R., Taine, L. and Battin, J. (1992) Confirmation of assignment of a locus for Rubinstein–Taybi syndrome gene to 16p13.3. *American Journal of Medical Genetics*, **44**, 126–8.

112 Petrij, F., Giles, R.H., Dauwerse, H.G., Saris, J.J., Hennekam, R.C.M., Masuno, M., Tommerup, N., van Ommen, G.J. *et al.* (1995) Rubinstein–Taybi syndrome caused by mutations in the transcriptional co-activator CBP. *Nature*, **376**, 348–51.

113 Coupry, I., Roudaut, C., Stef, M., Delrue, M.A., Marche, M., Burgelin, I., Taine, L., Cruaud, C. *et al.* (2002) Molecular analysis of the CBP gene in 60 patients with Rubinstein–Taybi syndrome. *Journal of Medical Genetics*, **39**, 415–21.

114 Bartsch, O., Schmidt, S., Richter, M., Morlot, S., Seemanova, E., Wiebe, G. and Rasi, S. (2005) DNA sequencing of CREBBP demonstrates mutations in 56% of patients with Rubinstein–Taybi syndrome (RSTS) and in another patient with incomplete RSTS. *Human Genetics*, **117**, 485–93.

115 Roelfsema, J.H., White, S.J., Ariyurek, Y., Bartholdi, D., Niedrist, D., Papadia, F., Bacino, C.A., den Dunnen, J.T. *et al.* (2005) Genetic heterogeneity in Rubinstein–Taybi syndrome: mutations in both the CBP and EP300 genes cause disease. *American Journal of Human Genetics*, **76**, 572–80.

116 Miller, R.W. and Rubinstein, J.H. (1995) Tumors in Rubinstein–Taybi syndrome. *American Journal of Medical Genetics*, **56**, 112–15.

117 Kitabayashi, I., Aikawa, Y., Yokoyama, A., Hosoda, F., Nagai, M., Kakazu, N., Abe, T. and Ohki, M. (2001) Fusion of MOZ and p300 histone acetyltransferases in acute monocytic leukemia with a t(8;22)(p11;q13) chromosome translocation. *Leukemia*, **15**, 89–94.

118 Iyer, N.G., Ozdag, H. and Caldas, C. (2004) p300/CBP and cancer. *Oncogene*, **23**, 4225–31.

119 Rothmund, A. (1868) Über Cataracte in Verbindung mit einer eigenthümlichen Hautdegeneration. *Graefe's Archive for Clinical and Experimental Ophthalmology*, **14**, 159–82.

120 Thomson, M.S. (1936) Poikiloderma congenitale. *The British Journal of Dermatology*, **48**, 221–34.

121 Wang, L.L., Levy, M.L., Lewis, R.A., Chintagumpala, M.M., Lev, D., Rogers, M. and Plon, S.E. (2001) Clinical manifestations in a cohort of 41 Rothmund–Thomson syndrome patients. *American Journal of Medical Genetics*, **102**, 11–17.

122 Kitao, S., Shimamoto, A., Goto, M., Miller, R.W., Smithson, W.A., Lindor, N.M. and Furuichi, Y. (1999) Mutations in RECQL4 cause a subset of cases of Rothmund–Thomson syndrome. *Nature Genetics*, **22**, 82–4.

123 Cumin, I., Cohen, J.Y., David, A., Mechinaud, F., Avet-Loiseau, H. and Harousseau, J.L. (1996) Rothmund–Thomson syndrome and osteosarcoma. *Medical and Pediatric Oncology*, **26**, 414–16.

124 Green, J.S. and Rickett, A.B. (1998) Rothmund–Thomson syndrome complicated by osteosarcoma. *Pediatric Radiology*, **28**, 48–50.

125 Borg, M.F., Olver, I.N. and Hill, M.P. (1998) Rothmund–Thomson syndrome and tolerance of chemoradiotherapy. *Australasian Radiology*, **42**, 216–18.

126 Piquero-Casals, J., Okubo, A.Y. and Nico, M.M. (2002) Rothmund–Thomson syndrome in three siblings and development of cutaneous squamous cell carcinoma. *Pediatric Dermatology*, **19**, 312–16.

127 Pujol, L.A., Erickson, R.P., Heidenreich, R.A. and Cunniff, C. (2000) Variable presentation of Rothmund–Thomson syndrome. *American Journal of Medical Genetics*, **95**, 204–7.

Part III
Site-Specific Aspects of Hereditary Tumors

5
Hereditary Brain Tumors

Christine Marosi

Summary

This chapter provides a comprehensive summary on hereditary brain tumor syndromes which are: Cowden syndrome/Lhermitte–Duclos syndrome, Li-Fraumen syndrome, Naevoid basal cell carcinoma syndrome (NBCCS)/Gorlin syndrome, Neurofibromatosis I, Neurofibromatosis II, Rhabdoid tumor predisposition syndrome, Tuberous sclerosis, Turcot syndrome, and Von Hippel–Lindau syndrome. They involve tumor suppressor genes and are inherited as autosomal dominant (AD) traits. Since most of the syndromes associated with brain tumors are also cancer family syndromes, the description is focused on the central nervous system (CNS) manifestations, and the reader is advised to also consider the Chapters 3 and 6 on family cancer syndromes and neurofibromatosis of this book.

5.1
Introduction and General Concepts

Generally brain tumors evoke an eccentric field of knowledge, dealing with dreadful disease entities which should best stay ignored. For the specialists involved in research or care of patients with central nervous system (CNS) tumors, it is a rapidly evolving, fascinating task on a striking multitude of different tumor entities, whose diagnosis and treatment encompasses a multitude of topics that involve many fields of basic science and clinical medicine. To mention only a few, working on brain tumors may consist of studying the embryonic development of the CNS, stem cell proliferation, tissue differentiation, angiogenesis, development of molecular and functional imaging tools, high end radiation therapies, diagnosis and management of CNS deficits, drug development, or psychosocial and palliative care.

Malignant brain tumors account for 1% of all cancers diagnosed in the developed countries, but still cause 2% of cancer deaths. In children, brain tumors are the most common or second common tumor diseases, mostly pilocytic or diffuse astrocytomas, medulloblastomas, and ependymomas, and constitute the first

Hereditary Tumors: From Genes to Clinical Consequences
Edited by Heike Allgayer, Helga Rehder and Simone Fulda
Copyright © 2009 WILEY-VCH Verlag GmbH & Co. KGaA, Weinheim
ISBN: 978-3-527-32028-8

cause of cancer deaths [1–6]. In adults, the most common brain tumors are astrocytomas, meningiomas, neurinomas, and ependymomas. There are more than 20 000 newly diagnosed patients with glioblastoma multiforme, the most common and most malignant brain tumor in adults, each year in the EU, 300 in Austria and 10 000 per year in the US [7–11].

Meningiomas, with an incidence of 6/100 000 inhabitants per year, are the most common benign tumors of the brain, probably the most common benign tumors causing symptoms, and requiring treatment. For almost all entities, there are no known risk factors, except previous skull irradiation, and heredity within a familial cancer syndrome with brain tumors. The proportion of hereditary brain tumors is unknown; in childhood brain tumors, it was an estimated 2% [12–14]. This is also the proportion estimated for adults by Hemminki and Li based at the Swedish Family-Cancer Database, covering all persons born in Sweden since 1932 and organized into families. They found that the standardized incidence ratios (SIR) for familial risk were increased for meningioma, astrocytomas, and hemangioblastomas. For children of affected parents, the SIR was 3.06 for meningiomas, 2.19 for astrocytoma, and 165 for hemangioblastomas, whereas the SIR was 4.41, 3.20, and 61 for the same tumors within siblings. Similar findings were presented for Utah [15, 16]. Hemmiki and Li suggest that many brain tumors, most probably those occurring in families with several histological entities, might represent yet unknown heritable conditions. Moreover, due to the improvement of diagnostic procedures in the last few years, there might be a considerable number of unreported cases of brain tumors, resulting in a significant loss of potential familial cases. The symptoms of CNS tumors are highly variable, according to tumor location. As soon as the tumor size increases over an individual tolerance level, symptoms of increased cranial or spinal pressure develop, consisting in headache, nausea, and vomiting, with a maximum in the morning hours and seizures. Diagnosis is established with magnetic resonance imaging with contrast enhancement, and needs to be confirmed by histology. The therapy of most tumor entities is now rapidly evolving in all the therapeutic modalities as the maximal feasible resection, radiation therapy, and chemotherapy. New therapeutic options using sophisticated radiation techniques or an increasing number of biologicals, are currently emerging.

5.2
Cowden Syndrome

Cowden syndrome is a multiple hamartoma syndrome [17] and probably the adult onset form of germline PTEN mutations. If it occurs with adult onset with dysplastic gangliocytoma of the cerebellum, it is called Lhermitte–Duclos disease [18–21].

The childhood onset form with macrocephaly, lipomas, pigmented maculae on the glans penis, developmental delay, and juvenile polyposis coli is called Bannayan–Riley–Ruvalcaba syndrome [22–29].

Incidence: 1 : 250 000

Involved gene: Germline mutation in PTEN

(A)   (B)

(C)

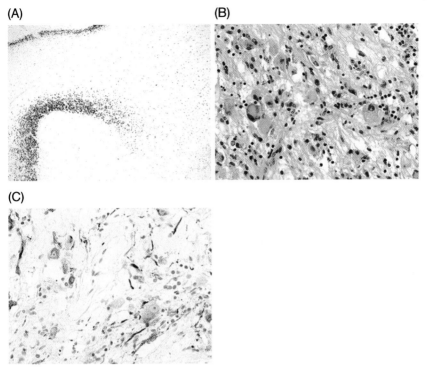

Figure 5.1 Lhermitte–Duclos disease: (A) Internal granular layer visualized by NeuN immunocytochemistry (brown ribbon). The transition into the tissue area with dysplastic gangliocytoma is associated with a dissolution of regular internal granular layer (×4). (B) A higher power view shows loose aggregates of dysplastic ganglion cells (HE ×40). (C) The dysplastic ganglion cells show strong immunoreactivity with anti-MAP2.

Chromosomal location: 10q23. Overexpression results in phosphatase – dependent cell cycle arrest at G1, or in apoptosis. Germline mutations involving exons 1–9 and the gene promoter have been found in 85% of all examined persons affected with Cowden syndrome.

Inheritance: Autosomal dominant (AD)

Definition: Multiple hamartomas involving tissues derived from all three germ cell layers. Most characteristic and pathognomonic for Cowden syndrome is the trichilemmoma.

Nervous system neoplasm: It is still unclear whether the cerebral manifestation of Cowden syndrome, the dysplastic gangliocytoma of the cerebellum (WHO grade I), is hamartomatous or neoplastic (Figure 5.1A–C shows Histological aspects of Lhremitte–Duclos disease.

The diffuse enlargement of the molecular and internal granular layers of the cerebellum with preservation of the cerebellar architecture is mostly diagnosed in adults who develop gait disturbances, dysmetria, and other cerebellar signs. The diagnosis is made by MRI. In 20% of cases, megalencephaly, heterotopic grey matter, hydrocephalus, mental retardation, seizures, and, very rarely, meningiomas and glioblastomas might also develop. As the CNS manifestations might precede other signs of Cowden disease, regular screening of Lhermitte–Duclos patients for the development of systemic cancers is recommended.

5.3
Li–Fraumeni Syndrome

Sarcoma family syndrome of Li and Fraumeni (cancer family syndrome).

Incidence: <1:10 million. 315 families reported from 1990 to 2005 in the IAR.C. Database (http://www.p53.iarc.fr) including 93 individuals with brain tumors (12.5%).

Involved gene: p53, germline mutation, mostly involving exons 5–8 with major hotspots in codons 175, 245, 248, and 273 (same hotspots as in sporadic brain tumors), resulting in missense mutations and complete loss of function of the p53 protein.

Chromosomal location: 17p13

Inheritance: AD

Nervous system neoplasm: Astrocytomas of any WHO grade (60% of brain tumors found in Li-Fraumeni patients), medulloblastomas, PNETS, all histopathologically indistinguishable from sporadic counterparts.

> *Several families showed a clustering of brain tumors. Analysis of the TP53 database showed that the occurrence of brain tumors was associated with missense mutations located in the DNA binding site of the p53 protein, essential for the contact with the minor groove of the DNA [30].*

CHEK2 is a gene coding for a protein involved in the G2 checkpoint control preventing cells with damaged DNA from entering mitosis. Despite anecdotal findings of CHEK2 mutations in several families with Li–Fraumeni syndrome or Li–Fraumeni-like syndrome (see Chapter 3 on family cancer syndromes), this mutation is not considered causative for other tumors occurring in the involved families, with the exception of breast cancers [31–35].

5.4
Naevoid Basal Cell Carcinoma Syndrome (NBCCS)

Gorlin syndrome, Gorlin–Gotz syndrome, fifth phacomatosis (cancer family syndrome).

Incidence: 1 : 57 000

Involved gene: PTCH gene; human homolog of a Drosophila segment polarity gene, which codes for a transmembrane protein that is expressed on many progenitor cells. The PTCH protein is a receptor for hedgehog proteins. Binding of hedgehog protein to PTCH releases the activity of another transmembrane protein, Smoothed, which ultimately is involved in the control of cell survival, differentiation, and proliferation. At least 130 mutations of PTCH have been reported associated with NBCCS [36–39].

Chromosomal location: 9q22.3

Inheritance: AD

Nervous system neoplasm: 10% of NBCCS patients develop early childhood medulloblastoma, mostly the desmoplastic variant, as early as before the age of 2 years. They have a better prognosis than sporadic medulloblastomas.

The occurrence of desmoplastic medulloblastoma before age 2 has been proposed as a major diagnostic criterion for NBCCS. As radiation induces multiple cutaneous basal cell carcinomas, it has been proposed to modify the treatment protocol for patients with medulloblastoma and Gorlin syndrome accordingly. The identification of NBCCS patients is suggested by the multiple developmental abnormalities in the affected patients, and might not consistently be confirmed by the identification of germline mutations within the PTCH gene.

5.5
Neurofibromatosis I

Neurofibromatosis Recklinghausen (Recklinghausen 1882), peripheral neurofibromatosis (see also Chapter 6 on neurofibromatosis).

Nervous system affection: It is characterized by cognitive disability with low average IQ (potentially related to the action of neurofibromin on microtubules), visual spatial orientation problems, and speech disorders (prevalence 30–60%). Seizures (prevalence 6%), hydrocephalus (prevalence 1–5%), primary progressive multiple sclerosis, and vascular malformations occur with higher prevalence in NF1 patients than in normal individuals. Gliomas occur in all parts of the brain, with a predilection for the ocular pathway, brainstem, and cerebellum (prevalence 2–3%). Optic pathway gliomas are most common in young children, as well as Lisch nodules (melanocytic dome shaped hamartomas, e.g. neurofibromas) of the iris [40] (prevalence 95%).

Cutaneous and subcutaneous neurofibromas, benign tumors arising from the Schwann cells of peripheral nerves, composed of Schwann cells, fibroblasts, perineural cells, mast cells, and embedded axons are the hallmark of NF1. The majority of neurofibromas express progesterone receptors, and their increase during pregnancy has been noted [41–43]. They may cause pain, itching, and neurological deficits, as well as severe disfigurement. The number and size of neurofibromas is highly variable among individuals, and might be associated with modifying genes.

Plexiform neurofibromas are found particularly subcutaneously in nearly 25% of patients, and by imaging techniques in about 50%. They consist of neurofibroma networks growing along nerves, involving multiple nerve branches and plexus.

Another complication is the malignant transformation into malignant peripheral nerve sheath tumors, a soft tissue sarcoma with poor prognosis, with a lifetime risk of 7–13% of affected patients [44].

Prognosis: The severity of the disease and the phenotype of an individual cannot be predicted so far.

5.6
Neurofibromatosis Type 2

Central neurofibromatosis (see also Chapter 6 on neurofibromatosis).

Incidence: 1 : 25 000

Involved gene: The NF2 gene spans 110 kb and contains 17 exons. It codes for merlin, a cytoskeleton-associated protein, with strong similarity to talin, moesin, ezrin, and radixin, which link actin to the cell membrane. NF2 functions as a tumor suppressor gene, and the germline mutations seen in NF2 patients are mostly point mutations with a potential hot spot in codon 57 of exon 2 [45–49].

Chromosomal location: 22q12

Inheritance: AD

Definition: The clinical diagnostic criteria for NF2 include either bilateral vestibular schwannoma, or a first-degree relative with NF2 and a vestibular schwannoma before the age of 30 years, or any two of the following: meningioma, schwannoma, glioma, and posterior subcapsular lens atrophy. The clinical course varies greatly within families and within the members of a given family. Figure 5.2A–C and Figure 5.3A and B illustrate Neurofibroamtosis II manifestations visualized in MRI and histology.

Nervous system neoplasms:
- Schwannomas, particularly vestibular schwannomas, are the diagnostic hallmark of the disease. In NF2 patients, they occur earlier than sporadic vestibular schwannomas. Other cranial nerves such as V and IX may also develop schwannomas, as well as the dorsal spinal roots. The schwannomas in NF2 patients are different from schwannomas in patients with sporadic disease, as they might entrap fibers of the eighth and seventh cranial nerve, thus showing a sort of "infiltrative" growth, and being less easily separable from the vestibular, acoustic, and facial nerve, either by surgery or by designing a radiation field, than sporadic schwannomas [50]. Besides the multiplicity of tumors and the

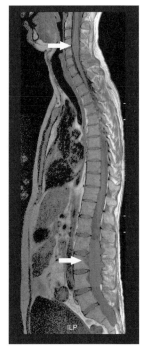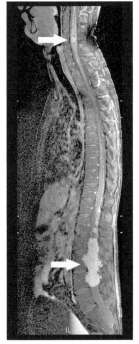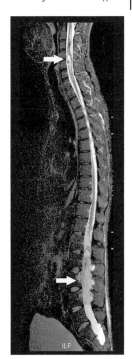

Figure 5.2 Sagittal T1-weighted, STIR, and T1-weighted contrast-enhanced images of intramedullary ependymoma in the cervical spinal cord (arrow), as well as intraspinal schwannoma at the lumbar level with scalloping of the adjacent vertebral bodies (arrow). After contrast media application, there is strong enhancement of both lesions.

(A) 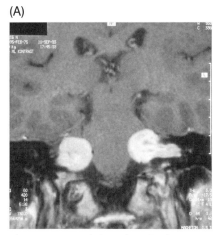 **(B)**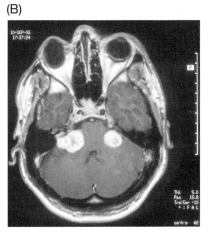

Figure 5.3 Coronal (A) and (B) Axial T1-SPIR contrast enhanced image of bilateral radicular schwannomas, and subcutaneous plexiform neurofibroma (arrows) with strong enhancement.

young age of affected patients, this particular feature of NF2-related schwannomas provides an additional explanation for the inferiority of treatment results as compared to patients with sporadic schwannomas. There are several series of patients with NF2-related vestibular schwannomas treated with Gamma Knife, showing that radiosurgery provides an acceptable treatment strategy for NF2 patients, allowing hearing preservation in a considerable number (36–43%), and the number of neuropathies observed (9%) compare favorably to the neuropathies observed after microsurgery, as stated by the team from Marseille [51–60].

- Meningiomas: half of the NF2 patients present with meningiomas, often multiple and recurrent. Although most meningiomas remain WHO I tumors, they have a higher mitotic index, and often show a more aggressive clinical behavior.

- Gliomas: most gliomas associated with NF2 are spinal intramedullary cauda equinae tumors, spinal ependymomas, or medullar gliomas.

- Rare nervous system lesions associated with NF2 consist of Schwannomatosis, a non-tumorous Schwann cell proliferation found in the dorsal roots of the spinal cord, meningiomatosis, plaque-like proliferations of meningiothelial cells, glial hamartomas, cerebral calcifications of the cortex, periventricular areas, plexus choroidei, and peripheral neuropathies.

Extraneural manifestations: Posterior lens opacity

5.7
Rhabdoid Tumour Predisposition Syndrome

Familial posterior fossa brain tumour syndrome of the infancy.

Incidence: rare, ≈3% of childhood brain tumors, ≈1/3 of patients with malignant rhabdoid tumors

Involved gene: INI1

Chromosomal location: 22q11.2

Inheritance: AD

Nervous system neoplasm: Atypical teratoid/rhabdoid tumors (AT/RT) are rapidly growing "blue tumors" in early childhood, rarely after the age of 6 years that bear a dismal prognosis [61–66]. There is a male preponderance of 1.3:1. The tumors can cause a wide variety of symptoms. Due to the rapid development of a mass lesion, children present with lethargy, headache, vomiting, failure to thrive, and cranial nerve palsy. In MRI, the tumors often show heterogeneous signal intensity, due to the presence of cysts and necrotic areas. AT/RTs are merely supratentorial and composed of histologically very diverse, primitive neuroepithelial, epithelial, and mesenchymal components with heterogeneously appearing cells, often with eccentrically placed nuclei and abundant cytoplasmatic inclusions, reminiscent of

(A) (B)

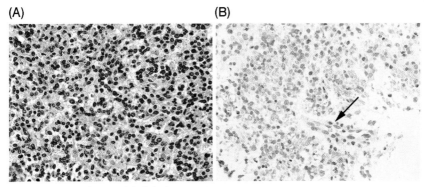

Figure 5.4 Atypical teratoid rhabdoid tumor (AT/RT):
(A) Prominent primitive neuroectodermal tumor component
(HE). (B) Loss of INI1 protein in tumor cells with retained
expression in intratumoural blood vessels (arrow).

rhabdoid cells. Loss of the nuclear staining of INI1, which is present in normal cells and endothelia, is a characteristic and sensitive diagnostic tool for AT/RTs [67]. Figure 5.4A and B illustrates histological features of RT/AT.

The germline status of all newly diagnosed patients with AT/RTs should be investigated for familial counseling.

Extraneural tumors: Similar, highly malignant rhabdoid tumors have been reported in the kidneys, (often bilateral), heart, soft tissue, head and neck, and liver.

5.8
Tuberous Sclerosis (TSC)

Pringle Bourneville disease (cancer family syndrome).

Incidence: 1:6000, previously probably under diagnosed.

Involved genes: Two genes are involved. In normal cells, the gene products of TSC1 and TSC2 heterodimerize inhibit the mTOR pathway. The TSC1 gene contains 23 exons and spans 45 kb. The gene product, hamartin, is a protein located in cytoplasmatic vesicles, and strongly expressed in brain, kidneys, and heart. The second gene, TSC2, codes for tuberin and contains 40 exons.

Chromosomal location: TSC1 9q34, TSC2 16p13.3

Inheritance: AD

Nervous system neoplasm: Subependymal giant cell astrocytoma (SEGA) is a benign, WHO grade I slowly growing neoplasm, mostly situated in the wall of the lateral ventricles, diagnosed within the first two decades of life, which occurs in 6–14% of all patients with TSC. It constitutes one of the major diagnostic criteria

(A)   (B)

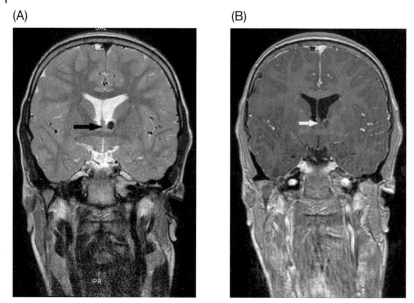

Figure 5.5 Tuberous sclerosis: (A) Coronal T2-weighted image of a calcified giant cell astrocytoma at the left foramen Monroe (arrow). (B) Coronal T1-weighted contrast enhanced image of a calcified giant cell astrocytoma at the left foramen Monroe with peripheral enhancement (arrow).

of TSC. Its prognosis is usually benign. Figure 5.5A and B shows a SEGA seen in MRI, Figure 5.6A and B histological aspects of SEGA.

The characteristic cortex lesions in the CNS are called tubers, constituted by developmental anomalies of the cortex with dysmorphic neurons, giant cells, and large astrocytes. Epilepsy occurs in 70–80% of patients with TSC [68]. There is a variety of other CNS lesions such as subcortical glioneural hamartomas, subependymal glial nodules, and subependymal giant cell astrocytomas. Figure 5.7A–C show tubera visualized by MRI, Figure 5.6C shows histological aspect of tubera,

Clinical manifestations have been divided into major and minor features, and in dubious cases genetic testing can be helpful.

5.9
Turcot Syndrome

Cancer family syndrome.

Incidence: very rare, 170 cases reported so far

Involved genes: Turcot syndrome 1: Mismatch repair associated genes. Turcot syndrome 2: familial polyposis coli gene.

(A)

(B)

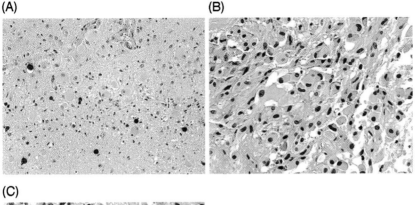

(C)

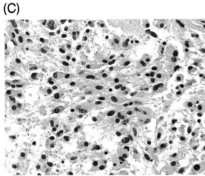

Figure 5.6 Tuberous sclerosis: histological features. (A, B) Histologicalal features of subependymal giant cell astrocytoma. Pleomorphic eosinophilic tumor cells ×40 (A), Elongated eosinophilic tumor cells ×40 (B). (C) Histology of cortical tuber. Numerous dysplastic cells with abundant eosinophilic cytoplasm (balloon cells), gliosis, and multiple calcifications (spherical dark-blue material) are visible ×40.

Chromosomal location: Turcot syndrome 1: Glioma polyposis syndrome seen in patients with a functional loss of one of the numerous DNA mismatch repair genes, namely MLH1 at 3p21.3, MSH2 at 2p16, MSH6/GTBP at 2p16, and PMS2 at 7p22. The latter is the most frequently reported genetic event in Turcot syndrome 1.

Turcot syndrome 2, the medulloblastoma polyposis syndrome, is related to the APC gene on 5q21.

Inheritance: AD

Definition: Subgroups of patients with hereditary colon cancer syndromes affected by CNS neoplasms.

Nervous system neoplasm: Association of glioblastomas with HNPCC (hereditary non-polyposis colorectal carcinoma, see Chapter 17 on Lynch syndrome (HNPCC)), usually before the age of 30 years. This is more than a decade earlier than sporadic glioblastomas. Thirty-eight percent of the patients with Turcot syndrome 1 show café-au-lait spots.

Turcot syndrome 2 combines medulloblastoma at a relatively late age of 10 years, with the familial adenomatous polyposis syndrome, with numerous small colon polyps and colon cancer in 20%. There are less skin lesions than in Turcot syndrome 1.

(A)

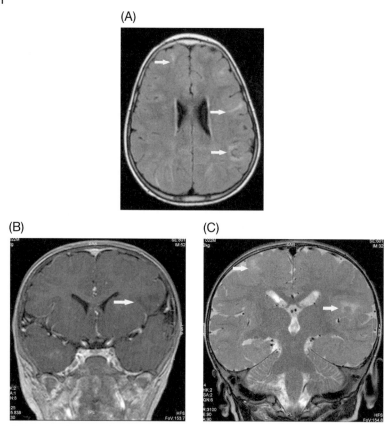

(B)   (C)

Figure 5.7 Tuberous sclerosis: tubera visualized by MRI magnet resonance tomography. (A) Axial flair image of subcortical hyperintense tubera (arrows). (B) Coronal T2-weighted image of hyperintense tubera (arrows). (C) Coronal T1-weighted contrast enhanced image of hypointense tubera without contrast media uptake (arrow).

Extraneural tumors: colorectal polyps and cancer.

5.10
von Hippel–Lindau Syndrome

Haemangioblastoma (cancer family syndrome).

Incidence: 1 : 40 000

Involved gene: The von Hippel–Lindau (VHL) gene, a tumor suppressor gene, composed of 3 exons and a coding sequence of 639 nucleotides. The alpha domain of the VHL protein forms a complex with different other proteins and provides ubiquitin-ligase activity, a step needed before proteasome-mediated degradation of cellular proteins [69–76]. The β domain of the VHL protein interacts with hypoxia-inducible factor alpha, which induces VEGF expression, and is related to the significantly increased microvascular density in VHL-associated neoplasms. Germline mutations are mostly missense mutations, but other forms of gene inactivation also occur.

Chromosomal location: 3p25–26

Inheritance: AD, VHL mutations can be identified in most cases.

Nervous system neoplasm: The characteristic VHL-associated haemangioblastomas are composed of neoplastic vascular and stromal cells in variable composition. In contrast to sporadic haemangioblastomas, they are often multiple and not exclusively located in the cerebellum, but also in the brain stem, spinal cord, or nerve roots.

They mostly occur in young adults with a mean age of less than 30 years. Multiple haemangioblastomas are a diagnostic hallmark of VHL syndrome. In haemangioblastomas, extramedullary haematopoiesis has been observed. There are four different subtypes of haemangioblastomas. The most frequent form is a macrocystic tumor, filled with a xanthochromatic fluid, and presenting as a dense red-colored parietal nodule. In the second category, the nodule is too small to be seen without a microscope. More rarely and mostly in spinal locations, the haemangioblastoma consists of a solid tumor, sometimes with internal cysts.

Acknowledgments

For providing the figures. I am very grateful to Daniela Prayer, Johannes Hainfellner, Negar Fakhrai, Gregor Kasprian, Christian Matula, Matthias Preusser, Ingeborg Fischer, and Marco Hassler, all at the Medical University Vienna, Vienna, Austria.

References

1 Dreifaldt, A.C., Carlberg, M. and Hardell, L. (2004) Increasing incidence rates of childhood malignant diseases in Sweden during the period 1960–1998. *European Journal of Cancer*, **40**, 1351–60.

2 Hemminki, K., Li, X., Vaittinen, P. and Dong, C. (2000) Cancers in the first-degree relatives of children with brain tumours. *British Journal of Cancer*, **83**, 407–11.

3 Kaatsch, P., Rickert, C.H., Kuhl, J., Schuz, J. and Michaelis, J. (2001) Population-based epidemiologic data on brain tumors in German children. *Cancer*, **92**, 3155–64.

4 Mutanen, P. and Hemminki, K. (2001) Childhood cancer and parental occupation in the Swedish Family-Cancer Database. *Journal of Occupational and Environmental Medicine*, **43**, 952–8.

5 Rickert, C.H., Probst-Cousin, S. and Gullotta, F. (1997) Primary intracranial neoplasms of infancy and early childhood. *Child's Nervous System*, **13**, 507–13.

6 Stegmaier, C., Muller, R., Semeniuk, E., Ziegler, H., Eisinger, B. and Stabenow, R. (2001) [Descriptive epidemiology in population based cancer registries using CNS tumors as an example]. *Zentralblatt fur Neurochirurgie*, **62**, 137–43.

7 Deorah, S., Lynch, C.F., Sibenaller, Z.A. and Ryken, T.C. (2006) Trends in brain cancer incidence and survival in the United States: Surveillance, Epidemiology, and End Results Program, 1973 to 2001. *Neurosurgical Focus*, **20**, E1.

8 Levin, V.A. (2007) Are gliomas preventable? *Recent Results in Cancer Research*, **174**, 205–15.

9 Norden, A.D. and Wen, P.Y. (2006) Glioma therapy in adults. *Neurologist*, **12**, 279–92.

10 Schwartzbaum, J.A., Fisher, J.L., Aldape, K.D. and Wrensch, M. (2006) Epidemiology and molecular pathology of glioma. *Nature Clinical Practice Neurology*, **2**, 494–503.

11 Semrad, T.J., O'Donnell, R., Wun, T., Chew, H., Harvey, D., Zhou, H. and White, R.H. (2007) Epidemiology of venous thromboembolism in 9489 patients with malignant glioma. *Journal of Neurosurgery*, **106**, 601–8.

12 Bondy, M.L., Lustbader, E.D., Buffler, P.A., Schull, W.J., Hardy, R.J. and Strong, L.C. (1991) Genetic epidemiology of childhood brain tumors. *Genetic Epidemiology*, **8**, 253–67.

13 Hemminki, K. and Li, X. (2003) Familial risks in nervous system tumors. *Cancer Epidemiology, Biomarkers and Prevention*, **12**, 1137–42.

14 Narod, S.A., Stiller, C. and Lenoir, G.M. (1991) An estimate of the heritable fraction of childhood cancer. *British Journal of Cancer*, **63**, 993–9.

15 Goldgar, D.E. (2002) Population aspects of cancer genetics. *Biochimie*, **84**, 19–25.

16 Goldgar, D.E., Easton, D.F., Cannon-Albright, L.A. and Skolnick, M.H. (1994) Systematic population-based assessment of cancer risk in first-degree relatives of cancer probands. *Journal of the National Cancer Institute*, **86**, 1600–8.

17 Weary, P.E., Gorlin, R.J., Gentry, W.C. Jr, Comer, J.E. and Greer, K.E. (1972) Multiple hamartoma syndrome

(Cowden's disease). *Archives of Dermatology*, **106**, 682–90.

18 Bignami, A. and De Matteis, A. (1956) Lhermitte–Duclos disease of the cerebellum (dysplastic ganglioneuroma). *Rivista di Anatomia Patologica e di Oncologia*, **11**, 523–38.

19 Chiofalo, M.G., Cappabianca, P., Del Basso De Caro, M.L. and Pezzullo, L. (2007) Lhermitte–Duclos disease. *Journal of Neuro-Oncology*, **82**, 183–5.

20 Demaerel, P., Van Calenbergh, F. and Wilms, G. (2003) Lhermitte-Duclos disease: a tumour or not a tumour. *Acta Neurologica Scandinavica*, **108**, 294–5.

21 Kumar, R., Vaid, V.K. and Kalra, S.K. (2007) Lhermitte–Duclos disease. *Child's Nervous System*, **23**, 729–32.

22 Arch, E.M., Goodman, B.K., Van Wesep, R.A., Liaw, D., Clarke, K., Parsons, R., McKusick, V.A. and Geraghty, M.T. (1997) Deletion of PTEN in a patient with Bannayan–Riley–Ruvalcaba syndrome suggests allelism with Cowden disease. *American Journal of Medical Genetics*, **71**, 489–93.

23 Buisson, P., Leclair, M.D., Jacquemont, S., Podevin, G., Camby, C., David, A. and Heloury, Y. (2006) Cutaneous lipoma in children: 5 cases with Bannayan–Riley–Ruvalcaba syndrome. *Journal of Pediatric Surgery*, **41**, 1601–3.

24 Fargnoli, M.C., Orlow, S.J., Semel-Concepcion, J. and Bolognia, J.L. (1996) Clinicopathologic findings in the Bannayan–Riley–Ruvalcaba syndrome. *Archives of Dermatology*, **132**, 1214–18.

25 Hendriks, Y.M., Verhallen, J.T., van der Smagt, J.J., Kant, S.G., Hilhorst, Y., Hoefsloot, L., Hansson, K.B., van der Straaten, P.J., Boutkan, H., Breuning, M.H. *et al.* (2003) Bannayan–Riley–Ruvalcaba syndrome: further delineation of the phenotype and management of PTEN mutation-positive cases. *Familial Cancer*, **2**, 79–85.

26 Lachlan, K.L., Lucassen, A.M., Bunyan, D.J. and Temple, I.K. (2007) Cowden Syndrome and Bannayan–Riley–Ruvalcaba syndrome represent one condition with variable expression and age-related penetrance: a clinical study of 42 individuals with PTEN mutations. *Journal of Medical Genetics*, **44**, 579–85.

27 Merg, A. and Howe, J.R. (2004) Genetic conditions associated with intestinal juvenile polyps. *American Journal of Medical Genetics Part C, Seminars in Medical Genetics*, **129**, 44–55.

28 Schaffer, J.V., Kamino, H., Witkiewicz, A., McNiff, J.M. and Orlow, S.J. (2006) Mucocutaneous neuromas: an under-recognized manifestation of PTEN hamartoma–tumor syndrome. *Archives of Dermatology*, **142**, 625–32.

29 Zhou, X.P., Waite, K.A., Pilarski, R., Hampel, H., Fernandez, M.J., Bos, C., Dasouki, M., Feldman, G.L., Greenberg, L.A., Ivanovich, J. *et al.* (2003) Germline PTEN promoter mutations and deletions in Cowden/Bannayan–Riley–Ruvalcaba syndrome result in aberrant PTEN protein and dysregulation of the phosphoinositol-3-kinase/Akt pathway. *American Journal of Human Genetics*, **73**, 404–11.

30 Olivier, M., Goldgar, D.E., Sodha, N., Ohgaki, H., Kleihues, P., Hainaut, P. and Eeles, R.A. (2003) Li-Fraumeni and related syndromes: correlation between tumor type, family structure, and TP53 genotype. *Cancer Research*, **63**, 6643–50.

31 Bachinski, L.L., Olufemi, S.E., Zhou, X., Wu, C.C., Yip, L., Shete, S., Lozano, G., Amos, C.I., Strong, L.C. and Krahe, R. (2005) Genetic mapping of a third Li–Fraumeni syndrome predisposition locus to human chromosome 1q23. *Cancer Research*, **65**, 427–31.

32 Nevanlinna, H. and Bartek, J. (2006) The CHEK2 gene and inherited breast cancer susceptibility. *Oncogene*, **25**, 5912–19.

33 Siddiqui, R., Onel, K., Facio, F., Nafa, K., Diaz, L.R., Kauff, N., Huang, H., Robson, M., Ellis, N. and Offit, K. (2005) The TP53 mutational spectrum and frequency of CHEK2*1100delC in Li-Fraumeni-like kindreds. *Familial Cancer*, **4**, 177–81.

34 Sodha, N., Houlston, R.S., Bullock, S., Yuille, M.A., Chu, C., Turner, G. and Eeles, R.A. (2002) Increasing evidence that germline mutations in CHEK2 do not cause Li–Fraumeni syndrome. *Human Mutation*, **20**, 460–2.

35 Walsh, T., Casadei, S., Coats, K.H., Swisher, E., Stray, S.M., Higgins, J.,

Roach, K.C., Mandell, J., Lee, M.K., Ciernikova, S. *et al.* (2006) Spectrum of mutations in BRCA1, BRCA2, CHEK2, and TP53 in families at high risk of breast cancer. *The Journal of the American Medical Association*, **295**, 1379–88.

36 de Meij, T.G., Baars, M.J., Gille, J.J., Hack, W.W., Haasnoot, K. and van Hagen, J.M. (2005) [From gene to disease: basal cell naevus syndrome]. *Nederlands Tijdschrift voor Geneeskunde*, **149**, 78–81.

37 Hasenpusch-Theil, K., Bataille, V., Laehdetie, J., Obermayr, F., Sampson, J.R. and Frischauf, A.M. (1998) Gorlin syndrome: identification of 4 novel germline mutations of the human patched (PTCH) gene. Mutations in brief no. 137. Online. *Human Mutation*, **11**, 480.

38 Ragge, N.K., Salt, A., Collin, J.R., Michalski, A. and Farndon, P.A. (2005) Gorlin syndrome: the PTCH gene links ocular developmental defects and tumour formation. *The British Journal of Ophthalmology*, **89**, 988–91.

39 Reifenberger, J. (2004) Hereditary tumor syndromes. Cutaneous manifestations and molecular pathogenesis of Gorlin and Cowden syndromes. *Hautarzt*, **55**, 942–51.

40 Lubs, M.L., Bauer, M.S., Formas, M.E. and Djokic, B. (1991) Lisch nodules in neurofibromatosis type 1. *The New England Journal of Medicine*, **324**, 1264–6.

41 Concolino, G., Liccardo, G., Conti, C., Panfili, C. and Giuffre, R. (1984) Hormones and tumours in central nervous system (CNS): steroid receptors in primary spinal cord tumours. *Neurological Research*, **6**, 121–6.

42 Fishbein, L., Zhang, X., Fisher, L.B., Li, H., Campbell-Thompson, M., Yachnis, A., Rubenstein, A., Muir, D. and Wallace, M.R. (2007) *In vitro* studies of steroid hormones in neurofibromatosis 1 tumors and schwann cells. *Molecular Carcinogenesis*, **46**, 512–23.

43 McLaughlin, M.E. and Jacks, T. (2003) Progesterone receptor expression in neurofibromas. *Cancer Research*, **63**, 752–5.

44 Evans, D.G., Baser, M.E., McGaughran, J., Sharif, S., Howard, E. and Moran, A. (2002) Malignant peripheral nerve sheath tumours in neurofibromatosis 1. *Journal of Medical Genetics*, **39**, 311–14.

45 Evans, D.G., Maher, E.R. and Baser, M.E. (2005) Age related shift in the mutation spectra of germline and somatic NF2 mutations: hypothetical role of DNA repair mechanisms. *Journal of Medical Genetics*, **42**, 630–2.

46 Jacoby, L.B., MacCollin, M., Parry, D.M., Kluwe, L., Lynch, J., Jones, D. and Gusella, J.F. (1999) Allelic expression of the NF2 gene in neurofibromatosis 2 and schwannomatosis. *Neurogenetics*, **2**, 101–8.

47 Legoix, P., Sarkissian, H.D., Cazes, L., Giraud, S., Sor, F., Rouleau, G.A., Lenoir, G., Thomas, G. and Zucman-Rossi, J. (2000) Molecular characterization of germline NF2 gene rearrangements. *Genomics*, **65**, 62–6.

48 Sanson, M., Marineau, C., Desmaze, C., Lutchman, M., Ruttledge, M., Baron, C., Narod, S., Delattre, O., Lenoir, G., Thomas, G. *et al.* (1993) Germline deletion in a neurofibromatosis type 2 kindred inactivates the NF2 gene and a candidate meningioma locus. *Human Molecular Genetics*, **2**, 1215–20.

49 Stemmer-Rachamimov, A.O., Ino, Y., Lim, Z.Y., Jacoby, L.B., MacCollin, M., Gusella, J.F., Ramesh, V. and Louis, D.N. (1998) Loss of the NF2 gene and merlin occur by the tumorlet stage of schwannoma development in neurofibromatosis 2. *Journal of Neuropathology and Experimental Neurology*, **57**, 1164–7.

50 Jaaskelainen, J., Paetau, A., Pyykko, I., Blomstedt, G., Palva, T. and Troupp, H. (1994) Interface between the facial nerve and large acoustic neurinomas. Immunohistochemical study of the cleavage plane in NF2 and non-NF2 cases. *Journal of Neurosurgery*, **80**, 541–7.

51 Kida, Y., Kobayashi, T., Tanaka, T. and Mori, Y. (2000) Radiosurgery for bilateral neurinomas associated with neurofibromatosis type 2. *Surgical Neurology*, **53**, 383–9. discussion 389–90.

52 Pellet, W., Regis, J., Roche, P.H. and Delsanti, C. (2003) Relative indications for radiosurgery and microsurgery for acoustic schwannoma. *Advances and Technical Standards in Neurosurgery*, **28**; 227–82; discussion 282–24.

53 Pellet, W. and Roche, P.H. (2004) [Microsurgery of vestibular schwannoma: persisting questions]. *Neurochirurgie*, **50**, 195–243.

54 Roche, P.H., Regis, J., Pellet, W., Thomassin, J.M., Gregoire, R., Dufour, H. and Peragut, J.C. (2000) Neurofibromatosis type 2. Preliminary results of gamma knife radiosurgery of vestibular schwannomas. *Neurochirurgie*, **46**, 339–53; discussion 354.

55 Roche, P.H., Robitail, S., Delsanti, C., Marouf, R., Pellet, W. and Regis, J. (2004) Radiosurgery of vestibular schwannomas after microsurgery and combined radio-microsurgery. *Neurochirurgie*, **50**, 394–400.

56 Roche, P.H., Robitail, S., Pellet, W., Deveze, A., Thomassin, J.M. and Regis, J. (2004) Results and indications of gamma knife radiosurgery for large vestibular schwannomas. *Neurochirurgie*, **50**, 377–82.

57 Roche, P.H., Robitail, S., Thomassin, J.M., Pellet, W. and Regis, J. (2004) Surgical management of vestibular schwannomas secondary to type 2 neurofibromatosis. *Neurochirurgie*, **50**, 367–76.

58 Rowe, J.G., Radatz, M., Walton, L. and Kemeny, A.A. (2002) Stereotactic radiosurgery for type 2 neurofibromatosis acoustic neuromas: patient selection and tumour size. *Stereotactic and Functional Neurosurgery*, **79**, 107–16.

59 Rowe, J.G., Radatz, M.W., Walton, L., Soanes, T., Rodgers, J. and Kemeny, A.A. (2003) Clinical experience with gamma knife stereotactic radiosurgery in the management of vestibular schwannomas secondary to type 2 neurofibromatosis. *Journal of Neurology, Neurosurgery, and Psychiatry*, **74**, 1288–93.

60 Subach, B.R., Kondziolka, D., Lunsford, L.D., Bissonette, D.J., Flickinger, J.C. and Maitz, A.H. (1999) Stereotactic radiosurgery in the management of acoustic neuromas associated with neurofibromatosis Type 2. *Journal of Neurosurgery*, **90**, 815–22.

61 Bhattacharjee, M., Hicks, J., Langford, L., Dauser, R., Strother, D., Chintagumpala, M., Horowitz, M., Cooley, L. and Vogel, H. (1997) Central nervous system atypical teratoid/rhabdoid tumors of infancy and childhood. *Ultrastructural Pathology*, **21**, 369–78.

62 Hilden, J.M., Meerbaum, S., Burger, P., Finlay, J., Janss, A., Scheithauer, B.W., Walter, A.W., Rorke, L.B. and Biegel, J.A. (2004) Central nervous system atypical teratoid/rhabdoid tumor: results of therapy in children enrolled in a registry. *Journal of Clinical Oncology*, **22**, 2877–84.

63 Kao, C.L., Chiou, S.H., Ho, D.M., Chen, Y.J., Liu, R.S., Lo, C.W., Tsai, F.T., Lin, C.H., Ku, H.H., Yu, S.M. and Wong, T.T. (2005) Elevation of plasma and cerebrospinal fluid osteopontin levels in patients with atypical teratoid/rhabdoid tumor. *American Journal of Clinical Pathology*, **123**, 297–304.

64 Meyers, S.P., Khademian, Z.P., Biegel, J.A., Chuang, S.H., Korones, D.N. and Zimmerman, R.A. (2006) Primary intracranial atypical teratoid/rhabdoid tumors of infancy and childhood: MRI features and patient outcomes. *AJNR. American Journal of Neuroradiology*, **27**, 962–71.

65 Packer, R.J., Biegel, J.A., Blaney, S., Finlay, J., Geyer, J.R., Heideman, R., Hilden, J., Janss, A.J., Kun, L., Vezina, G. *et al.* (2002) Atypical teratoid/rhabdoid tumor of the central nervous system: report on workshop. *Journal of Pediatric Hematology and Oncology*, **24**, 337–42.

66 Zimmerman, M.A., Goumnerova, L.C., Proctor, M., Scott, R.M., Marcus, K., Pomeroy, S.L., Turner, C.D., Chi, S.N., Chordas, C. and Kieran, M.W. (2005) Continuous remission of newly diagnosed and relapsed central nervous system atypical teratoid/rhabdoid tumor. *Journal of Neuro-Oncology*, **72**, 77–84.

67 Haberler, C., Laggner, U., Slavc, I., Czech, T., Ambros, I.M., Ambros, P.F., Budka, H. and Hainfellner, J.A. (2006) Immunohistochemical analysis of INI1 protein in malignant pediatric CNS tumors: Lack of INI1 in atypical teratoid/ rhabdoid tumors and in a fraction of primitive neuroectodermal tumors without rhabdoid phenotype. *The American journal of Surgical Pathology*, **30**, 1462–8.

68 Hottinger, A.F. and Khakoo, Y. (2007) Update on the management of familial central nervous system tumor syndromes. *Current Neurology and Neuroscience Reports*, **7**, 200–7.

69 Calzada, M.J., Esteban, M.A., Feijoo-Cuaresma, M., Castellanos, M.C., Naranjo-Suarez, S., Temes, E., Mendez, F., Yanez-Mo, M., Ohh, M. and Landazuri, M.O. (2006) von Hippel–Lindau tumor suppressor protein regulates the assembly of intercellular junctions in renal cancer cells through hypoxia-inducible factor-independent mechanisms. *Cancer Research*, **66**, 1553–60.

70 Iturrioz, X., Durgan, J., Calleja, V., Larijani, B., Okuda, H., Whelan, R. and Parker, P.J. (2006) The von Hippel-Lindau tumour–suppressor protein interaction with protein kinase Cdelta. *The Biochemical Journal*, **397**, 109–20.

71 Kamura, T., Brower, C.S., Conaway, R.C. and Conaway, J.W. (2002) A molecular basis for stabilization of the von Hippel–Lindau (VHL) tumor suppressor protein by components of the VHL ubiquitin ligase. *The Journal of Biological Chemistry*, **277**, 30388–93.

72 Lehman, N.L., van de Rijn, M. and Jackson, P.K. (2005) Screening of tissue microarrays for ubiquitin proteasome system components in tumors. *Methods in Enzymology*, **399**, 334–55.

73 Maxwell, P.H., Wiesener, M.S., Chang, G.W., Clifford, S.C., Vaux, E.C., Cockman, M.E., Wykoff, C.C., Pugh, C.W., Maher, E.R. and Ratcliffe, P.J. (1999) The tumour suppressor protein VHL targets hypoxia-inducible factors for oxygen-dependent proteolysis. *Nature*, **399**, 271–5.

74 Qi, H., Gervais, M.L., Li, W., DeCaprio, J.A., Challis, J.R. and Ohh, M. (2004) Molecular cloning and characterization of the von Hippel–Lindau-like protein. *Molecular CancerResearch*, **2**, 43–52.

75 Zagzag, D., Krishnamachary, B., Yee, H., Okuyama, H., Chiriboga, L., Ali, M.A., Melamed, J. and Semenza, G.L. (2005) Stromal cell-derived factor-1alpha and CXCR4 expression in hemangioblastoma and clear cell-renal cell carcinoma: von Hippel–Lindau loss-of-function induces expression of a ligand and its receptor. *Cancer Research*, **65**, 6178–88.

76 Zhang, N., Gong, K., Guo, H.F., Na, X., Wu, G., Yang, X.Y., Xin, D.Q. and Na, Y.Q. (2004) Mutation of von Hippel–Lindau gene and expression of vascular endothelial growth factor in sporadic clear cell renal cell carcinoma and their relationships to angiogenesis. *Zhonghua Yi Xue Za Zhi*, **84**, 1620–4.

6
Neurofibromatosis

Katharina Wimmer, Hildegard Kehrer-Sawatzki, and Eric Legius

Summary

The first scientific monograph on neurofibromatosis type 1 (NF1) was published 1882 by Friedrich Daniel von Recklinghausen, who coined the term "neurofi-broma" for the benign peripheral nerve sheath tumors that are typical for NF1. The leading feature of neurofibromatosis type 2 (NF2) are schwannomas of the vestibular nerve. The diagnostic criteria for NF1 and NF2 were formulated in 1987 by the National Institutes of Health (NIH) Consensus Development Conference Statement, and are still valid and widely used. Both disorders are caused by inactivating mutations in the respective genes and have an autosomal dominant pattern of inheritance. Recently, a third form of neurofibromatosis termed schwannomatosis has been described which is also, albeit rarely, inherited in an autosomal dominant fashion. Germline mutations in the tumor suppressor *INI1/ SMARCB1* may be responsible for some cases of familial schwannomatosis. In this chapter we summarize the current knowledge about clinical and genetic diagnosis, the molecular patho-mechanisms, and the clinical, in particular tumor manifestations of the three conditions.

6.1
Clinical Diagnosis

6.1.1
Neurofibromatosis Type 1

The incidence of NF1 [OMIM # 162200] is 1 in 2500–3000 worldwide. In adults and most children above the age of 8 years [1], the clinical diagnosis is straightforward using the criteria as defined by the NIH Consensus Development Conference Statement [2] (see Tables 6.1 and 6.2). The cardinal symptoms of NF1 are café-au-lait spots (CLS), axillary or inguinal freckling, neurofibromas, and Lisch nodules in the iris. The vast majority (95%) of small children with six and more CLS will develop NF1 [3]. Cranial T2-weighted magnetic resonance imaging

Hereditary Tumors: From Genes to Clinical Consequences
Edited by Heike Allgayer, Helga Rehder and Simone Fulda
Copyright © 2009 WILEY-VCH Verlag GmbH & Co. KGaA, Weinheim
ISBN: 978-3-527-32028-8

Table 6.1 Features and complications of NF1.

Feature	Frequency
Café-au-lait spots	>95%
Freckling	90%
Dermal neurofibroma	>95%
Lisch nodules (iris harmatomas)	95% (in adults)
Specific learning difficulties	30–65%
Macrocephaly	29–45%
Plexiform neurofibromas	~30%
Scoliosis	10%
Pseudarthrosis	rare
Optic pathway glioma	5–15% (symptomatic-asymptomatic)
Malignant peripheral nerve sheath tumor	8–13%
Juvenile myelo-monocytic leukemia	rare
Pheochromozytoma	rare

(MRI) scans show hyper-intense lesions named unidentified bright objects (UBOs) in up to 86% of NF1 children [4]. Cutaneous and subcutaneous neurofibromas present in over 95% of adult NF1 patients, usually starting to appear from puberty onwards.

Recently, a specific *NF1* mutation (c.2970–2972 delAAT) has been shown to be associated with a mild phenotype, and absence of cutaneous neurofibromas [5]. Furthermore, patients with a specific expression of NF1 such as familial spinal neurofibromatosis (SNF) have neurofibromas of multiple spinal nerve roots, which may be asymptomatic or cause neurological deficits, but they often lack cutaneous neurofibromas. Watson syndrome patients are another NF1 sub-type who present with pulmonary stenosis, cognitive impairment, and CLS, but only a few, if any, cutaneous neurofibromas. Mosaic or segmental NF1 patients, who commonly present with mild symptoms lacking cutaneous neurofibromas or CLS, or restriction of these features to only some body segments [6, 7], carry a somatic (postzygotic) *NF1* mutation that affects only a proportion of the body cells. If the manifestation of NF1 is restricted to mild cutaneous involvement, the clinical diagnosis may be difficult.

Furthermore, NF1-associated symptoms show an overlap with other conditions that warrant differential diagnosis. Some NF1 patients have facial and other characteristics reminiscent of Noonan syndrome. While Noonan patients carry mutations in the genes *PTPN11* (SHP2), *SOS1, KRAS,* or *RAF1,* patients with a Neurofibromatosis-Noonan (NF-Noonan) phenotype harbor *NF1* mutations [8]. Recently, a novel NF1-like syndrome caused by mutations in the *SPRED1* gene has been characterized [9]. The main clinical features of this disorder largely overlap with NF1, and include multiple CLS, axillary freckling, and macrocephaly. However, cutaneous neurofibromas, central nervous system tumors, and Lisch nodules have not been observed in patients with *SPRED1* mutations. In

Table 6.2 The criteria for clinical diagnosis NF1, NF2, and schwannomatosis.

NF1 according the NIH consensus statement [2]

Individuals should have two of the following:
- $\geq$ 6 Café-au-lait spots (diameter >0.5 cm before puberty and >1.5 cm after puberty)
- $\geq$ 2 neurofibromas of any type or one plexiform neurofibroma
- Axillary or inguinal freckling
- Optic pathway glioma
- $\geq$ 2 Lisch nodules (iris harmatoma)
- Specific bone lesions including pseudarthrosis of the tibia
- First-degree relative with NF1 (parent, child)

NF2 revised diagnostic criteria according to [12]
Individuals should have one of the following:
- Bilateral vestibular schwannomas
- First-degree relative with NF2 plus unilateral vestibular schwannoma or two of meningioma, schwannoma, glioma, neurofibroma, posterior subcapsular lens opacity
- Unilateral vestibular schwannoma plus two of the following: meningioma, schwannoma, glioma, neurofibroma , posterior subcapsular lens opacities
- Multiple meningiomas plus unilateral vestibular schwannomas or two of the following: schwannomas, glioma, neurofibroma, posterior subcapsular lens opacity

Schwannomatosis revised diagnostic criteria as given in [15]

Individuals should not fulfil the diagnostic criteria for NF2 or have any of the following:
- A vestibular schwannoma on MRI
- Constitutional NF2 mutation
- First-degree relative with NF2

Definite diagnosis schwannomatosis:
- Age > 30 years, and two or more non-intradermal schwannomas (at least one with histological confirmation)
- One schwannoma confirmed by histology and a first-degree relative who meets the above criteria

Possible schwannomatosis:
- Age > 30 years and two or more non-intradermal schwannomas (at least one with histological confirmation)
- Age > 45 years and no symptoms of eighth nerve dysfunction, and two or more non-intradermal schwannomas (at least one with histological confirmation)[a]
- Radiographic evidence of a schwannomas and a first-degree relative who meets the criteria for definite schwannomatosis

Segmental schwannomatosis:
- Meets criteria for definite or possible schwannomatosis but limited to one limb or five or fewer contiguous segments of the spine

a NF2 is unlikely in an individual who is >45 years and does not have eighth cranial nerve symptoms.

young patients presenting with signs of NF1 and haematological malignancies and/or malignant brain tumors, usually not belonging to the spectrum of NF1-associated tumors, a cancer predisposition syndrome that is caused by biallelic mutations in one of the mismatch repair (MMR) genes or the *BRCA2* gene, has to be considered (for review see [10]). Since these childhood cancer syndromes are autosomal recessively inherited, siblings also presenting with CLS will have the same high risk for childhood cancers and parents who do not show NF1 related features have an increased risk for HNPCC related malignancies or breast cancer during adult life, resulting from their heterozygous mutations in the respective genes.

Taken together, the clinical diagnosis of NF1 according the NIH criteria can readily be made in most patients above the age of 8 years. Diagnosis might be more difficult in younger patients without a family history. In patients with specific forms of NF1 (mosaic, segmental, spinal) or mild cutaneous NF1 features, molecular diagnosis (see Genetic Testing) may be of great help.

6.1.2
Neurofibromatosis Type 2

NF2 [OMIM # 101000] has an estimated birth incidence of about 1 in 25 000–33 000 [11]. The hallmark of NF2 is bilaterial vestibular schwannomas (VS). Since early recognition of NF2 is essential for optimal management, the originally stringent NIH criteria for NF2 have been revised to allow the inclusion of young NF2 patients lacking a family history of NF2 and bilateral VS [12] (see Table 6.2). Onset of the first disease manifestations varies largely from pre-pubertal childhood to the third decade of life, and depends on the nature of the *NF2* mutation (see also Genetic Testing), and on whether the mutation occurred in the germline or post-zygotically (mosaic mutation). In children, the first symptoms are usually cutaneous schwannomas, spinal tumors, meningiomas, posterior subcapsular lens opacities, or a mononeuropathy. Up to a third of the ~50% *de novo* NF2 cases are mosaic NF2 patients [13] who present with mild generalized disease including a later age of onset, or with clinical features localized to one area of the nervous system, most commonly unilateral VS and/or meningiomas [7]. The possibility of mosaic NF2 in such cases is raised by the diagnosis of a multifocal tumor. Differential diagnosis with schwannomatosis should be considered in patients who develop multiple schwannomas in the absence of VS.

6.1.3
Schwannomatosis

Schwannomatosis [OMIM # 162091] is a recently recognized third form of neurofibromatosis that is clearly distinct from NF2 [14]. Most importantly, schwannomatosis patients have multiple schwannomas confined mainly to spinal and peripheral nerves, but lack VS (Table 6.2). Nevertheless, a certain overlap of symptoms is seen in young NF2 patients [14]. Tumor presentation in schwannomatosis patients is characterized by pain rather than functional loss, which is more frequently seen in NF2 patients.

The prevalence of schwannomatosis is currently unknown, but it may be as high as NF2 [14–16]. It is estimated that 2.4–5.0% of all patients requiring schwannoma resection are schwannomatosis patients of whom a third have anatomically localized disease. Schwannomatosis is transmitted in an autosomal dominant fashion, but familial occurrence is inexplicably rare. The empirical risk of recurrence is less than 15%, but seems to increase up to 50% if the affected is already a familial case [14]. Low penetrance, mosaicism, and/or etiologic heterogeneity may be responsible for this low risk to pass on the disease to the next generation.

6.2
The Disease-Causing Genes

6.2.1
The NF1 Gene and Its Gene Product Neurofibromin

The *NF1* gene located at chromosome band 17q11.2 was cloned in 1990 [17, 18]. *NF1* is a classical tumor suppressor gene that leads to tumor formation by biallelic inactivation caused by germline and somatic mutations according to Knudson's two-hit hypothesis [19]. This has been confirmed in mouse models [20, 21] and in tumors of NF1 patients. Somatic inactivation of the wildtype allele has been shown in malignant peripheral nerve sheath tumors (MPNSTs) [22], juvenile myelomonocytic leukaemia (JMML) [23], astrocytomas [24], gastrointestinal stromal tumors [25], and pheochromocytomas [26]. Benign peripheral nerve sheath tumors consist of different cell types including Schwann cells (SCs), fibroblasts, mast cells, and axons. The development of culture conditions to selectively grow SC from neurofibromas *in vivo* [27] was instrumental in showing that only a proportion of SC in the neurofibromas carried a second hit in the *NF1* gene and not other cell types [28]. Transformation of a benign neurofibroma with biallelic *NF1* inactivation to a MPNST is accompanied by additional genetic and genomic alterations in genes such as p53, p16, or p27-Kip [29–31].

Non-neoplastic NF1 features have long been thought to be the result of *NF1* haplo-insufficiency. Recently, however, it has been shown that biallelic inactivation of *NF1* in melanocytes appears to be responsible for CLS formation [32], and loss of the wildtype allele has been observed also in pseudoarthrosis tissue of NF1 patients [33].

The NF1 gene codes for neurofibromin, a 280 kDa protein with a central domain showing similarities to the GTPase activating protein (GAP) family that functions as a negative regulator of Ras [34, 35] by catalyzing the transition of active GTP-bound Ras to inactive GDP-bound Ras. Ras plays an important role in cell survival, proliferation, and differentiation by transducing responses from growth factor receptors at the cell surface to several intracellular signaling molecules. The main Ras-dependent downstream pathway involved in NF1 is the mitogen activated

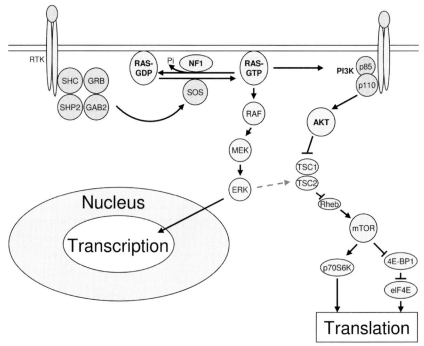

Figure 6.1 Neurofibromin is a negative regulator of cellular Ras and its downstream pathways Raf-MAPK-ERK, and PI3K-Akt-mTor.

protein kinase (MAPK) pathway including the kinases Raf, MEK1/2, and ERK1/2, which eventually alter the transcriptional program and the mammalian target of the rapamycin (mTOR) pathway (Figure 6.1). Aberrant mTOR activation is phosphatidylinositol-3-kinase (PI3K)-dependent and mediated by the phosphorylation and inactivation of the TSC2-encoded protein, tuberin, by AKT [36]. Taken together, increased Ras-GTP levels subsequent to loss of functional neurofibromin confer mitogen-induced cell proliferation by the Raf-MAPK-ERK and PI3K-Akt-mTOR axes. However, the Ras-GAP related domain (GRD) represents only a small proportion of the large *NF1* gene, hence it is conceivable that neurofibromin has also Ras-GAP-independent functions such as the regulation of intacellular cyclic AMP [37]. Furthermore, neurofibromin has been shown to associate with microtubules [38, 39] and with the actin-cytoskeleton upon phosphorylation by protein kinase C at phosphorylation sites contained in the cystein-rich domain [40].

6.2.2
The NF2 Gene and Its Gene Product Merlin

The *NF2* gene localized at 22q22.1 has been identified in 1993 [41, 42]. Biallelic mutations of *NF2* are the causal mechanism underlying all NF2 associated tumors (schwannomas, meningiomas, and ependymomas) as well as sporadic schwannomas, 50–60% of sporadic meningiomas, and a small proportion of sporadic ependymomas (reviewed in [43]). The *NF2* gene codes for Merlin (Moesin–Ezrin–Radixin-like-protein) that shows homology to members of the Ezrin–Radixin–Moesin (ERM) family. Merlin intcracts with components of adhesion-growth-factor-receptor complexes or signaling adaptors involved in vesicle trafficking, but none of these proteins has been shown to be necessary for Merlin-mediated tumor suppression. Therefore, it is assumed that the interaction partners function to recruit Merlin to various sub-cellular locations [44]. Merlin is involved in endocytic trafficking of membrane receptors, which commits these receptors to degradation in lysosomes. Thus, loss of Merlin function causes hyperactivation of pro-mitogenic signaling pathways. Furthermore, Merlin mediates contact inhibition in confluent cells by suppressing integrin-mediated recruitment of Rac to the plasma membrane. Merlin deficiency also leads to marked changes in the cell adhesion and in organization of the actin cytoskeleton most likely by Rac activation, thus promoting cell invasion. Taken together, Merlin seems to be involved in contact inhibition leading to neoplastic transformation, mitogenic signaling, and cell invasion, but the biochemical function of this protein is still elusive (reviewed in [44]).

6.2.3
INI1: The Familial Schwannomatosis Gene?

Several reports have shown biallelic NF2 gene inactivation in schwannomas of schwannomatosis patients [45, 46]. However, in a schwannomatosis patient, each schwannoma contains a completely different somatically acquired *NF2* mutation, usually in combination with loss of heterozygosity of the other *NF2* allele. This contrasts with NF2, where the same germline *NF2* mutation is found in every schwannoma in combination with a tumor specific somatic mutation in the other *NF2* allele. Moreover, linkage studies clearly excluded *NF2* from the candidate gene region mapped centromeric to the *NF2* locus on chromosome 22. This region harbors the *INI1* tumor suppressor gene. Recently, a father and his daughter, both affected with schwannomatosis, were shown to carry a truncating germline *INI1* mutation [47]. Taken together, the observation that a proportion of SCs of all tumors from these two patients showed loss of INI1 protein expression, and that silencing of the wildtype *INI1* allele was identified in 2/4 of their tumors, these findings indicate that *INI1* is the familial schwannomatosis gene in some families. However, further studies are needed to study the proportion of schwannomatosis patients and families with *INI1* germline mutations.

6.3
Genetic Testing

Adult NF1 patients usually fulfil the criteria for clinical diagnosis (Table 6.2). However, efficient and reliable genetic testing is very important for patients not fulfilling the NIH criteria, in particular young children with no family history of

NF1, patients with specific forms of NF1 (spinal NF, Noonan-NF), and patients in whom differential diagnosis is warranted. In particular, it is important to distinguish mild NF1 from the recently identified NF1-like syndrome caused by *SPRED 1* mutations [9], as well as to determine the genetic status of family members and to carry out prenatal or pre-implantation genetic diagnosis if desired. Mutation detection in the *NF1* gene is still a major task, due to: (i) the complex organization of this 57-exons gene; (ii) large parts of the 280-kb gene region are duplicated as pseudogenes in other regions of the genome; and (iii) the diverse spectrum of mutations ranging from large deletions, affecting the entire *NF1* locus and flanking genes (*NF1* micro-deletions) [48, 49], to minor-lesion mutations with a large number of unusual splicing mutations [50–52]. No single technique will identify all pathogenic lesions but comprehensive mutation analysis, applying a set of complementary techniques with a core assay that is based on the analysis of mRNA-transcripts of the *NF1* gene rather than genomic DNA, has shown to reach the highest mutation rates, identifying a clearly pathogenic lesion in 95% of non-founder NF1 patients fulfilling the criteria [51, 52].

In general, there is little genotype-phenotype correlation, and the clinical presentation can vary widely, even among members of a family carrying the same *NF1* mutation. So far the only exceptions are patients carrying a 3-bp deletion with a mild phenotype (see Clinical Diagnosis [5]), and the 5% NF1 patients with a micro-deletion who usually show a severe phenotype characterized by an early onset of neurofibromas, mild mental retardation, facial dysmorphism, childhood overgrowth [53], and an increased life-time risk of MPNSTs compared with the general NF1 population [54]. Of note, there are two major types of *NF1* micro-deletions, and patients carrying type-2 deletions, which are less frequent and slightly smaller than type-1 deletions, are mosaic cases in the first generation, while type-1 deletions are constitutional [55]. Owing to the mosaicism, type-2 deletion, patients frequently exhibit milder clinical manifestations [56], which have counseling implications, since the transmission of the type-2 deletion will lead to the severe *NF1* micro-deletion phenotype in the offspring who will carry the deletion constitutional. Conversely, the presence of a germline type-2 microdeletion in a severely affected child implies that one of the parents, in most of the cases the mother, is likely to carry the mutation in a mosaic state. This should be tested, to offer proper genetic counseling to the parents.

Whether the spectrum of *NF1* mutations in patients with SNF differs from that in classical NF1 patients is still under debate [57–60].

With improving therapeutic options for tumors arising in NF2 patients, testing is advocated in suspected NF2 patients and in individuals at risk for NF2. Reliable genetic testing is also relevant to carry out prenatal and pre-implantation genetic diagnosis if desired. Exon scanning techniques, including exon sequencing in combination with methods to identify DNA copy number alterations, achieve mutation rates of up to 91–100% in familial non-founder patients, but only about 60% in sporadic cases when analyzing blood lymphocytes [61, 62]. These figures reflect the fact that about 30% of sporadic NF2 patients are mosaic cases. Since the *NF2* mutation may be under-represented or absent in non-neoplatic tissue of these patients, it may escape detection when analyzing blood samples. However, recent reports show that analyzing material from multiple tumors can unambiguously identify the post-zygotic mosaic mutation in about 65% of these patients and, therefore, may significantly increase the mutation detection rates in founder NF2 patients [61, 62]. It is important to note that there is a risk of transmission of the mutation to the second generation for mosaic patients, and the clinical presentation is expected to be more severe in the offspring who will carry the mutation constitutionally. However, this risk is considerably reduced from $1:2$ to about $1:8$ for the offspring of mosaic patients [61].

Currently, *INI1* is the only gene for familial schwannomatosis. The analysis of a large number of schwannomatosis patients will uncover the frequency of *INI1* germline mutations in familial and sporadic schwannomatosis.

6.4
Clinical Manifestations

6.4.1
Tumors Arising in NF1 Patients

Neurofibromas that develop as focal cutaneous or subcutaneous lesions, spinal nerve root tumors, or plexiform neurofibromas, are typical for NF1, and almost all adult NF1 patients have neurofibromas.

Cutaneous neurofibromas usually start growing at puberty, and may increase in size and number throughout the entire lifetime. There have been no reports of cutaneous neurofibromas undergoing malignant transformation, and also subcutaneous neurofibromas rarely undergo malignant change [63].

Plexiform neurofibromas are thought to be congenital, and are present in about 30% of NF1 patients clinically, and in 50% by imaging. Plexiform neurofibromas develop along a nerve and involve multiple nerve branches. Growth of the tumor may cause pain and functional compromise. Plexiform neurofibromas are often highly vascularized and may cause soft tissue growth as well as bone hypertrophy. Removal is often challenging. Currently, there are several ongoing clinical trials to test the effects of different targeted therapies on the growth of plexiform neurofibromas, but the evidence so far is insufficient to conclude that any of these drugs are beneficial (for ongoing clinical trials see: http://www.ctf.org/research/nf1/. Plexiform and spinal neurofibromas have the risk of transforming into MPNSTs, which herald a poor prognosis.

MPNST develop in 8–13% NF1 patients during their lifetime [64]. Increased monitoring is recommended for NF1 patients who have plexiform neurofibroma and/or have been treated with radiotherapy, have a personal or family history of cancer, a *NF1* micro-deletion, high burden of internal neurofibromas, or neurofibromatous neuropathy [65]. Clinicians should be alerted when a patient develops unremitting pain, rapid increase in size of a plexiform neurofibroma, change in consistency from soft to hard, or a neurological deficit [66]. MRI should be

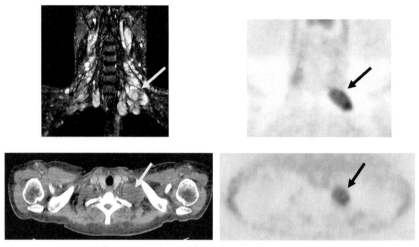

Figure 6.2 MRI (top left), CT-scan (lower left) and FDG-PET scan (top and lower right) images of a plexiform neurofibroma of the plexus brachialis, experiencing focal transformation to a malignant peripheral nerve sheath tumor (see arrows) in a patient carrying a *NF1* micro-deletion.

performed to locate the site, extent, and change in size of the plexiform neurofibroma, but it does not reliably detect malignant transformation. Fluorodeoxyglucose positron emission tomography (FDG-PET) has been shown as a sensitive and specific diagnostic tool to differentiate benign plexiform neurofibromas from MPNSTs. Furthermore, FDG-PET may also ensure that, in a heterogeneous lesion, the most active part of the tumor is biopsied. Therefore, FDG-PET constitutes a significant advance in the diagnosis of MPNST (see Figure 6.2) [67].

Optic pathway tumors (OPGs) are WHO grade I astrocytomas (i.e. pilocytic astrocytomas) that are seen in 15% of NF1 patients by imaging. However, only one-third of these tumors will cause clinical symptoms [68]. In general, OPGs in NF1 patients have a more indolent course than sporadic OPGs, which might at least partly be explained by the different genetic pathways involved [24, 69]. Treatment is recommended if there is clear evidence for tumor progression in symptomatic NF1-associated OPGs. Chemotherapy is the first-line therapy, and surgery is indicated only in cases with a large degree of proptosis and a blind or near-blind eye [70]. Radiotherapy should be avoided, since there are substantial risks of secondary malignancies in particular MPNSTs, cerebrovascular complications, and growth hormone deficiency after radiotherapy in NF1 patients (for review see [71]). It should be noted that signs of NF1 and malignant brain tumors in children, such as glioblastomas, are highly indicative of MMR-D syndrome, which should be considered as a differential diagnosis in such cases (see also Clinical Diagnosis NF1) [72].

Pheochromocytomas are catecholamine-secreting adrenal medulla tumors developing in 1–2% of NF1 patients. NF1 patients constitute approximately 3% of pheochromocytoma patients who occur also in conjunction with other inherited diseases, that is, multiple endocrine neoplasia type 2 (MEN2) (see Chapter 9 on hereditary medullary and familial nonmedullary thyroid crcinoma), von Hippel–Lindau disease, and hereditary pheochromocytoma and paraganglioma. NF1 associated pheochromocytomas are mainly adrenal tumors, of which 20% are multifocal and 12% are malignant [73]. The clinical presentation of pheochromocytoma includes hypertension and headaches, warranting a careful monitoring and examination in NF1 patients who also carry a higher risk for renal artery stenosis [74].

Juvenile myelomonocytic leukaemia (JMML) is a rare haematopoietic disorder of infancy and early childhood, for which NF1 patients have a 200 to 500-fold increased risk when compared to the general population. Therefore, about 11% of JMML patients have a clinical diagnosis of NF1 [75]. Of note, other haematological disorders, such as acute myeloid or lymphoid leukaemia, or lymphoma in young patients with CLS, are indicative of the recessive cancer predisposition syndrome, referred to as MMR-D syndrome here (see also Clinical Diagnosis NF1) [76]. Currently, allogenic haematopoietic stem cell transplantation is the only treatment modality for JMML, and offers a curative perspective for about 50% of patients.

Gastrointestinal stromal tumors (GISTs) are increasingly being recognized as belonging to the tumor spectrum of NF1 [25]. The interested reader is referred to Chapter 18 on GISTs in this book, which will discuss the underlying molecular events in NF1-associated GISTs, and the implications for treatment modalities, as well as the findings in patients with presumed intestinal neurofibromatosis [77].

Glomus tumors of the fingertips are also part of the NF1 tumor spectrum. The glomus organ in the fingertips is important for the thermo-perception and -regulation of the fingers. The presence of this small and nearly invisible tumor in NF1 patients can be very painful, especially in cold temperatures. The patients usually complain of pain for several years before the tumors are diagnosed and removed by simple surgery under local anaesthesia. It is important to realize that in NF1 patients, multiple fingertips can be affected [78].

For diagnosis and management of other clinical manifestations of NF1, we refer to guidelines given by Ferner and her colleagues [63].

6.4.2
Tumors Arising in NF2 Patients

Schwannomas are encapsulated tumors of pure SCs that usually do not experience malignant transformation. One in 1000 will be diagnosed with vestibular schwannoma (VS) in their lifetime, and about 7% of these patients have generalized or mosaic NF2 [11]. Pathologically, VS occurring in NF2 differ from sporadic tumors in that they are more lobular and have an increased meningothelial proliferation [79]. Other locations for schwannomas are the trigeminal nerve, the spinal nerve roots, and peripheral nerves with an estimated annual incidence of 1:4000 [16]. Approximately 13% of patients with spinal schwannomas have NF2 [80], and spinal-cord tumors have been reported in up to 90% of NF2 patients by neuroimaging, with the majority being asymptomatic [81].

There are three treatment options in VS of NF2 patients: (i) watchful waiting for tumors that are stable clinically and in neuroimaging; and (ii) microsurgery; or (iii) radiosurgery for large, symptomatic tumors. In general, so-called "gamma knife" radiosurgery seems to have better local tumor control rates, less hearing loss, and less involvement of facial nerves when compared to microsurgery (for review see [82]). Hence, recent reports also advocate radiation treatment for VS in NF2 patients, although they seem to profit less from this therapy than patients with sporadic unilateral tumors (for review see [15, 63]). Furthermore, since reports of an increased risk of malignant transformation and new primary tumors for irradiated as compared to unirradiated NF2 patients exists [71], physicians should exercise caution in strongly advocating radiation treatment for benign tumors in NF2, before valid long-term follow-up studies have been conducted [43, 83].

Meningiomas constitute up to 20–30% of all brain tumors and 5–15% of patients presenting with multiple meningiomas. Up to 20% of patients with multiple meningiomas may have NF2. Cranial meningiomas affecting 45% of NF2 patients are the major cause of mortality and morbidity (for review see [43]). MRI and surgery are the golden standard for enlarging or symptomatic tumors.

Ependymomas can be found in up to 6% of NF2 patients, usually in the brain-stem and upper cervical region. They remain quiescent for lengthy periods, but occasionally cause cord compression. In this case, complete resection or incomplete resection with low-grade adjuvant radiotherapy is recommended.

As for NF1, it is advisable that NF2 patients are treated in specialized centers which have a NF2 team, including a neurosurgeon, otolaryngologist, neurologist, geneticist, and audiologist [84]. NF2 patients now have realistic chances of having some serviceable hearing with an auditory brainstem implant [85]. Nevertheless, in discussing treatment options for NF2 patients, we always have to be aware that outcomes of surgery and radiosurgery are usually worse compared to spontaneous schwannomas and that the patient will usually develop multiple tumors.

6.5
Future Perspective/Translational Medicine

The Ras-MAPK pathway plays a central role for NF1-loss initiated tumor formation (see Section 6.2.1) and, hence appears to be a good target for therapeutic interventions. With the rationale to inhibit post-translational modifications, which are essential for normal Ras function, drugs that inhibit various enzymes responsible for the Ras farnesylation have been tested in clinical trials. Members of the statin family of drugs interfere with this modification by reducing the production of the lipid group donor, farnesyl pyrophosphate, an intermediate in the biosynthesis of cholesterol. Recently, statins have been discussed also as theraputics for non-neoplastic features of NF1, as lovastatin has been shown to rescue learning deficits in NF1 mouse models [86]. The effectiveness of lovastatin in improving learning difficulties of NF1 children is evaluated in ongoing clinical trials. Inhibitors of the farnesyl transferases (FTIs), such as lonarfarnib and tipifarnib, achieved promising results in preclinical trials. However, FTIs have shown only limited success in clinical trials. This may largely be explained by the fact that N- and K-Ras can alternatively be modified by geranylgeranyl transferases. Thus, even in the presence of FTIs, N- and K-Ras are able to function properly, at least to a certain degree. Furthermore, a drawback common to all therapeutic approaches interfering with the post-translational modification of Ras is the limited specificity of these drugs, since about 0.5% of all cellular proteins experience these modifications, and strong evidence supports the notion that the regulation of non-Ras targets at least contributes to the anti-cancer effects of these drugs (for review see [87]).

Downstream effectors and upstream activators of Ras may also be molecular targets for anti-tumor therapies in NF1. *In vivo* studies have shown that inhibitors of the downstream effectors of Ras, MEK1, 2, the p21-activated kinase (PAK), as well as PI3K and mTOR, are worth testing in clinical trials. The epidermal growth factor receptor (EGFR) expressed by MPNST cells, but absent from normal SCs, has been shown in different *in vivo* studies to be a promising target for anti-cancer drugs. Other members of the ErbB family of receptors such as ErbB2/neu may also serve as potential targets for therapies (for review see [87]) (see also Chapter 30 on molecular targeted therapy).

Viruses that are able to specifically infect and lyse cells with activated RAS signaling [88], the delivery of neurofibromin or parts of neurofibromin including the GAP-related domain to the cells, may be other potential treatment options.

Since there is strong evidence that also Merlin (the gene product of NF2) has an important role in growth factor receptor response, it is reasonable that the above-mentioned RAS/RAF/MEK, PI3K-AKT-mTOR pathways may also be targeted in NF2 associated tumors (for review see [43]).

References

1 DeBella, K., Szudek, J. and Friedman, J.M. (2000) Use of the national institutes of health criteria for diagnosis of neurofibromatosis 1 in children. *Pediatrics*, 105, 608–14.

2 National Institutes of Health Consensus Development Conference Statement (1988) Neurofibromatosis. Bethesda, Md., USA, July 13–15, 1987. *Neurofibromatosis*, 1, 172–8.

3 Korf, B.R. (1992) Diagnostic outcome in children with multiple café-au-lait spots. *Pediatrics*, 90, 924–7.

4 Rosenbaum, T., Engelbrecht, V., Krolls, W., van Dorsten, F.A., Hoehn-Berlage, M. and Lenard, H.G. (1999) MRI abnormalities in neurofibromatosis type 1 (NF1): a study of men and mice. *Brain and Development*, 21, 268–73.

5 Upadhyaya, M., Huson, S.M., Davies, M., Thomas, N., Chuzhanova, N., Giovannini, S., Evans, D.G., Howard, E., Kerr, B., Griffiths, S., Consoli, C., Side, L., Adams, D., Pierpont, M., Hachen, R., Barnicoat, A., Li, H., Wallace, P., Van Biervliet, J.P., Stevenson, D., Viskochil, D., Baralle, D., Haan, E., Riccardi, V., Turnpenny, P., Lazaro, C. and Messiaen, L. (2007) An absence of cutaneous neurofibromas associated with a 3-bp inframe deletion in exon 17 of the NF1 gene (c.2970–2972 delAAT): evidence of a clinically significant NF1 genotype-phenotype correlation. *American Journal of Human Genetics*, 80, 140–51.

6 Maertens, O., De Schepper, S., Vandesompele, J., Brems, H., Heyns, I., Janssens, S., Speleman, F., Legius, E. and

Messiaen, L. (2007) Molecular dissection of isolated disease features in mosaic neurofibromatosis type 1. *American Journal of Human Genetics*, **81**, 243–51.

7 Ruggieri, M. and Huson, S.M. (2001) The clinical and diagnostic implications of mosaicism in the neurofibromatoses. *Neurology*, **56**, 1433–43.

8 De Luca, A., Bottillo, I., Sarkozy, A., Carta, C., Neri, C., Bellacchio, E., Schirinzi, A., Conti, E., Zampino, G., Battaglia, A., Majore, S., Rinaldi, M.M., Carella, M., Marino, B., Pizzuti, A., Digilio, M.C., Tartaglia, M. and Dallapiccola, B. (2005) NF1 gene mutations represent the major molecular event underlying neurofibromatosis-Noonan syndrome. *American Journal of Human Genetics*, **77**, 1092–101.

9 Brems, H., Chmara, M., Sahbatou, M., Denayer, E., Taniguchi, K., Kato, R., Somers, R., Messiaen, L., De Schepper, S., Fryns, J.P., Cools, J., Marynen, P., Thomas, G., Yoshimura, A. and Legius, E. (2007) Germline loss-of-function mutations in SPRED1 cause a neuro-fibromatosis 1-like phenotype. *Nature Genetics*, **39**, 1120–6.

10 Felton, K.E., Gilchrist, D.M. and Andrew, S.E. (2007) Constitutive deficiency in DNA mismatch repair. *Clinical Genetics*, **71**, 483–98.

11 Evans, D.G., Moran, A., King, A., Saeed, S., Gurusinghe, N. and Ramsden, R. (2005) Incidence of vestibular schwannoma and neurofibromatosis 2 in the North West of England over a 10-year period: higher incidence than previously thought. *Otology and Neurotology*, **26**, 93–7.

12 Baser, M.E., Friedman, J.M., Wallace, A.J., Ramsden, R.T., Joe, H. and Evans, D.G. (2002) Evaluation of clinical diagnostic criteria for neurofibromatosis 2. *Neurology*, **59**, 1759–65.

13 Kluwe, L., Mautner, V., Heinrich, B., Dezube, R., Jacoby, L.B., Friedrich, R.E. and MacCollin, M. (2003) Molecular study of frequency of mosaicism in neurofibromatosis 2 patients with bilateral vestibular schwannomas. *Journal of Medical Genetics*, **40**, 109–14.

14 MacCollin, M., Chiocca, E.A., Evans, D.G., Friedman, J.M., Horvitz, R.,

Jaramillo, D., Lev, M., Mautner, V.F., Niimura, M., Plotkin, S.R., Sang, C.N., Stemmer-Rachamimov, A. and Roach, E.S. (2005) Diagnostic criteria for schwannomatosis. *Neurology*, **64**, 1838–45.

15 Hanemann, C.O. and Evans, D.G. (2006) News on the genetics, epidemiology, medical care and translational research of Schwannomas. *Journal of Neurology*, **253**, 1533–41.

16 Antinheimo, J., Sankila, R., Carpen, O., Pukkala, E., Sainio, M. and Jaaskelainen, J. (2000) Population-based analysis of sporadic and type 2 neurofibromatosis-associated meningiomas and schwannomas. *Neurology*, **54**, 71–6.

17 Viskochil, D., Buchberg, A., Xu, G., Cawthon, R., Stevens, J., Wolff, R., Culver, M., Carey, J., Copeland, N., Jenkins, N., White, R. and O'Connell, P. (1990) Deletions and a translocation interrupt a cloned gene at the neurofibromatosis type 1 locus. *Cell*, **62**, 187–92.

18 Wallace, M.R., Marchuk, D.A., Andersen, L.B., Letcher, R., Odeh, H.M., Saulino, A.M., Fountain, J.W., Brereton, A., Nicholson, J., Mitchell, A.L., Brownstein, B.H. and Collins, F.S. (1990) Type 1 neurofibromatosis gene: identification of a large transcript disrupted in three NF1 patients. *Science*, **249**, 181–6.

19 Knudson, A.G. Jr (1971) Mutation and cancer: statistical study of retinoblastoma. *Proceedings of the National Academy of Sciences of the United States of America*, **68**, 820–3.

20 Cichowski, K., Shih, T.S., Schmitt, E., Santiago, S., Reilly, K., McLaughlin, M.E., Bronson, R.T. and Jacks, T. (1999) Mouse models of tumor development in neurofibromatosis type 1. *Science*, **286**, 2172–6.

21 Jacks, T., Shih, T.S., Schmitt, E.M., Bronson, R.T., Bernards, A. and Weinberg, R.A. (1994) Tumor predisposition in mice heterozygous for a targeted mutation in Nf1. *Nature Genetics*, **7**, 353–61.

22 Legius, E., Marchuk, D.A., Collins, F.S. and Glover, T.W. (1993) Somatic deletion of the neurofibromatosis type 1 gene in a neurofibrosarcoma supports a tumor suppressor gene hypothesis. *Nature Genetics*, **3**, 122–6.

23 Shannon, K., O'Connell, P., Martin, G., Paderanga, D., Olson, K., Dinndorf, P. and McCormick, F. (1994) Loss of the normal NF1 allele from the bone marrow of children with type 1 neurofibromatosis and malignant myeloid disorders. *The New England Journal of Medicine*, **330**, 597–601.

24 Kluwe, L., Hagel, C., Tatagiba, M., Thomas, S., Stavrou, D., Ostertag, H., von Deimling, A. and Mautner, V.F. (2001) Loss of NF1 alleles distinguish sporadic from NF1-associated pilocytic astrocytomas. *Journal of Neuropathology and Experimental Neurology*, **60**, 917–20.

25 Maertens, O., Prenen, H., Debiec-Rychter, M., Wozniak, A., Sciot, R., Pauwels, P., De Wever, I., Vermeesch, J.R., de Raedt, T., De Paepe, A., Speleman, F., van Oosterom, A., Messiaen, L. and Legius, E. (2006) Molecular pathogenesis of multiple gastrointestinal stromal tumors in NF1 patients. *Human Molecular Genetics*, **15**, 1015–23.

26 Xu, W., Mulligan, L.M., Ponder, M.A., Liu, L., Smith, B.A., Mathew, C.G.P. and Ponder, B.A.J. (1992) Loss of *NFI* alleles in pheochromocytomas from patients with type I neurofibromatosis. *Genes Chromosomes Cancer*, **4**, 337–42.

27 Rosenbaum, T., Rosenbaum, C., Winner, U., Muller, H.W., Lenard, H.G. and Hanemann, C.O. (2000) Long-term culture and characterization of human neurofibroma-derived Schwann cells. *Journal of Neuroscience Research*, **61**, 524–32.

28 Serra, E., Rosenbaum, T., Winner, U., Aledo, R., Ars, E., Estivill, X., Lenard, H.G. and Lazaro, C. (2000) Schwann cells harbor the somatic NF1 mutation in neurofibromas: evidence of two different Schwann cell subpopulations. *Human Molecular Genetics*, **9**, 3055–64.

29 Kourea, H.P., Cordon-Cardo, C., Dudas, M., Leung, D. and Woodruff, J.M. (1999) Expression of p27(kip) and other cell cycle regulators in malignant peripheral nerve sheath tumors and neurofibromas: the emerging role of p27(kip) in malignant transformation of neuro-fibromas. *American Journal of Pathology*, **155**, 1885–91.

30 Kourea, H.P., Orlow, I., Scheithauer, B.W., Cordon-Cardo, C. and Woodruff, J.M. (1999) Deletions of the INK4A gene occur in malignant peripheral nerve sheath tumors but not in neurofibromas. *American Journal of Pathology*, **155**, 1855–60.

31 Legius, E., Dierick, H., Wu, R., Hall, B.K., Marynen, P., Cassiman, J.J. and Glover, T.W. (1994) TP53 mutations are frequent in malignant NF1 tumors. *Genes Chromosomes Cancer*, **10**, 250–5.

32 De Schepper, S., Maertens, O., Callens, T., Naeyaert, J.M., Lambert, J. and Messiaen, L. (2008) Somatic Mutation Analysis in NF1 Café-au-lait Spots Reveals Two NF1 Hits in the Melanocytes. *The Journal of Investigative Dermatology*, **128**, 1050–3.

33 Stevenson, D.A., Zhou, H., Ashrafi, S., Messiaen, L.M., Carey, J.C., D'Astous, J.L., Santora, S.D. and Viskochil, D.H. (2006) Double inactivation of NF1 in tibial pseudarthrosis. *American Journal of Human Genetics*, **79**, 143–8.

34 Martin, G.A., Viskochil, D., Bollag, G., McCabe, P.C., Crosier, W.J., Haubruck, H., Conroy, L., Clark, R., O'Connell, P., Cawthon, R.M., Innis, M.A. and McCormick, F. (1990) The GAP-related domain of the neurofibromatosis type 1 gene product interacts with ras p21. *Cell*, **63**, 843–9.

35 Xu, G., Lin, B., Tanaka, K., Dunn, D., Wood, D., Gesteland, R., White, R., Weiss, R. and Tamanoi, F. (1990) The catalytic domain of the neurofibromatosis type 1 gene product stimulates *ras* GTPase and complements *ira* mutants of S. cerevisiae. *Cell*, 835–44.

36 Johannessen, C.M., Reczek, E.E., James, M.F., Brems, H., Legius, E. and Cichowski, K. (2005) The NF1 tumor suppressor critically regulates TSC2 and mTOR. *Proceedings of the National Academy of Sciences of the United States of America*, **102**, 8573–8.

37 Dasgupta, B., Dugan, L.L. and Gutmann, D.H. (2003) The neurofibromatosis 1 gene product neurofibromin regulates pituitary adenylate cyclase-activating polypeptide-mediated signaling in astrocytes. *The Journal of Neuroscience*, **23**, 8949–54.

38 Gregory, P.E., Gutmann, D.H., Mitchell, A., Park, S., Boguski, M., Jacks, T., Wood,

D.L., Jove, R. and Collins, F.S. (1993) Neurofibromatosis type 1 gene product (neurofibromin) associates with micro-tubules. *Somatic Cell and Molecular Genetics*, **19**, 265–74.

39 Xu, H. and Gutmann, D.H. (1997) Mutations in the GAP-related domain impair the ability of neurofibromin to associate with microtubules. *Brain Research*, **759**, 149–52.

40 Mangoura, D., Sun, Y., Li, C., Singh, D., Gutmann, D.H., Flores, A., Ahmed, M. and Vallianatos, G. (2006) Phosphory-lation of neurofibromin by PKC is a possible molecular switch in EGF receptor signaling in neural cells. *Oncogene*, **25**, 735–45.

41 Rouleau, G.A., Merel, P., Lutchman, M., Sanson, M., Zucman, J., Marineau, C., Hoang-Xuan, K., Demczuk, S., Desmaze, C., Plougastel, B. *et al.* (1993) Alteration in a new gene encoding a putative membrane-organizing protein causes neuro-fibromatosis type 2. *Nature*, **363**, 515–21.

42 Trofatter, J.A., MacCollin, M.M., Rutter, J.L., Murrell, J.R., Duyao, M.P., Parry, D.M., Eldridge, R., Kley, N., Menon, A. G., Pulaski, K. *et al.* (1993) A novel moesin-, ezrin-, radixin-like gene is a candidate for the neurofibromatosis 2 tumor suppressor. *Cell*, **72**, 791–800.

43 Hanemann, C.O. (2008) Magic but treatable? Tumours due to loss of Merlin. *Brain*, **131**, 606–15.

44 Okada, T., You, L. and Giancotti, F.G. (2007) Shedding light on Merlin's wizardry. *Trends in Cell Biology*, **17**, 222–9.

45 Jacoby, L.B., MacCollin, M., Barone, R., Ramesh, V. and Gusella, J.F. (1996) Frequency and distribution of NF2 mutations in schwannomas. *Genes Chromosomes Cancer*, **17**, 45–55.

46 Kaufman, D.L., Heinrich, B.S., Willett, C., Perry, A., Finseth, F., Sobel, R.A. and MacCollin, M. (2003) Somatic instability of the NF2 gene in schwannomatosis. *Archives of Neurology*, **60**, 1317–20.

47 Hulsebos, T.J., Plomp, A.S., Wolterman, R.A., Robanus-Maandag, E.C., Baas, F. and Wesseling, P. (2007) Germline mutation of INI1/SMARCB1 in familial schwannomatosis. *American Journal of Human Genetics*, **80**, 805–10.

48 De Raedt, T., Brems, H., Lopez-Correa, C., Vermeesch, J.R., Marynen, P. and Legius, E. (2004) Genomic organization and evolution of the NF1 microdeletion region. *Genomics*, **84**, 346–60.

49 Jenne, D.E., Tinschert, S., Dorschner, M.O., Hameister, H., Stephens, K. and Kehrer-Sawatzki, H. (2003) Complete physical map and gene content of the human NF1 tumor suppressor region in human and mouse. *Genes Chromosomes Cancer*, **37**, 111–20.

50 Ars, E., Serra, E., García, J., Kruyer, H., Gaona, A., Lázaro, C. and Estivill, X. (2000) Mutations affecting mRNA splicing are the most common molecular defects in patients with neurofibromatosis type 1. *Human Molecular Genetics*, **9**, 237–47.

51 Messiaen, L., Callens, T., Mortier, G., Beysen, D., Vandenbroucke, I., Van Roy, N., Speleman, F. and De Paepe, A. (2000) Exhaustive mutation analysis of the NF1 gene allows identification of 95% of mutations and reveals a high frequency of unusual splicing defects. *Human Mutation*, **15**, 541–55.

52 Wimmer, K., Roca, X., Beiglbock, H., Callens, T., Etzler, J., Rao, A.R., Krainer, A.R., Fonatsch, C. and Messiaen, L. (2007) Extensive in silico analysis of NF1 splicing defects uncovers determinants for splicing outcome upon 5′ splice-site disruption. *Human Mutation*, **28**, 599–612.

53 Mensink, K.A., Ketterling, R.P., Flynn, H.C., Knudson, R.A., Lindor, N.M., Heese, B.A., Spinner, R.J. and Babovic-Vuksanovic, D. (2006) Connective tissue dysplasia in five new patients with NF1 microdeletions: further expansion of phenotype and review of the literature. *Journal of Medical Genetics*, **43**, e8.

54 De Raedt, T., Brems, H., Wolkenstein, P., Vidaud, D., Pilotti, S., Perrone, F., Mautner, V., Frahm, S., Sciot, R. and Legius, E. (2003) Elevated risk for MPNST in NF1 microdeletion patients. *American Journal of Human Genetics*, **72**, 1288–92.

55 Senger, C., Serra, E., Lazaro, C., Gilaberte, M., Wimmer, K., Mautner, V. and Kehrer-Sawatzki, H. (2007) Type 2 NF1 deletions are highly unusual by virtue of the absence of nonallelic homologous recombination hotspots and an apparent preference for female mitotic recombination. *American Journal of Human Genetics*, **81**, 1201–20.

56 Kehrer-Sawatzki, H., Kluwe, L., Sandig, C., Kohn, M., Wimmer, K., Krammer, U., Peyrl, A., Jenne, D.E., Hansmann, I. and Mautner, V.F. (2004) High frequency of mosaicism among patients with neurofibromatosis type 1 (NF1) with microdeletions caused by somatic recombination of the JJAZ1 gene. *American Journal of Human Genetics*, **75**, 410–23.

57 Ars, E., Kruyer, H., Gaona, A., Casquero, P., Rosell, J., Volpini, V., Serra, E., Lazaro, C. and Estivill, X. (1998) A clinical variant of neurofibromatosis type 1: familial spinal neurofibromatosis with a frameshift mutation in the NF1 gene. *American Journal of Human Genetics*, **62**, 834–41.

58 Kaufmann, D., Muller, R., Bartelt, B., Wolf, M., Kunzi-Rapp, K., Hanemann, C.O., Fahsold, R., Hein, C., Vogel, W. and Assum, G. (2001) Spinal neuro-fibromatosis without café-au-lait macules in two families with null mutations of the NF1 gene. *American Journal of Human Genetics*, **69**, 1395–400.

59 Kluwe, L., Tatagiba, M., Funsterer, C. and Mautner, V.F. (2003) NF1 mutations and clinical spectrum in patients with spinal neurofibromas. *Journal of Medical Genetics*, **40**, 368–71.

60 Messiaen, L., Riccardi, V., Peltonen, J., Maertens, O., Callens, T., Karvonen, S.L., Leisti, E.L., Koivunen, J., Vandenbroucke, I., Stephens, K. and Poyhonen, M. (2003) Independent NF1 mutations in two large families with spinal neuro-fibromatosis. *Journal of Medical Genetics*, **40**, 122–6.

61 Evans, D.G., Ramsden, R.T., Shenton, A., Gokhale, C., Bowers, N.L., Huson, S.M., Pichert, G. and Wallace, A. (2007) Mosaicism in neurofibromatosis type 2: an update of risk based on uni/bilaterality of vestibular schwannoma at presentation and sensitive mutation analysis including multiple ligation-dependent probe amplification. *Journal of Medical Genetics*, **44**, 424–8.

62 Kluwe, L., Nygren, A.O., Errami, A., Heinrich, B., Matthies, C., Tatagiba, M. and Mautner, V. (2005) Screening for large mutations of the NF2 gene. *Genes Chromosomes Cancer*, **42**, 384–91.

63 Ferner, R.E., Huson, S.M., Thomas, N., Moss, C., Willshaw, H., Evans, D.G., Upadhyaya, M., Towers, R., Gleeson, M., Steiger, C. and Kirby, A. (2007) Guidelines for the diagnosis and management of individuals with neurofibromatosis 1. *Journal of Medical Genetics*, **44**, 81–8.

64 Evans, D.G., Baser, M.E., McGaughran, J., Sharif, S., Howard, E. and Moran, A. (2002) Malignant peripheral nerve sheath tumours in neurofibromatosis 1. *Journal of Medical Genetics*, **39**, 311–4.

65 Ferner, R.E., Hughes, R.A., Hall, S.M., Upadhyaya, M. and Johnson, M.R. (2004) Neurofibromatous neuropathy in neurofibromatosis 1 (NF1). *Journal of Medical Genetics*, **41**, 837–41.

66 Ferner, R.E. and Gutmann, D.H. (2002) International consensus statement on malignant peripheral nerve sheath tumors in neurofibromatosis. *Cancer Research*, **62**, 1573–7.

67 Ferner, R.E., Golding, J.F., Smith, M., Calonje, E., Jan, W., Sanjayanathan, V. and O'Doherty, M. (2008) [18F]2-fluoro-2-deoxy-D-glucose positron emission tomography (FDG PET) as a diagnostic tool for neurofibromatosis 1 (NF1) associated malignant peripheral nerve sheath tumours (MPNSTs): a long-term clinical study. *Annals of Oncology*, **19**, 390–4.

68 Listernick, R., Darling, C., Greenwald, M., Strauss, L. and Charrow, J. (1995) Optic pathway tumors in children: the effect of neurofibromatosis type 1 on clinical manifestations and natural history. *The Journal of Pediatrics*, **127**, 718–22.

69 Wimmer, K., Eckart, M., Meyer-Puttlitz, B., Fonatsch, C. and Pietsch, T. (2002) Mutational and expression analysis of the NF1 gene argues against a role as tumor suppressor in sporadic pilocytic astro-cytomas. *Journal of Neuropathology and Experimental Neurology*, **61**, 896–902.

70 Listernick, R., Ferner, R.E., Liu, G.T. and Gutmann, D.H. (2007) Optic pathway gliomas in neurofibromatosis-1:

controversies and recommendations. *Annals of Neurology*, **61**, 189–98.

71 Evans, D.G., Birch, J.M., Ramsden, R.T., Sharif, S. and Baser, M.E. (2006) Malignant transformation and new primary tumours after therapeutic radiation for benign disease: substantial risks in certain tumor prone syndromes. *Journal of Medical Genetics*, **43**, 289–94.

72 Etzler, J., Peyrl, A., Zatkova, A., Schildhaus, H.-U., Ficek, A., Merkelbach-Bruse, S., Kratz, C.P., Attarbaschi, A., Hainfellner, J.A., Yao, S., Messiaen, L., Slavc, I. and Wimmer, K. (2008) RNA-based mutation analysis identifies an unusual MSH6 splicing defect and circumvents PMS2 pseudogene interference. *Hum Mutation*, **29**, 299–305.

73 Bausch, B., Borozdin, W. and Neumann, H.P. (2006) Clinical and genetic characteristics of patients with neurofibromatosis type 1 and pheochromocytoma. *The New England Journal of Medicine*, **354**, 2729–31.

74 Friedman, J.M., Arbiser, J., Epstein, J.A., Gutmann, D.H., Huot, S.J., Lin, A.E., McManus, B. and Korf, B.R. (2002) Cardiovascular disease in neurofibromatosis 1: report of the NF1 cardiovascular task force. *Genetics in Medicine*, **4**, 105–11.

75 Niemeyer, C.M. and Locatelli, F. (2006) Chronic myeloproliferative disorders, in *Childhood Leukemias* (ed. C.H. Pui), Cambridge University Press, New York, pp. 571–98.

76 Kratz, C.P., Niemeyer, C.M., Juttner, E., Kartal, M., Weninger, A., Schmitt-Graeff, A., Kontny, U., Lauten, M., Utzolino, S., Radecke, J., Fonatsch, C. and Wimmer, K. (2008) Childhood T-cell non-Hodgkin's lymphoma, colorectal carcinoma and brain tumor in association with café-au-lait spots caused by a novel homozygous PMS2 mutation. *Leukemia*, **22**, 1078–80.

77 de Raedt, T., Cools, J., Debiec-Rychter, M., Brems, H., Mentens, N., Sciot, R., Himpens, J., de Wever, I., Schoffski, P., Marynen, P. and Legius, E. (2006) Intestinal neurofibromatosis is a subtype of familial GIST and results from a dominant activating mutation in PDGFRA. *Gastroenterology*, **131**, 1907–12.

78 De Smet, L., Sciot, R. and Legius, E. (2002) Multifocal glomus tumours of the fingers in two patients with neurofibromatosis type 1. *Journal of Medical Genetics*, **39**, e45.

79 Sobel, R.A. (1993) Vestibular (acoustic) schwannomas: histologic features in neurofibromatosis 2 and in unilateral cases. *Journal of Neuropathology and Experimental Neurology*, **52**, 106–13.

80 Evans, D.G., Huson, S.M., Donnai, D., Neary, W., Blair, V., Newton, V. and Harris, R. (1992) A clinical study of type 2 neurofibromatosis. *The Quarterly Journal of Medicine*, **84**, 603–18.

81 Mautner, V.F., Lindenau, M., Baser, M.E., Hazim, W., Tatagiba, M., Haase, W., Samii, M., Wais, R. and Pulst, S.M. (1996) The neuroimaging and clinical spectrum of neurofibromatosis 2. *Neurosurgery*, **38**, 880–5. Discussion 885–6.

82 Mathieu, D., Kondziolka, D., Flickinger, J.C., Niranjan, A., Williamson, R., Martin, J.J. and Lunsford, L.D. (2007) Stereotactic radiosurgery for vestibular schwannomas in patients with neurofibromatosis type 2: an analysis of tumor control, complications, and hearing preservation rates. *Neurosurgery*, **60**, 460–8. discussion 468–70.

83 Ferner, R.E. (2007) Neurofibromatosis 1 and neurofibromatosis 2: a twenty first century perspective. *Lancet Neurology*, **6**, 340–51.

84 Evans, D.G., Baser, M.E., O'Reilly, B., Rowe, J., Gleeson, M., Saeed, S., King, A., Huson, S.M., Kerr, R., Thomas, N., Irving, R., MacFarlane, R., Ferner, R., McLeod, R., Moffat, D. and Ramsden, R. (2005) Management of the patient and family with neurofibromatosis 2: a consensus conference statement. *British Journal of Neurosurgery*, **19**, 5–12.

85 Shapiro, W.H., Golfinos, J.G., Cohen, N.L. and Roland, J.T. Jr, Kanowitz, S.J., (2004) Auditory brainstem implantation in patients with neurofibromatosis type 2. *Laryngoscope*, **114**, 2135–46.

86 Li, W., Cui, Y., Kushner, S.A., Brown, R.A., Jentsch, J.D., Frankland, P.W., Cannon, T.D. and Silva, A.J. (2005) The HMG-CoA reductase inhibitor lovastatin reverses the learning and attention deficits in a mouse model of neurofibromatosis type 1. *Current Biology*, **15**, 1961–7.

87 Dilworth, J.T., Kraniak, J.M., Wojtkowiak, J.W., Gibbs, R.A., Borch, R.F., Tainsky, M.A., Reiners, J.J. Jr and Mattingly, R.R. (2006) Molecular targets for emerging anti-tumor therapies for neurofibromatosis type 1. *Biochemical Pharmacology*, **72**, 1485–92.

88 Coffey, M.C., Strong, J.E., Forsyth, P.A. and Lee, P.W. (1998) Reovirus therapy of tumors with activated ras pathway. *Science*, **282**, 1332–4.

7
Retinoblastoma: The Prototypic Hereditary Tumor

Helen Dimaras and Brenda L. Gallie

Summary

As the first cancer to be described as a genetic disease, retinoblastoma represents the prototypic hereditary tumor. This childhood retinal cancer is initiated by the loss of the *RB1* tumor suppressor gene, which has important clinical implications, as highly sensitive mutation detection of mutant *RB1* alleles within families accurately identifies individuals at high risk for retinoblastoma and excludes those with normal *RB1* and thus directs costly and intense treatment and surveillance only to those who require it.

The unique molecular fingerprint of retinoblastoma can be correlated to clinical and histopathological stage. Loss of *RB1* initially leads to development of the benign tumor, retinoma. Further genetic insults are necessary for progression to malignancy, including gains of oncogenes *NMYC*, *KIF14*, *E2F3*, and/or *DEK*, and loss of tumor suppressor genes *CDH11* and $p75^{NTR}$.

7.1
Introduction

Retinoblastoma was recognized more than a century ago to be a heritable cancer. As soon as patients could be cured by surgical removal of the eye(s) affected by retinoblastoma, they survived to have children also affected by retinoblastoma [1]. However, only as genomic science came into the forefront was it recognized that retinoblastoma is not unique, but rather the prototype for the genetic disease called cancer [2, 3].

The retinoblastoma gene (*RB1*) was the first tumor suppressor gene to be identified [4]. Cytogenetically detectable large deletions of chromosome 13q14 pointed to the locus [5], and recognition that both alleles were mutated in the tumors [6] led to identification of the DNA fragment completely deleted from one tumor [7]. This clone turned out to be within an exon of *RB1* [4]. Clinical translation with precise identification of mutant alleles in each family has enhanced quality of

Hereditary Tumors: From Genes to Clinical Consequences
Edited by Heike Allgayer, Helga Rehder and Simone Fulda
Copyright © 2009 WILEY-VCH Verlag GmbH & Co. KGaA, Weinheim
ISBN: 978-3-527-32028-8

clinical care for affected children and decreased morbidity and healthcare costs for those removed from invasive clinical surveillance.

Although initially *RB1* loss was thought to cause retinoblastoma, it is now clear that retinoma is an *RB1*$^{-/-}$ premalignant precursor that often precedes the genomic changes observed with full malignancy. The somatic *RB1* second mutant allele in the tumor, and subsequent genomic signature of individual retinoblastoma tumors are now being explored for molecular monitoring for metastatic disease.

7.2
Clinical Features

The rare childhood retinal cancer retinoblastoma (OMIM#180200) affects between 1 in 22 000 to 1 in 15 000 children worldwide [8]. Parents commonly first observe a white reflection in pupil of the eye, called leukocoria (Figure 7.1A). At this early

(B)

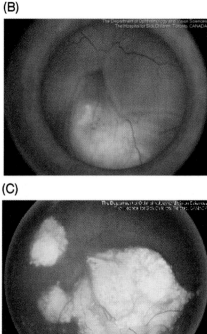

(A)

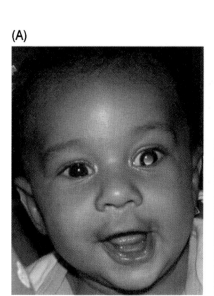

(C)

Figure 7.1 Child with leukocoria. (A) Retinoblastoma first is noted when leukocoria is noticed by parents, often now on digital images of the baby. (Image courtesy of Daisy's Eye Cancer Fund, www.daisyseyecancerfund.org). (B) Total retinal detachment is caused by calcified growing retinoblastoma. (C) After chemotherapy, calcified tumor remains but the retina is reattached; laser and cryotherapy will control residual and small recurrences.

stage, the tumor is usually contained within the eye and curable by surgery or combinations of treatments that may save the eye(s). One or both eyes may be independently affected. All children with bilateral retinoblastoma, and 15% of children with unilateral retinoblastoma have a constitutional *RB1* mutation that is commonly novel and not inherited, but heritable by future offspring. Rarely, the children with *RB1* constitutional mutations also develop intracranial tumors, called trilateral retinoblastoma. Eighty five percent of unilaterally affected children without a family history have no constitutional *RB1* mutation.

Worldwide, removal of the eye with advanced retinoblastoma is an excellent treatment to cure retinoblastoma, as long as the tumor has not spread outside the eye [9]. When one eye tumor is normal, removal of the affected eye is the most certain way to a cure. When both eyes are affected, removal of eyes threatening extraocular extension is recommended, but eyes with smaller and less invasive retinoblastoma can be treated by chemotherapy followed by cryotherapy and laser, or cryotherapy and laser alone for small tumors, eliminating the tumor and saving

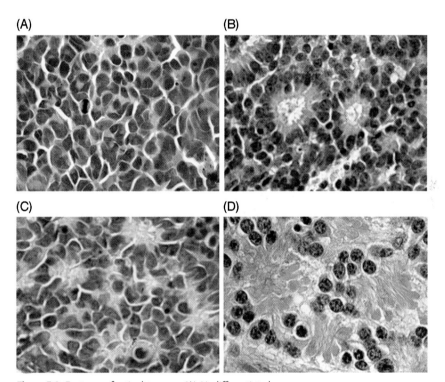

Figure 7.2 Features of retinal tumors. (A) Undifferentiated retinoblastoma consists of dense tissue with compact cells, nuclear moulding, and little cytoplasm. Differentiation in retinoblastomas takes the form of either (B) Flexner–Wintersteiner rosettes or (C) Homer Wright rosettes while retinomas specifically display (D) fleurettes.

at least one eye in many children (Figure 7.1B and C). There is room for better therapies that can save more eyes, and still avoid exposure of young children to high treatment-induced morbidity.

Retinoblastomas are composed of highly proliferative, often undifferentiated, basophilic cells with hyperchromatic nuclei and little cytoplasm [10]. The cells grow in a characteristic cobblestone pattern, the result of nuclear moulding [11, 12] (Figure 7.2A). Abundant mitoses, extensive necroses and highly characteristic calcification are commonly present. Growth of retinoblastoma in a perivascular ring forms "pseudorosettes", with the cells most distant from the blood supply demonstrating necrosis.

The most specific pattern of differentiation in retinoblastoma is the Flexner–Wintersteiner rosette [13] (Figure 7.2): a ring of cuboidal or wedge-shaped cells surround largely empty central lumen into which they extend small cytoplasmic projections [10]. Flexner–Wintersteiner rosettes are characteristic of retino-blastoma, but are also observed in pineoblastoma and medulloepithelioma [14]) where they may also represent an attempt at retinal differentiation. This theory is supported by electron microscopy (EM) studies that reveal retinal photoreceptor cell features [11] and hyaluronidase-resistant staining of the lumen, due to the presence of acid mucopolysaccaride, similar to the outer segments of photoreceptors [15].

The Homer Wright rosettes are commonly observed in retinoblastoma, repre-senting neuronal differentiation, as in many neural tumors. These rosettes show a central tangle of neuronal processes that intertwine and may force the cell bodies to the outer edges of the structure [14] (Figure 7.2C).

Fleurettes describe a linear arrangement of cells with bulbous processes of vari-able length, creating a structure that resembles the *Fleur-de-Lys,* from which its name is derived [11]. By EM, fleurettes display properties of retinal photoreceptor cells (Figure 7.2D). It was noted that the fleurette-rich portion of irradiated tumors changed very little, compared to the cell death and calcification of undifferentiated retinoblastoma, leading to the idea that fleurettes were "radiation resistant" [12]. Others suggested that fleurettes might actually result from the radiation, a type of forced differentiation, or regression. It is now clear that fleurettes are not a feature of proliferative retinoblastoma, but of the non-proliferative precursor, retinoma [16, 17].

7.3
Clinical Retinoma

After study of a number of adult, non-phthisical eyes that were considered to be spontaneously regressed retinoblastoma, it was suggested that they might actually be examples of spontaneously *arrested* retinoblastoma, and the term "retinoma" was proposed to describe these lesions [18]. Retinoma was clinically defined as an elevated, gray, translucent mass displaying calcification similar in appearance to cottage cheese, a hyperplastic pigment epithelium, and importantly, no evidence of regression [18]. Later, cases of retinoma were found to be associated with vitreous seeding [19], a feature previously thought to be specific only to malignant tumors.

Retinoma is rarely clinically observed (1.8% of retinoblastoma cases [18]) and treatment is not required since it is non-proliferative and usually poses no immediate threat to the affected individual's well-being. However, some cases of retinoma have been shown to progress to retinoblastoma [20–22], necessitating routine examination of retinoma-affected eyes. Specimens of retinoma are usually not available for histopathological assessment because they are enucleated only when they progress to retinoblastoma.

However, from rare cases of retinoma that were removed as therapy, the histopathological features were identified as abundant fleurettes without any type of rosettes, eosinophilic cytoplasm, rare foci of calcification, and a lack of mitoses and necroses were noted features of the same type of lesion as retinomas [23]. Using these histopathological features as markers, we recently showed that retinoma is present in 16% of eyes enucleated for retinoblastoma [16, 17].

7.4
Nature of Susceptible Retinal Cell

Key to understanding cancer is knowledge of the unique properties of the normal somatic cell that becomes susceptible to malignant transformation. Early histopathological studies of retinoblastoma suggested a glial cell of origin, hence the original name for the disease, "glioma of the retina". However, markers of numerous cell types are expressed by retinoblastoma. The cell of origin of retinoblastoma has a developmentally limited existence: before birth 50% of infants with an *RB1* mutant allele will already have one tumor, then develop more over the first years, but after about 3 years, new tumors stop emerging. Therefore a multipotent retinal progenitor cell is the best candidate for the retinoblastoma cell of origin, which would account for promiscuous expression of cell type markers in retinoblastoma.

7.5
Progression from Normal Retina to Retinoblastoma

7.5.1
Tumor Initiation: Bi-Allelic Inactivation of *RB1*

Individuals with heritable retinoblastoma (40% of cases) carry an *RB1* constitutional mutation (M1) and have lost the second allele (M2) in the emerging tumors [2, 3, 24]. Non-hereditary retinoblastoma tumors (50% of cases) also have somatic loss of both *RB1* alleles (M1/M2), but neither of these mutant alleles is detected in constitutional cells. Although M1 and M2 mutational events are necessary for

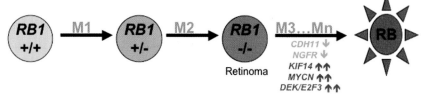

Figure 7.3 The molecular genetic progression of retina to retinoma and retinoblastoma. Retinoblastomas are initiated by the loss of both *RB1* alleles (M1 and M2). M1 commonly arises as a new mutation, unique in each family; M2 arises in each individual clone to initiate retinoma. Progression to retinoblastoma is driven by further events, M3-Mn, which provide selective advantage and increasing autonomy of cancer.

tumor initiation, they are not sufficient for malignant progression; further genetic insults (M3-Mn events) are required (Figure 7.3).

7.5.1.1 Types of *RB1* Mutations

The *RB1* gene is composed of 27 exons and the promoter region located on chromosome 13q14. The range of *RB1* mutations is great, as there is virtually an infinite number of ways to inactivate the gene. More than a thousand distinct *RB1* mutations have been identified [24, 25], including exonic and whole gene deletions (leading to frameshifts or loss of the entire gene, respectively) and point mutations (causing splicing defects, missense, or nonsense mutations) (Table 7.1). Clinical genetic tests can now identity 94% of mutant *RB1* alleles (www. retinoblastomasolutions.org) (Table 7.2). This knowledge enables precise screening of family members to determine their individual risk to develop retinoblastoma or transmit the dominant trait [26]. Clinical *RB1* mutation identification dramatically enhances care for families, since only children truly at risk for tumors, because of a constitutional *RB1* mutation, need clinical surveillance. Those children shown to not have the family's *RB1* mutant allele need no further examinations [24, 27].

7.5.1.2 Penetrance and Expressivity of *RB1* Mutations

The common *RB1* mutations result in no protein and show high penetrance and expressivity (multiple tumors) with 99% of persons at risk to develop retinoblastoma, usually in both eyes. Trilateral retinoblastoma is not associated with any particular constitutional *RB1* mutation type. Some families show low penetrance disease, related to *RB1* gene mutations (specific, splicing defects, promoter mutations, missense mutations) that permit some residual protein function [28], resulting in fewer tumors forming.

Low penetrance retinoblastoma also can result from mosaicism. The novel *RB1* mutation may occur in a multi-cell stage embryo, rather than in the initial germ cell. Such individuals will carry an *RB1* mutation in only a fraction of their cells. While only 4% of bilateral retinoblastoma patients show constitutional mosaicism,

Table 7.1 Types of *RB1* mutant alleles in blood of bilaterally affected probands, retinoblastoma tumors, and non-familial unilaterally affected probands who had constitutional mutant alleles found in blood. (Data from Retinoblastoma Solutions, January 2007).

Class of *RB1* mutation	Bilateral	Tumor alleles (250 × 2)	Unilateral germline
Small insertions/deletions	76 (23%)	55 (16%)	11 (16%)
Recurrent nonsense	79 (24%)	102 (29%)	18 (26%)
Other nonsense	49 (15%)	33 (9%)	3 (4%)
Splice	58 (17%)	40 (11%)	8 (12%)
Whole exon deletions/duplications	56 (17%)	73 (21%)	16 (24%)
Missense	13 (4%)	5 (1.5%)	11 (16%)
Regulatory	2 (<1%)	1	1 (1%)
Methylation promoter	0	41 (12%)	
Total (excluding LOH)		350	
LOH		150 alleles (60% of tumors) *179 alleles (71% of tumors)	
Total alleles	333	500	68

*Includes LOH due to deletion of one copy of the *RB1* gene.

25% of unilaterally affected individuals with no family history are now shown to be mosaic.

Later in life, individuals carrying a constitutional *RB1* mutant allele are at increased risk to develop other cancers [29–32] The relative risk (RR) to develop retinoblastoma due to a null constitutional *RB1* mutation is more than 40 000. The RR for trilateral retinoblastoma increased in the era of external beam radiation for intraocular disease to about 650, compared to 100 in the earlier part of the century [33–36]. The RR up to 30 for osteosarcoma and soft tissue sarcomas is radiation-dose dependent [37]. Melanoma, bladder, lung, and other cancers carry a risk greater for *RB1* mutation carriers than the normal population over a lifetime [31].

7.5.1.3 *RB1* Loss and Retinoma

Retinoma has been observed in individuals who carry one mutant *RB1* allele [18, 22, 38–42]. Retinoma is described to developing into retinoblastoma after an initial period of clinical dormancy [20–22]. Retinomas have been observed in parents and grandparents of children with retinoblastoma [41, 43–45], and in children with retinoblastoma in the same or opposite eye [22, 38, 44].

However, we observed 16% of eyes removed for retinoblastoma to contain non-proliferative retinoma adjacent to the retinoblastoma. We have shown absence of

Table 7.2 Sensitivity to find *RB1* mutant alleles in clinical samples (blood for bilateral and familial retinoblastoma, tumor if available for unilateral retinoblastoma with no family history). Of all identified germline *RB1* mutations the fraction in which the proband is mosaic differs for bilaterally affected probands (3%) and unilaterally affected probands (25%). (Data from Retinoblastoma Solutions, September 2007).

	Number of families studied	Mutations fully identified	Sensitivity	Germline	Germline mosaic (% of all germline)
Bilateral	397	374	94.2%	NA	11(3%)
Unilateral blood + family history	25	23	92%		NA
Isolated unilateral with tumor	346	317	91.6%	45 (13%)	11/44 (25%)
Total sensitivity	768	714	92.9%		
Isolated unilateral with NO tumor (blood)	152	20	NA	20 (13.2%)	5/20 (25%)
Total analyzed	920				

functional protein product of the *RB1* (pRB) gene with the identical M2 mutant alleles in retinomas and the adjacent retinoblastomas, indicating clonal progression from retina (normal or M1) to retinoma to *RB1* with identical M1 and M2 [16, 17].

The rarity of clinically observed retinoma indicates that malignant progression is a rapid and highly likely transition. The rare cases of retinoma that do not progress must be arrested in some manner. Unlike retina and retinoblastoma, retinoma expresses p16^{INK4a} [16, 17], a protein involved in regulating cellular arrest, or senescence, upon oncogenic stimulation [46–48]. It is possible that a reversal of the senescent state in retinoma, by disruption of the p16^{INK4a} pathway, could promote the progression to retinoblastoma from retinoma, as observed in gastrointestinal cancer [49] and melanoma [50].

7.5.2
Tumor Progression: Post-*RB1* Genomic Changes in Retinoblastoma

Most retinoblastoma tumors contain gross genomic changes in addition to *RB1* loss (M3-Mn), as identified by comparative genomic hybridization (CGH) [51–58].

Common regions of gain and loss were identified at chromosomal arm 1q31-32 (>47% gain) [59], 2p24 (30% gain) [53], 6p22 (44% gain) [53], and 16q22 (31% loss) [60]. These chromosomal regions were narrowed using Quantitative Multiplex Polymerase Chain Reaction (QM-PCR) to identify candidate oncogenes and tumor suppressor genes that may contribute to tumor progression in *RB1*[-/-] cells [61]. In addition to genes identified by genomic gains and losses, other important events have been identified by the candidate gene approach.

7.5.2.1 Genomic Gain at Chromosome 1q
QM-PCR on chromosome 1 identified a minimal region of gain at 1q32.1 [59]. This region contained 12 genes, but expression analysis of all 12 pointed to *KIF14* (Gene ID: 9928) as a potential oncogene, as its expression by quantitative real-time Reverse Transcription Polymerase Chain Reaction (qRT-PCR) was up to 1000-fold higher in retinoblastoma compared to unaffected retina. KIF14 is a mitotic kinesin [62], and its overexpression in tumors may cause overactive cell division that contributes to the expansion of tumor cells. Further data implicating *KIF14* as a potent oncogene are correlation of expression level with higher tumor grade and worse outcome in lung [63] and breast cancers [64], and genomic amplification in one retinoblastoma [65].

Another gene implicated at chromosome 1 is *MDM4*, an inhibitor of the transcriptional activity of p53. MDM4 is gained in a subset of retinoblastoma tumors [66]. Further study is required to discover if one or both candidate genes on 1q are important for retinoblastoma progression.

7.5.2.2 Genomic Gain of 2p: *NMYC*
The commonly gained chromosomal arm 2p was narrowed to 2p24, known to harbor the neuroblastoma oncogene *NMYC* (Gene ID: 4613) [67]. As with neuroblastoma, the Y79 retinoblastoma cell line displayed *NMYC* amplification. *NMYC* has been assumed to be the retinoblastoma 2p oncogene [68, 69]. Further study of the potential function of overexpression of *NMYC* or other 2p genes, in retinoblastoma, is required.

7.5.2.3 Genomic Gain at Chromosome 6p
The gain at chromosome 6p was first identified as an isochromosome [51] and the most common region of gain later narrowed down to 6p22 [53]. Initial studies pinpointed a novel kinesin, coined RBKIN (*KIF13A*, Gene ID: 63971), as a potential oncogene at this site [70]. However, subsequent studies identified *DEK* (Gene ID: 7913) and *E2F3* (Gene ID: 1871) as candidate oncogenes, because they are expressed at higher levels in retinoblastoma than retina [58, 71]. How DEK and E2F3 might function when overexpressed in retinoblastoma is unclear. E2F3 is involved in cell cycle entry [72, 73], thus it could play a role in the enhanced proliferation of tumor cells. On the other hand, DEK, a nuclear protein [74] with diverse functions including chromatin remodeling [75], mRNA splicing [76], and transcription regulation [77], has been implicated as an oncogene in many cancers,

including leukemia, where the gene is translocated [78]. Recently, E2F3 was found to regulate *DEK* [79], thus the two may be acting cooperatively to enhance tumorigenesis in the retina. Evidence supporting this comes from targeted disruption of either gene by siRNA in retinoblastoma cell lines with 6p22 gain; knockdown of DEK causes considerable cell death, and knockdown of either DEK or E2F3 decreases cellular growth rates [80].

7.5.2.4 Genomic Loss at Chromosome 16q

Chromosome 16 loss was narrowed to region 16q22, containing two potential tumor suppressor genes, *CDH11* (Gene ID: 1009) and *CDH13* (Gene ID: 1012) [60]. Subsequent expression analysis identified *CDH11* as the potential tumor suppressor gene as it was expressed in the retina but either decreased or was not expressed in 91% of retinoblastoma studied, unlike *CDH13* which was ubiquitously expressed [60] and not mutated in retinoblastoma tumors [81]. *CDH11* belongs to the cadherin family of proteins, which are thought to function in cellular adhesion [82], thus its loss in retinoblastoma could contribute to vitreous seeding, the most difficult kind of intraocular retinoblastoma to treat. Furthermore, data from a murine model of retinoblastoma indicates *CDH11* loss could lead to increased rates of tumor proliferation [83], implying a multi-faceted role for *CDH11* as a retinoblastoma tumor suppressor.

7.5.2.5 Cell Death Regulator p53

The default process in many tissues, that lose *RB1* expression, is cell death. However, in the retina, loss of *RB1* commonly progresses to cancer. It was logical to assume then, that a defect in a cell death pathway was responsible for the survival of the mutant $RB1^{-/-}$ cells. Early on, scientists pinpointed the well-known cell death regulator p53 (Gene ID: 7157) as a candidate tumor suppressor in retinoblastoma, however no strong evidence has emerged to support this hypothesis. Rare retinoblastoma cells do show detectable levels of p53, however this does not suggest mutant protein, as radiation of retinoblastoma cell lines shows normal upregulation of p53. Furthermore, no p53 mutations have been detected in either cell lines or primary retinoblastoma tumors. This does not exclude the possibility that a defect exists elsewhere in the p53 regulatory pathway.

7.5.2.6 *NGFR/p75^NTR*

The *p75^NTR* neurotrophin receptor (*NGFR*, Gene ID: 4804) was identified as a potential retinoblastoma tumor suppressor, considering its role in developmental retinal cell death. Indeed, p75^NTR was found to be expressed in normal retina and retinoma, but lost in retinoblastoma [84]. In a murine model of retinoblastoma, p75^NTR was lost as tumors progressed, which correlated with a decrease in apoptosis [84]. Indeed, mice with complete inactivation of p75^NTR, at the onset of retinoblastoma development, developed larger tumors than controls [17].

7.6
Conclusions

The loss of both *RB1* alleles in a susceptible developing retinal cell results in failure of normal differentiation and the formation of retinoma with distinctive non-proliferative fleurette formation. Commonly retinoma progresses to malignant retinoblastoma, with the addition of genomic imbalance proto-oncogenes and tumor suppressor genes. Specifically, gain of *KIF14, DEK*, and *E2F3*, and loss of *CDH11* and p75^{NTR} expression differentiate retinoblastoma from retinoma, excellent targets for future therapeutic intervention.

RB1 clinical mutation detection has achieved 94% sensitivity to find each family's *RB1* mutant allele(s) in tumor or constitutional cells. This permits accurate determination of which infants have high risk for retinoblastoma, who then receive intense surveillance to control emerging tumors early, and which infants do not carry the family's *RB1* mutant allele and need no further intervention. Such precise health care has excellent outcomes and costs less than conventional surveillance of all untested at-risk infant relatives and frees resources to optimize care for the children with retinoblastoma. The distinctive genomic fingerprint of the retinoblastoma in each child also is an opportunity for high sensitivity molecular surveillance for metastases.

References

1 Albert, D.M. (1987) Historic review of retinoblastoma. *Ophthalmology*, **94** (6), 654–62.

2 Comings, D.E. (1973) A general theory of carcinogenesis. *Proceedings of the National Academy of Sciences of the United States of America*, **70** (12), 3324–8.

3 Knudson, A.G. (1971) Mutation and cancer: statistical study of retinoblastoma. *Proceedings of the National Academy of Science of the United States of America*, **68** (4), 820–3.

4 Friend, S.H., Bernards, R., Rogelj, S., Weinberg, R.A., Rapaport, J.M., Albert, D.M. and Dryja, T.P. (1986) A human DNA segment with properties of the gene that predisposes to retinoblastoma and osteosarcoma. *Nature*, 16–22; **323** (6089), 643–6.

5 Yunis, E., Zuniga, R. and Ramirez, E. (1981) Retinoblastoma, gross internal malformations, and deletion 13q14 leads to q31. *Human Genetics*, **56** (3), 283–6.

6 Cavenee, W.K., Dryja, T.P., Phillips, R.A., Benedict, W.F., Godbout, R., Gallie, B.L., Murphree, A.L., Strong, L.C. and White, R.L. (1983) Expression of recessive alleles by chromosomal mechanisms in retinoblastoma. *Nature*, **305** (5937), 779–84.

7 Dryja, T.P., Rapaport, J.M., Joyce, J.M. and Petersen, R.A. (1986) Molecular detection of deletions involving band q14 of chromosome 13 in retinoblastomas. *Proceedings of the National Academy of Science of the United States of America*, **83** (19), 7391–4.

8 MacCarthy, A., Draper, G.J., Steliarova-Foucher, E. and Kingston, J.E. (2006) Retinoblastoma incidence and survival in European children (1978–1997). Report from the Automated Childhood Cancer Information System project. *European Journal of Cancer*, **42** (13), 2092–102.

9 Gallie, B.L., Zhao, J., Vandezande, K., White, A. and Chan, H.S. (2007) Global issues and opportunities for optimized retinoblastoma care. *Pediatric Blood and Cancer*, **49** (7 Suppl), 1083–90.

10 Ts'o, M.O., Fine, B.S. and Zimmerman, L.E. (1969) The Flexner-Wintersteiner rosettes in retinoblastoma. *Archives of Pathology*, **88** (6), 664–71.

11 Ts'o, M.O., Fine, B.S. and Zimmerman, L.E. (1970) The nature of retinoblastoma. II. Photoreceptor differentiation: an electron microscopic study. *American Journal of Ophthalmology*, **69** (3), 350–9.

12 Ts'o, M.O., Zimmerman, L.E. and Fine, B.S. (1970) The nature of retinoblastoma. I. Photoreceptor differentiation: a clinical and histopathologic study. *American Journal of Ophthalmology*, **69** (3), 339–49.

13 Wintersteiner, H. (1897) *Die Neuro-pithelioma Retinae. Eine Anatomische und Klinische Studie*, Dentisae, Leipzig.

14 Wippold, F.J.2nd and Perry, A. (2006) Neuropathology for the neuroradiologist: rosettes and pseudorosettes. *American Journal of Neuroradiology*, **27** (3), 488–92.

15 Zimmerman, L.E. (1985) Retinoblastoma and retinocytoma, in *Ophthalmic Pathology: An Atlas and Textbook*, 3rd edn (ed. W.H. Spencer), W.B. Saunders Company, Philadelphia, pp. 1292–348.

16 Dimaras, H., Khetan, V., Halliday, W., Orlic, M., Prigoda, N.L., Piovesan, B., Marrano, P., Corson, T.W., Eagle, R.C. Jr., Squire, J.A. and Gallie, B.L. (2008) Loss of RB1 induces non-proliferative retinoma: increasing genomic instability correlates with progression to retinoblastoma. *Human Molecular Genetics*, **17** (10), 1363–72.

17 Dimaras, H. (2007) *The Molecular Progression from Retina through Retinoma to Retinoblastoma and the Role of the P75NTR Neurotrophin Receptor*, University of Toronto, Toronto.

18 Gallie, B.L., Ellsworth, R.M., Abramson, D.H. and Phillips, R.A. (1982) Retinoma: spontaneous regression of retinoblastoma or benign manifestation of the mutation? *British Journal of Cancer*, **45** (4), 513–21.

19 Lueder, G.T., Heon, E. and Gallie, B.L. (1995) Retinoma associated with vitreous seeding. *American Journal of Ophthal-mology*, **119** (4), 522–3.

20 Eagle, R.C. Jr , Shields, J.A., Donoso, L. and Milner, R.S. (1989) Malignant transformation of spontaneously regressed retinoblastoma, retinoma/ retinocytoma variant. *Ophthalmology*, **96** (9), 1389–95.

21 Balmer, A., Munier, F. and Gailloud, C. (1991) Retinoma. Case studies. *Ophthalmic Paediatrics and Genetics*, **12** (3), 131–7.

22 Santos, C.M., Shields, C.L., Shields, J.A. and Eagle, R.C. Jr, Singh, A.D., (2000) Observations on 17 patients with retinocytoma. *Archives of Ophthalmology*, **118** (2), 199–205.

23 Margo, C., Hidayat, A., Kopelman, J. and Zimmerman, L.E. (1983) Retinocytoma. A benign variant of retinoblastoma. *Archives of Ophthalmology*, **101**, 1519–31.

24 Richter, S., Vandezande, K., Chen, N., Zhang, K., Sutherland, J., Anderson, J., Han, L., Panton, R., Branco, P. and Gallie, B. (2003) Sensitive and efficient detection of RB1 gene mutations enhances care for families with retinoblastoma. *American Journal of Human Genetics*, **72** (2), 253–69.

25 Valverde, J.R., Alonso, J., Palacios, I. and Pestana, A. (2005) RB1 gene mutation up-date, a meta-analysis based on 932 reported mutations available in a searchable database. *BMC Genetics*, **6**, 53.

26 Albrecht, P., Ansperger-Rescher, B., Schuler, A., Zeschnigk, M., Gallie, B. and Lohmann, D.R. (2005) Spectrum of gross deletions and insertions in the RB1 gene in patients with retinoblastoma and association with phenotypic expression. *Human Mutation*, **26** (5), 437–45.

27 Houdayer, C., Gauthier-Villars, M., Lauge, A., Pages-Berhouet, S., Dehainault, C., Caux-Moncoutier, V., Karczynski, P., Tosi, M., Doz, F., Desjardins, L., Couturier, J. and Stoppa-Lyonnet, D. (2004) Comprehensive screening for constitutional RB1 mutations by DHPLC and QMPSF. *Human Mutation*, **23** (2), 193–202.

28 Lohmann, D. and Gallie, B.L. (2007) Retinoblastoma, in GeneReviews at GeneTests: Medical Genetics Information Resource (database online) Copyright (ed. C. Dolan), University of Washington, Seattle, 1997–2007. Available at http:// wwwgenetests.org.

29 Eng, C., Li, F.P., Abramson, D.H., Ellsworth, R.M., Wong, F.L., Goldman, M.B., Seddon, J. and Boice, J.D. (1993) Mortality from second tumors among long-term survivors of retinoblastoma.

Journal of the National Cancer Institute, **85** (*14*), 1121–8.

30 Draper, G.J., Sanders, B.M. and Kingston, J.E. (1986) Second primary neoplasms in patients with retinoblastoma. *British Journal of Cancer*, **53** (*5*), 661–71.

31 Fletcher, O., Easton, D., Anderson, K., Gilham, C., Jay, M. and Peto, J. (2004) Lifetime risks of common cancers among retinoblastoma survivors. *Journal of the National Cancer Institute*, **96** (*5*), 357–63.

32 Tucker, M.A., Abramson, D.H., Seddon, J.M., Tarone, R.E. and Fraumeni, J.F. Jr, Kleinerman, R.A., (2007) Risk of soft tissue sarcomas by individual subtype in survivors of hereditary retinoblastoma. *Journal of the National Cancer Institute*, **99** (*1*), 24–31.

33 De Potter, P., Shields, C.L. and Shields, J.A. (1994) Clinical variations of trilateral retinoblastoma: a report of 13 cases. *Journal of Pediatric Ophthalmology and Strabismus*, **31** (*1*), 26–31.

34 Kivela, T. (1999) Trilateral retinoblastoma: a meta-analysis of hereditary retinoblastoma associated with primary ectopic intracranial retinoblastoma. *Journal of Clinical Oncology*, **17** (*6*), 1829–37.

35 Lueder, G.T., Judisch, G.F. and Wen, B.C. (1991) Heritable retinoblastoma and pinealoma. *Archives of Ophthalmology*, **109** (*12*), 1707–9.

36 Paulino, A.C. (1999) Trilateral retinoblastoma: is the location of the intracranial tumor important? *Cancer*, **86** (*1*), 135–41.

37 Wong, F.L., Boice, J.D. Jr , Abramson, D.H., Tarone, R.E., Kleinerman, R.A., Stovall, M., Goldman, M.B., Seddon, J.M., Tarbell, N., Fraumeni, J.F. Jr and Li, F.P. (1997) Cancer incidence after retinoblastoma. Radiation dose and sarcoma risk. *JAMA*, **278** (*15*), 1262–7.

38 Keith, C.G. and Webb, G.C. (1985) Retinoblastoma and retinoma occurring in a child with a translocation and deletion of the long arm of chromosome 13. *Archives of Ophthalmology*, **103** (*7*), 941–4.

39 Yilmaz, S., Horsthemke, B. and Lohmann, D.R. (1998) Twelve novel RB1 gene mutations in patients with hereditary retinoblastoma. Mutations in brief no. 206. Online. *Human Mutation*, **12** (*6*), 434.

40 Munier, F.L., Thonney, F., Balmer, A., Heon, E., Pescia, G. and Schorderet, D.F. (1996) Sex mutation ratio in retinoblastoma and retinoma: relevance to genetic counseling. *Klin Monatsbl Augenheilkd*, **208** (*5*), 400–3.

41 Sampieri, K., Hadjistilianou, T., Mari, F., Speciale, C., Mencarelli, M.A., Cetta, F., Manoukian, S., Peissel, B., Giachino, D., Pasini, B., Acquaviva, A., Caporossi, A., Frezzotti, R., Renieri, A. and Bruttini, M. (2006) Mutational screening of the RB1 gene in Italian patients with retinoblastoma reveals 11 novel mutations. *Journal of Human Genetics*, **51** (*3*), 209–16.

42 Theodossiadis, P., Emfietzoglou, I., Grigoropoulos, V., Moschos, M. and Theodossiadis, G.P. (2005) Evolution of a retinoma case in 21 years. *Ophthalmic Surgery, Lasers and Imaging*, **36** (*2*), 155–7.

43 Messmer, E.P., Richter, H.J., Hopping, W., Havers, W. and Alberti, W. (1987) Non-ocular, malignant secondary tumor following spontaneous healing of a retinoblastoma ("retinoma", "retinocytoma"). *Klinische Monatsblätter für Augenheilkünde*, **191** (*4*), 299–303.

44 Marrakchi, S., Bouguila, H., Ghorbal, M., Ben Osman, N., Munier, F. and Ayed, S. (1995) Regressive bilateral retinoblastoma. Clinical and genetic study. Apropos of a case. *Journal Francais D'ophtalmologie*, **18** (*5*), 390–5.

45 Kiratli, H. and Bilgic, S. (2006) Multiple bilateral retinomas. A case study. *Journal Francais D'ophtalmologie*, **29** (*1*), 58–60.

46 Collado, M., Gil, J., Efeyan, A., Guerra, C., Schuhmacher, A.J., Barradas, M., Benguria, A., Zaballos, A., Flores, J.M., Barbacid, M., Beach, D. and Serrano, M. (2005) Tumour biology: senescence in premalignant tumours. *Nature*, **436** (*7051*), 642.

47 Braig, M., Lee, S., Loddenkemper, C., Rudolph, C., Peters, A.H., Schlegelberger, B., Stein, H., Dorken, B., Jenuwein, T. and Schmitt, C.A. (2005) Oncogene-induced senescence as an initial barrier in lymphoma development. *Nature*, **436** (*7051*), 660–5.

48 Braig, M. and Schmitt, C.A. (2006) Oncogene-induced senescence: putting the brakes on tumor development. *Cancer Research*, **66** (*6*), 2881–4.

49 Sabah, M., Cummins, R., Leader, M. and Kay, E. (2004) Loss of heterozygosity of chromosome 9p and loss of p16INK4A expression are associated with malignant gastrointestinal stromal tumors. *Modern Pathology*, **17** (*11*), 1364–71.

50 Radhi, J.M. (1999) Malignant melanoma arising from nevi, p53, p16, and Bcl-2: expression in benign versus malignant components. *Journal of Cutaneous Medicine and Surgery*, **3** (*6*), 293–7.

51 Squire, J., Phillips, R.A., Boyce, S., Godbout, R., Rogers, B. and Gallie, B.L. (1984) Isochromosome 6p, a unique chromosomal abnormality in retinoblastoma: verification by standard staining techniques, new densitometric methods, and somatic cell hybridization. *Human Genetics*, **66** (*1*), 46–53.

52 Mairal, A., Pinglier, E., Gilbert, E., Peter, M., Validire, P., Desjardins, L., Doz, F., Aurias, A. and Couturier, J. (2000) Detection of chromosome imbalances in retinoblastoma by parallel karyotype and CGH analyses. *Genes Chromosomes and Cancer*, **28** (*4*), 370–9.

53 Chen, D., Gallie, B.L. and Squire, J.A. (2001) Minimal regions of chromosomal imbalance in retinoblastoma detected by comparative genomic hybridization. *Cancer Genetics and Cytogenetics*, **129** (*1*), 57–63.

54 Herzog, S., Lohmann, D.R., Buiting, K., Schuler, A., Horsthemke, B., Rehder, H. and Rieder, H. (2001) Marked differences in unilateral isolated retinoblastomas from young and older children studied by comparative genomic hybridization. *Human Genetics*, **108** (*2*), 98–104.

55 Lillington, D.M., Kingston, J.E., Coen, P.G., Price, E., Hungerford, J., Domizio, P., Young, B.D. and Onadim, Z. (2003) Comparative genomic hybridization of 49 primary retinoblastoma tumors identifies chromosomal regions associated with histopathology, progression, and patient outcome. *Genes Chromosomes and Cancer*, **36** (*2*), 121–8.

56 van der Wal, J.E., Hermsen, M.A., Gille, H.J., Schouten-Van Meeteren, N.Y., Moll, A.C., Imhof, S.M., Meijer, G.A., Baak, J.P. and van der Valk, P. (2003) Comparative genomic hybridisation divides retinoblastomas into a high and a low level chromosomal instability group. *Journal of Clinical Pathology*, **56** (*1*), 26–30.

57 Zielinski, B., Gratias, S., Toedt, G., Mendrzyk, F., Stange, D.E., Radlwimmer, B., Lohmann, D.R. and Lichter, P. (2005) Detection of chromosomal imbalances in retinoblastoma by matrix-based comparative genomic hybridization. *Genes Chromosomes and Cancer*, **43** (*3*), 294–301.

58 Grasemann, C., Gratias, S., Stephan, H., Schuler, A., Schramm, A., Klein-Hitpass, L., Rieder, H., Schneider, S., Kappes, F., Eggert, A. and Lohmann, D.R. (2005) Gains and overexpression identify DEK and E2F3 as targets of chromosome 6p gains in retinoblastoma. *Oncogene*, **24** (*42*), 6441–49.

59 Corson, T. and Gallie, B. (2005) KIF14 is a candidate oncogene in the 1q minimal region of genomic gain in retinoblastoma. *Proceedings of the 15th Meeting of the International Society for Genetic Eye Disease, the 12th International Retinoblastoma Symposium, and the 12th International Congress of Ocular Oncology, Whistler*, 15.

60 Marchong, M.N., Chen, D., Corson, T.W., Lee, C., Harmandayan, M., Bowles, E., Chen, N. and Gallie, B.L. (2004) Minimal 16q genomic loss implicates cadherin-11 in retinoblastoma. *Molecular Cancer Research*, **2** (*9*), 495–503.

61 Corson, T.W. and Gallie, B.L. (2007) One hit, two hits, three hits, more? Genomic changes in the development of retinoblastoma. *Genes Chromosomes and Cancer*, **46** (*7*), 617–34.

62 Gruneberg, U., Neef, R., Li, X., Chan, E.H., Chalamalasetty, R.B., Nigg, E.A. and Barr, F.A. (2006) KIF14 and citron kinase act together to promote efficient cytokinesis. *The Journal of Cell Biology*, **172** (*3*), 363–72.

63 Corson, T.W., Zhu, C.Q., Lau, S.K., Shepherd, F.A., Tsao, M.S. and Gallie, B.L. (2007) KIF14 messenger RNA expression is independently prognostic for outcome in lung cancer. *Clinical Cancer Research*, **13** (*11*), 3229–34.

64 Corson, T.W. and Gallie, B.L. (2006) KIF14 mRNA expression is a predictor of grade and outcome in breast cancer. *International Journal of Cancer*, **119** (*5*), 1088–94.

65 Bowles, E., Corson, T.W., Bayani, J., Squire, J.A., Wong, N., Lai, P.B. and Gallie, B.L. (2007) Profiling genomic copy number changes in retinoblastoma beyond loss of RB1. *Genes Chromosomes and Cancer*, **46** (*2*), 118–29.

66 Laurie, N.A., Donovan, S.L., Shih, C.S., Zhang, J., Mills, N., Fuller, C., Teunisse, A., Lam, S., Ramos, Y., Mohan, A., Johnson, D., Wilson, M., Rodriguez-Galindo, C., Quarto, M., Francoz, S., Mendrysa, S.M., Guy, R.K., Marine, J.C., Jochemsen, A.G. and Dyer, M.A. (2006) Inactivation of the p53 pathway in retinoblastoma. *Nature*, **444** (*7115*), 61–6.

67 Brodeur, G.M. and Saylors, R.L. (1991) Neuroblastoma, retinoblastoma, and brain tumors in children. *Current Opinion in Oncology*, **3** (*3*), 485–96.

68 Squire, J., Goddard, A.D., Canton, M., Becker, A., Phillips, R.A. and Gallie, B.L. (1986) Tumour induction by the retinoblastoma mutation is independent of N-*myc* expression. *Nature*, **322** (*6079*), 555–7.

69 Squire, J.A., Thorner, P.S., Weitzman, S., Maggi, J.D., Dirks, P., Doyle, J., Hale, M. and Godbout, R. (1995) Co-amplification of MYCN and a DEAD box gene (DDX1) in primary neuroblastoma. *Oncogene*, **10** (*7*), 1417–22.

70 Chen, D., Pajovic, S., Duckett, A., Brown, V.D., Squire, J.A. and Gallie, B.L. (2002) Genomic amplification in retinoblastoma narrowed to 0.6 megabase on chromosome 6p containing a kinesin-like gene, RBKIN. *Cancer Research*, **62** (*4*), 967–71.

71 Orlic, M., Spencer, C.E., Wang, L. and Gallie, B.L. (2006) Expression analysis of 6p22 genomic gain in retinoblastoma. *Genes Chromosomes and Cancer*, **45** (*1*), 72–82.

72 Adams, M.R., Sears, R., Nuckolls, F., Leone, G. and Nevins, J.R. (2000) Complex transcriptional regulatory mechanisms control expression of the E2F3 locus. *Molecular and Cellular Biology*, **20** (*10*), 3633–9.

73 Leone, G., Nuckolls, F., Ishida, S., Adams, M., Sears, R., Jakoi, L., Miron, A.

and Nevins, J.R. (2000) Identification of a novel E2F3 product suggests a mechanism for determining specificity of repression by Rb proteins. *Molecular and Cellular Biology*, **20** (*10*), 3626–32.

74 Kappes, F., Burger, K., Baack, M., Fackelmayer, F.O. and Gruss, C. (2001) Subcellular localization of the human proto-oncogene protein DEK. *The Journal of Biological Chemistry*, **276** (*28*), 26317–23.

75 Alexiadis, V., Waldmann, T., Andersen, J., Mann, M., Knippers, R. and Gruss, C. (2000) The protein encoded by the proto-oncogene DEK changes the topology of chromatin and reduces the efficiency of DNA replication in a chromatin-specific manner. *Genes and Development*, **14** (*11*), 1308–12.

76 McGarvey, T., Rosonina, E., McCracken, S., Li, Q., Arnaout, R., Mientjes, E., Nickerson, J.A., Awrey, D., Greenblatt, J., Grosveld, G. and Blencowe, B.J. (2000) The acute myeloid leukemia-associated protein, DEK, forms a splicing-dependent interaction with exon-product complexes. *The Journal of Cell Biology*, **150** (*2*), 309–20.

77 Campillos, M., Garcia, M.A., Valdivieso, F. and Vazquez, J. (2003) Transcriptional activation by AP-2alpha is modulated by the oncogene DEK. *Nucleic Acids Research*, **31** (*5*), 1571–5.

78 von Lindern, M., Breems, D., van Baal, S., Adriaansen, H. and Grosveld, G. (1992) Characterization of the translocation breakpoint sequences of two DEK-CAN fusion genes present in t(6;9) acute myeloid leukemia and a SET-CAN fusion gene found in a case of acute undifferentiated leukemia. *Genes Chromosomes and Cancer*, **5** (*3*), 227–34.

79 Carro, M.S., Spiga, F.M., Quarto, M., Di Ninni, V., Volorio, S., Alcalay, M. and Muller, H. (2006) DEK Expression is controlled by E2F and deregulated in diverse tumor types. *Cell Cycle*, **5** (*11*), 1202–7.

80 Orlic, M. (2007) *Identification of the 6p22 Oncogene in Retinoblastoma*, University of Toronto.

81 Gratias, S., Rieder, H., Ullmann, R., Klein-Hitpass, L., Schneider, S., Boloni, R., Kappler, M. and Lohmann, D.R. (2007) Allelic loss in a minimal region on

chromosome 16q24 is associated with vitreous seeding of retinoblastoma. *Cancer Research*, **67** (*1*), 408–16.

82 Gumbiner, B.M. (1996) Cell adhesion: the molecular basis of tissue architecture and morphogenesis. *Cell*, **84** (*3*), 345–57.

83 Marchong, M. (2007) *Identification of CDH11 as a Candidate Tumor Suppressor in Retinoblastoma and Characterization of its Role in Retina and Retinoblastoma*, University of Toronto.

84 Dimaras, H., Coburn, B., Pajovic, S. and Gallie, B.L. (2006) Loss of p75 neurotrophin receptor expression accompanies malignant progression to human and murine retinoblastoma. *Molecular Carcinogenesis*, **45** (*5*), 333–43.

8
Hereditary Cancer in the Head and Neck

Barbara Wollenberg

Summary

Several studies have been conducted to investigate genetic mechanisms in cancer origin and pathogenesis, in head and neck cancer. The idea behind this was to detect specific chromosomal defects in normal cells of cancer patients and their first degree relatives, to intensify the possibilities for prevention or early detection, if not even new therapeutic strategies, for these cancers. Up to the current state of knowledge, there is clear evidence that Head and Neck Squamous Cell Cancer (HNSCC) is directly or indirectly caused by environmental factors, predominantly smoking (active or passive), and in a second step due the immunosuppressive effect of alcohol. It is difficult to depict the increased relative risk of first degree relatives (about 3 to 5 times) to develop HNSCC from familial habits, as so far there is no evidence for a shared genetic event that could be responsible for a cancerous origin. Nevertheless, there are several genetic factors that are clearly altering the genetic susceptibility for HNSCC, for example, the capacity for detoxifying the consumption of noxious substances, or the frequency of the presence of fragile sites. Future studies will be necessary to clarify the issue of familial origin of HNSCC.

8.1
Familial Factors in Head and Neck Squamous Cell Cancer (HNSCC)

Head and neck cancer is the sixth most frequent entity of cancer and therefore a major cause of morbidity and mortality. The most frequent type of cancer in the head and neck with about 90% of the cases is Squamous Cell Cancer (HNSCC) presenting in four different grades of histologic differentiation. Current treatment options cover primarily surgical procedures, radiation, chemotherapy, and combinations thereof. Survival options depend on the tumor stage (lymphatic spread) upon initial diagnosis. Five year survival rates of stage III and IV cancers remain poor, with an overall survival of about 30%.

Hereditary Tumors: From Genes to Clinical Consequences
Edited by Heike Allgayer, Helga Rehder and Simone Fulda
Copyright © 2009 WILEY-VCH Verlag GmbH & Co. KGaA, Weinheim
ISBN: 978-3-527-32028-8

Up to the current state of knowledge, there is clear evidence that HNSCC is directly or indirectly caused by environmental factors, predominantly smoking (active or passive), and in a second step due the immunosuppressive effect of alcohol. Although many shared genetic events in the development of a smoking- as well as non-smoking induced head and neck cancers have been identified, very little is known about hereditary components, and there are no reliable data on a familial increased frequency or germline associated origin of this cancer type [1].

Sporadic HNSCC occur at a much higher incidence, nevertheless revealing a possible familial clustering with a suggested autosomal dominant mode of inheritance in oral HNSCC [2].Three other case cohort studies showed that first degree relatives and siblings of patients with HNSCC have an increased incidence of HNSCC (relative risk 3.5 and 14.6, respectively) of respiratory and upper digestive tract malignancies relative to control subjects [3, 4]. The study of Copper *et al.* found that a family history of head and neck cancer was more common in patients with oral and pharyngeal cancer than in those with laryngeal cancer, but these differences were not significant, possibly due to the small sizes of the subgroups [4]. Finally, Day *et al.* found no increased risk of cancer in the first degree relatives of patients with oral or pharyngeal cancer [5]. Given these differing results of patient cohort studies, larger as well as specific studies of individual head and neck cancer sites are needed to further elucidate the question of a familial origin of HNSCC–especially since the familial predisposition for HNSCC interferes with the familial habits and exposure to strong environmental risk factors such as smoking or alcohol consumption [6].

8.2
Interactions of Genetic and Environmental Factors

From a molecular point of view, there are nonetheless many host or genetic factors that may lead to altered genetic pathways involved in the genesis and expansion of HNSCC, and there are most likely familiar factors which are very important in determining the individual susceptibility to head and neck cancer. Molecular epidemiology studies may be used to further uncover the relevant interactions between genetic and environmental factors.

8.2.1
Metabolizing Enzyme Polymorphism

Since not all persons with heavy smoking or drinking habits develop HNSCC, different abilities to detoxify electrophilic carcinogens have been assumed, based on inherited polymorphisms in metabolizing enzymes, such as *N*-acetyltransferase, cytochrome P450, the glutathione S-transferases, and others [7]. These enzymes display a high degree of genetic polymorphism, and these polymorphisms have been linked to an altered risk of lung, bladder, and colon cancer [8]. To date, the role of several different DNA polymorphisms in detoxification or tumor suppressor genes have been examined in small case-control studies of HNSCC. However, results of these studies have often been conflicting due to the relatively small number of patients and controls included, or the lack of proper controls for other environmental exposures that are also risk factors for HNSCC [9].

Dominant Mendelian inheritance patterns and the occurrence of HNSCC in young patients with little or no exposure to carcinogens is suggestive of a single heritable genetic defect that directly predisposes individuals to cancer, which cannot be explained by polymorphisms or metabolizing enzymes.

8.3
Mutagenicity, Genetic Susceptibility and Tumor Suppressor Genes

8.3.1
Mutagenicity in Bleomycin Assays

In vitro mutagenicity assays have been focused on determining the familial predisposition for HNSCC. In order to detect mutagen sensitivity, patients with cancers of the upper aerodigestive tract were tested for chromosomal sensitivity to bleomycin. Mutagen sensitivity was defined as the presence of one or more breaks per cell [3], The results showed an increased ratio of chromosomal breaks for patients with a family history of any cancer in a first degree relative, and an even higher ratio if there were two or more relatives involved [10]. The ratio also increased in patients with multiple primary head and neck neoplasms [11, 12].

8.3.2
Multiple Primary Cancers

Multiple primary tumors are frequent in the head and neck region [5]. According to the hypothesis of Slaughter, damage to epithelial cells in the upper aerodigestive tract following exposure of the common carcinogens are ubiquitous, and could involve several different locations at the same time in the sense of a "field cancerization" [13]. Foulkes *et al.* could show that the risk for HNSCC in relatives of patients with multiple primary tumors was significantly increased, also suggesting an inherited susceptibility contributing to the risk of multiple primary tumors in the head and neck [12, 14].

8.3.3
Relationship between the Genetic Susceptibility to HNSCC
and the Presence of Common Fragile Sites

Smoking causes chromosomal damage and fragile chromosomal sites. Tobacco smoke contains several severe carcinogens such as benzopyrene, benzopyrene diol epoxide, dimethylsulfate, and dimethylnitrosamine. These carcinogens especially attack 3p14 and 3 p21 sites [15, 16]. Oncogenetic tree models for tumor progression of HNSCC from CGH data using branching and distance-based tree models predicted that + 3q21–29 was the most important early chromosomal event, and −3p, which occurred after + 3q21–29, was also an important chromosomal event for all subsites of HNSCC [17].

There are studies that believe that mutagen associated chromosomal aberrations are not random, but reflect the inherited genetic susceptibility of specific loci to damage by carcinogens. Those studies support the idea that fragile sites might be the unstable factors in the human genome and that their appearance could not only be affected by the environmental factors such as those mentioned above, but also by some genetic factors such as tumor suppressor genes and mismatch repair genes. In conclusion, the generation of fragile sites may be playing an important role in the genetic tendency to head and neck cancer [18].

8.3.4
Germline Mutations of Tumor Suppressor Gene p16INK4a (p16)

Familial mutations in p16 have been focused on as possibly being associated with HNSCC in patients without exposure to carcinogens [19]. Functionally, p16 acts as a regulator of the retinoblastoma gene product and controls cell cycle progression, resulting in a major impact on tumor progression. P16 inactivation has been proven to occur through several mechanisms, including homozygous deletion, point mutation, and promoter methylation [20]. Somatic mutations of p16 are frequently associated with multiple tumor types including HNSCC, non-small lung cancer, oesophageal cancer, and bladder cancer [21]. Germline mutations of p16 have been associated with familial melanoma and familial pancreatic adenocarcinoma (II) [22] (see Chapter 20 "Pancreatic Cancer" and Chapter 24 "Malignant Melanoma").

In HNSCC, alterations of the p16/CDK-cyclin D/Rb pathway are present in almost 80% of the cases, making it the most commonly altered gene in HNSCC [20, 23].

In a report on a family with an unusually high incidence of HNSCC suggesting a dominant Mendelian inheritance pattern, a germline mutation within the p16 gene was found [24]. It remains open whether these studies are representative enough to establish HNSCC as a familial cancer and as a new clinical entity caused by germline mutations of the p16 gene.

8.4
Familial Nasopharyngeal Carcinoma

Nasopharyngeal cancer (NPC) is a frequent malignancy in Southeast Asia, with an incidence of 10–53 cases per 100000. The incidence is equally high in Eskimos in Alaska and Greenland, as well as in Tunisians [25]. A clear etiology for NPC is still lacking. In general, NPC is thought to be the result of both genetic susceptibility and environmental factors such as carcinogens and infection with Epstein Barr Virus (EBV). Familial Clustering of NPC has been observed in Chinese people [26, 27], but also in patients that are not of Chinese origin [27]. The relative risk of NPC in first degree relatives was about 8.0. Familial NPC is usually poorly differentiated, and mostly associated with elevated levels of antibodies to EBV. The serum levels of antibodies can help to screen for patients at high risk for the development of NPC. Nevertheless, epidemiologic studies suggest that most of the familial aggregation of NPC derives from inherited susceptibility [28]. The molecular genetic basis of nasopharyngeal carcinomas, however, remains unknown, but there is evidence for the linkage of these tumors to chromosome 3p.

References

1 Suárez, C., Rodrigo, J.P., Ferlito, A., Cabanillas, R., Shaha, A.R. and Rinaldo, A. (2006) Tumours of familial origin in the head and neck. *Oral Oncology*, **42** (10), 965–78.

2 Ankathil, R., Matthew, A., Joseph, F. and Nair, M.K. (1996) Is oral cancer susceptibility inherited? *European Journal of Cancer. Part B, Oral Oncology*, **32B**, 63–7.

3 Bondy, M.L., Spitz, M.R., Halabi, S., Fueger, J.J., Schantz, S.P. and Sample, D. (1993) Association between family history of cancer and mutagen sensitivity in upper aerodigestive tract cancer patients. *Cancer Epidemiology, Biomarkers and Prevention*, **2**, 103–6.

4 Foulkes, W.D., Brunet, J.S., Kowalski, L.P. Narod, S.A. and Franco, E.L. (1995) Family history of cancer is a risk factor for squamous cell carcinoma of the head and neck in brazil–a case control study. *International Journal of Cancer*, **63**, 769–73.

5 Day, G.L. and Blot, W.J. (1992) Second primary tumors in patients with oral cancer. *Cancer*, **70**, 14–9.

6 Copper, M.P., Jovanovic, A., Nauta, J.J., Braakhuis, B.J., de Vries, N. and van der Waal, C. (1995) Role of genetic factors in the etiology of squamous cell cancer in the head and neck. *Archives of Otolaryngology–Head and Neck Surgery*, **121**, 157–60.

7 Gonzalez, M.V., Alvarez, V., Pello, M.F., Menendez, M.J., Suarez, C. and Coto, E. (1998) Polymorphism of Acetyltransferase-2, gluthatione

S-transferase-M1, and cytochromes P450IIE1 in the susceptibility of HNSCC. *Journal of Clinical Pathology*, **51**, 294–8.

8 Raunio, H. (1999) Diagnosis of polymorphisms in carcinogen activating and inactivating enzymes and cancer susceptibility–a review. *Gene*, **159** (1), 113–21.

9 McWilliams, J.E., Evans, A.J., Beer, T.M., Andersen, P.E., Cohen, J.I., Everts, E.C. and Henner, W.D. (2000) Genetic polymorphisms in head and neck cancer risk. *Head and Neck*, **22**, 609–17.

10 Cloos, J., Reid, C.B., Snow, G.B. and Braakhuis, B.J. (1996) Mutagen sensitivity: enhanced risk assessment of squamous cell carcinoma. *European Journal of Cancer*, **6**, 367–72.

11 Spitz, M.R., Hoque, A., Trizna, Z., Schantz, S.P., Amos, C.I., King, T.M., Bondy, M.L., Hong, W.K., and Hsu, T.C. (1994) Mutagen sensitivity as a risk factor for second malignant tumors following malignancies of the upper aerodigestive tract. *Journal of the National Cancer Institute* **86**(22), 1681–4.

12 Cloos, J., Leemanns, C.R., van der Sterre, M.L., Kuik, D.J., Snow, G.B. and Braakhuis, B.J. (2000) Mutagen sensitivity as a biomarker for second primary tumors after head and neck squamous cell cancer. *Cancer Epidemiology, Biomarkers and Prevention*, **7**, 713–7.

13 Slaughter, D.P., Southwick, H.W. and Smejkal, W. (1953) Field cancerization in oral stratified squamous epithelium. *Cancer*, **6**, 963–8.

14 Foulkes, W.D., Brunet, J.S., Sieh, W., Black, M.J., Shenouda, G. and Narod, S.A. (1996) Familial risks of squamous cell carcinoma of the head and neck: a retrospective case-control study. *BMJ*, **313**, 716–21.

15 Yunis, JJ. and Soreng, A.L. (1984) Constitutive fragile sites and cancer. *Science*, **226**, 1199–204.

16 Wu, X.F., Hsu, T.C., Annegers, J.F., Amos, C.I., Fueger, J.J. and Spitz, M.R. (1995) A case-control study of nonrandom distribution of bleomycin-induced chromatiod breaks in lymphocytes of lung cancer patients. *Cancer Research*, **55**, 557–61.

17 Huang, Q., Yu, G.P., McCormick, S.A., Mo, J., Datta, B., Mahimkar, M., Lazarus, P., Schäffer, A.A., Desper, R. and Schantz, S.P. (2002) Genetic differences detected by comparative genomic hybridization in head and neck squamous cell carcinomas from different tumor sites: construction of oncogenetic trees for tumor progression. *Genes Chromosomes Cancer*, **34** (2), 224–33.

18 Egeli, Ü., Özkan, L., Tunca, B., Kahraman, S., Cecener, G., Ergül, E. and Engin, K. (2000) The relationship between genetic susceptibility to head and neck cancer with the expression of common fragile sites. *Head and Neck*, **22**, 591–8.

19 Yarbrough, W.G., Aprelikova, O., Pei, H., Olshan, A.F. and Liu, E.T. (1996) Familial tumor syndrome associated with a germline non-functional p16INK4a allele. *Journal of the National Cancer Institute*, **88**, 1489–91.

20 Reed, A.L., Califano, J., Cairns, P., Westra, W.H., Jones, R.M. and Koch, W. (1996) High frequency of p16 inactivation in head and neck squamous cell carcinoma. *Cancer Research*, **56**, 3630–3.

21 Kamb, A., Gruis, N.A., Weaver-Feldhaus, J., Liu, Q., Harshman, K. and Tavtigian, S.V. (1994) A cell cycle regulator potentially involved in genesis of many tumour types. *Science*, **264**, 436–40.

22 Kamb, A., Shattuck-Eidens, D., Eeles, R., Liu, Q., Gruis, N.A. and Ding, W. (1994) Analysis of the p16 gene (CDKN2) as a candidate for the chromosome 9p melanoma susceptibility locus. *Nature Genetics*, **8**, 23–6.

23 Okami, K., Reed, A.L., Cairns, P., Koch, W.M., Westra, W.H. and Wehage, S. (1999) Cyclin D1 amplification is independent of p16 inactivation in head and neck squamous cell carcinoma. *Oncogene*, **18**, 3541–5.

24 Yu, K.K., Zanation, A.M., Moss, J.R. and Yarbrough, W.G. (2002) Familial head and neck cancer: molecular analysis of a new entity. *Laryngoscope*, **112**, 1587–93.

25 Chan, A.T.C., Leo, P.M.L. and Johnson, P.J. (2002) Nasopharyngeal carcinoma. *Annals of Oncology*, **13**, 1007–15.

26 Jia, W.H., Feng, B.J., Xu, Z.L., Zhang, X.S., Huang, P. and Huang, L.X. (2004) Familial risk and clustering of nasopharyngeal carcinoma in Guandong, China. *Cancer*, **101**, 363–9.

27 Zeng, Y.X. and Jia, W.H. (2002) Familial nasopharyngeal Carcinoma. *Seminars in Cancer Biology*, **12**, 443–50.

28 Friborg, J., Wohlfahrt, J., Koch, A., Storm, H., Olsen, O.R. and Melbye, M. (2005) Cancer susceptibility in nasopharyngeal carcinoma families – a population based cohort study. *Cancer Research*, **65**, 8567–72.

9
Hereditary Medullary and Familial Non-Medullary Thyroid Carcinoma

Theresia Weber

Summary

Hereditary medullary thyroid carcinoma (MTC) and familial nonmedullary thyroid carcinoma (FNMTC) account for approximately 20 and 5%, respectively, of all patients with medullary and papillary thyroid carcinoma (PTC). For MTC, a germ-line mutation of the rearranged during transfection (*RET*) proto-oncogene associated with multiple endocrine neoplasia 2A was described in 1993. Mutations of the *RET* proto-oncogene, localized on chromosome 10q11.2, are inherited in an autosomal dominant pattern. Genetic testing for *RET* proto-oncogene mutations enables identification of individuals at risk of developing MTC. For carriers of intermediate or high-risk *RET* oncogene mutations, prophylactic thyroidectomy is recommended during childhood. For symptomatic MTC, thyroidectomy and systematic compartment-oriented cervicocentral and cervicolateral neck dissection provides the best results for biochemical cure.

FNMTC is mostly found in patients with PTC. The genetic inheritance of FNMTC remains unknown, but it is believed to follow an autosomal dominant pattern with incomplete penetrance. In FNMTC families, some of the members are affected by thyroid carcinoma, while others present with non-malignant multinodular goiter. As seen in patients with hereditary MTC, hereditary PTC tends to be multifocal and bilateral. The biological behavior of FNMTC tends to be more aggressive than the sporadic form. In FNMTC, cervical lymph node involvement and distant metastases are found more frequently than in sporadic PTC. Surgery for FNMTC includes total thyroidectomy, and a prophylactic central neck dissection (level VI).

9.1
Introduction

Thyroid carcinoma is an uncommon malignancy. For the U.S. population, the life-time risk of being diagnosed with thyroid carcinoma is about 1% [1].

Hereditary Tumors: From Genes to Clinical Consequences
Edited by Heike Allgayer, Helga Rehder and Simone Fulda
Copyright © 2009 WILEY-VCH Verlag GmbH & Co. KGaA, Weinheim
ISBN: 978-3-527-32028-8

Approximately 33550 new cases of thyroid carcinoma were diagnosed in the United States in 2007. The estimated death rate from thyroid carcinoma was 2320 persons [2].

Papillary (PTC) and follicular thyroid carcinomas (FTC) develop from thyroid follicular cells. PTC is the most common form of thyroid cancer with the best prognosis, especially in patients younger than 45 years. PTC may be induced by previous radiation to the head and neck, as demonstrated after the nuclear accident in Chernobyl in 1986. Younger age at the time of the nuclear accident (≤8 years) was associated with more aggressive tumors, more lymph node involvement, and distant metastases [3]. Ten-year survival rates for PTC are more than 90% [4, 5].

FTC occurs mostly in elder patients and develops more frequently hematogenic metastases in the lungs and bones. The minimal-invasive form of FTC has an excellent prognosis. Other forms of FTC, such as highly invasive FTC, Hurthle cell carcinomas, or insular carcinomas, show an extensive invasion of blood vessels, develop distant metastases more frequently, have higher mortality rates [6, 7], and show a lower I^{131} uptake [8], which is essential for radioiodine ablation. Ten-year survival rates for FTC are about 85 and 76% for Hurthle cell carcinomas, respectively [4].

Only about 5% of all thyroid carcinomas are medullary thyroid carcinomas (MTC). MTC originates from the neuroendocrine parafollicular or calcitonin-producing cells (C-cells). The highest number of C-cells in the thyroid gland is found in the upper poles. C-cells secrete calcitonin, which is the most sensitive and specific marker for MTC. Routine measurement of calcitonin in patients with thyroid nodules is recommended by some authors [9] to detect MTC. Regional lymphatic spread occurs in early stages into the lymph nodes around the trachea, the oesophagus, the jugular chain, and the upper mediastinum [10]. MTC is found in a sporadic and three hereditary forms. Sporadic MTC accounts for approximately 80% of all cases of the disease. The remaining 20% are inherited tumor syndromes, such as endocrine neoplasia type 2A (MEN 2A), MEN 2B, or familial MTC (FMTC). Overall, 10-year survival rates for MTC are 83 to 87% [9, 11].

9.2
Hereditary Medullary Thyroid Carcinoma

In 1957 MTC was described for the first time by Hazard, Hawk, and Crile [12]. Familial forms of MTC (Table 9.1) are inherited in an autosomal-dominant pattern. In MEN 2A, patients develop multifocal, bilateral MTC associated with neoplastic C-cell hyperplasia. Approximately 40% of these patients develop pheochromocytomas, which may be bilateral. In 10 to 20% of the patients with MEN 2A, primary hyperparathyroidism, mostly caused by a hyperplasia of all four parathyroid glands, is found. In MEN 2B, all patients develop neural gangliomas in the mucosa of the digestive tract, including lips and tongue [13]. Other associated

Table 9.1 Clinical features of sporadic and hereditary MTC.

	MTC	Inheritance pattern	Associated diseases
Sporadic MTC	Unifocal	None	None
MEN 2A	Multifocal, bilateral	Autosomal dominant	Pheochromocytoma Primary hyperparathyroidism
MEN 2B	Multifocal, bilateral	Autosomal dominant	Pheochromocytoma Mucosal neuromas Megacolon Muscoskeletal abnormalities
FMTC	Multifocal, bilateral	Autosomal dominant	None

diseases are skeletal abnormalities and megacolon. MEN 2B syndrome has a very early onset of MTC in infants. In FMTC, MTC is found without other endocrinopathies [14].

Recently, after genetic examination of living relatives, Neumann *et al.* [15] demonstrated that the 18-year-old female patient mentioned in the first description of pheochromocytoma in the literature in 1886, had multiple endocrine neoplasia type 2.

9.2.1
Genetic Testing for MEN 2A, MEN 2B and FMTC

In 1993, Mulligan *et al.* [16] and Donis-Keller *et al.* [17] described a germline mutation of the *RET (rearranged during transfection)* proto-oncogene associated with multiple endocrine neoplasia 2A. The *RET* proto-oncogene, localized on chromosome 10q11.2, encodes a transmembrane receptor for a neurotrophic factor with tyrosine kinase activity. In MEN 2A and FMTC, mutations have been identified mostly in the cysteine-rich extracellular domains of exons 10, 11, and 13. In MEN 2B, mutations are found within the intracellular exons 14–16. Mutations affecting the extracellular domain of the *RET* oncogene are located in exon 10 (codons 609, 611, 618, and 620) and exon 11 (codons 630 and 634). Mutations affecting the intracellular domain are found for exons 13 (codons 768, 790, and 791), exon 14 (codon 804), exon 15 (codon 891), and exon 16 (codon 918). Overall, mutations of the *RET* proto-oncogene are found in up to 95% of kindreds with MEN 2A. According to the *NCCN (National Comprehensive Cancer Nerwork) Clinical Practice Guidelines in Oncology* [18], genetic testing for *RET* proto-oncogene mutations should be encouraged in all newly-diagnosed patients with MTC, as well as for screening children and adults in known kindreds with inherited MTC. At least two independently obtained blood samples should be tested in different laboratories to minimize the likelihood of false results, which are described as 3 to 5% [19].

Table 9.2 Risk-group assessment of hereditary MTC according
to the localization of the mutation.

Author	Low risk (Codons)	Intermediate risk (Codons)	High risk (Codons)
Brandi et al. (2001)[a] [20]	609, 768, 790, 791, 804, 891	611, 618, 620, 634	883, 918, 922
Machens et al. (2001)[b] [21]	768, 804	611, 620, 790	618, 634
Yip et al. (2003)[a] [22]	609, 804, 891	611, 618, 620, 634	918
Gimm et al. (2004)[b] [23]	768, 791	620, 790, 891	611, 618
Frank-Raue et al. (2006)[b] [24]	790, 791, 804, 891	618, 620, 630, 634	Not included

a   Publication presents the results of MEN 2A and MEN 2B.
b   Publication presents the results of MEN 2A only.

9.2.2
Genotype-Phenotype-Correlation

The most common form of hereditary MTC is a mutation in codon 634, which is
responsible for 85% of all hereditary MTC in MEN 2A. With this mutation, an
almost 100% genotype-phenotype correlation is described. Other mutations (Table
9.2), as for example, mutations in codon 790/791 (Figure 9.1), show a various
penetrance [25]. Carriers of RET mutations in codon 634 not only have a higher
penetrance of developing MTC, but have a higher risk of developing pheochromocytomas and hyperparathyroidism, as compared to carriers of other mutations of
the extracellular domain of the RET proto-oncogene [26–28].
    Studies on larger series of patients with hereditary MTC classified the various
mutations of the RET proto-oncogene in groups with low, intermediate, and high
risk of developing MTC (Table 9.2). The various mutations of the RET proto-
oncogene not only differ in the aggressiveness and prognosis of hereditary MTC,
but also in age of manifestation of the tumor. The EUROMEN study [29] showed
that carriers of mutations affecting the extracellular domain of the RET proto-
oncogene significantly differed in age of manifestation of MTC. In carriers of
extracellular mutations, lymph node-negative MTC developed significantly earlier
than in carriers of intracellular mutations (10.2 versus 16.6 years).

9.2.3
Surgical Management for Hereditary MTC

Surgery for hereditary MTC has completely changed with the constantly increasing
knowledge of the different forms and mutations of the disease. S.A. Wells Jr. was

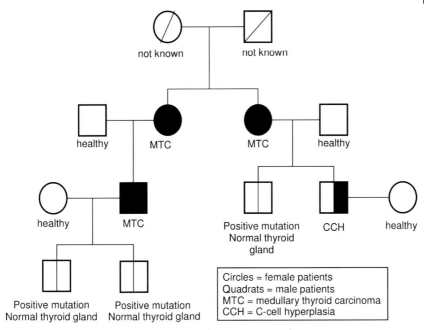

Figure 9.1 Pedigree of a family with FMTC and a mutation in codon 790.

the first surgeon to translate the results of molecular testing for mutations of the *RET* proto-oncogene into surgery. In 1994, he published the first results of thyroidectomy in 13 carriers of mutations of the extracellular domain of the *RET* proto-oncogene [30]. Each of the resected thyroid glands showed either neoplastic C-cell hyperplasia or MTC. Postoperative stimulated calcitonin levels (Pentagastrin test) were within the normal range in all of the patients. About 6 to 11% of patients without a family history of hereditary MTC carry a germline mutation in *RET*, leading to the identification of new kindreds [31, 32]. The detection of a *RET* oncogene mutation helps to identify family members at risk of developing MTC, which might be cured by prophylactic surgery at an early stage of the disease. The *NCCN Practice Guidelines in Oncology* [18] recommend that "even with patients who have apparently sporadic disease, the possibility of MEN 2 should dictate that a *RET* proto-oncogene mutation is proven to be absent, or that hyperparathyroidism and pheochromocytoma should be excluded preoperatively".

Thyroidectomy in carriers of *RET* mutations without preoperative evidence of MTC is called prophylactic thyroidectomy. In addition, it may be combined with systematic cervicocentral lymphadenectomy. Table 9.3 shows a selection of publications on the results of prophylactic surgery in hereditary MTC. An ongoing discussion exists about the best time for prophylactic surgery. The youngest patient with a mutation in codon 918, reported in the literature with MTC was 9 months old [29]. MTC with lymph node involvement in MEN 2 B was found in a 2.7 year-old patient [37] and distant metastases in a 5-year-old patient [38]. In MEN 2A and

Table 9.3 Results of prophylactic thyroidectomy in gene carriers of hereditary MTC.

Author (year)	Number of patients	Histopathology	Biochemical cure
Wells et al. (1994) [30]	13	7 MTC, 6 CCH	100%
Skinner et al. (1996) [33]	14	11 MTC, 3 CCH	96%
Frank-Raue et al. (1997) [34]	11	6 MTC, 5 CCH	100%
Dralle et al. (1998)[a] [35]	75	46 MTC, 29 CCH	96%
Niccoli-Sire et al. (1999)[a] [36]	71	66 MTC, 5 CCH	76%
Skinner et al. (2005) [37]	50	33 MTC, 17 CCH or normal thyroid gland	62%
Frank-Raue et al. (2006) [24]	46	26 MTC, 18 CCH, 2 normal thyroid gland	83%

a Multicenter trial.

FMTC, the youngest patient with MTC was 1 year old [39] and the youngest patient with lymph node metastases was 5 years old [40]. Distant metastases were not found before the age of 22 years [38]. The onset of MTC in carriers for low risk mutations (codons 768, 790, 791, and 891) is even later than for the intermediate risk group as mentioned above. Only one 6-year-old patient with a mutation in codon 804 developed metastatic MTC and died from this disease at the age of 12 years [41].

The international consensus statement of 2001 [20] recommends thyroidectomy for gene carriers of *RET* proto-oncogene mutations within the first year of life for MEN 2B (mutations in codons 883, 918, and 922), and before the age of 5 years for MEN 2A and intermediate or high risk mutations (codons 609, 611, 618, 620, 630, and 634). For patients with low-risk mutations (codons 768, 790, 791, 804, and 891), thyroidectomy should be performed before the age of 10 years, with one reported exception of one child with a fatal course of MTC at 6 years [29, 42]. In long-term studies [24, 43], prophylactic thyroidectomy for hereditary MTC provides excellent results with biochemical cure rates (= normalization of basal and stimulated calcitonin levels) of 62 to 83%. Additional lymph node dissection is recommended for carriers of the highest risk mutations in codon 918 (MEN 2B syndrome). For high-risk mutations in codon 634, lymphadenctomy is recommended from the age of 5 years, and at 10 years for mutations in codons 609, 611, 618, 620, and 630 [42].

For symptomatic hereditary and sporadic MTC with elevated calcitonin levels, thyroidectomy and systematic compartment-oriented cervicocentral and cervicolateral neck dissection [44, 45] is recommended by the German Cancer Society [46]. The *NCCN Guidelines for Thyroid Carcinoma* [18] recommend a central neck dissection (level VI) for patients with MEN 2A and an increased stimulated calcitonin level. A cervicolateral lymph node dissection (levels II to V) is suggested for MTC ≥1 cm or larger in diameter, ≥0.5 cm for MEN 2B, or patients with positive lymph nodes in the central compartment. The problem of the latter recommendation is, however, that lymph node metastases may occur only in the cervicolateral, but not in the central compartment of the neck (so-called skip metastases). Machens *et al.* [47] found a frequency of 21.3% of skip metastases in patients with MTC. In contrast to the results of prophylactic surgery in carriers of *RET* proto-oncogene mutations, a normalization of basal and stimulated calcitonin levels is achieved in patients with symptomatic MTC in experienced centers in 40 to 49% of the cases [11, 48–50]. Biochemical cure rates for MTC strongly depend on the presence of regional lymph node metastases. Ukkat *et al.* [50] described normal basal and stimulated calcitonin levels in 89% of the patients without lymph node involvement, as compared to only 27% of the patients with involved nodes. If more than 10 lymph nodes are involved, biochemical cure of MTC seems almost to be impossible [51].

In persistent or recurrent MTC, the chance for biochemical cure is regarded as small. Even in very specialized centers of endocrine surgery, only in 28% of these patients [52] basal and stimulated calcitonin levels decreased into the normal range.

9.2.4
Postoperative Management and Prognosis of Medullary Thyroid Carcinoma

Measurement of basal and stimulated serum calcitonin is considered to be the best postoperative assessment for residual disease or tumor recurrence in MTC. During the first years postoperatively, serum calcitonin should be measured every 6 months. Neck ultrasound of the thyroid bed and cervical lymph nodes should also be performed. In patients with MEN 2A or 2B syndromes, annual screening for pheochromocytoma or hyperparathyroidism is recommended.

If postoperative calcitonin levels remain elevated or increase, and residual disease in the neck is unlikely, a CT scan of the chest and the abdomen or MRI may help to detect distant metastases. Since liver metastases of MTC are usually very small, Quayle *et al.* [53] recommend the use of diagnostic laparoscopy to confirm this diagnosis. Giraudet *et al.* [54] recently evaluated 55 consecutive patients with persistent elevated calcitonin levels, and concluded that the most efficient imaging work-up for depicting MTC tumor sites would consist of a neck ultrasound, chest CT, liver MRI, bone scintigraphy, and axial skeleton MRI.

Despite the early progression into the cervical lymph nodes, the prognosis of MTC is considered to be favorable. For MTC, 10-year survival rates are described between 83 to 87% [9, 11] and therefore regarded to be very satisfactory, even if biochemical cure rates tend to be much lower.

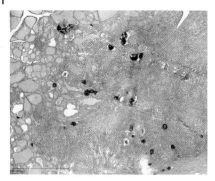 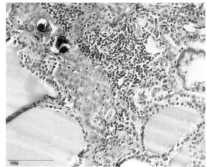

Figure 9.2 37 year-old patient with FNMTC and a multifocal papillary thyroid carcinoma with multiple characteristic interspensed PSAmmon bodies in the left thyroid lobe (PT1N1MO). (Prof. Dr. T.F.E. Barth, Department of Pathology, University of Ulm, Germany).

9.3
Familial Nonmedullary Thyroid Carcinoma

Familial nonmedullary thyroid carcinoma (FNMTC) is defined by the presence of thyroid carcinomas of follicular origin in two or more first-degree relatives without another familial syndrome. Familial syndromes associated with PTC are Gardner's syndrome, familial adenomatous polyposis [55], the Carney complex [56], and Cowden's syndrome [57]. FNMTC accounts for about 5.0 to 6.2% [58–60] of all nonmedullary thyroid cancers (NMTC). In a hospital-based case control study, Pal *et al.* [60] described the relative risk for NMTC as 10-fold higher in relatives of cancer patients than in the control group. Histologically, PTC is found in more than 90% of the FNMTC cases [61] (Figure 9.2a and b). Benign thyroid disorders, such as multinodular goiter and Hashimoto's thyroiditis, are found frequently in patients with FNMTC and their relatives.

The genetic inheritance of FNMTC remains unknown, but is believed to follow an autosomal dominant pattern with incomplete penetrance and variable expressivity [58–60, 62, 63]. Canzian *et al.* [64] identified a gene located on chromosome 19q13.2, named TCO1 (thyroid tumors with cell oxyphilia), which was detected in a French family with multinodular goiter and oxyphilic PTCs. In 2001 [65], TCO1 was found in a British family with FNMTC.

In patients with FNMTC, most PTCs tend to be multifocal and bilateral [59, 61, 66, 67]. FNMTC shows more extracapsular and vascular invasion [59, 61, 66] and an early lymph node involvement [59, 67]. Lupoli *et al.* [59] described 2 of 7 patients with familial papillary microcarcinoma (8 and 10 mm in diameter), who developed local recurrence, and another patient with pulmonary metastases who died from FNMTC. Several studies [59, 61, 66–68] report that the biological behavior of FNMTC is more aggressive than the sporadic form. Triponez *et al.* [69] described that the cumulative survival was significantly shorter for families with three or more affected family members, as compared to families with only two affected members.

Surgery for FNMTC should consist of total thyroidectomy, regardless of the size of the tumor. Even small lesions less than 1 cm in diameter can be associated with multifocal disease, vascular invasion, lymph node metastases, and local recurrence. A prophylactic central neck dissection is recommended in patients with FNMTC [70]. If there are suspicious lymph nodes in the lateral compartment of the neck, an additional cervicolateral modified-radical lymphadenectomy should be performed.

When two or more family members of kindreds with FNMTC have been identified, one of the most important considerations is how to screen patients at risk for FNMTC. Since familial thyroid carcinomas are often very small, neck ultrasound provides the best results to detect and describe thyroid nodules as well as pathologically enlarged lymph nodes. Uchino *et al.* [67] found at least one thyroid nodule in 52% of symptom-free family members of patients with FNMTC. Ten percent (15/149) of these individuals were subsequently diagnosed with thyroid cancer. The average tumor diameter was 9.1 mm (3–21 mm).

References

1 Ries, L.A.G., Eisner, M.P., Kosary, C.L. et al. (eds) (2004) *SEER Cancer Statistics Review, 1975-2001*, National Cancer Institute, Bethesda, MD, http://seer.cancer.gov/csr/1975–2001/.

2 Jemal, A., Siegel, R., Ward, E., Murray, T., Xu, J. and Thun, M.J. (2007) Cancer Statistics. *CA: A Cancer Journal for Clinicians*, **57**, 43–66.

3 Farahati, J., Demidchik, E.P., Biko, J. and Reiners, C. (2000) Inverse association between age at the time of radiation exposure and extent of disease in cases of radiation-induced childhood thyroid carcinoma in Belarus. *Cancer*, **88**, 1470–6.

4 Hundahl, S.A., Fleming, I.D., Fremgen, A.M. and Menck, H.R. (1998) A National Cancer Data Base report on 53 856 cases of thyroid carcinoma treated in the United States, 1985–1995. *Cancer*, **83**, 2638–48.

5 Passler, C., Scheuba, C., Prager, G., Kaczirek, K., Kaserer, K., Zettinig, G. and Niederle, B. (2004) Prognostic factors of papillary and follicular thyroid cancer: differences in an iodine-replete endemic goiter region. *Endocrine-Related Cancer*, **11**, 131–9.

6 Lopez-Penabad, L., Chiu, A.C., Hoff, A.O., Schultz, P., Gaztambide, S.,

Ordonez, N.G. and Sherman, S.I. (2003) Prognostic factors in patients with Hürthle cell neoplasms of the thyroid. *Cancer*, **97**, 1186–94.

7 Kushchayeva, Y., Duh, Q.-Y., Kebebew, E. and Clark, O.H. (2004) Prognostic indications for Hürthle cell cancer. *World Journal of Surgery*, **28**, 1266–70.

8 Samaan, N.A., Schultz, P.N., Haynie, T.P. and Ordonez, N.G. (1985) Pulmonary metastasis of differentiated thyroid carcinoma: treatment results in 101 patients. *The Journal of Clinical Endocrinology and Metabolism*, **60**, 376–80.

9 Elisei, R., Bottici, V., Luchetti, F., Di Coscio, G., Romei, C., Grasso, L., Miccoli, P., Iacconi, P., Basolo, F., Pinchera, A. and Pacini, F. (2004) Impact of routine measurement of serum calcitonin on the diagnosis and outcome of medullary thyroid cancer: experience in 10 864 patients with nodular thyroid disorders. *The Journal of Clinical Endocrinology and Metabolism*, **89**, 163–8.

10 Moley, J.F. and DeBenedetti, M.K. (1999) Patterns of nodal metastases in palpable medullary thyroid carcinoma: Recommendations for extent of node dissection. *Annals of Surgery*, **229**, 880–8.

11 Quayle, F.J., Benveniste, R., DeBenedetti, M.K., Wells, S.A. and Moley, J.F. (2004)

Hereditary medullary thyroid carcinoma in patients greater than 50 years old. *Surgery*, **136**, 1116–21.

12 Hazard, J., Hawk, W. and Crile, G. (1959) Medullary (solid) carcinoma of the thyroid–a clinicopathologic entity. *The Journal of Clinical Endocrinology and Metabolism*, **19**, 152–8.

13 O'Riordain, D.S., O'Brien, T., Crotty, T.B., Gharib, H., Grant, C.S. and van Heerden, J.A. (1995) Multiple endocrine neoplasia type 2B: more than an endocrine disorder. *Surgery*, **118**, 936–42.

14 Farndon, J.R., Leight, G.S., Dilley, W.G., Baylin, S.G., Smallridge, R.C., Harrison, T.S. and Wells, S.A. Jr (1986) Familial medullary thyroid carcinoma without associated endocrinopathies: A distinct clinical entity. *British Journal of Surgery*, **73**, 278–81.

15 Neumann, H.P., Vortmeyer, A., Schmidt, D., Werner, M., Erlic, Z., Cascon, A., Bausch, B., Januszewicz, A. and Eng, C. (2007) Evidence of MEN-2 in the original description of classic pheochromocytoma. *The New England Journal of Medicine*, **357**, 1311–5.

16 Mulligan, L.M., Gardner, E., Smith, B.A., Mathew, C.G. and Ponder, B.A. (1993) Genetic events in tumour initiation and progression in multiple endocrine neoplasia type 2. *Genes Chromosomes Cancer*, **6**, 166–77.

17 Donis-Keller, H., Dou, S., Chi, D., Carlson, K.M., Toshima, K., Lairmore, T. C., Howe, J.R., Moley, J.F., Goodfellow, P. and Wells, S.A. Jr (1993) Mutations in the RET proto-oncogene are associated with MEN 2A and FMTC. *Human Molecular Genetics*, **2**, 851–6.

18 NCCN Clinical Practice Guidelines in Oncology (2006) Thyroid Carcinoma in www.nccn.org.

19 Gagel, R.F., Cote, G.J. and Martins Bugalho, M.J. (1995) Boyd, A.E. 3rd, Cummings, T., Goepfert, H., Evans, D.B., Cangir, A., Khorana, S. and Schultz, P.N. (1995) Clinical use of molecular information in the management of multiple endocrine neoplasia type 2A. *Journal of Internal Medicine*, **238**, 333–41.

20 Brandi, M.L., Gagel, R.F., Angeli, A., Bilezikian, J.P., Beck-Peccoz, P., Bordi, C., Conte-Devolx, B., Falchetti, A., Gheri, R.G., Libroia, A. *et al.* (2001) Guidelines for diagnosis and therapy of MEN type 1 and type 2. *The Journal of Clinical Endocrinology and Metabolism*, **86**, 5658–71.

21 Machens, A., Gimm, O., Hinze, R., Hoppner, W., Boehm, B.O. and Dralle, H. (2001) Genotype-phenotype correlations in hereditary medullary thyroid carcinoma: oncological features and biochemical properties. *The Journal of Clinical Endocrinology and Metabolism*, **86**, 1104–9.

22 Yip, L., Cote, G.J., Shapiro, S.E., Ayers, G.D., Herzog, C.E., Sellin, R.V., Sherman, S.I., Gagel, R.F., Lee, J.E. and Evans, D.B. (2003) Multiple endocrine neoplasia type 2: evaluation of the genotype-phenotype relationship. *Archives of Surgery*, **138**, 409–16.

23 Gimm, O., Ukkat, J., Niederle, B.E., Weber, T., Thanh, P.N., Brauckhoff, M., Niederle, B. and Dralle, H. (2004) Timing and extent of surgery in patients with familial medullary thyroid carcinoma/ multiple endocrine neoplasia 2A-related RET mutations not affecting codon 634. *World Journal of Surgery*, **28**, 1312–6.

24 Frank-Raue, K., Buhr, H., Dralle, H., Klar, E., Senninger, N., Weber, T., Rondot, S., Hoppner, W. and Raue, F. (2006) Long-term outcome in 46 gene carriers of hereditary medullary thyroid carcinoma after prophylactic thyroidectomy: impact of individual *RET* genotype. *European Journal of Endocrinology*, **155**, 229–236.

25 Fitze, G., Schierz, M., Bredow, J., Saeger, H.D., Roesner, D. and Schackert, H.K. (2002) Various penetrance of familial medullary thyroid carcinoma in patients with *RET* proto-oncogene codon 790/791 germline mutations. *Annals of Surgery*, **236**, 570–5.

26 Eng, C., Clayton, D., Schuffenecker, I., Lenoir, G., Cote, G., Gagel, R.F., van Amstel, K.H., Lips, C.J., Nishisho, I. and Takai, S.I. (1996) The relationship between specific *RET* proto-oncogene mutations and disease phenotype in multiple endocrine neoplasia type 2. *JAMA*, **276**, 1575–9.

27 Frank-Raue, K., Hoppner, W., Frilling, A., Kotzerke, J., Dralle, H., Haase, R., Mann, K., Seif, F., Kirchner, R., Rendl, J., Deckart, H.F., Ritter, M.M., Hampel, R., Klempa, J., Scholz, G.H. and Raue, F.

(1996) Mutations of the *RET* protooncogene in German multiple endocrine neoplasia families: relation between genotype and phenotype. *The Journal of Clinical Endocrinology and Metabolism*, **81**, 1780–3.

28 Heshmati, H.M., Gharib, H., Khosla, S., Abu-Lebdeh, H.S., Lindor, N.M. and Thibodeau, S.N. (1997) Genetic testing in medullary thyroid carcinoma syndromes: mutation types and clinical significance. *Mayo Clinic proceedings*, **72**, 430–6.

29 Machens, A., Niccoli-Sire, P., Hoegel, J., Frank-Raue, K., van Vroonhoven, T.J., Roeher, H.D., Wahl, R.A., Lamesch, P., Raue, F., Conte-Devolx, B. and Dralle, H. (2003) Early malignant progression of hereditary medullary thyroid carcinoma. *The New England Journal of Medicine*, **349**, 1517–25.

30 Wells, S.A. Jr, Chi, D.D., Toshima, K., Dehner, L.P., Coffin, C.M., Dowton, S.B., Ivanovich, J.L., DeBenedetti, M.K., Dilley, W.G., Moley, J.F. *et al.* (1994) Predictive DNA testing and prophylactic thyroidectomy in patients at risk for multiple endocrine neoplasia type 2A. *Annals of Surgery*, **220**, 237–47.

31 Wohllk, N., Cote, G.J., Bugalho, M.M.J., Ordonez, N., Evans, D.B., Goepfert, H., Khorana, S., Schultz, P., Richards, C.S. and Gagel, R.F. (1996) Relevance of *RET* proto-oncogene mutations in sporadic medullary thyroid carcinoma. *The Journal of Clinical Endocrinology and Metabolism*, **81**, 3740–5.

32 Berndt, I., Reuter, M., Saller, B., Frank-Raue, K., Groth, P., Grussendorf, M., Raue, F., Ritter, M.M. and Hoppner, W. (1998) A new hot spot for mutations in the *RET* proto-onocogene causing familial medullary thyroid carcinoma and multiple endocrine neoplasia type 2A. *The Journal of Clinical Endocrinology and Metabolism*, **83**, 770–4.

33 Skinner, M.A. and DeBenedetti, M.K., Moley, J.F., Norton, J.A. and Wells, S.A. Jr (1996) Medullary thyroid carcinoma in children with multiple endocrine neoplasia types 2A and 2B. *Journal of Pediatric Surgery*, **31**, 177–82.

34 Frank-Raue, K., Hoppner, W., Buhr, H., Herfarth, C. and Raue, F. (1997) Results and follow-up in eleven MEN 2A gene carriers after prophylactic thyroidectomy. *Experimental and Clinical Endocrinology and Diabetes*, **105** (Suppl. 4), 76–8.

35 Dralle, H., Gimm, O., Simon, D., Frank-Raue, K., Görtz, G., Niederle, B., Wahl, R. A., Koch, B., Walgenbach, S., Hampel, R., Ritter, M.M., Spelsberg, F. *et al.* (1998) Prophylactic thyroidectomy in 75 children and adolescents with hereditary medullary thyroid carcinoma: German and Austrian experience. *World Journal of Surgery*, **22**, 744–51.

36 Niccoli-Sire, P., Murat, A., Baudin, E., Henry, J.-F., Proye, C., Bigorgne, J.-C., Bstandig, B., Modigliani, E., Morange, S., Schlumberger, M. and Conte-Devolx, B. (1999) Early or prophylactic thyroidectomy in MEN 2/FMTC gene carriers: results of 71 thyroidectomized patients. *European Journal of Endocrinology*, **141**, 468–74.

37 Leboulleux, S. Travagli, J.P., Caillou, B., Laplanche, A., Bidart, J.M., Schlumberger, M. and Baudin, E. (2002) Medullary thyroid carcinoma as part of a multiple endocrine neoplasia type 2B syndrome. Influence of the stage on the clinical course. *Cancer*, **94**, 44–50.

38 Machens, A., Holzhausen, H.J., Thanh, P.N. and Dralle, H. (2003) Malignant progression from C-cell hyperplasia to medullary thyroid carcinoma in 167 carriers of *RET* germline mutations. *Surgery*, **134**, 425–31.

39 Machens, A., Schneyer, U., Holzhausen, H.J., Raue, F. and Dralle, H. (2004) Emergence of medullary thyroid carcinoma in a family with the Cys630Arg *RET* germline mutation. *Surgery*, **136**, 1083–7.

40 Gill, J.R., Reyes-Mugica, M., Iyengar, S., Kidd, K.K., Touloukian, R.J., Smith, C., Keller, M.S. and Kenel, M. (1996) Early presentation of metastatic medullary carcinoma in multiple endocrine neoplasia, type IIA: implications for therapy. *The Journal of Pediatrics*, **129**, 459–64.

41 Frohnauer, M.K. and Decker, R.A. (2000) Update on the MEN 2A c804 RET mutation: is prophylactic thyroidectomy indicated? *Surgery*, **128**, 1052–8.

42 Machens, A. and Dralle, H. (2007) Genotype-phenotype based surgical concept of hereditary medullary thyroid

carcinoma. *World Journal of Surgery*, **31**, 957–68.

43 Skinner, M.A., Moley, J.F., Dilley, W.G., Owzar, K., DeBenedetti, M.K. and Wells S.A. Jr (2005) Prophylactic thyroidectomy in multiple endocrine neoplasia type 2A. *The New England Journal of Medicine*, **353**, 1105–13.

44 Tisell, L.-E., Hansson, G., Jansson, S. and Salander, H. (1986) Reoperation in the treatment of asymptomatic metastasizing medullary thyroid carcinoma. *Surgery*, **99**, 60–6.

45 Dralle, H., Damm, I., Scheumann, G.F.W., Kotzerke, J., Kupsch, E., Geerlings, H. and Pichlmayr, R. (1994) Compartment-oriented microdissection of regional lymph nodes in medullary thyroid carcinoma. *Surgery Today*, **24**, 112–21.

46 AWMF: maligne Schilddrüsentumoren. Dt. Krebsgesellschaft, kurzgefasste interdisziplinäre Leitlinien, 3. Auflage 2002, aktualisierte Version 10/2003.

47 Machens, A., Holzhausen, H.J. and Dralle, H. (2004) Skip metastases in thyroid cancer leaping the central node compartment. *Archives of Surgery*, **139**, 43–5.

48 Kebebew, E., Ituarte, P.H., Siperstein, A.E., Duh, Q.-Y. and Clark, O.H. (2000) Medullary thyroid carcinoma: clinical characteristics, treatment, prognostic factors, and comparison of staging systems. *Cancer*, **88**, 1139–48.

49 Weber, T., Schilling, T., Frank-Raue, K., Colombo-Benkmann, M., Hinz, U., Ziegler, R. and Klar, E. (2001) Impact of modified radical neck dissection on biochemical cure in medullary thyroid carcinomas. *Surgery*, **130**, 1044–9.

50 Ukkat, J., Gimm, O., Brauckhoff, M., Bilkenroth, U. and Dralle, H. (2004) Single center experience in primary surgery for medullary thyroid carcinoma. *World Journal of Surgery*, **28**, 1271–4.

51 Machens, A., Gimm, O., Ukkat, J., Hinze, R., Schneyer, U. and Dralle, H. (2000) Improved prediction of calcitonin normalization in medullary thyroid carcinoma patients by quantitative lymph node analysis. *Cancer*, **88**, 1909–15.

52 Moley, J.F., Wells, S.A., Dilley, W.G. and Tisell, L.E. (1993) Reoperation for recurrent or persistent medullary thyroid cancer. *Surgery*, **114**, 1090–6.

53 Quayle, F.J. and Moley, J.F. (2005) Medullary thyroid carcinoma: including MEN 2A and MEN 2B syndromes. *Journal of Surgical Oncology*, **89**, 122–9.

54 Giraudet, A.L., Vanel, D., Leboulleux, S., Aupérin, A., Dromain, C., Chami, L., Tovo, N.N., Lumbroso, J., Lassau, N., Bonniaud, G. *et al.* (2007) Imaging medullary thyroid carcinoma with persistent elevated calcitonin levels. *The Journal of Clinical Endocrinology and Metabolism*, **28**, 4185–90. Epub ahead of print.

55 Soravia, C., Sugg, S.L., Berk, T., Mitri, A., Cheng, H., Gallinger, S., Cohen, Z., Asa, S.L. and Bapat, B.V. (1999) Familial adenomatous polyposis-associated thyroid cancer: a clinical, pathological, and molecular genetics study. *The American Journal of Pathology*, **154**, 127–35.

56 Stratakis, C.A., Courcoutsakis, N.A., Abati, A., Filie, A., Doppman, J.L., Carney, J.A. and Shawker, T. (1997) Thyroid gland abnormalities in patients with the syndrome of spotty skin pigmentation, myxomas, endocrine overactivity, and schwannomas (Carney complex). *The Journal of Clinical Endocrinology and Metabolism*, **82**, 2037–43.

57 Marsh, D.J., Dahia, P.L.M., Caron, S., Kum, J.B., Frayling, I.M., Tomlinson, I.P., Hughes, K.S., Eeles, R.A., Hodgson, S.V., Murday, V.A., Houlston, R. and Eng, C. (1998) Germline PTEN mutations in Cowden syndrome-like families. *Journal of Medical Genetics*, **35**, 881–5.

58 Stoffer, S.S., Van Dyke, D.L., Bach, J.V., Szpunar, W. and Weiss, L. (1986) Familial papillary carcinoma of the thyroid. *American Journal of Medical Genetics*, **25**, 775–82.

59 Lupoli, G., Vitale, G., Caraglia, M., Fittipaldi, M.R., Abbruzzese, A., Tagliaferri, P. and Bianco, A.R. (1999) Familial papillary thyroid microcarcinoma: a new clinical entity. *Lancet*, **353**, 637–9.

60 Pal, T., Vogl, F.D., Chappuis, P.O., Tsang, R., Brierley, J., Renard, H., Sanders, K., Kantemiroff, T., Bagha, S., Goldgar, D.E., Narod, S.A. and Foulkes, W.D. (2001) Increased risk for nonmedullary thyroid cancer in the first degree relatives of prevalent cases of nonmedullary thyroid cancer: a hospital-based study. *The Journal of Clinical Endocrinology and Metabolism*, **86**, 5307–12.

61 Loh, K.C. (1997) Familial nonmedullary thyroid carcinoma: a meta-review of case series. *Thyroid*, **7**, 107–13.

62 Burgess, J.R., Duffield, A., Wilkinson, S.J., Ware, R., Greenaway, T.M., Percival, J. and Hoffman, L. (1997) Two families with an autosomal dominant inheritance pattern for papillary carcinoma of the thyroid. *The Journal of Clinical Endocrinology and Metabolism*, **82**, 345–8.

63 Sturgeon, C. and Clark, O.H. (2005) Familial nonmedullary thyroid cancer. *Thyroid*, **15**, 588–93.

64 Canzian, F., Amati, P., Harach, H.R., Kraimps, J.L., Lesueur, F., Barbier, J., Levillain, P., Romeo, G. and Bonneau, D. (1998) A gene predisposing to familial thyroid tumors with cell oxyphilia maps on chromosome 19p13.2. *American Journal of Human Genetics*, **63**, 1743–8.

65 Bevan, S., Pal, T., Greenberg, C.R., Green, H., Wixey, J., Bignell, G., Narod, S.A., Foulkes, W.D., Stratton, M.R. and Houlston, R.S. (2001) A comprehensive analysis of MNG1, TCO1, fPTC, PTEN, TSHR, and TRKA in familial nonmedullary thyroid cancer: confirmation of linkage to TCO1. *The Journal of Clinical Endocrinology and Metabolism*, **86**, 3701–4.

66 Grossman, R.F., Tu, S.H., Duh, Q.-Y., Siperstein, A.E., Novosolov, F. and Clark, O.H. (1995) Familial nonmedullary thyroid cancer. An emerging entity that warrants aggressive treatment. *Archives of Surgery*, **130**, 892–7.

67 Uchino, S., Noguchi, S., Yamashita, H., Murakami, T., Watanabe, S., Ogawa, T., Tsuno, A. and Shuto, S. (2004) Detection of asymptomatic differentiated thyroid carcinoma by neck ultrasonographic screening for familial nonmedullary thyroid carcinoma. *World Journal of Surgery*, **28**, 1099–102.

68 Alsanea, O., Wada, N., Ain, K., Wong, M., Taylor, K., Ituarte, P.H., Treseler, P.A., Weier, H.U., Freimer, N., Siperstein, A.E. *et al.* (2000) Is familial non-medullary thyroid carcinoma more aggressive than sporadic thyroid cancer? A multicenter series. *Surgery*, **128**, 1043–51.

69 Triponez, F., Wong, M., Sturgeon, C., Caron, N., Ginzinger, D.G., Segal, M.R., Kebebew, E., Duh, Q.-Y. and Clark, O.H. (2006) Does familial non-medullary thyroid cancer adversely affect survival? *World Journal of Surgery*, **30**, 787–93.

70 Sippel, R.S., Caron, N.R. and Clark, O.H. (2007) An evidence-based approach to familial nonmedullary thyroid cancer: screening, clinical management, and follow-up. *World Journal of Surgery*, **31**, 924–33.

10
Lung Tumors

Sarah Danson, M Dawn Teare, and Penella Woll

Summary

Whilst the hereditary components of many tumors are well described, this is not the case for thoracic malignancies and much work is ongoing in this area. A strong family history is rare but there is increasing evidence that testing for polymorphisms, especially for genes involved in detoxification and DNA repair, may one day be used to identify those at risk of lung cancer. In those that develop lung cancer, polymorphism status could be combined with tumor characteristics to design customized treatment regimens.

10.1
Introduction

Lung cancer is one of the commonest forms of cancer, with an incidence of over a million new cases annually worldwide. Lung cancer contributes to one-third of cancer deaths, with only 2% of patients surviving 5 years from diagnosis. Cigarette smoking accounts for over 85% of lung cancers. However, some people are life-long heavy smokers and never develop the disease; conversely, a significant proportion of people who develop lung cancer have never smoked [1]. Passive smoking increases the risk in non-smokers by about 20% [2], and it is uncertain in what proportion of non-smokers this may be the attributable factor. There do appear to be other factors influencing the development of the disease, such as asbestos exposure, air pollutants, radiation exposure, dietary factors, and immunosuppression. Possible genetic reasons for increased lung cancer susceptibility will be discussed in this chapter. The patterns of lung cancer in families and candidate polymorphisms are detailed. Other areas of interest are that women are more susceptible, dose-for-dose, to the adverse effects of tobacco smoke [3], and that there may be a genetic contribution to nicotine addiction, treatment response, and treatment toxicity.

Hereditary Tumors: From Genes to Clinical Consequences
Edited by Heike Allgayer, Helga Rehder and Simone Fulda
Copyright © 2009 WILEY-VCH Verlag GmbH & Co. KGaA, Weinheim
ISBN: 978-3-527-32028-8

10.2
Familial Aggregation Studies of Lung Cancer

Many reports have described clustering of lung cancer cases in families. The risk of lung cancer in first-degree relatives of lung cancer patients is raised 1.3-fold to 3-fold compared to controls, after allowing for tobacco use [4–6]. Segregation analyses have revealed evidence that the familial aggregation is likely due to co-inheritance of few genetic factors [7, 8], though some have found evidence of clustering due to environmental effects only [9]. There are also associations with increased risk of other tumors, such as breast cancer [10, 11] and other smoking related cancers [12]. Some cancer syndrome families, such as those with retino-blastoma gene mutations or Li Fraumeni syndrome, are at increased risk of lung cancer [13].

The main evidence cited against lung cancer having a high heritable component is based on a review of twin studies and cancer [14]. When comparing monozygote (MZ) and dyzygote (DZ) twin risk of lung cancer in five studies, the DZ twins frequently had a higher risk than the MZ twins, which is not expected if a strong genetic component exists. However, though an interesting trend, these studies relied on small numbers and within individual studies the risks for MZ and DZ twins were generally not significantly different. The strongest evidence to date for a high heritable component comes from a population based study in Iceland [15]. Researchers were able to link all records on 2756 lung cancer cases diagnosed between 1950 and 2002 to their extensive genealogical database. They found significantly raised risks of lung cancer in first-, second-, and third-degree relatives. By also studying the risk of lung cancer but using smoker probands, they were able to show that the raised risks in relatives were significantly higher than expected for smoking alone. They also confirmed higher familial risks in relatives of early onset cases.

The evidence from familial aggregation studies for the involvement of major susceptibility genes in lung cancer suggests a similar contribution to that observed for other common cancers, such as breast and prostate. The lack of family-based linkage studies in lung cancer is partly due to the difficulty in collecting sufficiently large families because the prognosis is so poor. The largest linkage study reported to date, using 52 families, found evidence of a major lung cancer gene mapping to chromosome 6q23–25 [16]. This work was done on the most powerful collection available of family-based material through a large consortium and thus far has not been confirmed.

Progress in mapping major genes in lung cancer has been slow because of the difficulty in collecting sufficient family-based material. However, research into the genetic epidemiology of other common cancers has revealed a likely role for common low penetrance alleles. Such low penetrance genetic effects are more efficiently detected through candidate gene association studies requiring large samples of unrelated cases and controls, and this type of study has been possible in lung cancer. A review of these studies follows.

10.3
Polymorphisms

Many candidate single nucleotide polymorphisms (SNPs) have been identified for lung cancer and the best documented are summarized in Table 10.1. We will discuss those that appear to be of most importance in detail.

10.3.1
Detoxification Genes

Detoxification genes metabolise a wide range of carcinogens. The most important detoxification gene for lung cancer seems to be cytochrome P450 CYP1A1. CYP1A1 is a phase I enzyme which metabolises polycyclic aromatic hydrocarbons in cigarette smoke. Polymorphisms in CYP1A1 lead to increased metabolism of these hydrocarbons, producing more of the highly reactive metabolites. Polymorphisms in CYP1A1 have been associated with an increased risk of lung cancer by some [18, 19], but others have not confirmed this [20]. Others have reported that polymorphisms in CYP1A1 are associated with the development of lung cancer in "low risk groups": that is younger people, defined as those below 45 years of age (MspI), never smokers (462 Val), and women (462 Val) [21–24]. CYP1A1 polymorphisms may occur in association with null genotypes of glutathione-S-transferase (GST) M1 and GSTT1, which are involved in the detoxification of diol epoxide metabolites that are the breakdown products of polycyclic aromatic hydrocarbons [21, 22]. Other members of the cytochrome P450 superfamily metabolize 60% of prescribed drugs and are important in drug toxicity, for example, toxicity associated with non-steroidal anti-inflammatory drugs, proton pump inhibitors, and the cytotoxic agents, ifosfamide, cyclophosphamide, and paclitaxel [25]. However, the significance of CYP1A1 in drug toxicity is uncertain. The correlation between other CYP family members and lung cancer susceptibility is less clear. CYP1B1 is associated with increased lung cancer susceptibility in Caucasians who have never smoked [26]. The CYP3A4*1B allele has been linked to an increased SCLC risk and this risk is eight-fold in women smokers [27]. Interestingly, CYP2A6 mediates approximately 90% of the inactivation of nicotine to cotinine and CYP2A6 polymorphism is thought to predispose to nicotine addiction [28].

NAD(P)H-quinone oxidoreductase 1 (NQO1, also known as DT-diaphorase) is a phase II enzyme involved in the detoxification of quinones, whether they are environmental, dietary, or cytotoxic. The detoxification step bypasses the formation of free radicals and so protects tissues against mutagens, carcinogens, and cytotoxics. There are conflicting data about whether the NQO1*2 polymorphism is increased in those with lung cancer [29, 30]. The NQO1*2 polymorphism may also be associated with an increased risk of chemotherapy-related myeloid leukemia, including those leukemias associated with abnormalities in chromosomes 5 and 7 [31], greater likelihood of carcinogen-induced skin and visceral tumors [32], and higher susceptibility to quinone toxicity [33].

Table 10.1 Candidate SNPs for lung cancer (from literature search, with majority from [17]).

Detoxification

CYP1A1, CYP1B1, CYP3A4, CYP2A6	NAT
GSTM1, GSTT1	MEH
NQO1	EPHX1
MPO	

DNA repair

ERCC1, ERCC6	Serine hydroxymethyltransferase
XPD (ERCC2)	GPX1
XRCC1, XRCC4, XRCC5	hOGG1
BRCA2	CHD1L
MSH4, MSH5	

Others

BARD1	POP1
DATF1	IGFBP5
THBS1	GRIK1
Interleukins (IL-1A, IL-1B, IL-13)	IL17RB
MMPs (MMP1–3, MMP12)	MS4A6A
p53	SETDB2
MDM2	DHX16
ABCB1, ABCC2	PHACS
BAT3, BAT4	GUCY2D
CAMKK1	GH1
AKAP9, AKAP10	ITGA7
NRIP1	SERPINI2
PPAT	RB1CC1
DKK3	TBX10
GHR	CFTR
DUSP23	ATF1
PYCRL	TNC
AKR7A3	PLCD1
SULT1E1	TLR1
HIF1AN	HUS1B
ITGA11	FGFRL1
CER1	PTPN13
WLN	GHR4
GTFRE1	GPR68
CDH12	FASN
ZNF624, ZNF24, ZNF600	PFAS
COL12A1	EPX
SFTPD	APOH
GPAM	

Myeloperoxidase (MPO) is a lysosomal protein in white blood cells that can transform environmental precarcinogens into highly reactive intermediaries [25]. The MPO-463A polymorphism has been associated with a decreased risk of lung cancer [34]; this reduction may principally occur in SCLC [35].

N-acetyltransferases (NATs) conjugate environmental and dietary toxins and drugs, such as the anti-tuberculosis drug isoniazid. Slow conjugators are at increased risk of both drug toxicity and the development of cancer, including bladder cancer and colorectal carcinoma [25]. With regard to smoking, it is hypothesized that rapid acetylators detoxify arylamines in cigarette smoke more effectively so that fewer free radicals are left to initiate carcinogenesis. Individuals with a combined NAT1 fast/NAT2 slow genotype have been shown to have a significantly elevated risk of adenocarcinoma of the lung (two-fold) compared with other genotype combinations [36].

10.3.2
DNA Repair Genes

DNA repair is critical to protect the integrity of DNA against environmental factors, including carcinogens in cigarette smoke. The most important part of this is the nucleotide excision repair (NER) pathway, which is involved in tobacco-related adduct clearance and resistance to cisplatin.

Excision repair cross-complementing 1 (ERCC1) is a major component of the NER pathway and there is a growing body of evidence that ERCC1 mRNA levels in tumors are important in NSCLC, possibly through ERCC1 stabilizing mRNA [37, 38]. ERCC1 polymorphisms, such as C8092A, may predict for increased survival in NSCLC patients treated with platinum-based chemotherapy [39]. Others disagree, saying that ERCC6 is associated with lung cancer risk, whereas ERCC1 and ERCC3 are not [40].

Xeroderma pigmentosum D (XPD), also known as ERCC2, encodes for a DNA helicase and is also part of the NER repair pathway. Both the XPD 751Gln and 312Asn polymorphisms are associated with increased lung cancer risk [41, 42]. The 312Asn polymorphism results in significantly reduced survival in advanced NSCLC, and a non-significant trend towards treatment response with gemcitabine-cisplatin chemotherapy [43].

X-ray cross complementing group 1 (XRCC1) is a member of the base excision repair (BER) pathway. It acts as a scaffold protein through physical interaction with ligase III and poly(ADP-ribose) polymerase. The XRCC1 280His polymorphism is associated with an increased risk of lung cancer [44]. Patients with NSCLC and the XRCC1 399 Gln polymorphism may have a longer median survival time after platinum-based chemotherapy than those without the polymorphism [45].

10.3.3
Others

Polymorphisms implicated in lung cancer risk in apoptosis-related genes include BRCA1 associated RING domain 1 (BARD1) and death associated transcription factor 1 (DATF1). Further genes involved in the growth hormone/insulin-like growth factor pathway, which regulates cellular proliferation and apoptosis, may also be involved [17].

Angiogenic activity may be influenced by polymorphisms in pro-angiogenic and anti-angiogenic proteins [46]. The N700S polymorphism of the anti-angiogenic molecule, thrombospondin (THBS1) is associated with lung cancer [17].

A dysregulated inflammatory response to tobacco-induced lung damage may promote carcinogenesis. Polymorphisms in the genes encoding interleukin (IL)-1A and IL-1B are linked with increased lung cancer risk [47].

MMPs are a family of more than 20 proteolytic enzymes that degrade the extracellular matrix. The MMP1 G-1607GG, MMP2 C-1306T, and MMP3 6A-1171–5A polymorphisms increase the risk of lung cancer, especially in heavy and current smokers [48–50]. Neutrophil elastase activates MMPs; polymorphisms in the promotor region are implicated in lung cancer development [51].

The p53 tumor suppressor gene can be mutated in all types of cancer. Several polymorphisms in the p53 gene have been reported but the significance of these at the present time is poorly understood [40]. Mutations in p53 may co-exist with other gene polymorphisms, such as XRCC1 399Gin variant [52]. Mouse double minute 2 (MDM2) is a negative regulator of p53. The SNP polymorphism of MDM2 is associated with a 1.27-fold increased risk of lung cancer and it is postulated that it may modify the time of tumor onset and prognosis [53].

10.4
Genome Wide Association Studies

Technological advances have enabled the leap from candidate gene association studies, where only several polymorphisms within a gene are considered by genome-wide association (GWA) panels consisting of up to 500 000 SNP markers. These studies require thousands of cases and controls and provide a means of identifying the strongest effects followed up by replication studies often using common marker platforms. Early results from these studies for other common diseases are promising. At the moment these studies focus on the use of SNPs but other forms of genome-wide variation such as copy number variants will be considered in future designs. As mentioned earlier, a large-scale genetic association study considering variation within 871 candidate genes reported evidence for association with variants in genes in the GH-IGF axis [17]. These results need confirmation from larger panels of SNPs and GWAs.

10.5
Other Thoracic Tumors

This chapter has focused on lung cancer as the data for other thoracic tumors are limited. Mesothelioma is an infrequently occurring tumor but its incidence is increasing and its prognosis is also poor. Familial clustering of mesothelioma has been documented but the relevance of hereditary susceptibility is uncertain, as most family members have a shared asbestos exposure, due to work or home contamination [54, 55]. It has been suggested that hereditary mesothelioma occurs in those with connective tissue disorders, such as Ehlers–Danlos syndrome and Marfan's syndrome [56, 57]. Thymoma is even rarer and at this time there are no known hereditary characteristics.

10.6
Future Directions

Further work on polymorphisms in lung cancer should be performed, following leads from the large GWA studies, in the setting of large prospective studies, as these results will be meaningful for the general population. Such an approach will likely involve testing the interaction between multiple polymorphisms [58], as single polymorphisms tend to be associated with an increased risk of less then ten-fold. It will be necessary to incorporate new candidate polymorphisms as they are described.

With these results, it may be possible to reduce the lung cancer risk in susceptible individuals through appropriate interventions, such as smoking cessation and chemoprevention. For example, slow conjugators could be treated with drugs to increase conjugation. In addition, the importance of SNPS on treatment response and toxicity must be clarified for those treated with radiotherapy and novel agents, as well as cytotoxic chemotherapy.

10.7
Conclusions

Much work is ongoing to try and determine the importance of hereditary factors in lung cancer. As with other common malignancies, a strong family history is rare but there is increasing evidence that testing for polymorphisms, especially in those genes involved in detoxification and DNA repair, may one day be used to identify those at risk of lung cancer. In those that develop lung cancer, polymorphism status could be combined with information from tumors to design customized treatment regimens.

References

1 Parkin, D.M., Bray, F., Ferlay, J. and Pisani, P. (2002) Global cancer statistics, 2002. *CA: A Cancer Journal for Clinicians*, 55, 74–108.

2 Takagi, H., Sekino, S., Kato, T., Matsuno, Y. and Umemoto, T. (2006) Revisiting evidence of lung cancer and passive smoking: adjustment for publication bias by means of "trim and fill" algorithm. *Lung Cancer*, 51, 245–6.

3 International Early Lung Cancer Action Program Investigators (2006) Women's susceptibility to tobacco carcinogens and survival after diagnosis of lung cancer. *JAMA*, 296, 180–4.

4 Ooi, W.L., Elston, R.C., Chen, V.W., Bailey-Wilson, J.E. and Rothschild, H. (1986) Increased familial risk for lung cancer. *Journal of the National Cancer Institute*, 76, 217–22.

5 Etzel, C.J., Amos, C.I. and Spitz, M.R. (2003) Risk for smoking-related cancer among relatives of lung cancer patients. *Cancer Research*, 63, 8531–5.

6 Matikidou, A., Eisen, T., Bridle, H., O'Brien, M., Mutch, R. and Houlston, R.S. (2005) Case-control study of familial lung cancer risks in UK women. *International Journal of Cancer*, 116, 445–50.

7 Sellers, T.A., Potter, J.D., Bailey-Wilson, J.E., Rich, S.S., Rothschild, H. and Elston, R.C. (1992) Lung cancer detection and prevention: evidence for an inter-action between smoking and genetic predisposition. *Cancer Research*, 52, 2694–7.

8 Xu, H., Spitz, M.R., Amos, C.I. and Shete, S. (2005) Complex segregation analysis reveals a multigene model for lung cancer. *Human Genetics*, 116, 121–7.

9 Yang, P., Schwartz, A.G., McAllister, A.E., Aston, C.E. and Swanson, G.M. (1997) Genetic analysis of families with nonsmoking lung cancer probands. *Genetic Epidemiology*, 14, 181–97.

10 Schwartz, A.G., Siegfried, J.M. and Weiss, L. (1999) Familial aggregation of breast cancer with early onset lung cancer. *Genetic Epidemiology*, 17, 274–84.

11 Gorlova, O.Y., Weng, S.F., Zhang, Y., Amos, C.I. and Spitz, M.R. (2007) Aggregation of cancer among relatives of never-smoking lung cancer patients. *International Journal of Cancer*, 121, 111–8.

12 Chen, C.J., Liang, K.Y., Chang, A.S. *et al.* (1991) Effects of hepatitis B virus, alcohol drinking, cigarette smoking and familial tendency on hepatocellular carcinoma. *Hepatology*, 13, 398–406.

13 Sanders, B.M., Jay, M., Draper, G.J. and Roberts, E.M. (1989) Non-ocular cancer in relatives of retinoblastoma patients. *British Journal of Cancer*, 60, 358–65.

14 Risch, N. (2001) The genetic epidemiology of cancer; interpreting family and twin studies and their implications for molecular genetic approaches. *Cancer Epidemiology Biomarkers and Prevention*, 10, 733–41.

15 Jonsson, S., Thorsteinsdottir, U., Gudbjartsson, D.F. *et al.* (2004) Familial risk of lung carcinoma in the Icelandic population. *JAMA*, 292, 2977–83.

16 Bailey-Wilson, J.E., Amos, C.I., Pinney, S.M. *et al.* (2004) A major lung cancer susceptibility locus maps to chromosome 6q23–25. *American Journal of Human Genetics*, 73, 460–74.

17 Rudd, M.F., Webb, E.L., Matakidou, A. *et al.* (2006) Variants in the GH-IGF axis confer susceptibility to lung cancer. *Genome Research*, 16, 693–701.

18 Vineis, P., Veglia, F., Anttila, S. *et al.* (2004) CYP1A1, GSTM1 and GSTT1 polymorphisms and lung cancer: a pooled analysis of gene-gene interactions. *Biomarkers*, 9, 298–305.

19 Vineis, P., Veglia, F., Benhamou, S. *et al.* (2003) CYP1A1 T3810C polymorphism and lung cancer: a pooled analysis of 2451 cases and 3358 controls. *International Journal of Cancer*, 104, 650–7.

20 Houlston, R.S. (2000) CYP1A1 polymorphisms and lung cancer risk. *Pharmacogenetics*, 10, 105–14.

21 Taioli, E., Gaspari, L., Benhamou, S. *et al.* (2003) Polymorphisms in CYP1A1, GSTM1, GSTT1 and lung cancer below the age of 45 years. *International Journal of Epidemiology*, 32, 60–3.

22 Hung, R.J., Boffetta, P., Brockmoller, J. *et al.* (2003) CYP1A1 and GSTM1 genetic polymorphisms and lung cancer risk in Caucasian non-smokers: a pooled analysis. *Carcinogenesis*, **24**, 875–82.

23 Le Marchand, L., Guo, C., Benhamou, S. *et al.* (2003) Pooled analysis of the CYP1A1 exon 7 polymorphism and lung cancer (United States). *Cancer Causes Control*, **14**, 339–46.

24 Siegfried, J.M. (2001) Women and lung cancer: does ostrogen play a role?. *The Lancet Oncology*, **2**, 506–13.

25 Cascorbi, I. (2006) Genetic basis of toxic reactions to drugs and chemicals. *Toxicology Letters*, **162**, 16–28.

26 Wenzlaff, A.S., Cote, M.L., Bock, C.H. *et al.* (2005) CYP1A1 and CYP1BIX1 polymorphisms and risk of lung cancer among never smokers: a population-based study. *Carcinogenesis*, **26**, 2207–12.

27 Dally, H., Edler, L., Jager, B. *et al.* (2003) The CYP3A4*1B allele increases risk for small cell lung cancer: effect of gender and smoking dose. *Pharmacogenetics*, **13**, 607–18.

28 Arinami, T., Ishiguro, H. and Onaivi, E.S. (2000) Polymorphisms in genes involved in neurotransmission in relation to smoking. *European Journal of Pharmacology*, **410**, 215–26.

29 Rosvold, E.A., Mcglynn, K.A., Lustbader, E.D. and Buetow, K.H. (1995) Identification of an NAD(P)H: quinone oxidoreductase polymorphism and its association with lung cancer and smoking. *Pharmacogenetics*, **5**, 199–206.

30 Yin, L., Pu, Y., Liu, T.-Y., Tung, Y.-H., Chen, K.-W. and Lin, P. (2001) Genetic polymorphisms of NAD(P)H quinone oxidoreductase, CYP1A1 and microsomal epoxide hydrolase and lung cancer risk in Nanjing. *China Lung Cancer*, **33**, 133–41.

31 Larson, R.A., Wang, Y., Banerjee, M. *et al.* (1999) Prevalence of the inactivating 609C–>T polymorphism in the NAD(P)H:quinone oxidoreductase (NQO1) gene in patients with primary and therapy-related myeloid leukemia. *Blood*, **94**, 803–7.

32 Jaiswal, A.K. (2000) Regulation of genes encoding NAD(P)H:quinone oxido-

reductases. *Free Radical Biology and Medicine*, **29**, 254–62.

33 Radjendirane, V., Joseph, P., Lee, Y.H. *et al.* (1998) Disruption of the DT-diaphorase (NQO1) gene in mice leads to increased menadione toxicity. *The Journal of Biological Chemistry*, **273**, 7382–9.

34 Van Schooten, F.J., Boots, A.W., Knappen, A.M. *et al.* (2004) Myeloperoxidase (MPO)-463G->A reduces MPO activity and DNA adduct levels in bronchoalveolar lavages of smokers. *Cancer Epidemiology, Biomarkers and Prevention*, **13**, 828–33.

35 Dally, H., Gassner, K., Jager, B. *et al.* (2002) Myeloperoxidase (MPO) genotype and lung cancer histologic types: the MPO-463 A allele is associated with reduced risk for small cell lung cancer in smokers. *International Journal of Cancer*, **102**, 530–5.

36 Wikman, H., Thiel, S., Jager, B. *et al.* (2001) Relevance of N-acetyltransferase 1 and 2 (NAT1, NAT2) genetic polymorphisms in non-small cell lung cancer susceptibility. *Pharmacogenetics*, **11**, 157–68.

37 Lord, R.V., Brabender, J., Gandara, D. *et al.* (2002) Low ERCC1 expression correlates with prolonged survival after cisplatin plus gemcitabine chemotherapy in non-small cell lung cancer. *Clinical Cancer Research*, **8**, 2286–91.

38 Cobo, M., Isla, D., Massuti, B. *et al.* (2007) Customizing cisplatin based on quantitative excision repair cross-complementing 1 mRNA expression: a phase III trial in non-small cell lung cancer. *Journal of Clinical Oncology*, **25**, 2747–54.

39 Zhou, W., Gurubhagavatula, S., Liu, G. *et al.* (2004) Excision repair cross-complementation group 1 polymorphism predicts overall survival in advanced non-small cell lung cancer patients treated with platinum-based chemotherapy. *Clinical Cancer Research*, **10**, 4939–43.

40 Kiyohara, C., Otsu, A., Shirakawa, T., Fukuda, S. and Hopkin, J.M. (2002) Genetic polymorphisms and lung cancer susceptibility: a review. *Lung Cancer*, **37**, 241–56.

41 Kiyohara, C. and Yoshimasu, K. (2007) Genetic polymorphisms in the nucleotide excision repair pathway and lung cancer risk: a meta-analysis. *International Journal of Medical Sciences*, **4**, 59–71.

42 Hu, Z., Wei, Q., Wang, X. and Shen, H. (2004) DNA repair gene XPD polymorphism and lung cancer risk. *Lung Cancer*, **46**, 1–10.

43 Camps, C., Sarries, C., Rig, B. *et al.* (2003) Assessment of nucleotide excision repair XPD polymorphisms in the peripheral blood of gemcitabine/ cisplatin-treated advanced non-small-cell lung cancer patients. *Clinical Lung Cancer*, **4**, 237–41.

44 Ratnasinghe, D., Yao, S.X., Tangrea, J.A. *et al.* (2001) Polymorphisms of the DNA repair gene XRCC1 and lung cancer risk. *Cancer Epidemiology, Biomarkers and Prevention*, **10**, 119–23.

45 Giachino, D.F., Ghio, P., Regazzoni, S. *et al.* (2007) Prospective assessment of XPD Lys751Gin and XRCC1 Arg399Gin single nucleotide polymorphisms in lung cancer. *Clinical Cancer Research*, **13**, 2876–81.

46 Balasubramanian, S.P., Brown, N.J. and Reed, M.W. (2002) Role of genetic polymorphisms in tumour angiogenesis. *British Journal of Cancer*, **87**, 1057–65.

47 Engels, E.A., Wu, X., Gu, J., Dong, Q., Liu, J. and Spitz, M.R. (2007) Systematic evaluation of genetic variants in the inflammation pathway and risk of lung cancer. *Cancer Research*, **67**, 6520–7.

48 Zhu, Y., Spitz, M.R., Lei, L., Mills, G.B. and Wu, X. (2001) A single nucleotide polymorphism in the matrix metalloproteinase-1 promotor enhances lung cancer susceptibility. *Cancer Research*, **61**, 7825–9.

49 Yu, C., Pan, K., Xing, D., Liang, L. and Lin, D. (2002) Correlation between a single polymorphism in the matrix metalloproteinase-2 promotor and risk of lung cancer. *Cancer Research*, **62**, 6430–3.

50 Fang, S., Jin, X., Wang, R. *et al.* (2005) Polymorphisms in the MMP1 and MMP3 promotor and non-small cell lung carcinoma in north China. *Carcinogenesis*, **26**, 481–6.

51 Taniguchi, K., Yang, P., Jett, J. *et al.* (2002) Polymorphisms in the promotor region of the neutrophil elastase gene are associated with lung cancer development. *Clinical Cancer Research*, **8**, 1115–20.

52 Casse, C., Hu, Y.C. and Ahrendt, S.A. (2003) The XRCC1 codon 399 Gin is associated with adenine to guanine p53 mutations in non-small cell lung cancer. *Mutation Research*, **528**, 19–27.

53 Wilkening, S., Bermejo, J.L. and Hemminki, K. (2007) MDM2 SNP309 and cancer risk: a combined analysis. *Carcinogenesis*, **28**, 2262–7 (epub ahead of print).

54 Bianchi, C., Brollo, A., Ramani, L., Bianchi, T. and Giarelli, L. (2004) Familial mesothelioma of the pleura – a report of 40 cases. *Industrial Health*, **42**, 235–9.

55 Martensson, G., Larsson, S. and Zettergren, L. (1984) Malignant mesothelioma in two pairs of siblings: is there a hereditary predisposing factor? *European Journal of Respiratory Diseases*, **65**, 179–84.

56 Bisconti, M., Bisetti, A. and Bidoli, P. (2000) Malignant mesothelioma in subjects with Marfan's syndrome and Ehlers-Danlos syndrome: only an apparent association? *Respiration*, **67**, 223–8.

57 Musti, M., Cavone, D., Aalto, Y., Scattone, A., Serio, G. and Knuutila, S. (2002) A cluster of familial malignant mesothelioma with del(9p) as the sole chromosomal anomaly. *Cancer Genetics and Cytogenetics*, **138**, 73–6.

58 Yang, M., Choi, Y., Hwangbo, B. and Lee, J.S. (2007) Combined effects of genetic polymorphisms in six selected genes on lung cancer susceptibility. *Lung Cancer*, **57**, 135–42.

11
Hereditary Breast Cancer

Rita Katharina Schmutzler

Summary

Multidisciplinary counseling enables patients to make an informed decision on molecular genetic testing of the *BRCA1* and *BRCA2* breast cancer susceptibility genes. The offer of molecular genetic testing and preventive options depend on pedigree analysis and risk calculation. It is generally agreed that a mutation detection risk of ≥10% is a prerequisite for coverage by regular health care. In the GC-HBOC, the pseudonymous documentation of 5500 families (up to January 2008) in a centralized database has led to the compilation of empirically-based inclusion criteria with an overall mutation detection rate of 25%. Preventive options exist that reduce morbidity and mortality in *BRCA* mutation carriers and should be offered to these women in tertiary care centers. Chances and risks have to be discussed in detail in order to allow the counselee an individual and sustainable shared decision. The next challenges will be: (1) the introduction of new molecular targets into treatment and medical prevention of *BRCA* associated tumors; and (2) the identification of low penetrance genes and the understanding of their concerted action that may play a pivoral role in the development of the majority of breast cancers.

11.1
Introduction

Breast cancer is the most common form of cancer among women in Western countries. While 10% of all women fall ill with an average age of 63, a small group of women have a much higher risk of 60 to 85% of contracting the disease with an average age of 45.

The reason is usually hereditary and mostly caused by a mutation in the susceptibility genes *BRCA1* or *BRCA2*. Population-based surveys have proven that every 500th–2500th woman (0.04–0.2%) in the general population carries such a predisposing mutation and every 20th women who is affected by breast cancer.

Hereditary Tumors: From Genes to Clinical Consequences
Edited by Heike Allgayer, Helga Rehder and Simone Fulda
Copyright © 2009 WILEY-VCH Verlag GmbH & Co. KGaA, Weinheim
ISBN: 978-3-527-32028-8

In a further 15%, familial clustering suggests the impact of mutations in as yet unknown genes that may be transmitted by a complex genetic trait.

Women at increased risk can be identified by predictive molecular genetic analysis that should be preceded by interdisciplinary and non-directive counseling. Prophylactic surgery, preventive drugs, and intensified surveillance can all be considered as preventive measures. Recent data suggest that *BRCA*-associated tumors require different chemotherapeutic regimes compared to sporadic tumors.

In the course of a cooperative research project supported by the German Cancer Aid, a comprehensive prevention concept for women at high risk was established and evaluated in 12 university-based interdisciplinary centers in Germany from 1997 to 2004 [1]. This concept became part of the regular health care in 2005.

In the following, the characteristics of hereditary breast cancer, the current prevention concept, and the recommendations of the GC-HBOC will be detailed.

11.2
Genetic Background

11.2.1
High Penetrance Genes

In about 50% of high risk families, mutations in the breast cancer genes *BRCA1* (breast cancer gene) or *BRCA2* are detected [1, 2]. In a further 40 to 45% of hereditary ailments, mutations in breast cancer genes not yet identified are considered causal. The remaining hereditary breast cancer cases (5–10%) occur in association with rare syndromes that are covered in more detail by other chapters of this book.

11.2.1.1 **BRCA1**
The *BRCA1* gene is located on the long arm of chromosome 17 (17q21) and consists of 22 encoding exons (a total of 24 exons) that generate a protein of 1863 amino acids [3]. So far, over 2000 unique mutations have been documented in this gene worldwide [4]. Numerous individual amino acid exchanges or putative splice changes of uncertain significance have also been identified. These unclassified variants (UCVs) require further investigations, for example, by functional assays, structure-based assessment, or a multifactorial likelihood-ratio model [5–7]. However, classification is cumbersome, as the majority of UCVs occur only one to three times.

In many populations, specific mutation spectra have been described [8, 9]. A mutation profile for the German population was drafted by the GC-HBOC on the basis of 5500 families tested (unpublished data). Founder mutations were identified that had been found in other Caucasian populations, as well as popula-

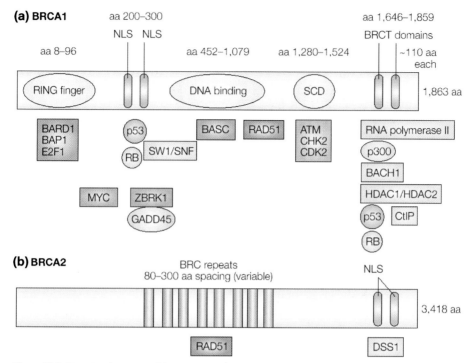

Figure 11.1 Functional regions of the *BRCA1* and *BRCA2* genes. (Reprinted from [11] with permission from Macmillan Publishers Ltd, 2004).

tion-specific changes [1]. These results now permit targeted pre-screening of potential mutation carriers.

Much has been learned about the function of the BRCA1 protein (Figure 11.1a). It interacts with a range of proteins involved in DNA repair by homologous recombination, and is hence responsible for the integrity of the genome [10]. Other functions of the BRCA1 protein, such as cell cycle regulation, ubiquitination, and chromatine remodeling, are probably also associated with DNA repair (Figure 11.2) [11].

11.2.1.2 BRCA2

The *BRCA2* gene is located on the long arm of chromosome 13 (13q13.1) and consists of 26 encoding exons (total 27 exons) responsible for forming a protein from 3418 amino acids [12]. Over 1000 different pathogenic mutations have been found [4]. Even more UCV have been found in the *BRCA2* compared to the *BRCA1* gene.

Although the BRCA2 protein is not as intensively characterized as the BRCA1 protein, it is clear that it also plays a role in DNA repair. It directly binds to RAD51 and initiates homologous recombination in concert with other binding partners Figure 11.1 [10]. *BRCA2* was found to be identical with the *FAND1* gene, one of the genes responsible for Fanconi anaemia, an autosomal recessive disorder which is characterized by radiation sensitivity, skeleton anomalies, abnormal skin pigmentation, dwarf stature, and microophthalmia [13]. Interestingly, while biallelic mutations of *BRCA2* are thus found to be viable, knockout mice provide evidence that biallelic mutations of *BRCA1* are embryonically lethal [14].

11.2.2
Low Penetrance Genes

Due to the failure of linkage analysis in *BRCA1/2*-negative families a polygenic inherited trait is the most plausible explanation, that is, the interaction of many genes of low penetrance. Some genes have already been identified by a candidate gene approach, while high density SNP (single nucleotide polymorphisms) arrays allow genome-wide association (GWA) studies that may reveal novel genes. For the latter approach, high risk families constitute an enriched sample set that enables the use of a reasonable sample size [15, 16].

11.2.2.1 CHEK2
The CHEK2 protein (checkpoint kinase 2), which regulates the cell cycle, interacts directly with the BRCA1 protein. An international CHEK2 consortium identified a truncating mutation in exon 10 in approximately 5% of *BRCA1/2*-negative families, whereas it was found in only 1% of healthy controls [17]. Examination of the complete *CHEK2* gene in *BRCA1/2*-negative families from Germany revealed lower mutation frequencies in the healthy and the ill. A new truncating mutation was also identified that is not associated with any increased breast cancer risk [18]. No diagnostics involving this gene are therefore currently offered. *CHEK2* may, however, play a role as part of a polygenic inheritance trait.

11.2.2.2 ATM
The ATM protein is instantly activated after inducing DNA damage by radiation and interacts with the CHEK2 protein (Figure 11.2). Compound heterozygosity in the *ATM* gene localized at chromosomal band 11q23.2 leads to the rare Ataxia teleangiectasia (AT) syndrome. Patients develop progressive cerebral ataxia and have a greatly increased risk of malignant tumors, especially lymphomas. Heterozygous carriers of an *ATM* mutation have a five-fold increased risk of developing breast cancer [19]. Although about 0.7% of the female population are heterozygous carriers to date, only a few families have been identified in which pathogenic mutations in the *ATM* gene are clearly associated with breast cancer. Research is still required to ascertain the pathogenic significance of missense mutations in the *ATM* gene [20, 21].

11.2.2.3 PALP2
PALP2 encodes for a BRCA2 interacting protein, which is involved in nuclear localization and stability of BRCA2. Biallelic *PALP2* mutations have been detected in a subset of Fanconi anaemia patients and *PALP2* was subsequently found to

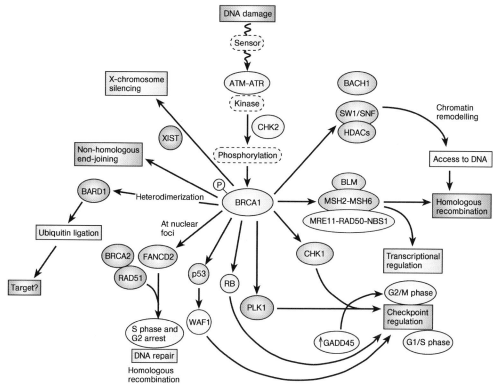

Figure 11.2 Complex and interaction partners of the *BRCA1* and *BRCA2* genes. (Reprinted from [11] with permission from Macmillan Publishers Ltd, 2004).

be identical with *FANCN* [22]. A single association study suggests a two- to three-fold higher risk in individuals with familial breast cancer compared to healthy controls, which needs further validation [23]. As is true for *CHEK2* and *ATM*, incomplete segregation in affected individuals was observed, which seems to be typical for low penetrance genes.

Besides these, multiple susceptibility alleles with low allele frequencies have been identified that also confer moderate risk increases [24–28].

11.2.3
Genome-Wide Association Studies

The hypothesis free GWA approach has recently led to the identification of novel breast cancer susceptible loci [29, 30]. Four of these loci harbor potential causative genes, that is, *FGFR2, TNRC9, MAP3K1*, and *LSP1*. None of these genes appear to be involved in signal transduction pathways that have previously been linked to breast cancer. Although the minor allele frequencies are high (>25%), the per allele odds ratios only range from 1.07 to 1.26. Therefore, predictive genetic testing for these variants does not seem to be justified at the moment. Future studies may unravel the interaction of multiple of these risk alleles and non-genetic risk factors that may finally enter the clinical arena.

11.3
Risk Calculation

Mutations in the *BRCA1* or *BRCA2* gene are transmitted by an autosomal dominant trait. Proof of a mutation associated with the disease means that first-degree relatives, that is, children and siblings, have a 50% risk of inheriting the mutation. Therefore, patients seeking advice are motivated to advise their relatives of the availability of tumour-genetic counseling.

Determining the individual genetic risk for hereditary breast and/or ovarian cancer requires thorough pedigree analysis. It must cover a complete family tree over at least three generations, diagnosis of all tumors in all relatives, age at initial diagnosis for all tumor patients in the family, and age and gender of all affected and unaffected relatives. Also, reproductive and lifestyle factors as well as earlier breast biopsies are considered. The data are used to calculate the individual risk by various models involving different risk weightings.

The epidemiological model most frequently used by clinicians is the Gail model. It is based on data obtained in a case-control study of the participants in a major mammography study (BCDDP study) carried out between 1973 and 1980 in the United States [31]). In addition to reproductive factors and earlier breast biopsies, the number of first-degree relatives with breast cancer is included in the risk calculation. The model was used in a modified form for the U.S. tamoxifen prevention study (NSABP-P1). The Gail model is suitable for estimating a moderate breast cancer risk based on mainly non-genetic factors.

The Clause tables are used as a genetic model. This data are based on a case-control study that was part of the U.S. Cancer and Steroid Hormone Study (CASH) carried out between 1980 and 1982 [32]. The model focuses primarily on breast and ovarian cancer cases among the mothers and sisters of those seeking advice. It is suitable for calculating the risk, given moderate hereditary factors. In large families with many affected women, however, the risk may be underestimated.

The genetic model was developed further by Parmigiani *et al.* [33]. They developed a computer program (BRCAPRO, Cyrillic) that calculates the probability of a *BRCA* gene mutation based on the Bayes theorem. First- and second-degree affected relatives, prevalence and penetration of *BRCA1* and *BRCA2* mutations, relationships between patients, age at diagnosis, and age of healthy relatives are allowed for to calculate the likelihood of heterozygosity and disease risk. The Tyrer–Cuzick model merges genetic and personal risk factors [34].

Within the GC-HBOC a heterozygous probability of at least 20% or a life-time risk of at least 30% according to BRCAPRO is considered a high hereditary disposition. This complies in essence with international guidelines, for example [35]. In such cases preventive measures are offered, even if genetic testing of an index case is not informative.

11.4
Clinical and Histopathological Characteristics

BRCA1 mutation carriers recruited by familial risk criteria have a risk of approximately 80% to develop breast cancer and a risk of approximately 55% to develop ovarian cancer throughout their lifetimes. *BRCA2* mutation carriers contract the disease later in life and have a risk of approximately 85% for breast cancer and a 25% for ovarian cancer throughout their lifetimes. [36]. However, studies based on cases unselected for family history resulted in lower risk estimates [37].

The risk of contralateral breast cancer is significantly higher too, and depends on the age of primary cancer [38]. Forty percent of cases with first breast cancer before the age of 50 develop a contralateral breast cancer. After menopause this risk falls to 12%. The risk is also higher for carriers of a *BRCA1* (43%) than for carriers of a *BRCA2* (35%) mutation, and can be reduced by ovarectomy or tamoxifen [39].

For those with a *BRCA1* mutation there is an increased risk of stomach, kidney, pancreas, uterus cancer, and leukemia. For those with a *BRCA2* mutation, colon, stomach, pancreas, and prostate cancer as well as melanomas are considered associated tumors [40, 41]. Absolute risks have not yet been finally evaluated.

BRCA1 associated tumors in particular show histopathological characteristics. They are often of the medullary sub-type and present with lymphocyte infiltration and pushing margins. They are usually hormone receptor-negative, Her2/neu negative, and poorly differentiated [42]. The histopathology can hence lead to speculate on a *BRCA1* origin.

There are indications that the prognostic significance of the axillary lymph node status in *BRCA*-associated tumors is less reliable compared to sporadic tumors [43]. Moreover, *in vitro* and retrospective analyses suggest that these tumors have a different chemo-sensitivity range and respond especially well to platinum-containing regimens [44, 45]. These data provide the rational for ongoing prospective randomized trials elaborating the most efficacious chemotherapeutic regimes for *BRCA*-associated tumors.

Exciting data have recently been presented suggesting that *BRCA* associated tumors can be specifically targeted by poly(ADP-ribose)polymerase (PARP1), an enzyme that is essential for base excision repair. During cell division, inhibition of PARP1 leads to the conversion of single strand breaks into double-strand breaks in the replication forks. In BRCA-deficient cells these defects cannot be repaired by homologous recombination, hence leading to apoptosis [46, 47]. These results open the potential for targeted therapeutic options in the future, that are currently evaluated in clinical studies.

11.5
Clinical Management

The preventive measures available for the general population are inadequate for women with hereditary risk of developing breast and/or ovarian cancer. Mammography screening generally starts at the age of 50 when half of the *BRCA1* mutation carriers of the current birth cohort are already affected by breast cancer. The early age makes mammography in particular unsuitable as the sole screening measure since it has a high rate of false-negatives given the typical dense parenchyma of younger breasts.

11.5.1
Ovarectomy

Prospective and retrospective cohort studies show that bilateral prophylactic salpingo-oophorectomy (BPSO) reduces the risk of ovarian cancer in *BRCA* mutation carriers by more than 90% [48, 49]. The remaining risk of breast cancer is also significantly reduced to 50% and remains in about the same range after low hormonal add-back [50]. It has recently been demonstrated that BPSO reduces overall mortality by 70% [51]. BPSO is hence recommended by the GC-HBOC in certain circumstances (Table 11.1).

Detailed histological processing by reference pathologists is advised that may reveal preneoplasias or early carcinomas so that the time of surgery can be optimized in the future. As reported by international centres, BPSO is also well accepted in Germany by over 50% of the mutation carriers.

11.5.2
Mastectomy

Retrospective and prospective cohort studies demonstrate that breast cancer risk in *BRCA* mutation carriers is greatly reduced by bilateral prophylactic mastectomy (BPM) [52]. To achieve the best preventive effect, bilateral mastectomy should include removal of the pectoralis fascia, the mamillary areola complex, and the lobus axillaris. Simultaneous reconstruction should routinely be offered. The guidelines from the GC-HBOC are outlined in Table 11.1. Interestingly, the acceptance for BPM varies greatly among countries and seems to depend on both cultural influences and the availability of screening programs. In Germany, where women at high risk have access to a structured surveillance program within the normal medical services, BPM is chosen by less than 10% of mutation carriers.

11.5.3
Prevention Using Drugs

No reliable data yet exist for hereditary breast cancer. Retrospective genetic analysis of the affected women in the NSABP P1 study indicated that tamoxifen has a protective effect in women with a *BRCA2* mutation [53]. This is supported by the reduction in contralateral secondary carcinomas under tamoxifen treatment [39]. However, *in vitro* data suggest that in the absence of *BRCA1*, breast cancer development can be promoted by an agonistic activity of tamoxifen [54, 55]. Currently women at risk are offered participation in the Europe-wide IBIS II study in which an aromatase inhibitor is employed.

Table 11.1 Bilateral prophylactic salpingo-oophorectomy and bilateral prophylactic mastectomy: Indications and surgery.

Bilateral prophylactic salpingo-oophorectomy (BPSO)

Indications
Completed family planning and age over 35 years or 5 years before earliest disease age in the family and, interdisciplinary counselling[a] and proven mutation in the *BRCA1* or *BRCA2* gene or heterozygosity risk ≥ 20% or lifelong risk ≥ 30% given an uninformative genetic test.[b,c]

Surgery
Laparoscopic extirpation of the ovaries and fallopian tubes with peritoneal sampling and lavage.

Bilateral prophylactic mastectomy (BPM)

Indications
Age over 25 years or 5 years before earliest disease age in the family, interdisciplinary counseling[a] and proven mutation in the *BRCA1* or *BRCA2* gene or heterozygosity risk ≥ 20% or lifelong risk ≥ 30% given an uninformative genetic test.[b,c]

Surgery
Complete mastectomy incl. the mamilla areola complex. Simultaneous reconstruction should be offered.

---

a Before any prophylactic surgery is undertaken, gynaecological, human genetic, and psycho-oncological counseling to clarify the individual risk of contracting the disease, the risk reduction to be expected, and the patient's motivational circumstances, is recommended.
b Uninformative molecular genetic diagnosis exists if the index case in the family has no mutation in the *BRCA1* or *BRCA2* gene, or no mutation clearly relevant to the illness (unclassified variant, UCV). In such cases, no predictive analysis is carried out on the healthy relatives. If no index patient is available, a predictive genetic test may be offered in case the counselee would opt for prophylactic surgery, if a deleterious mutation is detected.
c There is as yet no data on mortality reduction through secondary prophylactic surgery for patients already diseased.

11.5.4
Structured Surveillance

Many prospective cohort studies have been undertaken to prove the benefits of intensive surveillance in *BRCA* mutation carriers and women at high risk, starting around 25 to 30 years of age. All studies, including ours, confirmed low sensitivity of mammography in this young risk group [56–62]. The GC-HBOC therefore established a structured surveillance program that includes sonography, mammography, and MRI (Table 11.2). MRI examination leads to an improved detection rate of early breast cancer stages [62–64]. As Kriege *et al.* [64] showed that 18% of the screen detected carcinomas were only visible by mammography, it still remains an obligatory part of the screening program. Also, recent data suggest a benefit of high-resolution sonography as an interval examination, in case one takes into consideration the specific imaging criteria of *BRCA1* associated tumors that fre-

Table 11.2 The GC-HBOC structured surveillance program.

Target groups
Age over 25 years or 5 years before earliest disease age in the family and proven mutation in
the *BRCA1* or *BRCA2* gene or heterozygosity risk ≥ 20% or lifelong risk ≥ 30% given an
uninformative genetic test.[a]

Examinations/tests
Regular self-examination of the breasts after instruction[b] by a doctor
Regular medical examination of the breasts and ovaries every 6 months
Ultrasound examination of the breasts (min. 7.5 MHz) every 6 months
Mammography every 12 months[b]
Magnetic resonance tomography (MRT) of the breasts every 12 months[c]

---

a Uninformative molecular genetic diagnosis exists if the index case in the family has no mutation
   in the *BRCA1* or *BRCA2* gene, or no mutation clearly relevant to the illness (unclassified variant
   (UCV)). In such cases, no predictive analysis is carried out on the healthy relatives.
b Starting at the age of 30.
c MRT is usually carried out until involution of the gland parenchyma (ACR1 or 2).

quently resemble criteria of fibroadenomas [65]. Optimal screening intervals and
the optimal combination of imaging modalities are still not certain. Moreover, data
on mortality reduction are still missing. Taking together, after the identification
of the right risk genes BRCA1 and BRCA2 a decade ago, we now enter a second
era of genetic discovery of low penetrance genes that may be relevant for the vast
majority of breast cancer. Effective preventive strategies have been established for
BRCA1/2 mutation carriers. With the identification of low penetrance genes, risk-
adjusted prevention programs may become feasible. The recent development of
the molecular targets for BRCA1/2 associated tumors is exiting and may further
improve the well-being of such burdened women.

References

1 German Consortium for Hereditary
  Breast and Ovarian Cancer (2002)
  Comprehensive analysis of 989 patients
  with breast or ovarian cancer provides
  BRCA1 and *BRCA2* mutation profiles
  and frequencies for the German
  population. *International Journal of
  Cancer*, **97**, 472–80.
2 Frank, T.S., Deffenbaugh, A.M., Reid,
  J.E., Hulick, M., Ward, B.E., Lingenfelter,
  B., Gumpper, K.L. *et al.* (2002) Clinical
  characteristics of individuals with
  germline mutations in *BRCA1* and
  BRCA2: analysis of 10 000 individuals.
  Journal of Clinical Oncology, **20**, 1480–90.
3 Miki, Y., Swensen, J., Shattuck-Eidens, D.,
  Futreal, P.A., Harshman, K., Tavtigian, S.,
  Liu, Q., Cochran, C. *et al.* (1994) A strong
  candidate for the breast and ovarian cancer
  susceptibility gene *BRCA1*. *Science*, **266**,
  66–71.
4 BIC database http://www.nhgri.nih.
  gov/intramural_research/labtransfer/bic.
5 Carvalho, M.A., Couch, F.J. and Monteiro,
  A.N.A. (2007) Functional assays for
  BRCA1 and *BRCA2*. *J. Biocel.*, **39**,
  298–310.
6 Mirkovic, N., Marti-Renom, M.A., Weber,
  B.L., Sali, A. and Monteiro, A.N. (2004)
  Structure-based assessment of missense

mutations in human *BRCA1*: implications for breast and ovarian cancer predisposition. *Cancer Research*, **64**, 3790–7.

7 Goldgar, D.E., Douglas, F.E., Deffenbaugh, A.M., Monteiro, A.N.A., Tavtigian, S.V., Couch, F.J. and BIC Steering Committee (2004) Integrated evaluation of DNA sequence variants of unknown clinical significance: application to *BRCA1* and *BRCA2*. *American Journal of Human Genetics*, **75**, 535–44.

8 Tonin, P., Weber, B., Offit, K., Couch, F., Rebbeck, T.R., Neuhausen, S., Godwin, A.K., Daly, M. *et al.* (1996) Frequency of recurrent *BRCA1* and *BRCA2* mutations in Ashkenazi Jewish breast cancer families. *Nature Medicine*, **2**, 1179–83.

9 Syrjäkoski, K., Vahteristo, P., Eerola, H., Tamminen, A., Kivinummi, K., Sarantaus, L., Holli, K., Blomqvist, C. *et al.* (2000) Population-based study of *BRCA1* and *BRCA2* mutations in 1035 unselected Finnish breast cancer patients. *Journal of the National Cancer Institute*, **92**, 1529–31.

10 Venkitaraman, A.R. (2004) Tracing the network connecting BRCA and Fanconi anaemia proteins. *Nature Reviews. Cancer*, **4**, 266–76.

11 Narod, S.A. and Foulkes, W.D. (2004) BRCA1 and BRCA2: 1994 and beyond. *Nature Reviews. Cancer*, **4**, 665–76.

12 Wooster, R., Bignell, G., Lancaster, J., Swift, S., Seal, S., Mangion, J., Collins, N., Gregory, S. *et al.* (1995) Identification of the breast cancer susceptibility gene *BRCA2*. *Nature*, **378**, 789–92.

13 Howlett, N.G., Taniguchi, T., Olson, S., Cox, B., Waisfisz, Q., De Die-Smulders, C., Persky, N., Grompe, M. *et al.* (2002) Biallelic inactivation of *BRCA2* in Fanconi anaemia. *Science*, **297**, 606–9.

14 Hakem, R., de la Pampa, J.L., Sirard, C., Mo, R., Woo, M., Hakem, A., Wakeham, A., Potter, J. *et al.* (1996) The tumor suppressor gene *BRCA1* is required for embryonic cellular proliferation in the mouse. *Cell*, **85**, 1009–23.

15 Houlston, R.S. and Peto, J. (2002) The future of association studies of common cancers. *Human Genetics*, **112**, 434–5.

16 Houlston, R.S. and Peto, J. (2004) The search for low-penetrance cancer susceptibility alleles. *Oncogene*, **23**, 6471–6.

17 Meijers-Heijboer, H., van den Ouweland, A., Klijn, J., Wasielewski, M., de Snoo, A., Oldenburg, R., Hollestelle, A., Houben, M. *et al.* (2002) Low penetrance susceptibility to breast cancer due to CHEK2 del1100delC in noncarriers of *BRCA1* and *BRCA2* mutations. *Nature Genetics*, **31**, 55–9.

18 Dufault, M.R., Betz, B., Wappenschmidt, B., Hofmann, W., Bandick, K., Golla, A., Pietschmann, A., Nestle-Krämling, C. *et al.* (2004) Limited relevance of the *CHEK2* gene in hereditary breast cancer. *International Journal of Cancer*, **110**, 320–5.

19 Teraoka, S.N., Malone, K.E., Doody, D.R., Suter, N.M., Ostrander, E.A., Daling, J.R. and Concannon, P. (2001) Increased frequency of *ATM* mutations in breast carcinoma patients with early onset disease and ovarian cancer. *Cancer*, **93**, 479–87.

20 Thorstenson, Y.R., Roxas, A., Kroiss, R., Jenkins, M.A., Yu, K.M., Bachrich, T., Muhr, D., Wayne, T.L. *et al.* (2003) Contributions of *ATM* mutations to familial breast and ovarian cancer. *Cancer Research*, **63**, 3325–33.

21 Renwick, A., Thompson, D., Seal, S., Kelly, P., Chagtai, T., Ahmed, M., North, B., Jayatilake, H. *et al.* (2006) *ATM* mutations that cause ataxia-telangiectasia are breast cancer susceptibility alleles. *Nature Genetics*, **38**, 873–5.

22 Reid, S., Schindler, D., Hanenberg, H., Barker, K., Hanks, S., Kalb, R., Neveling, K., Kelly, P. *et al.* (2006) Biallelic mutations in PALBIX2 cause Fanconi anemia subtype FA-N and predispose to childhood cancer. *Nature Genetics*, **39**, 162–4.

23 Rahmann, N., Seal, S., Thompson, D., Kelly, P., Renwick, A., Elliot, A., Reid, S., Spanova, K. *et al.* (2007) PALBIX2, which encodes a BRCA2-interacting protein, is a breast cancer susceptibility gene. *Nature Genetics*, **39**, 165–7.

24 Burwinkel, B., Wirtenberger, M., Klaes, R., Schmutzler, R.K., Grzybowska, E., Forsti, A., Frank, B., Bermejo, J.L. *et al.* (2005) Association of NCOA3 polymorphisms with breast cancer risk. *Clinical Cancer Research*, **15**, 2169–74.

25 Frank, B., Hemminki, K., Wappenschmidt, B., Meindl, A., Klaes, R., Schmutzler, R.K., Bugert, P., Untch, M. *et al.* (2005) Association of the CASP10 V410I variant with reduced familial breast cancer risk and interaction with the CASP8 D302H variant. *Carcinogenesis*, **27**, 606–9.

26 Frank, B., Bermejo, J.L., Hemminki, K., Klaes, R., Bugert, P., Wappenschmidt, B., Schmutzler, R.K. and Burwinkel, B. (2005) Re: association of a common variant of the *CASP8* gene with reduced risk of breast cancer. *Journal of the National Cancer Institute*, **97**, 1012–13.

27 Wilkening, S., Bermejo, J.L., Burwinkel, B., Klaes, R., Wappenschmidt, B., Schmutzler, R.K., Meindl, A., Bugert, P. *et al.* (2006) The single nucleotide polymorphism IVS+309 in MDM2 does not affect risk of familial breast cancer. *Cancer Research*, **66**, 646–8.

28 Tchatchou, S., Wirtenberger, M., Hemminki, K., Sutter, C., Meindl, A., Wappenschmidt, B., Kiechle, M., Bugert, P. *et al.* (2007) Aurora kinases A and B and familial breast cancer risk. *Cancer Letters*, **247**, 266–72.

29 Easton, D.F., Pooley, K.A., Dunning, A.M., Pharaoah, P.D., Thompson, D., Ballinger, D.G., Struewing, J.P., Morrison, J. *et al.* (2007) Genome-wide association study identifies novel breast cancer susceptibility loci. *Nature*, **28**, 1–9.

30 Hunter, D.J., Kraft, P., Jacobs, K.B., Cox, D.G., Yeager, M., Hankinson, S.E., Wacholder, S., Wang, Z. *et al.* (2007) A genome-wide association study identifies alleles in FGFR2 associated with risk of sporadic postmenopausal breast cancer. *Nature Genetics*, 1–5, DOI: 10.1038.

31 Gail, M.H. and Benichou, J. (1994) Epidemiology and biostatistics program of the National Cancer Institute. *Journal of the National Cancer Institute*, **86**, 573–5.

32 Claus, E.B., Schildkraut, J.M., Thompson, W.D. and Risch, N.J. (1996) The genetic attributable risk of breast and ovarian cancer: *American Cancer Society*, **20**, 2318–24.

33 Parmigiani, G., Berry, D.A. and Aguilar, O. (1998) Determining carrier probabilities for breast cancer-susceptibility genes BRCA1 and BRCA2. *American Journal of Human Genetics*, **62**, 145–58.

34 Tyrer, J., Duffy, S.W. and Cuzick, J. (2003) A breast cancer prediction model incorporating familial and personal risk factors. *Statistics in Medicine*, **23**, 1111–30.

35 NICE, N.H.S.Clinical Guideline 14 (2004) and 41 (2006) The classification and care of women at risk of familial breast cancer in primary, secondary and tertiary care.

36 King, M.C. and Marks, J.H. and Mandell, J.B. for the New York Breast Cancer Study Group (2003) Breast and ovarian cancer risks due to inherited mutations in BRCA1 and BRCA2. *Science*, **302**, 643–6.

37 Antoniou, A., Pharoah, P.D., Narod, S., Risch, H.A., Eyfjord, J.E., Hopper, J.L., Loman, N., Olsson, H. *et al.* (2003) Average risks of breast and ovarian cancer associated with BRCA1 or BRCA2 mutations detected in case series unselected for family history: a combined analysis of 22 studies. *American Journal of Human Genetics*, **72**, 1117–30.

38 Verhoog, L.C., Brekelmans, C.T.M., Seynaeve, C., Meijers-Heijboer, E.J., Klijn, J.G. *et al.* (2000) Contralateral breast cancer risk is influenced by the age at onset in BRCA1-associated breast cancer. *British Journal of Cancer*, **83**, 384–6.

39 Metcalfe, K., Lynch, H.T., Ghadirian, P., Tung, N., Olivotto, I., Warner, E., Olopade, O.I., Eisen, A. *et al.* (2004) Contralateral breast cancer in BRCA1 and BRCA2 mutation carriers. *Journal of Clinical Oncology*, **22**, 2328–35.

40 Risch, H.A., McLaughlin, J.R., Cole, D.E., Rosen, B., Bradley, L., Kwan, E., Jack, E., Vesprini, D.J. *et al.* (2001) Prevalence and penetrance of germline BRCA1 and BRCA2 mutations in a population series of 649 women with ovarian cancer. *American Journal of Human Genetics*, **68**, 700–10.

41 Thompson, D., Easton, D.F. and Breast Cancer Linkage Consortium (2002) Cancer incidence in BRCA1 mutation carriers. *Journal of the National Cancer Institute*, **94**, 1358–65.

42 Lakhani, S.R., Jacquemier, J., Sloane, J.P., Gusterson, B.A., Anderson, T.J., van de Vijver, M.J., Farid, L.M., Venter, D. *et al.* (1998) Multifactorial analysis of differences between sporadic breast cancers and

cancers involving *BRCA1* and *BRCA2* mutation. *Journal of the National Cancer Institute*, **90**, 1138–45.

43 Robson, M.E., Chappuis, P.O., Satagopan, J., Wong, N., Boyd, J., Goffin, J.R., Hudis, C., Roberge, D. *et al.* (2003) A combined analysis of outcome following breast cancer: differences in survival based on *BRCA1/BRCA2* mutation status and administration of adjuvant treatment. *Breast Cancer Research*, **6**, R8–17.

44 Quinn, J.E., Kennedy, R.D., Mullan, P.B., Gilmore, P.M., Carty, M., Johnston, P.G. and Harkin, D.P. (2003) BRCA1 functions as a differential modulator of chemotherapy-induced apoptosis. *Cancer Research*, **63**, 6221–8.

45 Byrski, T., Gronwald, J., Huzarski, T., Grzybowska, E., Budryk, M., Stawicka, M., Mierzwa, T., Szwiec, M. *et al.* (2007) Response to neo-adjuvant chemotherapy in women with BRCA1-positive breast cancers. *Breast Cancer Research and Treatment*, 1–8. DOI: 10.1007.

46 Bryant, H.E., Schultz, N., Thomas, H.D., Parker, K.M., Flower, D., Lopez, E., Kyle, S., Meuth, M. *et al.* (2005) Specific killing of BRCA2-deficient tumours with inhibitors of poly(ADP-ribose) polymerase. *Nature*, **434**, 913–17.

47 Farmer, H., McCabe, N., Lord, C.J., Tutt, A.N., Johnson, D.A., Richardson, T.B., Santarosa, M., Dillon, K.J. *et al.* (2005) Targeting the DNA repair defect in *BRCA* mutant cells as a therapeutic strategy. *Nature*, **434**, 917–21.

48 Kauff, N.D., Satagopan, J.M., Robson, M.E., Scheuer, L., Hensley, M., Hudis, C.A., Ellis, N.A., Boyd, J. *et al.* (2002) Risk-reducing salpingo-oophorectomy in women with a *BRCA1* or *BRCA2* mutation. *New England Journal of Medicine*, **346**, 1609–15.

49 Rebbeck, T.R., Lynch, H.T., Neuhausen, S.L., Narod, S.A., Van't Veer, L., Garber, J.E., Evans, G., Isaacs, C. *et al.* (2002) Prophylactic oophorectomy in carriers of *BRCA1* or *BRCA2* mutations. *New England Journal of Medicine*, **346**, 1616–22.

50 Rebbeck, T.R., Friebel, T., Wagner, T., Lynch, H.T., Garber, J.E., Daly, M.B., Isaacs, C., Olopade, O.I. *et al.* (2005) Effect of short-term hormone replacement therapy on breast cancer risk reduction after bilateral prophylactic oophorectomy in *BRCA1* and *BRCA2* mutation carriers: the PROSE Study Group. *Journal of Clinical Oncology*, **23**, 7804–10.

51 Domchek, S.M., Friebel, T.M., Neuhausen, S.L., Wagner, T., Evans, G., Isaacs, C., Garber, J.E., Daly, M.B. *et al.* (2006) Mortality after bilateral salpingo-oophorectomy in *BRCA1* and *BRCA2* mutation carriers: a prospective cohort study. *The Lancet Oncology*, **7**, 223–9.

52 Meijers-Heijboer, H., van Geel, B., van Putten, W.L., Henzen-Logmans, S.C., Seynaeve, C., Menke-Pluymers, M.B., Bartels, C.C., Verhoog, L.C. *et al.* (2001) Breast cancer after prophylactic bilateral mastectomy in women with a *BRCA1* or *BRCA2* mutation. *New England Journal of Medicine*, **345**, 159–64.

53 King, M.C., Wieand, S., Hale, K., Lee, M., Walsh, T., Owens, K., Tait, J., Ford, L. *et al.* (2001) Tamoxifen and breast cancer incidence among women with inherited mutations in *BRCA1* and *BRCA2*: National Surgical Adjuvant Breast and Bowel Project (NSABP-P1) breast cancer prevention trial. *The Journal of the American Medical Association*, **286**, 2251–6.

54 Jones, L.P., Li, M., Halama, E.D., Ma, Y., Lubet, R., Grubbs, C.J., Deng, C.X., Rosen, E.M. *et al.* (2005) Promotion of mammary cancer development by tamoxifen in a mouse model of *BRCA1*-mutation-related breast cancer. *Oncogene*, **24**, 3554–62.

55 Jones, L.P., Tilli, M.T., Assefnia, S., Torre, K., Halama, E.D., Parrish, A., Rosen, E.M. and Furth, P.A. (2007) Activation of estrogen signalling pathways collaborates with loss of *BRCA1* to promote development of ER(-positive mammary preoplasis and cancer. *Oncogene*, 1–9, DOI: 10.1038.

56 Brekelmans, C.T., Seynaeve, C., Bartels, C.C., Tilanus-Linthorst, M.M., Meijers-Heijboer, E.J., Crepin, C.M., van Geel, A.A., Menke, M. *et al.* (2001) Effectiveness of breast cancer surveillance in *BRCA1/2* gene mutation carriers and women with high familial risk. *Journal of Clinical Oncology*, **19**, 924–30.

57 Gui, G.P.H., Hogben, R.K.F., Walsh, G., Hern, R.A. and Eeles, R. (2001) The

incidence of breast cancer from screening women according to predicted family history risk: does annual clinical examination add to mammography? *European Journal of Cancer*, **37**, 1668–73.

58 Kollias, J., Sibbering, D.M. and Blamey, R.W. (1998) Screening women aged less than 50 years with a family history of breast cancer. *European Journal of Cancer*, **34**, 878–83.

59 Lalloo, F., Boggis, C.R., Evans, D.G., Shenton, A., Threlfall, A.G. and Howell, A. (1998) Screening by mammography, women with a family history of breast cancer. *European Journal of Cancer*, **34**, 937–40.

60 Scheuer, L., Kauff, N., Robson, M., Kelly, B., Barakat, R., Satagopan, J., Ellis, N., Hensley, M. *et al.* (2002) Outcome of preventive surgery and screening for breast and ovarian cancer in *BRCA* mutation carriers. *Journal of Clinical Oncology*, **20**, 1260–8.

61 Tilanus-Linthorst, M.M., Bartels, C.C., Obdeijn, A.I. and Oudkerk, M. (2000) Earlier detection of breast cancer by surveillance of women at familial risk. *European Journal of Cancer*, **36**, 514–19.

62 Kuhl, C.K., Schmutzler, R.K., Leutner, C.C., Kempe, A., Hocke, A., Wardelmann, E., Maringa, M., Krebs, D. and Schild, H. (2000) Breast MR imaging screening in 192 women proved or suspected to be carriers of a breast cancer susceptibility gene: preliminary results. *Radiology*, **215**, 267–79.

63 Warner, E., Plewes, D.B., Shumak, R.S., Catzavelos, G.C., Di Prospero, L.S., Yaffe, M.J., Goel, V., Ramsay, E. *et al.* (2001) Comparison of breast magnetic resonance imaging, mammography, and ultrasound for surveillance of women at high risk for hereditary breast cancer. *Journal of Clinical Oncology*, **19**, 3524–31.

64 Kriege, M., Brekelmans, C.T., Boetes, C., Besnard, P.E., Zonderland, H.M., Obdeijn, I.M., Manoliu, R.A., Kok, T. *et al.* (2004) Efficacy of MRI and mammography for breast-cancer screening in women with a familial or genetic predisposition. *New England Journal of Medicine*, **351**, 427–37.

65 Rhiem, K., Flucke, U. and Schmutzler, R.K. (2006) BRCA1 associated breast carcinomas frequently present with benign sonographic features. *American Journal of Roentgenology*, **186**, E11–12.

12
Hereditary Ovarian and Endometrial Cancer

Marion Kiechle

Summary

Five percent of endometrial and ovarian carcinomas are based on a genetic pre-disposition. Most of the hereditary ovarian cancers (HOC) occur due to deleterious mutations in *BRCA1* or *BRCA2*. Hereditary endometrial cancer (HEC) mainly occurs within the Lynch syndrome or hereditary non-polyposis colon cancer (HNPCC) and is based on mutations in the mismatch repair genes (*MLH1, MSH2, MSH6*). Besides the positive family history for further endometrial or colon carci-nomas in the case of HEC, or further ovarian carcinomas and breast cancer cases in the case of HOC, the clinical feature is the relatively young age of onset, which is under the age of 50 for HEC, and under the age of 55 for HOC. The most effec-tive prevention strategies are prophylactic surgical procedures.

12.1
Epidemiology

Epithelial ovarian cancer is the sixth most common malignant tumor in women and has the worst prognosis of all malignant tumors of the genitourinary tract. The 5-year survival rate is low (40%) and has not improved dramatically over the last 20 years, which is thought to be related to the advanced stage of the disease at presentation. The life-time risk for European women without any family history is low (1.25–1.6%). Ninety-five percent of ovarian cancers occur sporadically and 5% are based on a genetic predisposition. If a first-degree relative is diagnosed with ovarian cancer, the life-time risk increases to 5% [1]. The following family constellations fulfill the criteria for hereditary ovarian cancer (HOC):

- Women with a personal history of both breast and ovarian cancer;

- Women with ovarian cancer and a close relative with breast cancer at ≤50 or ovarian cancer at any age;

- At least two women with ovarian cancer in a family;

- Women from families with multiple cases of colorectal adenocarcinomas with early onset (under the age of 50) together with ovarian or endometrial cancer, hereditary non-polyposis colon cancer (HNPCC);

- Women from families with germline mutations of *BRCA1* or *BRCA2,* mismatch repair genes (*MLH1, MSH2*) or *PT53.*

Endometrial cancer is the most common gynecological cancer with a life-time risk of 2.7%. The disease has an excellent 5-year survival rate of 85% due to early clinical disease presentation. Epidemiological studies have shown a significantly increased risk of several different cancers (mainly colon cancer, but also cancer of the ovaries, stomach, pancreas, and urothelium) in first-degree relatives of women with endometrial cancer, indicating a genetic component in some women, which is estimated to be 5%. The majority of hereditary endometrial cancer (HEC) occurs in HNPCC families which are clinically identified by the Amsterdam criteria (see Chapter 17 on Lynch syndrome (HNPCC)). The following modified Bethesda criteria help to identify more HNPCC-associated hereditary endometrial carcinomas or atypical HNPCC families:

- Women diagnosed with endometrial cancer under the age of 50;

- Women with endometrial cancer and a first-degree relative with a HNPCC-associated malignancy (cancer of the colon, rectum, stomach, uroepithelium, ovary, skin) in a family;

- Two first-degree relatives with endometrial cancer and/or HNPCC associated malignancy (one under age 45) and/or colorectal adenoma under age 40;

- Women with endometrial or ovarian cancer with a synchronous or metachronous colon or HNPCC associated tumor at any age.

12.2
Genetic Background

Approximately 95% of hereditary ovarian cancers are based on mutations in *BRCA1* or *BRCA2* (Table 12.1). The penetrance rates reported in the literature

Table 12.1 Susceptibility genes in HOC and HEC.

Genes	HOC (%)	HEC (%)
BRCA1	75	5
BRCA2	10	–
P53	2	–
Mismatch repair genes: *MSH2, MLH1, MSH6*	8	85
Unknown	5	10

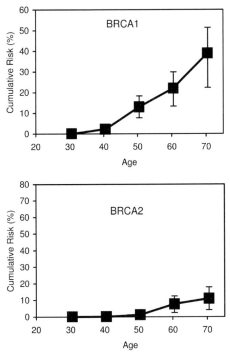

Figure 12.1 Cumulative life-time risk for ovarian cancer in *BRCA1* and *BRCA2* mutation carriers.

vary, depending on the analyzed population and gene mutation. The largest meta-analysis comprises 22 studies including 8000 *BRCA1* and 2 mutation carriers [2]. The cumulative life-time risk for *BRCA1* mutation carriers to develop ovarian cancer is 39 to 46%. Estimations for the life-time risk for *BRCA2* mutation carriers to develop ovarian cancer are much lower compared to *BRCA1* and are reported to be 10 to 27% (Figure 12.1). The basic life-time risk for a woman to develop ovarian cancer is significantly lower and is estimated to be 1 to 2% until the age of 70. The median age of onset for hereditary ovarian cancer is lower compared to sporadic cases. Regarding *BRCA* mutation carriers, the risk for ovarian cancer increases tremendously up from the age of 40, which should be considered for prophylactic procedures (Figure 12.1).

Besides the increased risk for breast and ovarian cancer in *BRCA1* mutation carriers, there is also an increased risk for colon (2x) and prostate (2x) and possibly also for endometrial and cervical cancer [3, 4]. In families with *BRCA2* mutations there are increased risks for male breast cancer (15x), prostate (4x), and pancreatic cancer (3x) [3, 5].

The vast majority of HEC is based on mutations in the mismatch repair genes and occur within the Lynch syndrome or HNPCC. The most commonly affected genes are *MLH1* and *MSH2*, followed by *MSH6*. Germline *MSH6* mutations have been reported in several families with multiple members affected with endometrial cancer. In families with atypical HNPCC, in which endometrial cancer was the leading feature, mainly germline mutations were identified in the *MSH6* gene. It appears from a number of studies that highly penetrant endometrial cancer genes other than HNPCC genes are unlikely to exist, or may be extremely rare. If a site-specific HEC syndrome exists, it results from inherited susceptibility rendered by one or several polymorphic alleles, each acting with relatively low penetrance [6].

The mismatch repair genes show highly penetrant autosomal dominant inheritance. In females, the life-time risk of endometrial cancer by 70 is 40 to 60% with an equally high risk for colon cancer, and a life- time risk of ovarian cancer of 9 to 12%. Most of the inherited endometrial carcinomas occur under the age of 50 (median age 48). In unselected patients with endometrial cancer under the age of 50, the rate of detectable germline mutations in the mismatch repair genes is between 5.2 and 9% [7].

12.3
Phenotype

Regarding the phenotype of hereditary ovarian cancer, three different syndromes can be distinguished:

1. The breast and ovarian cancer syndrome is the most common and accounts for 90% of all hereditary ovarian cancer cases. It is inherited in an autosomal dominant pattern and based on deleterious mutations of the genes *BRCA1* located on chromosome 17q21, and *BRCA2* located on chromosome 13q12. The probability of detecting a *BRCA1* or two germline mutation increases with the number of breast and ovarian cancer cases in a family and younger ages of onset.

2. HOC as well as HEC are also common in females from families with HNPCC, based on mutations in the mismatch repair genes, such as *MLH1* (chromosome 3p21) or *MSH2* (chromosome 2p15).

3. Germline mutations of p53 located on chromosome 17p13 are very rare (<1% of all hereditary tumor syndromes). The so-called Li-Fraumeni syndrome (see Chapter 3 on family cancer syndromes) leads to a heterogeneous occurrence of multiple malignant diseases (osteo- and soft tissue sarcomas, brain tumors, leukemia, breast cancer, lung cancer, prostate cancer, pancreatic cancer, colon cancer, ovarian cancer), which can develop very early during childhood.

Further susceptibility genes or gene clusters are assumed for HOC, since not in all families mutations of the above-mentioned genes are found [8].

The histology and the survival rates of HOC based on *BRCA1/2* mutations are not as well analyzed as the *BRCA1/2* associated breast cancer cases (see Chapter 11 on hereditary breast cancer) [9]. Nevertheless, it was published that *BRCA1-*

associated ovarian cancer cases show a higher grading and a higher percentage of solid tumor components compared to sporadic ovarian cancer. Moreover, higher rates of somatic p53 mutations were found in *BRCA1* positive ovarian carcinomas [7]. Several studies revealed a larger number of serous adenocarcinomas in HOC (89%) compared to cases without any family history of ovarian cancer [11–13]. There is first evidence that *BRCA1* induced ovarian carcinomas show a different protein expression profile as compared to *BRCA2* positive or sporadic cases [12].

Some retrospective studies came to the conclusion that the *BRCA1/2* mutational status might have an impact on survival. *BRCA1* mutation carriers seem to have a shorter survival rate. The 5-year survival rate of patients with epithelial *BRCA1* positive ovarian cancer was calculated to be 21% and for patients with *BRCA2* mutations 25%. This was significantly lower compared to the survival rate of 45% of the patients with sporadic ovarian cancer [14]. Further larger and prospective studies have to be conducted before patients can be counseled regarding a prognostic difference between hereditary and sporadic ovarian cancer.

Most of the HECs occur within the HNPCC or Lynch syndrome (see Chapter 17 on Lynch syndrome (HNPCC)). HNPCC families are usually identified clinically by their family history of colorectal cancer (Amsterdam criteria) rather than endometrial or ovarian cancer. However, in about 10%, atypical HNPCC families are reported in which endometrial cancer is the leading feature.

Except for a younger age of onset, so far there is no evidence that HECs have a different histopathology, clinical appearance, or survival rate. However, in a recent cohort study of 100 women with endometrial cancer under the age of 50, it was shown that a low body mass index is associated with a higher risk of having a deleterious mismatch repair mutation [7].

12.4
Clinical Management

So far there is no difference in the clinical management between sporadic and hereditary ovarian and endometrial cancer. The standard surgical procedure in primary ovarian cancer is a maximal tumor debulking and an adjuvant chemotherapy with six intravenous courses of platinum and paclitaxel. Women with endometrial cancer will receive a hysterectomy and salpingo-oophorectomy, a stage dependent pelvic and para-aortal lymphadenectomy, and a stage dependent adjuvant radiation therapy. In selected cases, a primary radiation therapy is also possible.

So far, there is no evidence for a different therapy response of hereditary ovarian and endometrial cancer compared to the sporadic counterparts. However, the knowledge of the normal functions of the BRCA1/2 proteins in DNA repair (see Chapter 11 on hereditary breast cancer) suggests that tumors with mutations in the *BRCA* genes might be particularly sensitive to platinum-based drugs, which induce cross-linking between DNA molecules. In an ongoing clinical trial with patients suffering from advanced *BRCA1/2* positive carcinomas, carboplatin will be compared with docetaxel for response and time to progression. Moreover, a new drug known as Poly(ADP-Ribose) polymerase (PARP)-inhibitor is currently applied to cancer patients with *BRCA1* and two mutations in a multi-center trial. PARP inhibitors selectively kill cells in which DNA repair is absent due to mutations in the *BRCA1* or *BRCA2* gene [6].

12.5
Prevention Strategies

12.5.1
Primary Prevention

12.5.1.1 Prophylactic Salpingo-Oophorectomy (BPSO)
Prospective and retrospective cohort studies show that bilateral prophylactic salpingo-oophorectomy (BPSO) reduces the risk of ovarian cancer in *BRCA* mutation carriers by more than 90% [15, 16], and also reduces mortality by 70% [17]. BPSO is hence recommended by the GC-HBOC under certain circumstances (see Table 12.1, Chapter 11 on hereditary breast cancer). The standard procedure is a laparoscopic extirpation of the ovaries and fallopian tubes with peritoneal samples and lavage. The whole abdomen should be carefully examined since there is a risk of 3% for the development of an extra ovarian carcinomatosis of the peritoneum. Detailed histological processing of the ovaries is recommended that may reveal pre-neoplastic lesions or early carcinomas so that an adequate adjuvant therapy can be given. The time of surgery can be optimized in the future. BPSO is a well-accepted procedure by over 50% of the mutation carriers in Germany.

For patients from HNPCC families, a prophylactic hysterectomy with bilateral salpingo-oophorectomy is a highly effective strategy for preventing endometrial and ovarian cancer. In a retrospective study of 315 women with germline mutations of *MLH1, MSH2,* and *MSH6*, none of the women with prophylactic surgery revealed endometrial cancer. The median age of surgery was 42 with a follow-up time of 13 years for the surgery group, and 7.4 years for the control group [18].

12.5.1.2 Prevention Using Drugs
It is well-known that oral contraceptives (OC) have a protective effect on the development of sporadic ovarian cancer [19]. A retrospective analysis of *BRCA1* and *BRCA2* mutation carriers also shows a protective effect of OC on the occurrence of ovarian cancer, depending on the duration of usage: the use of OC for 6 or more years leads to a risk reduction of 60% [20]. Based on the small numbers of retrospectively analyzed *BRCA1/2* mutation carriers, the lack of prospective data and contradictory results of another study [21], OC cannot

be generally recommended for the prevention of ovarian cancer. It has also been considered that by using OC the risk for breast cancer increases [22]. For this reason, only low-dose estrogen and progesterone OC should be given to *BRCA1/2* mutations carriers.

For endometrial cancer, there is an ongoing clinical study to identify whether intrauterine progestagens, delivered using the MIRENA intrauterine contraceptive device, can reduce the risk of endometrial cancer in women with HNPCC mutations [6].

12.5.2
Secondary Prevention (Structured Surveillance)

Based on the increased risk for breast and ovarian cancer, women with *BRCA1* and *BRCA2* mutations should take part in a structured surveillance program (Chapter 11 on hereditary breast cancer). A gynecological examination including vaginal sonography of the ovaries, uterus, and endometrium should be performed every six months. However, even with the additional measurement of the tumor marker CA 12-5, the program failed to detect ovarian carcinomas at an early stage.

The appropriate surveillance method for endometrial cancer is still discussed, and some would argue that, given the relatively early presentation with symptoms and the relatively good prognosis, active surveillance is not warranted. Surveillance methods have included transvaginal ultrasound, Pipelle aspiration, and hysteroscopy. The detection rates for endometrial cancer using the Pipelle method were 97 and 91% in post- and pre-menopausal women, respectively [6].

References

1 Kiechle, M. and Meindl, A. (2006) Das familiäre Mamma- und Ovarialkarzinom. *Geburtsh Frauenheilk*, **66**, 1–4.

2 Antoniou, A., Pharoah, P.D., Narod, S. et al. (2003) Average risks of breast and ovarian cancer associated with *BRCA1* or *BRCA2* mutations detected in case Series unselected for family history: a combined analysis of 22 studies. *American Journal of Human Genetics*, **72**, 1117–30.

3 Ford, D., Easton, D.F., Bishop, D.T., Narod, S.A., Goldgar, D.E. and Breast Cancer Linkage Consortium (1994) Risks of Cancer in *BRCA1* mutation carriers. *Lancet*, **343**, 692–5.

4 Thompson, D. and Easton, D.F. (2002) Cancer incidence in *BRCA1* mutation carriers. *Journal of the National Cancer Institute*, **94**, 1358–65.

5 Ford, D., Easton, D.F. and Peto, J. (1995) Estimates of the gene frequency of *BRCA1* and its contribution to breast and ovarian cancer incidence. *American Journal of Human Genetics*, **57**, 1457–62.

6 Gardiner, C. (2007) Family history of gynecological cancers. *Obstetrics, Gynecology and Reproductive Medicine*, **17**, 356–61.

7 Lu, K., Schorge, J.O., Rodabaugh, K.J., Daniels, M.S., Sun, C.C., Soliman, P.T., White, K.G., Luthra, R., Gershenson, D.M. and Broaddus, R.R. (2007) Prospective determination of prevalence of Lynch syndrome in young women with endometrial cancer. *Journal of Clinical Oncology*, **25**, 5158–64.

8 Antoniou, A.C., Gayther, S.A., Stratton, J.F., Ponder, B.A. and Easton, D.F. (2000)

Risk models for familial ovarian and breast cancer. *Genetic Epidemiology*, **18**, 173–90.

9 Lakhani, S.R., Gusterson, B.A., Jacquemier, J. *et al.* (2000) The pathology of familial breast cancer: histological features of cancers in families not attributable to mutations in *BRCA1* or *BRCA2*. *Clinical Cancer Research*, **6**, 782–9.

10 Moslehi, R., Chu, W., Karlan, B. *et al.* (2000) *BRCA1* and *BRCA2* mutation analysis of 208 Ashkenazi Jewish women with ovarian cancer. *American Journal of Human Genetics*, **66**, 1259–72.

11 Chang, J., Fryatt, I., Ponder, B., Fisher, C. and Gore, M.E. (1995) A matched control study of familial epithelial ovarian cancer: patient characteristics, response to chemotherapy and outcome. *Annals of Oncology*, **6**, 80–2.

12 Johannsson, O.T., Idvall, I., Anderson, C. *et al.* (1997) Tumour biological features of *BRCA1* induced breast and ovarian cancer. *European Journal of Cancer*, **33**, 362–71.

13 Rubin, S.C., Benjamin, I., Behbakht, K. *et al.* (1996) Clinical and pathological features of ovarian cancer in women with germline mutations of *BRCA1*. *New England Journal of Medicine*, **335**, 1413–16.

14 Pharoah, P.D.P., Easton, D.F., Stockton, D.L., Gayther, S.A. and Ponder, B.A.J. (1999) Survival in familial *BRCA1* and *BRCA2* associated epithelial ovarian cancer. *Cancer Research*, **59**, 868–71.

15 Rebbeck, T.R., Lynch, H.T., Neuhausen, S.L. *et al.* (2002) Prophylactic oophorectomy in carriers of *BRCA1* or *BRCA2* mutations. *New England Journal of Medicine*, **346**, 1616–22.

16 Kauff, N.D., Satagopan, J.M., Robson, M.E. *et al.* (2002) Risk-reducing salpingo-oophorectomy in women with a *BRCA1* or *BRCA2* mutation. *New England Journal of Medicine*, **346**, 1609–15.

17 Domchek, S.M., Friebel, T.M., Neuhausen, S.L., Wagner, T., Evans, G., Isaacs, C., Garber, J.E., Daly, M.B. *et al.* (2006) Mortality after bilateral salpingo-oophorectomy in *BRCA1* and *BRCA2* mutation carriers: a prospective cohort study. *The Lancet Oncology*, **7**, 223–9.

18 Schmeler, K., Lynch, H.T., Chen, L.M., Munsell, M.F., Solima, P.T., Clark, M.B., Damiels, M.S., White, K.G., Boyd-Rogers, S.G., Conrad, P.G., Yang, K.Y., Rubin, M.M., Sun, C.C., Slomovitz, B.M., Gershenson, D.M. and Lu, K.H. (2006) Prophylactic surgery to reduce the risk of gynecologic cancers in the Lynch syndrome. *New England Journal of Medicine*, **354**, 261–9.

19 Whittemore, A.S., Harris, R. and Itnyre, J. (1992) Characteristics relating to ovarian cancer risk: collaborative analysis of 12 U.S. case-control studies. II. Invasive epithelial ovarian cancers in white women. Collaborative Ovarian Cancer Group. *American Journal of Epidemiology*, **136**, 1184–203.

20 Narod, S.A., Risch, H., Moslehi, R. *et al.* (1998) Oral contraceptives and the risk of hereditary ovarian cancer. *New England Journal of Medicine*, **339**, 424–8.

21 Modan, B., Hartge, P., Hirsh-Yechezkel, G. *et al.* (2001) Parity, oral contraceptives, and the risk of ovarian cancer among carriers and noncarriers of a *BRCA1* or *BRCA2* mutation. *New England Journal of Medicine*, **345**, 235–40.

22 Grabrick, D.M., Hartmann, L.C., Cerhan, J.R. *et al.* (2000) Risk of breast cancer with oral contraceptive use in women with a family history of breast cancer. *The Journal of the American Medical Association*, **284**, 1791–8.

13
Prostate Cancer

Raphaela Waidelich

Summary

There is considerable evidence that both genetics and environment play a role in the origin and evolution of prostate cancer (PC). At least 22 genes show evidence of being involved in the origin and/or progression of PC. However, studies to assess the nature of familial aggregation of PC show conflicting results. Few, if any, genes that are reproducibly associated with increased risk for PC across different study populations have been identified, emphasizing the heterogeneous nature of this disease. Analyzing defined sets of families with common origin, and using the co-occurrence of other cancers in HPC families, are promising strategies for developing genetically homogeneous data for reducing locus heterogeneity problems associated with studying complex traits.

13.1
Epidemiology

Prostate cancer (PC) is the fourth most common male malignant neoplasm worldwide. Its incidence and mortality vary widely between countries and ethnic populations [1]. The lowest yearly incidence rates occur in Asia (1.9 cases per 100 000), and the highest in Scandinavia and North America [2]. Mortality is highest in Sweden (23 per 100 000 per year) and lowest in Asia (<5 per 100 000 per year in Singapore, Japan, and China) [2].

There is considerable evidence that both genetics and environment play a role in the origin and evolution of the disease. Asian Americans have a lower PC incidence than white or African Americans. However, Japanese and Chinese men in the United States have a higher risk to develop PC and to die of it than their relatives in Japan and China [3]. PC incidence and mortality have increased in Japan as the country has become more westernized [4]. In addition, access to and quality of healthcare, accuracy of cancer registries, and penetrance of prostate specific antigen (PSA) screening influence the worldwide and ethnic variations in PC incidence and mortality [1].

Hereditary Tumors: From Genes to Clinical Consequences
Edited by Heike Allgayer, Helga Rehder and Simone Fulda
Copyright © 2009 WILEY-VCH Verlag GmbH & Co. KGaA, Weinheim
ISBN: 978-3-527-32028-8

13.2
Phenotypes of Prostate Cancer

For investigative purposes, PC is divided into three phenotypes: sporadic, familial, and hereditary. Sporadic cancers occur in individuals with a negative family history. Familial PC is defined as cancer in a man with one or more affected relatives. As a subset of the hereditary form, hereditary PC (HPC) has been defined as a cluster of three or more affected relatives within a nuclear family or the occurrence of PC in three generations or two or more affected family members with an age at onset of 55 years or younger [5]. While sporadic cancers account for about 85% of PC, about 15% are familial or hereditary [6].

The clinical phenotype of PC is complex and heterogeneous. Association between early age of diagnosis and familial PC is well documented in the literature [7–11]. Forty-three percent of early-onset PCs (men 55 years of age or younger) are hereditary, but only 9% of PCs occurring by the age of 85 years [6].

Controversy exists concerning the differences between hereditary and sporadic PC with respect to clinical features, pathological characteristics, and outcome.

Some studies report that the outcome after radical prostatectomy [11] or definitive external beam radiation therapy is similar in patients with or without a family history of PC [12, 13]. In contrast, other studies report that men with a history of PC in first-degree relatives have a higher likelihood of biochemical failure [8] and 5-year distant failure after radical prostatectomy [14] or radiation therapy [15]. Grönberg showed that PC in families associated with the HPC1 locus on chromosome 1q24–25 may more often be poorly differentiated and at an advanced stage at diagnosis [16]. A few studies have reported more favorable pathological features (lower mean Gleason score [17] and lower proportion of positive surgical margins, perineural infiltration, and lymph node metastases [18] in familial cases.

The conflicting results of these population-based studies may be caused by two major problems: First, PC is a common disease. Therefore, analyses of the phenotype of HPC may be biased by the fact that many PC cases in families with HPC are phenocopies, that is, they are diagnosed as PC although they are not mutation carriers. For example, almost 10% of mutation non-carriers among men in Swedish HPC families have clinical PC [9]. Second, men with a family history of PC are more inclined to undergo rectal examination and PSA tests at an earlier age [19].

13.3
Genetics

13.3.1
Hereditary Transmission

Evidence for PC susceptibility genes that segregate in families has been consistently provided by multiple segregation studies [20]. However, studies to assess the nature of familial aggregation of PC produce conflicting results. The majority of segregation analyses support an autosomal dominant inheritance mode [6, 21–25]. Analyzing Australian families affected by PC, Cui *et al.* [26] report autosomal dominant inheritance in younger-onset families, and recessive or X-linked inheritance in older-onset families. Also, multifactorial [27] and codominant [28] models have been suggested. Recently, Pakkanen et al. [29] reported that the inheritance of PC in the Finnish population is best explained by a Mendelian recessive model with a significant paternal regressive coefficient that is indicative of a polygenic multifactorial component.

13.3.2
PC Susceptibility Genes

Despite the large number of studies of HPC, few, if any, genes that are reproducibly associated with an increased risk for PC across different study populations have been identified, emphasizing the heterogeneous nature of this disease [30]. One of the major difficulties in studying PC is genetic heterogeneity, possibly due to multiple, incompletely penetrant PC-susceptibility genes [31]. At least 22 genes show evidence of being involved in the origin and/or progression of PC (Table 13.1).

Of the known susceptibility genes, ribonuclease L (2′,5′-oligoisoadenylate synthetase-dependent) (RNASEL) is the best characterized. RNASEL encodes a ribonuclease that mediates the antiviral and apoptotic activities of interferons. It is a latent enzyme, expressed in nearly every mammalian cell type. Its activation requires its binding to a small oligonucleotide, 2–5 A, a series of unique 5′-triphosphorylated oligoadenylates with 2′-5′ phosphodiester bonds [33]. This gene is a candidate for the HPC1 allele [34]. Grönberg investigated phenotypic characteristics of families potentially linked to the HPC1 locus on chromosome 1q24–25 [16]. In this study, families that provide evidence for segregation of an altered HPC1 gene showed three characteristics: younger age at diagnosis, higher-grade tumors, and more advanced-stage disease. A variety of inactivating and missense mutations of RNASEL have been identified in families with HPC [35]. However, results of studies investigating the role of these mutations are conflicting. Casey et al. [36] determined that the RNASEL variant Arg462Gnl has three times less enzymatic activity than the wildtype, and is significantly associated with PC risk (P = 0.007). The single nucleotide polymorphism R462Q, resulting from an arginine to glutamine substitution, is suggested to be associated with an increased risk of PC [36]. Several studies showed that men with cell lines with this allelic variant have reduced RNASEL activity leading to deficient apoptosis [34, 35, 37]. A truncating mutation, E265X, was found in 5 (4.3%) of the 116 patients from Finnish families with HPC. This was significantly higher than the frequency of E265X in controls. The highest mutation frequency was found in patients from families with four or more affected members [38]. In contrast to these findings, large-scale case-control studies performed by Wiklund [39] and Daugherty [40] provided evidence against a major role of RNASEL in PC etiology in Sweden and the United States, respectively.

Table 13.1 Genes showing evidence to be involved in the origin and/or progression of PC (from Online Mendelian Inheritance in Man. Available at: www.nci.nlm.nih.gov [32]).

Title/s	Symbol/s	Gene map locus
eph tyrosine kinase 3 (ephrin receptor EphB2)PC/brain cancer susceptibility	*EPHB2, EPHT3, DRT, ERK, PCBC, CAPB*	1p36.1-p35
Ribonuclease L (2′,5′-oligoisoadenylate synthetase-dependent)	*RNASEL, RNS4, PRCA1, HPC1*	1q25
PC, hereditary 8 / Predisposing for PC	*HPC8 / PCAP*	1q42.2-q43
PC, hereditary 5	*HPC5*	3p26
PC, hereditary, 4	*HPC4*	7p11-q21
Mitotic arrest-deficient 1, yeast, homolog-like 1	*MAD1L1, TXBP181*	7p22
Macrophage scavenger receptor	*MSR1*	8p22
PC, hereditary, 10	*HPC10*	8q24
Kruppel-like factor-6	*KLF6, COPEB, BCD1, ZF9*	10p15
Phosphatase and tensin homolog (mutated in multiple advanced cancers 1)	*PTEN, MMAC1*	10q23.31
MAX-interacting protein 1	*MXI1*	10q25
CD82 antigen	*CD82, SAR2, KAI1, ST6*	11p11.2
Breast cancer-2, early onset	*BRCA2, FANCD1*	13q12.3
PC, hereditary, 7	*HPC7*	15q12
Cadherin-1 (E-cadherin; uvomorulin)	*CDH1, UVO, LCAM, ECAD*	16q22.1
AT motif-binding factor 1	*ATBF1*	16q22.3-q23.1
PC, hereditary, 9	*HPC9*	17q21-q22
elaC, *E. coli*, homolog 2	*ELAC2, HPC2*	17p11
PC, hereditary, 3	*HPC3*	20q13
PC, hereditary 6	*HPC6*	22q12
Checkpoint kinase 2, S. pombe, homolog of (RAD53, S. cerevisiae, homolog of)	*CHEK2, RAD53, CHK2, CDS1, LFS2*	22q12.1
Androgen receptor (dihydrotestosterone receptor)	*AR, DHTR, TFM, SBMA, KD, SMAX1*	Xq11-q12
PC, hereditary, X-linked	*HPCX*	Xq27-q28

Two other PC susceptibility loci are suggested as being linked to different regions on chromosome 1: EPH receptor B2 (EPHB2) at 1p36.1–p35, and predisposing for PC gene (PCAP, also known as HPC2), located at 1q42.2–43 [41]. Mutational inactivation of the EPHB2 gene has been implicated in the progression and metastasis of PC [42]. A case-control association analysis showed that the K1019X mutation in the EphB2 gene differs in frequency between African American and European American men, is associated with an increased risk for PC in African American men with positive family history, and may be a genetic risk factor for PC in African Americans [43]. Homogeneity analysis indicated that PCAP is the most frequent known locus predisposing to HPC in Southern and Western Europe [44]. Also, the HSD3 gene family at 1p13 coding for 3beta-hydroxysteroid dehydrogenases is hypothesized to have a role in PC susceptibility [45, 46].

Performing linkage analysis, Rokman et al. [47] conclude that 3p26 is likely to contain a predisposing gene for Finnish HPC, although no disease-segregating variants were found in two candidate genes in the region.

In an attempt to reduce locus heterogeneity, Friedrichsen *et al.* [48] performed a genome-wide linkage scan for PC susceptibility genes with 36 Jewish families. The strongest signal was a significant linkage peak at 7q11–21, with a nonparametric linkage (NPL) score of 3.01 (P = 0.0013).

Tsukasaki *et al.* [49] found a relatively high frequency of heterozygous mutations in the MAD1L1 gene (located on 7p22) in cases of PC, either in cell lines or in tissue specimens. One of the mutations was a 175C-T transition in the MAD1L1 gene leading to a missense arg59-to-cys (R59C) substitution.

Chromosome 8p is commonly deleted in many cancers, including colon, breast, ovarian, liver, lung, bladder, and head and neck cancer. Deletion of sequences from chromosome 8p is the most common deletion event in the genome of prostate tumors [50]. Despite the overwhelming evidence for 8p deletions, few specific genes have been consistently implicated as prostate tumor suppressor genes in this region. One of the major obstacles in the identification of tumor suppressor genes at 8p is the broad size of the deleted regions, which is affected by the resolution of methods used to detect deletions. In the largest genome-wide linkage analysis, Xu *et al.* found suggestive evidence for linkage at 8p21 among 1233 PC families [31]. Combining the results from their somatic deletion study and germline linkage study, Chang and co-workers [51] found overlapping results, implicating consensus regions at 8p21.3 between 20.6 and 23.7 Mb, and 8p23.1 between 9.8 and 11.2 Mb. In a study that estimated the frequency of DNA copy number alterations in the PC genome based upon all published comparative genomic hybridization studies of PCs, Sun and co-workers [52] found that one-third of 891 PCs had a deletion at 8p21.3 At least 37 known protein-coding genes are located at the 8p21.3 consensus region. Some of these genes, including NKX3.1, have been associated with HPC. Macrophage scavenger receptor 1 (MSR1) is one of the major candidate PC susceptibility genes [53]. Xu *et al.* [53] found a nonsense mutation, arg293 to ter (R293X), in the MSR1 gene in 6 different HPC families of European descent, and an asp174-to-tyr (D174Y) in 4 African American HPC families, respectively. However, follow-up studies to confirm the gene's relevance for PC came to conflicting results [54, 55].

Carriers of germline mutations in the BRCA2 gene are known to be at high risk of breast and ovarian cancers [56, 57]. Several epidemiologic studies have reported that carriers of germline mutations in the BRCA2 gene have an increased risk of PC, with the highest risk observed in men diagnosed at earlier ages. However, studies of the contribution of BRCA2 mutations to the etiology of HPC have been inconsistent. Edwards [58] reports that the relative risk of developing PC by age 56 years from a deleterious germline BRCA2 is 23-fold. In 940 Ashkenazi Israelis with PC, Giusti *et al.* [59] tested DNA obtained from paraffin sections for the 3 Jewish founder mutations: 185delAG and 5382insC in BRCA1, and 6174delT in BRCA2. They estimated that there is a two-fold increase in BRCA mutation-related PC among Ashkenazi Israelis. No evidence was found in the Seattle-based Prostate Cancer Genetic Research Study for an association between BRCA2 mutations and susceptibility to HPC [60]. A genome-wide linkage scan on 71 families with 2 or more men suffering from aggressive PC showed statistically significant evidence for linkage at chromosome 15q12, with a LOD score of 3.49 (genome-wide $p = 0.005$) [61].

Sun *et al.* [62] report that ATBF1, mRNA is abundant in normal prostates but more scarce in approximately half of PCs tested. They narrowed the region of deletion at 16q22 to 861 kb containing ATBF1 and conclude that loss of ATBF1 is one mechanism that defines the absence of growth control in PC.

Jonsson *et al.* [63] analyzed the association between the −160C/A promoter polymorphism and the risk of sporadic, familial, and hereditary PC in Sweden. They found no significant association between the A-allele, and sporadic or familial PC. However, risk of hereditary cancer was increased among heterozygote CA carriers, and particularly among homozygote AA carriers, indicating that the −160 single nucleotide polymorphism in CDH1 is a low-penetrant PC susceptibility gene that might explain a proportion of familial and notably HPC.

A linkage scan on 1233 PC families from the International Consortium for Prostate Cancer Genetics found suggestive evidence for a linkage to chromosome 17q21–22 (HLOD = 1.99) [31]. Combined linkage analysis of PC on 24 chromosome 17 markers using 453 families from the University of Michigan Prostate Cancer Genetics Project and Johns Hopkins University groups showed that the evidence for linkage is stronger in the subsets of families with 4 or more confirmed PC cases, or families having PC cases with an average age of diagnosis of 65 years or younger [64].

The HPC susceptibility gene ELAC2 on chromosome 17p was the first PC susceptibility gene characterized by positional cloning [65]. ElAC homolog 2 (*E. coli*) (ELAC2), located at 17p11.2 was found to possess an important transcriptional scaffold function for ELAC2 in TGF-beta/Smad signaling mediated growth arrest [66]. Two common missense variants (a ser-to-leu change at amino acid 217 (S217L) and an ala-to-thr change at amino acid 541 (A541T)) have been reported in the gene. However, epidemiologic analyses come to conflicting results. In studies performed in Japan, a leu allele at codon 217 [67] and also a thr allele at

541 in HPC2/ELAC2 [68] indicate a strong significance in the predisposition of sporadic PC. In a European-American population, ELAC2 217L and RNASEL 541E are associated with metastatic sporadic disease [69]. However, in a population-based study in Australia, there was no evidence that either ELAC2 polymorphism is associated with PC or PSA level [70]. Results of a study at the Mayo Clinic [71] suggest that alterations in the ELAC2 gene play a limited role in genetic suscepti-bility to HPC. The absence of ELAC2 mutations and lack of association between polymorphisms in ELAC2 and PC led Shea et al. [72] to conclude that ELAC2 does not contribute significantly to the elevated prevalence of PC in Afro-Caribbean males of Tobago.

Conducting a genome-wide search on 162 North American families with 3 or more members affected by PC, Berry et al. [73] found evidence for a linkage to chromosome 20q13. The strongest evidence of linkage was evident with the pedi-grees having less than five family members affected with PC, a later average age of diagnosis, and no male-to-male transmission. These findings were confirmed by Zheng et al. [74] who genotyped 16 markers spanning approximately 95 cm on chromosome 20 in 159 HPC families. However, Bock et al. [75], who studied 172 unrelated families affected by PC, using 17 polymorphic markers across a 98.5 cm segment of chromosome 20 (that contains the candidate region), did not find sta-tistically significant support for the existence of a PC-susceptibility locus HPC20 at 20q13.

Combining linkage data from a total of 1233 families and focusing on subsets of families that are more likely to segregate highly penetrant mutations, including families with large numbers of affected individuals or early age at diagnosis, Xu et al. [31] identified strong evidence for linkage at 22q12, with an LOD score of 3.57. In 14 high-risk Utah pedigrees, Camp et al. [76] identified a 881 538-bp inter-val at 22q12.3, between D22S1265 and D22S277 as the most likely region that contains the 22q PC predisposition gene.

In response to DNA damage, eukaryotic cells use a system of checkpoint con-trols to delay cell-cycle progression [77]. CHEK2 (gene map locus 22q12.1) has been identified as a downstream affecter of the ATM-dependent DNA damage checkpoint pathway [78]. Mutations in CHEK2 have been associated with Li-Fraumeni syndrome 2 (Li-Fraumeni-like syndrome) [79] (see Chapters 3 and 5 on family cancer syndromes and hereditary brain tumors). There is evidence that mutations in *CHEK2* may contribute to both sporadic PC and HPC risk [80] through the reduction of CHEK2 activation in response to DNA damage and/or oncogenic stress [81].

Linkage to Xq27–28 was observed in a combined study population of 360 PC fam-ilies collected at 4 independent sites in North America, Finland, and Sweden [82], a finding consistent with results of previous population-based studies suggesting an X-linked mode of HPC inheritance. Baffoe-Bonnie et al. [83] reduced the HPCX critical locus to a region flanked by markers between "D3S2390" and "bG82i1.0".

Mutations of Kruppel-like factor-6 (KLF6) [84], Phosphatase and tensin (PTEN) homolog (mutated in multiple advanced cancers 1) [85], MAX-interacting protein 1 (MXI1) [86], CD82 antigen (KAI1) [87], and androgen receptor (AR) [88] also have been shown to be associated with PC initiation and/or progression. Whether these mutations are linked to HPC still has to be determined.

13.4
Prevention and Early Detection

As PC rarely causes symptoms early in the course of the disease, its early diagnosis relies on a combination of digital rectal examination and PSA. Screening efforts in the past decade have resulted in a marked downward stage migration [89]. Given the long natural history of low-stage PC detected in 1990s (the so-called "PSA era"), additional observation time is necessary to determine whether early detection also reduces mortality [1]. Although the value of PC screening remains controversial, men who present for periodic health examinations should be made aware of PC early detection by digital rectal examination and PSA [89]. The optimum timing of early detection measures has not been determined. There is strong evidence, however, that men with a family history of PC should be offered PC early detection at a younger age [90] than the general population, for example at the age of 40 years.

As the specific causes of PC initiation and progression are not yet known, the current body of evidence is insufficient to make a routine recommendation of any drug or diet for the prevention of PC [1]. 5-alpha-reductase inhibitors [91], the antioxidants selenium and vitamin E [92], soy [93], lycopenes [94], and other nutritional supplements are currently under study as potential chemo-preventive agents.

13.5
Therapy

Therapy of PC depends on tumor stage. Radical prostatectomy still remains the "gold standard" to treat localized PC. Alternatively, external or interstitial radiotherapy (brachytherapy) provide local tumor control. Watchful waiting is a reasonable option in patients with a life expectancy of less than ten years and clinically localized, well-differentiated, or moderately differentiated PC [95]. Hormone therapy (especially hormone deprivation) is the treatment of choice for metastatic disease. These guidelines currently also apply to patients with a suspected hereditary/familial component of the disease.

13.6
Future Aspects

HPC is a genetically heterogeneous disease. One of the major problems with population-based linkage studies is the widely varying ethnic background of the populations within different studies. Analyzing defined sets of families with common origin, for reducing locus heterogeneity problems associated with studying complex traits, may be useful [48]. Data presented by Friedrichsen and co-workers [48] support the concept that the optimal approach for mapping highly penetrant PC genes is to focus efforts on families that most likely segregate these types of genes, specifically families with large numbers of young PC cases. It was this type of approach that ultimately led to the successful identification of the breast cancer susceptibility gene *BRCA1* [96].

Using the co-occurrence of other cancers in HPC families is another promising strategy for developing genetically homogeneous datasets that can enhance the ability to identify susceptibility loci using linkage analysis. A genome-wide scan of HPC families with primary kidney cancer [97] showed suggestive genetic linkage to chromosome 11p11.2–q12.2. In 12 HPC families with the co-occurrence of adenocarcinoma of the pancreas, non-parametric linkage analysis for a prostate/pancreas cancer susceptibility phenotype was performed using 441 genome-wide micro-satellite markers. Despite the lack of statistically significant findings, four chromosomal regions, (2q, 16q, 17q, and 21q), showed suggestive linkage results in this scan [98].

Another interesting aspect is to screen unaffected men in families with HPC [99].

One of the major causes for the difficulty in mapping PC genes is the reduced statistical power due to multiple susceptibility genes, incomplete penetrance, and high rates of sporadic PC in the general population. To overcome these obstacles is the challenge of future research on HPC.

References

1 Klein, E., Platz, E. and Thompson, I. (2007) Epidemiology, etiology, and prevention of prostate cancer, in *Campbell-Walsh Urology* (eds A. Wein, L. Kavoussi, A. Novick, A. Partin and C. Peters), Saunders Elsevier, Philadelphia, pp. 2854–73.

2 Quinn, M. and Babb, P. (2002) Patterns and trends in prostate cancer incidence, survival, prevalence and mortality. Part I: international comparisons. *BJU International*, **90** (*2*), 162–73.

3 Muir, C., Nectoux, J. and Staszewski, J. (1991) The epidemiology of prostatic cancer. Geographical distribution and time-trends. *Acta Oncologica*, **30**, 133–40.

4 Landis, S., Murray, T., Bolden, S. and Wingo, P. (1999) Cancer statistics. *CA: A Cancer Journal for Clinicians*, **49**, 8–31.

5 Carter, B., Bova, G., Beaty, T., Steinberg, G., Childs, B. and Isaacs, W. (1993) Hereditary prostate cancer: epidemiologic and clinical features. *The Journal of Urology*, **150**, 797–802.

6 Carter, B., Beaty, T., Steinberg, G., Childs, B. and Walsh, P. (1992) Mendelian inheritance of familial prostate cancer. *Proceedings of the National Academy of Sciences of the United States of America*, **89**, 3367–71.

7 Grönberg, H., Xu, J., Smith, J., Carpten, J., Isaacs, S., Freiije, D., Bova, G., Danber, J. *et al.* (1997) Early age at diagnosis in families providing evidence of linkage to the hereditary prostate cancer locus (HPC1) on chromosome 1. *Cancer Research*, **57** (*21*), 4707–9.

8 Kupelian, P., Katcher, J., Levin, H., Zippe, C. and Klein, E. (1996) Correlation of

clinical and pathologic factors with rising prostate-specific antigen profiles after radical prostatectomy alone for clinically localized prostate cancer. *Urology*, **48** (*2*), 249–60.

9 Bratt, O., Damber, J., Emanuelsson, M. and Grönberg, H. (2002) Hereditary prostate cancer: clinical characteristics and survival. *The Journal of Urology*, **167** (*6*), 2423–6.

10 Paiss, T., Herkommer, K., Bock, B., Heinz, H., Vogel, W., Kron, M., Kuefer, R., Hautmann, R. *et al.* (2003) Association between the clinical presentation and epidemiological features of familial prostate cancer in patients selected for radical prostatectomy. *European Urology*, **43**, 615–21.

11 Roehl, K., Loeb, S., Antenor, J., Corbin, N. and Catalona, W. (2006) Characteristics of patients with familial versus sporadic prostate cancer. *The Journal of Urology*, **176** (*6*), 2438–42.

12 Azzouzi, A.R., Valeri, A., Cormier, L., Fournier, G., Mangin, P. and Cussenot, O. (2003) Familial prostate cancer cases before and after radical prostatectomy do not show any aggressiveness compared with sporadic cases. *Urology*, **61** (*6*), 1193–7.

13 Hanus, M., Zagars, G. and Pollack, A. (1999) Familial prostate cancer: outcome following radiation therapy with or without adjuvant androgen ablation. *International Journal of Radiation Oncology, Biology, Physics*, **43** (*2*), 379–83.

14 Kupelian, P., Klein, E., Witte, J., Kupelian, V. and Suh, J. (1997) Familial prostate cancer: a different disease? *The Journal of Urology*, **158** (*6*), 2197–201.

15 Kupelian, P., Kupelian, V., Witte, J., Macklis, R. and Klein, E. (1997) Family history of prostate cancer in patients with localized prostate cancer: an independent predictor of treatment outcome. *Journal of Clinical Oncology*, **15** (*4*), 1478–80.

16 Grönberg, H., Isaacs, S., Smith, J., Carpten, J., Bova, G., Freije, D., Xu, J., Meyers, D. *et al.* (1997) Characteristics of prostate cancer in families potentially linked to the hereditary prostate cancer 1 (HPC1) locus. *The Journal of the*

American Medical Association, **278** (*15*), 1251–2.

17 Keetch, D., Humphrey, P., Smith, D., Stahl, D. and Catalona, W. (1996) Clinical and pathological features of hereditary prostate cancer. *The Journal of Urology*, **155** (*6*), 1841–3.

18 Sacco, E., Prayer-Galetti, T., Pinto, F., Ciaccia, M., Fracalanza, S., Betto, G. and Paganoet, F. (2005) Familial and hereditary prostate cancer by definition in an Italian surgical series: clinical features and outcome. *European Urology*, **47** (*6*), 761–8.

19 Norrish, A., McRae, C., Cohen, R. and Jackson, R. (1999) A population-based study of clinical and pathological prognostic characteristics of men with familial and sporadic prostate cancer. *BJU International*, **84** (*3*), 311–15.

20 Schaid, D. (2004) The complex genetic epidemiology of prostate cancer. *Human Molecular Genetics*, **13**, 103–21.

21 Grönberg, H., Damber, L., Damber, J.E. and Iselius, L. (1997) Segregation analysis of prostate cancer in Sweden: support for dominant inheritance. *American Journal of Epidemiology*, **146**, 552–7.

22 Schaid, D., McDonnell, S., Blute, M. and Thibodeau, S. (1998) Evidence for autosomal dominant inheritance of prostate cancer. *American Journal of Human Genetics*, **62** (*6*), 1425–38.

23 Verhage, B., Baffoe-Bonnie, A., Baglietto, L., Smith, D., Bailey-Wilson, J., Beaty, T., Catalona, W. and Kiemeney, L. (2001) Autosomal dominant inheritance of prostate cancer: a confirmatory study. *Urology*, **57** (*1*), 97–101.

24 Conlon, E., Goode, E., Gibbs, M., Stanford, J., Badzioch, M., Janer, M., Kolb, S., Hood, L. *et al.* (2003) Oligogenic segregation analysis of hereditary prostate cancer pedigrees: Evidence for multiple loci affecting age at onset. *International Journal of Cancer*, **105**, 630–5.

25 Valeri, A., Briollais, L., Azzouzi, R., Fournier, G., Mangin, P., Berthon, P., Cussenot, O. and Demenais, F. (2003) Segregation analysis of prostate cancer in France: evidence for autosomal dominant inheritance and residual brother–brother dependence. *Annals of Human Genetics*, **67**, 125–37.

26 Cui, J., Staples, M., Hopper, J., English, D., McCredie, M. and Giles, G. (2001) Segregation analyses of 1476 population-based Australian families affected by prostate cancer. *American Journal of Human Genetics*, **68**, 1207–18.

27 Gong, G., Oakley-Girvan, I., Wu, A., Kolonel, L.N., John, E., West, D.W., Felberg, A., Gallagher, R. *et al.* (2002) Segregation analysis of prostate cancer in 1719 white, African–American and Asian–American families in the United States and Canada. *Cancer Causes Control*, **13**, 471–82.

28 Baffoe-Bonnie, A., Kiemeney, L., Beaty, T., Bailey-Wilson, J., Schnell, A., Sigvaldsson, H., Olafsdottir, G., Tryggvadottir, L. et al. (2002) Segregation analysis of 389 Icelandic pedigrees with breast and prostate cancer. *Genet Epidemiology*, **23**, 349–63.

29 Pakkanen, S., Baffoe-Bonnie, A., Matikainen, M., Koivisto, P., Tammela, T., Deshmukh, S., Ou, L., Bailey-Wilson, J. *et al.* (2007) Segregation analysis of 1546 prostate cancer families in Finland shows recessive inheritance. *Human Genetics*, **121**, 257–67.

30 Easton, D., Schaid, D., Whittemore, A. and Isaacs, W. (2003) Where are the prostate cancer genes? A summary of eight genome-wide searches. *Prostate*, **57**, 261–9.

31 Xu, J., Dimitrov, L., Chang, B., Adams, T., Turner, A., Meyers, D., Eeles, R., Easton, D., Foulkes, W. *et al.* (2005) A Combined genome-wide linkage scan of 1233 families for prostate cancer-susceptibility genes conducted by the International Consortium for Prostate Cancer Genetics. *American Journal of Human Genetics*, **77**, 219–29.

32 Online Mendelian Inheritance in Man. Available at: www.nci.nlm.nih.gov.

33 Bisbal, C. and Silverman, R.H. (2007) Diverse functions of RNase L and implications in pathology. *Biochimie*, **89**, 789–98.

34 Carpten, J., Nupponen, N., Isaacs, S., Sood, R., Robbins, C., Xu, J., Faruque, M., Moses, T. *et al.* (2002) Germline mutations in the ribonuclease L gene in families showing linkage with HPC1. *Nature Genetics*, **30** (*2*), 181–4.

35 Xiang, Y., Wang, Z., Murakami, J., Plummer, S., Klein, E.A., Carpten, J.D., Trent, J.M., Isaacs, W.B. *et al.* (2003) Effects of RNase L mutations associated with prostate cancer on apoptosis induced by 2′,5′-oligoadenylates. *Cancer Research*, **63** (*20*), 6795–801.

36 Casey, G., Neville, P., Plummer, S., Xiang, Y., Krumroy, L., Klein, E., Catalona, W., Nupponen, N. *et al.* (2002) RNASEL Arg462Gln variant is implicated in up to 13% of prostate cancer cases. *Nature Genetics*, **32** (*4*), 581–3.

37 Malathi, K., Paranjape, J.M., Ganapathi, R. and Silverman, R.H. (2004) HPC1/RNASEL mediates apoptosis of prostate cancer cells treated with 2′,5′-oligo-adenylates, topoisomerase I inhibitors, and tumor necrosis factor-related apoptosis-inducing ligand. *Cancer Research*, **64** (*24*), 9144–51.

38 Rökman, A., Ikonen, T., Seppälä, E.H., Nupponen, N., Autio, V., Mononen, N., Bailey-Wilson, J., Trent, J. *et al.* (2002) Germline alterations of the RNASEL gene, a candidate HPC1 gene at 1q25, in patients and families with prostate cancer. *American Journal of Human Genetics*, **70**, 1299–304.

39 Wiklund, F., Jonsson, B., Brookes, A., Strömqvist, L., Adolfsson, J., Emanuelsson, M., Adami, H., Augustsson-Balter, K. *et al.* (2004) Genetic analysis of the RNASEL gene in hereditary, familial, and sporadic prostate cancer. *Clinical Cancer Research*, **10** (*21*), 7150–6.

40 Daugherty, S., Hayes, R., Yeager, M., Andriole, G., Chatterjee, N., Huang, W., Isaacs, W. and Platz, E. (2007) RNASEL Arg462Gln polymorphism and prostate cancer in PLCO. *Prostate*, **67**, 849–54.

41 Berthon, P., Valeri, A., Cohen-Akenine, A., Drelon, E., Paiss, T., Wöhr, G., Latil, A., Millasseau, P. *et al.* (1998) Predisposing gene for early-onset prostate cancer, localized on chromosome 1q42.2-43. *American Journal of Human Genetics*, **62**, 1416–24.

42 Huusko, P., Ponciano-Jackson, D., Wolf, M., Kiefer, J., Azorsa, D., Tuzmen, S., Weaver, D., Robbins, C. *et al.* (2004) Nonsense-mediated decay microarray analysis identifies mutations of EPHB2 in

human prostate cancer. *Nature Genetics*, **36** (*9*), 979–83.

43 Kittles, R., Baffoe-Bonnie, A., Moses, T., Robbins, C., Ahaghotu, C., Huusko, P., Pettaway, C., Vijayakumar, S. *et al.* (2007) A common nonsense mutation in EphB2 is associated with prostate cancer risk in African American men with a positive family history. *Journal of Medical Genetics*, **43**, 507–11.

44 Cancel-Tassin, G., Latil, A., Valeri, A., Mangin, P., Fournier, G., Berthon, P. and Cussenot, O. (2001) PCAP is the major known prostate cancer predisposing locus in families from south and west Europe. *European Journal of Human Genetics*, **9**, 135–42.

45 Guerini, V., Sau, D., Scaccianoce, E., Rusmini, P., Ciana, P., Maggi, A., Martini, P., Katzenellenbogen, B. *et al.* (2005) The Androgen derivative 5α-androstane-3ß,17ß-diol inhibits prostate cancer cell migration through activation of the estrogen receptor ß subtype. *Cancer Research*, **65** (*12*), 5445–53.

46 Chang, B., Zheng, S., Hawkins, G., Isaacs, S., Wiley, K., Turner, A., Carpten, J., Bleeker, E. *et al.* (2002) Joint effect of *HSD3B1* and *HSD3B2* genes is associated with hereditary and sporadic prostate cancer susceptibility. *Cancer Research*, **62** (*6*), 1784–9.

47 Rökman, A., Baffoe-Bonnie, A.B., Gillanders, E., Fredriksson, H., Autio, V., Ikonen, T., Gibbs, K.D. Jr, Jones, M. *et al.* (2005) Hereditary prostate cancer in Finland: fine-mapping validates 3p26 as a major predisposition locus. *Human Genetics*, **116**, 43–50.

48 Friedrichsen, D., Stanford, J., Isaacs, S., Janer, M., Chang, B., Deutsch, K., Gillanders, E., Kolb, S. *et al.* (2004) Identification of a prostate cancer susceptibility locus on chromosome 7q11-21 in Jewish families. *Proceedings of the National Academy of Sciences of the United States of America*, **101**, 1939–44.

49 Tsukasaki, K., Miller, C., Greenspun, E., Eshaghian, S., Kawabata, H.., Fujimoto, T., Tomonaga, M., Sawyers, C. *et al.* (2001) Mutations in the mitotic check point gene, MAD1L1, in human cancers. *Oncogene*, **20**, 3301–5.

50 Dong, J. (2001) Chromosomal deletions and tumor suppressor genes in prostate cancer. *Cancer and Metastasis Reviews*, **20**, 173–93.

51 Chang, B., Liu, W., Sun, J., Dimitrov, L., Li, T., Turner, A., Zheng, S., Isaacs, W. *et al.* (2007) Integration of somatic deletion analysis of prostate cancers and germline linkage analysis of prostate cancer families reveals. *Two Small Consensus Regions for Prostate Cancer Genes at 8p Cancer-Research*, **67** (*9*), 4098–103.

52 Sun, J., Liu, W., Adams, Tamara S. , Sun, T.S., , Li, J., , Turner, X., , Chang, A.R., , B. *et al.* (2007) DNA copy number alterations in prostate cancers: a combined analysis of published CGH studies. *The Prostate*, **67** (*7*), 692–700.

53 Xu, J., Zheng, S., Komiya, A., Mychaleckyj, J., Isaacs, S., Hu, J., Sterling, D., Lange, E. *et al.* (2002) Germline mutations and sequence variants of the macrophage scavenger receptor 1 gene are associated with prostate cancer risk. *Nature Genetics*, **32**, 321–5.

54 Wang, L., McDonnell, S., Cunningham, J., Hebbring, S., Jacobsen, S., Cerhan, J., Slager, S., Blute, M. *et al.* (2003) No association of germline alteration of MSR1 with prostate cancer risk. *Nature Genetics*, **35**, 128–9.

55 Maier, C., Vesovic, Z., Bachmann, N., Herkommer, K., Braun, A., Surowy, H., Assum, G., Paiss, T. *et al.* (2006) Germline mutations of the MSR1 gene in prostate cancer families from Germany. *Human Mutation*, **27** (*1*), 98–102.

56 Breast Cancer Linkage Consortium56. (1997) Pathology of familial breast cancer: differences between breast cancers in carriers of BRCA1 and BRCA2 mutations and sporadic cases. *Lancet*, **349**, 1505–10.

57 Boyd, J., Sonoda, Y., Federici, M.G., Bogomolniy, F., Rhei, E., Maresco, D.L., Saigo, P.E., Almadrones, L.A. *et al.* (2000) Clinicopathologic features of BRCA-linked and sporadic ovarian cancer. *The Journal of the American Medical Association*, **283** (*17*), 2260–5.

58 Edwards, S.M., Kote-Jarai, Z., Meitz, J., Hamoudi, R., Hope, Q., Osin, P., Jackson, R., Southgate, C. *et al.* (2003) Two percent of men with early-onset prostate cancer harbor germline mutations in the BRCA2 gene. *American Journal of Human Genetics*, **72** (*1*), 1–12.

59 Giusti, R., Rutter, J., Duray, P., Freedman, L., Konichezky, M., Fisher-Fischbein, J., Greene, M., Maslansky, B. *et al.* (2003) A two-fold increase in BRCA mutation related prostate cancer among Ashkenazi Israelis is not associated with distinctive histopathology. *Journal of Medical Genetics*, **40**, 787–92.

60 Agalliu, I., Kwon, E., Zadory, D., McIntosh, L., Thompson, J., Stanford, J. and Ostrander, E. (2007) Germline mutations in the BRCA2 gene and susceptibility to hereditary prostate cancer. *Clinical Cancer Research*, **13** (*3*), 839–43.

61 Lange, E., Ho, L., Beebe-Dimmer, J., Wang, Y., Gillanders, E., Trent, J., Lange, L., Wood, D. *et al.* (2006) Genome-wide linkage scan for prostate cancer susceptibility genes in men with aggressive disease: significant evidence for linkage at chromosome 15q12. *Human Genetics*, **119**, 400–7.

62 Sun, X., Frierson, H., Chen, C., Li, C., Ran, Q., Otto, K., Cantarel, B., Vessella *et al.* (2005) Frequent somatic mutations of the transcription factor ATBF1 in human prostate cancer. *Nature Genetics*, **37** (*4*), 407–12.

63 Jonsson, B., Adami, H., Hägglund, M., Bergh, A., Göransson, I., Stattin, P., Wiklund, F. and Grönberg, H. (2004) 160C/A polymorphism in the E-cadherin gene promoter and the risk of hereditary, familial, and sporadic prostate cancer. *International Journal of Cancer*, **109**, 348–52.

64 Lange, E., Robbins, C., Gillanders, E., Zheng, S., Xu, J., Wang, Y., White, K., Chang, B. *et al.* (2007) Fine-mapping the putative chromosome 17q21–2 prostate cancer susceptibility gene to a 10 cm region based on linkage analysis. *Human Genetics*, **121**, 49–55.

65 Tavtigian, S., Simard, J., Teng, D., Abtin, V., Baumgard, M., Beck, A., Camp, N., Carillo, A. *et al.* (2001) A candidate prostate cancer susceptibility gene at chromosome 17p. *Nature Genet*, **27**, 172–80.

66 Noda, D., Itoh, S., Watanabe, Y., Inamitsu, M., Dennler, S., Itoh, F.,

Koike, S., Danielpour, D. *et al.* (2006) ELAC2, a putative prostate cancer susceptibility gene product, potentiates TGF-beta/Smad-induced growth arrest of prostate cells. *Oncogene*, **25** (*41*), 5591–600.

67 Takahashi, H., Lu, W., Watanabe, M., Katoh, T., Furusato, M., Tsukino, H., Nakao, H., Sudo, A. *et al.* (2003) Ser217Leu polymorphism of the HPC2/ELAC2 gene associated with prostatic cancer risk in Japanese men. *International Journal of Cancer*, **107**, 224–8.

68 Yokomizo, A., Koga, H., Kinukawa, N., Tsukamoto, T., Hirao, Y., Akaza, H., Mori, M. and Naito, S. (2004) HPC2/ELAC2 polymorphism associated with Japanese sporadic prostate cancer. *Prostate*, **61**, 248–52.

69 Noonan-Wheeler, F.C., Wu, W., Roehl, K.A., Klim, A., Haugen, J., Suarez, B.K. and Kibel, A.S. (2006) Association of hereditary prostate cancer gene polymorphic variants with sporadic aggressive prostate carcinoma. *Prostate*, **66**, 49–56.

70 Severi, G., Giles, G.G., Southey, M.C., Tesoriero, A., Tilley, W., Neufing, P., Morris, H., English, D.R. *et al.* (2003) ELAC2/HPC2 polymorphisms, prostate-specific antigen levels, and prostate cancer. *Journal of the National Cancer Institute*, **95** (*11*), 818–24.

71 Wang, L., McDonnell, S.K., Elkins, D.A., Slager, S.L., Christensen, E., Marks, A.F., Cunningham, J.M., Peterson, B.J. *et al.* (2001) Role of HPC2/ELAC2 in hereditary prostate cancer. *Cancer Research*, **61** (*17*), 6494–9.

72 Shea, P., Ferrell, R., Patrick, A., Kuller, L. and Bunker, C. (2002) ELAC2 and prostate cancer risk in Afro-Caribbeans of Tobago. *Human Genetics*, **111**, 398–400.

73 Berry, R., Schroeder, J.J., French, A.J., McDonnell, S.K., Peterson, B.J., Cunningham, J.M., Thibodeau, S.N. and Schaid, D.J. (2000) Evidence for a prostate cancer-susceptibility locus on chromosome 20. *American Journal of Human Genetics*, **67**, 82–91.

74 Zheng, S., Xu, J., Isaacs, S., Wiley, K., Chang, B., Bleecker, E., Walsh, P., Trent, J. *et al.* (2001) Evidence for a prostate cancer linkage to chromosome 20 in 159

hereditary prostate cancer families. *Human Genetics*, **108**, 430–5.

75 Bock, C., Cunningham, J., McDonnell, S., Schaid, D., Peterson, B., Pavlic, R., Schroeder, J., Klein, J. *et al.* (2001) Analysis of the prostate cancer-susceptibility locus HPC20 in 172 families affected by prostate cancer. *American Journal of Human Genetics*, **68**, 795–801.

76 Camp, N., Farnham, J. and Cannon-Albright, L. (2006) Localization of a prostate cancer predisposition gene to an 880-kb region on chromosome 22q12.3 in Utah high-risk pedigrees. *Cancer Research*, **66** (*20*), 10205–12.

77 Blasina, A., de Weyer, I., Laus, M., Luyten, W., Parker, A. and McGowan, C.A. (1999) Human homologue of the checkpoint kinase Cds1 directly inhibits Cdc25 phosphatase. *Current Biology*, **9** (*1*), 1–10.

78 Chaturvedi, P., Eng, W., Zhu, Y., Mattern, M., Mishra, R., Hurle, M., Zhang, X., Annan, R. *et al.* (1999) Mammalian Chk2 is a downstream effector of the ATM-dependent DNA damage checkpoint pathway. *Oncogene*, **18**, 4047–54.

79 Bell, D., Varley, J., Szydlo, T., Kang, D., Wahrer, D., Shannon, K., Lubratovich, M., Verselis, S. *et al.* (1999) Heterozygous germ line hCHK2 mutations in Li-Fraumeni syndrome. *Science*, **286**, 2528–31.

80 Dong, X., Wang, L., Taniguchi, K., Wang, X., Cunningham, J.M., McDonnell, S.K., Qian, C., Marks, A.F. *et al.* (2003) Mutations in CHEK2 associated with prostate cancer risk. *American Journal of Human Genetics*, **72**, 270–80.

81 Wu, X., Dong, X., Liu, W. and Chen, J. (2006) Characterization of CHEK2 mutations in prostate cancer. *Human Mutation*, **27**, 742–7.

82 Xu, J., Meyers, D., Freije, D., Isaacs, S., Wiley, K., Nusskern, D., Ewing, C., Wilkens, E. *et al.* (1998) Evidence for a prostate cancer susceptibility locus on the X chromosome. *Nature Genetics*, **20** (*2*), 175–9.

83 Baffoe-Bonnie, A., Smith, J., Stephan, D., Schleutker, J., Carpten, J., Kainu, T.,

Gillanders, E., Matikainen, M. *et al.* (2005) A major locus for hereditary prostate cancer in Finland: localization by linkage disequilibrium of a haplotype in the HPCX region. *Human Genetics*, **117**, 307–16.

84 Narla, G., Heath, K., Reeves, H., Li, D., Giono, L., Kimmelman, A., Glucksman, M., Narla, J. *et al.* (2001) KLF6, a candidate tumor suppressor gene mutated in prostate cancer. *Science*, **294**, 2563–6.

85 Cairns, P., Okami, K., Halachmi, S., Halachmi, N., Esteller, M., Herman, J.G., Jen, J., Isaacs, W.B. *et al.* (1997) Frequent inactivation of PTEN/MMAC1 in primary prostate cancer. *Cancer Research*, **57** (*22*), 4997–5000.

86 Prochownik, E., Eagle Grove, L., Deubler, D., Zhu, X., Stephenson, R., Rohr, L., Yin, X. and Brothman, A.R. (1998) Commonly occurring loss and mutation of the MXI1 gene in prostate cancer. *Genes Chromosomes Cancer*, **22**, 295–304.

87 Kim, J.H., Kim, B., Cai, L., Choi, H.J., Ohgi, K.A., Tran, C., Chen, C., Chung, C.H. *et al.* (2005) Transcriptional regulation of a metastasis suppressor gene by Tip60 and beta-catenin complexes. *Nature*, **434** (*7035*), 921–6.

88 Mononen, N., Syrjakoski, K., Matikainen, M., Tammela, T.L., Schleutker, J., Kallioniemi, O.P., Trapman, J. and Koivisto, P.A. (2000) Two percent of Finnish prostate cancer patients have a germline mutation in the hormone-binding domain of the androgen receptor gene. *Cancer Research*, **60** (*22*), 6479–81.

89 Carter, H., Allaf, M. and Partin, A. (2007) Diagnosis and staging of prostate cancer, in *Campbell-Walsh Urology* (eds A. Wein, L. Kavoussi, A. Novick, A. Partin and C. Peters), Saunders Elsevier, Philadelphia, pp. 2912–31.

90 Nieder, A., Taneja, S., Zeegers, M. and Ostrer, H. (2003) Genetic counseling for prostate cancer risk. *Clinical Genetics*, **63** (*3*), 169–76.

91 Lazier, C., Thomas, L., Douglas, R., Vessey, J. and Rittmaster, R. (2004) Dutasteride, the dual 5a-reductase inhibitor, inhibits androgen action and promotes cell death in the LNCaP prostate cancer cell line. *Prostate*, **58**, 130–44.

92 Klein, E., Thompson, I., Lippman, S., Goodman, P., Albanes, D., Taylor, P., and Coltman, C. (2001) Select: the next prostate cancer prevention trial. *The Journal of Urology*, **166**, 1311–15.

93 Cohen, L., Zhao, Z., Pittman, B. and Scimeca, J. (2003) Effect of soy protein isolate and conjugated linoleic acid on the growth of Dunning R-3327-AT-1 rat prostate tumors. *Prostate*, **54**, 169–80.

94 Kucuk, O., Sarkar, F., Sakr, W., Djuric, Z., Pollak, M., Khachik, F., Li, Y., Banerjee, M. *et al.* (2001) Phase II randomized clinical trial of lycopene supplementation before radical prostatectomy. *Cancer Epidemiology Biomarkers & Prevention*, **10**, 861–8.

95 Eastham, J. and Scardino, P. (2007) Expectant management of prostate cancer, in *Campbell-Walsh Urology* (eds A. Wein, L. Kavoussi, A. Novick, A. Partin and C. Peters), Saunders Elsevier, Philadelphia, pp. 2947–55.

96 Hall, J., Lee, M., Newman, B., Morrow, J., Anderson, L., Huey, B., and King and M. (1990) Linkage of early-onset familial breast cancer to chromosome 17q21. *Science*, **250**, 1684–9.

97 Johanneson, B., Deutsch, K., McIntosh, L., Friedrichsen-Karyadi, D., Janer, M., Kwon, E., Iwasaki, L., Hood, L. *et al.* (2007) Suggestive genetic linkage to chromosome 11p11.2-q12.2 in hereditary prostate cancer families with primary kidney cancer. *Prostate*, **67** (7), 732–42.

98 Pierce, B., McIntosh, -L, Friedrichsen-Karyadi, D., Deutsch, K., Hood, L., Ostrander, E., Austin, M. and Stanford, J. (2007) Genomic scan of 12 hereditary prostate cancer families having an occurrence of pancreas cancer. *Prostate*, **67** (4), 410–15.

99 Bratt, O., Damber, J., Emanuelsson, M. and Grönberg, H. (2002) Hereditary prostate cancer: clinical characteristics and survival. *The Journal of Urology*, **167**, 2423–6.

14
Wilms and Rhabdoid Tumors of the Kidney

Brigitte Royer-Pokora

Summary

Wilms tumor (WT) is an embryonal tumor of the kidney, attributed to an aberrant proliferation of early metanephric kidney cells. It can arise from more than one developmental error, and therefore many genes have been implicated in WT. Deletion of the *WT1* gene, having a function in the development of kidneys and gonads, is observed in patients with the WT-aniridia-urogenital abnormalities-mental retardation syndrome (WAGR), whereas intragenic mutations are found in 10 to 15% of patients with sporadic WT. Germline mutations in this gene are found in patients with urogenital abnormalities (GU), isolated nephrotic syndrome (NS), Denys–Drash syndrome (DDS), Frasier syndrome (FS), but rarely in familial WT. Patients with *WT1* germline mutations have a high risk for unilateral WT as well as synchronous or metachronous bilateral WT (BWT), which might even occur later in life. An increased WT risk is also observed in some overgrowth syndromes, especially in Beckwith–Wiedeman syndrome (BWS), where dysregulated expression of imprinted genes at chromosome 11p15 occurs. Here, the loss of imprinting (LOI) of the growth promoting *IGF2* gene plays an important role, as this is observed in a large proportion of WT. In addition, WT can be associated with several malformation syndromes or familial diseases.

Survival for WT has improved steadily and is now approaching 90%. However, other non-WT renal childhood cancers are associated with substantial mortality. This is a heterogeneous group including renal-cell carcinoma, clear cell carcinoma, (congenital) mesoblastic nephroma, rhabdoid tumor, and renal medullary carcinoma. The malignant rhabdoid tumor (MRT) of the kidney was originally thought to be an unfavorable subtype of WT. It is a rare but aggressive malignancy, representing 2% of pediatric renal tumors. A high proportion occurs under the age of 2 years, and there is a male predominance. Much progress on the genetics of this tumor has occurred in the past few years, and inactivation of a tumor suppressor gene, *SNF5/INI1,* on the long arm of chromosome 22 has been found. This gene encodes a subunit of the chromatin-remodeling complex SWI/SNF, regulating the expression of many genes.

Hereditary Tumors: From Genes to Clinical Consequences
Edited by Heike Allgayer, Helga Rehder and Simone Fulda
Copyright © 2009 WILEY-VCH Verlag GmbH & Co. KGaA, Weinheim
ISBN: 978-3-527-32028-8

14.1
Wilms Tumor

Wilms tumor (WT) is observed at a frequency of $1:10\,000$ in newborn babies. Approximately 1 to 2% of the patients have a hereditary form of the tumor with autosomal dominant inheritance and variable penetrance. Knudson's "two-hit" model (see Chapter 2 on the genetic background of hereditary tumor disease) for the development of tumors in children describes that two successive mutations ("hits") are necessary for the uncontrolled division of the cells in a tumor [1]. Only one hit is necessary for tumor development in the hereditary form, as one allele is already mutant in all cells. Therefore, a tumor develops earlier in life and is more often bilateral than in the sporadic type, where both mutations have to occur in the same somatic cell (two hits).

Somatic and germline mutations in *WT1* (see below) have been found in WT, as well as tumor specific alterations in various other genes. Often, *WT1* mutations are associated with β-*Catenin (CTNNB1)* mutations, defining a genetic subset of WT. This subset, which recently was called the ideal type I WT [2], is characterized by stromal type histology with rhabdomyogenesis, early onset of WT, and GU abnormalities in males [2, 3]. WTs from patients with WT-aniridia-urogenital abnormalities-mental retardation syndrome(WAGR) and Denys–Drash syndrome (DDS) belong to this subtype of tumors. Embryonal remnants in the kidney, the nephrogenic rests (NR), are known precursor lesions for WT. Two classes of NR can be distinguished, the perilobar NR (PLNR) and the intralobar NR (ILNR), which differ in their location in the kidney: PLNR are found in the periphery and ILNR usually deep in the renal parenchyma [4]. Kidneys with WT of the ideal Type I often contain ILNRs, and it was postulated that these occur early in nephrogenesis. The tumors arising from ILNR show a broader spectrum of differentiation with heterologous elements, such as rhabdomyoblasts, cartilage, fat, and bone.

Patients with germline *WT1* mutations have a high risk of developing WT, often as bilateral WT (BWT) and independent secondary tumors [3]. We have recently shown that the recurrent tumors, which developed after one year in both kidneys of a patient with a germline *WT1* mutation and bilateral tumors, were new independent tumors. The molecular genetic analyses showed that the two primary and two secondary tumors had, besides the first *WT1* mutation, LOH for 11p13. The analysis of *CTNNB1* showed that all four tumors had different mutations in this gene, a molecular proof of their independent genesis and the high selection pressure for *CTNNB1* mutations in these tumors. In these WTs, three hits occurred; the first is a germline *WT1* mutation, the second LOH of the *WT1* wildtype allele, and the third a *CTNNB1* mutation [5].

Our study of 117 patients with *WT1* germline mutations revealed a substantial variation in the age of onset, bilaterality, and associated anomalies depending on the type of *WT1* alteration [3]. A correlation of the distribution of unilateral versus bilateral tumors with the type of mutation as well as with the position of the mutation in the *WT1* gene is shown in Figure 14.1.

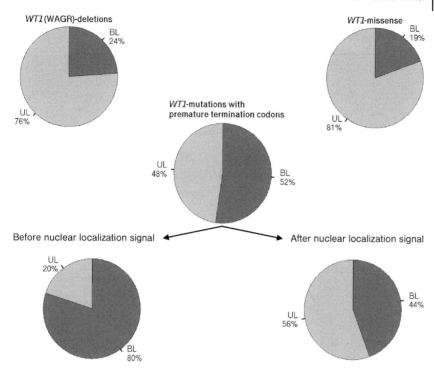

Figure 14.1 Unilateral and bilateral tumors in patients with different *WT1* germline mutations, and correlation to the position of the mutation in the gene. Data are based on 21 patients with WAGR syndromes or *WT1* deletions, 32 with missense mutations, and 68 with mutations resulting in a premature termination codon (modified from ref. [3]). The *WT1* gene has a nuclear localization signal (NLS) from codon 267 to 326. The percentage of bilateral tumors is even higher in patients with a mutation resulting in a stop codon before the NLS.

Another subset of WTs is associated with PLNRs and epigenetic alterations in the 11p15 region, and this has been termed the ideal type II WT [2]. A type II WT is characterized by a limited nephrogenic differentiation with mostly blastemal or epithelial type histology, a later age of tumor onset, and heavier birthweight, and is observed in patients with overgrowth syndromes such as BWS and hemihypertrophy. Tumors in this group have a higher proportion of either loss of imprinting (LOI) of genes located in 11p15, or chromosome 11 uniparental disomy (UPD) [6]. In these tumors, a loss of the maternal allele is observed, which indicates epigenetic and imprinting defects, and involves the telomeric imprinting domain (*IGF2*) and the centromeric imprinted domain (*LIT1*, antitranscript of the *K LQT*1 gene) [7]. In these cases, aberrant expression of the *IGF2* gene, encoding a fetal growth factor being expressed only from the paternal allele during embryonal development, most likely is an important factor for the development of this type of WT.

Besides tumor specific *CTNNB1* mutations, somatic alterations of another recently discovered gene, *WTX*, are found in approximately 10 to 20% of WT [8]. Interestingly, *WTX* resides on the X chromosome, which undergoes X inactivation in females and therefore only one hit is necessary to inactivate the one functional copy of this gene. Alterations of *CTNNB1* are found in ideal Type I WT and are associated with *WT1* mutations, whereas *WTX* alterations were not observed together with mutations in *WT1*. Therefore, tumors with *WTX* alterations may define a third subset of WTs, or may be part of the ideal Type II tumors.

Tumor-specific genetic alterations are not discussed further in this review focusing on hereditary tumors.

14.2
The *WT1* Gene and Its Functions

The *WT1* gene consists of ten exons and encodes a transcription factor with four zinc-finger (ZF) motifs, of which numerous isoforms are known [9]. Figure 14.2 shows the current status and complexity of the *WT1* gene. The *WT1* expression pattern in fetal kidneys and various cells of the genital system points to its specific role in the early urogenital development, and in kidney differentiation. In the developing kidney, the expression is seen first in the condensing metanephritic blastema, the highest expression occurring in the podocytes of the early glomerulus at a time when the cells pass through their strongest proliferation phase. In adults, *WT1* is only found in podocytes of the kidney, the Sertoli cells of the testis, and in the epithelial cells of the follicles of the ovaries.

WT1 transcript

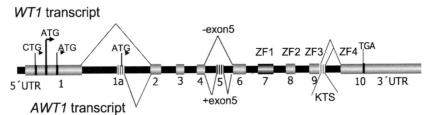

AWT1 transcript

Figure 14.2 Complex structure of the *WT1* gene. The 10 exons of *WT1* are shown with the alternative exon 1a in intron 1. The *WT1* transcript has three alternative translation start sites, an upstream in-frame CTG, the regular ATG start site (labeled with a thick arrow), and an in-frame downstream ATG, leading to a shorter protein. Exon 5 and the "KTS" amino acid sequence at the end of exon 9 are labeled in a striped pattern, and alternative usage of these sequences is found in all isoforms. In addition, transcription from an alternative promotor in intron 1, and production of the *AWT1* transcript, results in a shorter protein with a different amino terminus.

Expression of *WT1* during early development is associated with the conversion of mesenchymal cells to epithelial structures, implicating its function in epithelial differentiation.

14.3
Function of the *WT1* Gene in the Development of the Kidneys and the Formation of Tumors

At present it is still not entirely clear how mutations, or the loss of the WT1 protein activity, contribute to tumor formation. An essential role for *WT1* in the course of normal kidney development has been demonstrated by studies of *wt1* knockout mice, which do not develop metanephritic kidneys and die prior to birth [10]. The *WT1* negative metanephritic mesenchyme dies by apoptosis, demonstrating that the presence of *WT1* is necessary for the survival of these cells. In agreement with these observations, RNAi experiments in kidney organ cultures confirmed that *WT1*, apart from its function as a differentiation factor, has a function as survival factor in kidney development [11].

Taken together, these observations suggest that cells lacking *WT1* activity cannot survive. Recent analyses have shown that most tumors with *WT1* loss due to mutations at the same time have *CTNNB1* mutations [12] (and Uschkereit and Royer-Pokora, unpublished results). During the conversion of mesenchymal cells to epithelial structures in the kidney, interactive processes between different cell types involving WNT signaling play important roles. During WNT signal activation, the β-catenin protein is stabilized, and together with transcription factors of the TCF family activates WNT target genes. At the beginning of epithelial differentiation, cell division activity will be reduced; this phase is accompanied by increased *WT1* expression, and simultaneous downregulation of the WNT signaling pathway. In tumors lacking *WT1* and having a stabilizing *CTNNB1* mutation, the constitutively activated WNT signaling pathway might function as survival factor, and the cells remain in a proliferative phase.

WTs without *WT1* mutations usually show a strong expression of the WT1 protein. In these tumors, the continuous expression of WT1 might promote their growth, suggesting an oncogenic effect of high *WT1* levels.

14.4
Wilms Tumor-Associated Syndromes

In the following, several syndromes and genetic diseases are presented, which are associated with an increased risk of WT. Due to space limitation, I refer to review articles for a more detailed description of these different syndromes. The clinical care of these patients, as well as suggested surveillance guidelines for early recognition of tumors, was recently published in two comprehensive reviews by Scott *et al.* [13, 14].

14.5
WT1 Gene Associated Syndromes

14.5.1
Aniridia and WAGR Syndrome

Sporadic aniridia (AN), the congenital absence of parts or the entire iris, occurs at a frequency of 1:100000. Familial AN is inherited as an autosomal dominant disease, and is due to germline mutations in the *PAX6* gene. In 7.5/1000 WT patients, AN is observed. The risk for WT in sporadic AN patients is about 6%. When AN appears in conjunction with WT, GU, and mental retardation, a WAGR-syndrome is present, usually with a cytogenetically detectable deletion of chromosome 11p13. However, submicroscopic deletions may also be present, at least covering the *WT1* and *PAX6* genes, which are 647 kB apart.

The deletion of an entire copy of the *WT1* gene in male WAGR patients usually leads to mild forms of GU, such as hypospadias and/or maldescended testis. A detailed clinical description of WAGR patients and their clinical surveillance can be found in Fischbach *et al.* [15]. Breslow *et al.* [16] analyzed 64 WAGR patients and found that the risk of synchronous or metachronous BWT was 17.2%, while BWT in non-WAGR patients occurred in 6.4%. Another important observation was that these patients, 11 to 27 years after the WT diagnosis, have a 53% risk of renal failure [16]. Exact numbers for the tumor risk of WAGR patients are currently not available.

Therefore, it is recommended to examine newborns with sporadic AN for the presence of a *WT1* deletion, which confers a substantial risk for WT. Submicroscopic deletions may be identified by fluorescence-*in-situ*-hybridization or, more recently, by MLPA. An intragenic mutation in the *PAX6* gene confirms an isolated form of AN, and the patients have a normal population risk for WT.

14.5.2
Genitourinary Anomalies (GU) and Isolated Nephrotic Syndrome (NS)

Male patients with germline *WT1* mutations often have GU anomalies, including kidney abnormalities, hypospadias, and maldescended testis. The presentation of GU is highly variable, and male patients with germline *WT1* mutations without GU were described. GU can be attributed to the functional loss of one *WT1* allele, called haploinsufficiency. Male patients with GU may have either deletions of the entire gene (as in WAGR), or of single exons or mutations in *WT1* that lead to premature protein truncation. In the majority of cases these are *de-novo*-mutations; however, some cases are known with transmission from an unaffected parent [17]. Missense mutations in *WT1* such as those found in DDS patients usually lead to a more severe GU phenotype (see Section 14.5.3).

A WT develops only if at least the second *WT1* allele has been inactivated. Patients with a *WT1* germline mutation have a risk of at least 50% of developing a WT.

Isolated NS leading to terminal renal failure prior to the third year of life may also be due to a germline *WT1* mutation. In male patients this may be associated with GU, whereas in female individuals this is not easily attributed to *WT1*. In most NS cases, the histology is a diffuse mesangial sclerosis (DMS); however, in exceptional cases, this might also be a focal-segmental glomerulosclerosis (FSGS). Patients with early onset terminal kidney failure often have *WT1* missense mutations in the ZF region and the analysis can be initiated with this segment of the gene. When finding a *WT1* mutation there is a high risk for the development of a WT. The clinical care of these patients should be the same as for DDS patients (see Section 14.5.3).

14.5.3
Denys–Drash Syndrome (DDS)

This combination of GU, NS, and WT is usually due to a germline *WT1* missense mutation in exons 8 or 9 (ZF2 and 3). In karyotypic male patients, the GU is highly variable, ranging from hypospadias to female external genitalia and streak gonads, leading to pseudohermaphroditism masculinus. Some XX individuals may have gonadal dysgenesis, but the majority have normal external female genitalia, and attract attention at first by an isolated NS only. The early appearance of NS in patients with *WT1* missense mutations suggests that these act in a dominant negative fashion for normal renal function. However, a WT only develops if the second allele has been inactivated, and this explains why not every patient with DDS develops a WT.

The incidence for WT with over 90% is so high that, at present, in cases of acute terminal renal failure often a prophylactic bilateral nephrectomy is performed, preventing the development of a WT. It is recommended to examine male patients with GU and early NS, as well as female patients with early NS, for *WT1* mutations. In patients with *WT1* missense mutations, the percentage of BWT is lower (19%) than in patients with deletions (24%) or mutations leading to premature protein truncation (52%) (Figure 14.1). The percentage of bilateral tumors increases to 80% when the mutation results in a stop codon at an amino acid before codon 267, which is the position for a nuclear localization.

14.5.4
Frasier-Syndrome (FS)

FS is characterized by NS associated with gonadal dysgenesis and a risk for gonadoblastoma, but a low risk for WT. The NS is typically an FSGS, leading to renal failure later in life than in DDS patients. In XY individuals, sex reversal is common. Patients with FS have germline mutations in intron 9 of the *WT1* gene, leading to altered splicing and loss or reduction of the +KTS isoform. This shows that a correct ratio of the + and −KTS *WT1* isoforms is necessary for normal male genital development.

14.6
Non-*WT1* Gene Associated Syndromes

14.6.1
Overgrowth Syndromes

Patients with several overgrowth syndromes have an increased risk of malignancy including WT; however, the risk seems to be low. Some overgrowth syndromes with a specific WT risk are briefly described in the following.

Beckwith–Wiedemann syndrome (BWS) patients have a risk between 4 and 21% of developing embryonal tumors, where WT is the most frequent. Characteristics of BWS are prenatal and postnatal overgrowth, macroglossia, abdominal wall defects, ear creases and pits, neonatal hypoglycaemia, and hemihypertrophy. More than 80% of the cases are sporadic; in the familial cases, an autosomal dominant inheritance with varying expressivity and reduced penetrance has been observed. BWS is genetically heterogeneous and caused by the deregulation of imprinted genes, located in close proximity at chromosome 11p15.

The maternal/paternal expression of these genes is regulated by two imprinting centres [7]. An increased tumor risk of BWS has been observed when the activity of growth promoting genes such as *IGF2* is increased; however, this is not the case when germline mutations in the *P57* gene are present [7]. This demonstrates that the analysis of the underlying molecular alterations in BWS is important, in order to identify those individuals with an increased tumor risk.

Perlman syndrome is another rare autosomal-recessive overgrowth syndrome with a high neonatal mortality. Of the 21 cases with Perlman syndrome described, 7 had developed a WT. WT was also observed in patients with the Simpson–Golabi–Behmel–Syndrome (SGBS). SGBS is due to mutations or deletions in the *glypican3 (GPC3)* gene on Xq26. Up to now, 3 out of 35 SGBS-patients with identified *GPC3* mutations had developed a WT.

14.6.2
Familial Wilms Tumors

Studies of some large families with WT in several generations did not show linkage to *WT1*. An autosomal dominant WT predisposition gene has been mapped to 17q21 (*FWT1*), but the causative gene has not been identified so far. In *FWT1*, the penetrance for WT is approximately 30%, and no LOH of 17q was observed in the tumors, therefore *FWT1* might not function as a classical tumor suppressor gene. Another peculiarity of *FWT1* is the fact that the tumors occur late (medium age of diagnosis: 6 years) and present at a higher stage than sporadic WT. In other families, neither a linkage to chromosome 17q nor 19q has been discovered so that, still, another familial WT gene has to be postulated.

14.6.3
Tumor Predisposition Syndromes

WT can also be observed in families with other genetic tumor predisposition syndromes, such as neurofibromatosis (*NF1*), hyperparathyroidism-jaw-syndrome *(HPT-JT, HRPT2, parafibromin)*, and Li–Fraumeni-syndrome (*TP53*). WT also appears in patients with Blooms syndrome (BS), an autosomal recessive disease with pre- and postnatal growth delay, teleangiectases, sun sensitivity, hyperpigmentation, and predisposition for malignant tumors. BS cells show an increased rate of somatic crossover, caused by biallelic inactivation of the *BLM* gene, a DNA helicase. This leads to hemizygosity and homozygosity of parts of the genome, and in consequence to the functional inactivation of tumor suppressor genes.

In Mulibrey nanism (MUL), a rare autosomal-recessive disease involving various tissues of mesodermal origin, WT has been observed. MUL is characterized by growth retardation, distinctive facial features, and hepatomegaly. This is due to mutations of the *TRIM37* gene, an ubiquitin E3 ligase. It occurs hardly anywhere else but in the Finnish population with a frequency of 1:40000. WT has been observed in 2 out of 40 MUL patients.

Recently, there have been reports on families where several children had different tumor illnesses; for instance, in one family one child had myeloid leukemia, one WT, and one medulloblastoma. It turned out that these children had biallelic *BRCA2* mutations, and this corresponds to the Fanconi anaemia (FA) subgroup D1 [18]. FA is an autosomal recessive disorder characterized by short stature, radial ray defects, and bone marrow failure. Heterozygous constitutional mutations in *BRCA2* predispose to breast and ovarian cancers, however not to childhood cancers. Children from these rare families with biallelic inactivation of *BRCA2* show spontaneous chromosome breaks in their cells, but have less of the typical stigmata for FA. The tumor spectrum includes a high risk for WT and brain tumors. Often, the bi-allelically affected children developed their tumors prior to their parents who, as carriers of *BRCA2* mutations, also have an increased tumor risk as adults.

WT also rarely occurs in patients with mosaic variegated aneuploidy, which is characterized by constitutional mosaicism for losses and gains of whole chromosomes, and is based on a mutation in *BUB1B*, a spindle control gene. An increased risk is also observed in patients with trisomy 13 and 18 [13].

14.6.4
Malignant Renal Rhabdoid Tumor (MRR)

A detailed clinical and pathological description of the various forms of non-WT renal tumors can be found in [19]. MRR was originally classified as an unfavorable subtype of WT with a rhabdomyosarcomatoid histological pattern. It is a rare and aggressive kidney tumor occurring in early infancy. Occasionally, separate tumors outside of the kidney may occur, most frequently CNS tumors, now called atypical teratoid-rhabdoid tumors. Both types of tumors show inactivation of the *hSNF5/INI1* gene on 22q11, and many are constitutional changes of one allele [20]. The second allele may be inactivated by different mechanisms in primary renal tumors and primary tumors of the CNS, indicating their independent origin. Biallelic inactivation of this gene has been observed in sporadic renal rhabdoid tumors and in choroid plexus tumors, medulloblastoma, and neuroectodermal tumors.

The *hSNF5/INI1* gene is a core subunit of the chromatin-remodeling complex SWI/SNF. This complex alters histone-DNA interactions in an ATP dependent process, thereby regulating (activating or repressing) many genes [21]. The complex consists of approximately 10 subunits, and loss of the activity of some of these genes is found in many human cancers. Mice with a reversibly inactivating conditional allele of *Snf5* have a highly penetrant cancer predisposition phenotype, and 100% of the mice develop T-cell lymphoma and rhabdoid tumors after a short latency period [22]. It is of interest that these mice develop a limited spectrum of tumors only. In these mice it was also observed that loss of *Snf5* expression results in death of many cell types, therefore the normal function is required for survival of all non-malignant cells. An explanation for this contradiction may be that loss of *Snf5* results in a change of the epigenetic state of a cell leading to cell death, unless additional mutations occur which lead to the development of cancer [22].

The genomic location of the *hSNF5/INI1* gene at 22q11 is at the same position of micro-deletions in 22q11.2, found in patients with DiGeorge/Velocardiofacial syndrome (DGS/VCFS). These micro-deletions occur with a frequency of 1/3000 to 1/5000 in newborns, and are associated with a variable expression of neonatal hypocalcemia, various heart defects, abnormal faces with ear abnormalities, hypoplasia, or absence of the thymus (resulting in immune defects) and the parathyroid. The children may be of short stature and present with mild to moderate learning difficulties. The phenotype is highly variable, this in part being explained by different sizes and positions of the deletions. A common deleted region of 3 Mb proximal of the *hSNF5/INI1* gene has been defined, but patients with deletions entirely outside of this region were also identified [23]. In addition, micro-duplications of the same genomic region have been observed. The 22q11.2 genomic segment contains many low-copy repeats, which have about 95% sequence homology and appear to cause aberrant recombinations leading to deletions or duplications.

Wieser *et al.* described a patient with a 22q11 micro-deletion syndrome phenotype who developed a rhabdoid tumor of the kidney [24]. The cytogenetic and molecular studies of this patient revealed a complex rearrangement of the band q11 on the paternal chromosome 22, involving a micro-duplication and a micro-deletion telomeric of the duplicated segment. The deletion extended beyond the previously identified common deleted region, and included the *hSNF5/INI1* gene. In the tumor, the second allele of the gene was inactivated by a frameshift mutation [24]. In addition, using high-density single nucleotide polymorphism array analysis, five patients with malignant rhabdoid tumors (MRT) and germline deletions of 22q11.2, including the *INI1* locus, were recently described. In two patients, phenotypic findings were suggestive, but non-conclusive for the DGS/VCFS syndrome. The molecular studies of these two patients revealed a more distally located deletion outside of the typically deleted segment. The other three patients had smaller deletions including the *INI1* gene, and they had two or more primary tumors [25]. The mechanism leading to deletions in these patients could be similar to those found in DGS/VCFS syndrome patients, involving aberrant recombination events of low copy repeat sequences.

The variable phenotype observed in these patients makes it difficult to decide who should be screened for *INI1* deletions. However, modern FISH techniques using a BAC probe covering the *INI1* locus, or newer techniques such as MLPA, could be used in the future to identify 22q11 micro-deletion patients with an increased risk of MRR.

14.7
Micro-Deletion Syndromes and Tumor Risk

WT and MRR now have a common feature: both may occur in patients with micro-deletion syndromes. A tumor risk is only observed if the respective tumor suppressor gene resides within the deleted segment. Therefore, molecular studies defining the endpoints of the deletions are warranted in these cases to identify patients with an increased tumor risk, and to start surveillance programs for early tumor detection.

14.8
Recommendations for Genetic Counseling and Therapy

For patients with the diseases and syndromes described above, who are open to a (presymptomatic) molecular analysis and have not yet developed a tumor, genetic counseling is recommended prior to the molecular test. It would also be highly desirable that patients who have already presented with a tumor are counseled before a molecular genetic analysis is performed, and that the possible results and their consequences are explained to them or their parents.

In Europe and North America most children with Wilms tumors can be cured with current treatment protocols. In North America this involves primary resection of the tumor after clinical and imaging assessment. This is followed by chemotherapy with two or three drugs: dactinomycin, vincristine, and doxorubicin. Only in patients with relapses, four other drugs may be added: cyclophsophamide, ifosfamide, carboplatin, and etoposide [26]. Most European studies, which are mainly organized by the Société International d'Oncologie Pédiatrique (SIOP), focus on developing stage specific strategies after prenephrectomy chemotherapy. This involves delaying staging and histopathological diagnosis until after surgery [26]. Postoperative chemotherapy is based on stage of the disease and response to therapy.

Treatment for malignant renal rhabdoid tumor (MRR) remains investigational. No accepted standard therapy has been established for this disease. Enrollment of patients on clinical trials is strongly encouraged. In MRR, primary tumor surgery is followed by chemotherapy. Using initially the same drugs as in WT, dactinomycin, vincristine, and doxorubicin, the survival rate for MRR was only 23%. Currently cyclophosphamide-carboplatin-etoposide (CCE) alternating with VDC is the main treatment in the childrens oncology group COGstudy. In addition, radiation therapy may be used if there is CNS involvement [27].

References

1 Knudson, A.G. (1971) *Proceedings of the National Academy of Sciences of the United States of America*, **68**, 820–3.

2 Breslow, N.E., Beckwith, J.B., Perlman, E.J. and Reeve, A.E. (2006) *Pediatric Bood and Cancer*, **47**, 260–7.

3 Royer-Pokora, B., Beier, M., Henzler, M., Alam, R., Schumacher, V., Weirich, A. and Huff, V. (2004) *American Journal of Medical Genetics*, **127A**, 249–57.

4 Beckwith, J.B., Kiviat, N.B. and Bonadio, J.F. (1990) *Pediatric Pathology*, **10**, 1–36.

5 Uschkereit, C., Perez, N., de Torres, C., Küff, M., Mora, J. and Royer-Pokora, B. (2007) *Journal of Medical Genetics*, **44**, 393–6.

6 Fukuzawa, R. and Reeve, A.E. (2007) *Journal of Pediatric Hematology Oncology*, **29**, 589–94.

7 Weksberg, R., Shuman, C. and Smith, A.C. (2005) *American Journal of Medical Genetics Part C (Seminars in Medical Genetics)*, **137C**, 12–23.

8 Rivara, M.N., Kim, W.J., Wells, J., Driscoll, D.R., Brannigan, B.W., Kim, J. C., Feinberg, A.P., Gerald, W.L., Vargas, S.O., Chin, L., Iafrate, A.J., Bell, D.W. and Haber, D.A. (2007) *Science*, **315**, 642–5.

9 Hohenstein, P. and Hastie, N.D. (2006) *Human Molecular Genetics*, **15**, R196–201.

10 Kreidberg, J.A., Sariola, H., Loring, J.M., Maeda, M., Pelletier, J., Housman, D. and Jaenisch, R. (1993) *Cell*, **74**, 679–69.

11 Davies, J.A., Ladomery, M., Hohenstein, P., Michael, L., Shafe, A., Spraggon, L. and Hastie, N. (2004) *Human Molecular Genetics*, **13**, 235–46.

12 Maiti, S., Alam, R., Amos, C.I. and Huff, V. (2000) *Cancer Research*, **60**, 6288–92.

13 Scott, R.H., Walker, L., Olsen, O.E., Levitt, G., Kenney, I., Maher, E., Owens, C.M., Pritchard-Jones, K., Craft, A. and Rahman, N. (2006) *Archives of Disease in Childhood*, **91**, 995–9.

14 Scott, R.H., Stiller, C.A., Walker, L. and Rahman, N. (2006) *Journal of Medical Genetics*, **43**, 705–14.

15 Fischbach, B.V., Trout, K.L., Lewis, J., Luis, C.A. and Sika, M. (2005) *Pediatrics*, **116**, 984–8.

16 Breslow, E., Norris, R., Norkool, P.A., Kang, T., Beckwith, J.B., Perlman, E.J., Ritchey, M.L., Green, D.M. and Nichols, K.E. (2003) *Journal of Clinical Oncology*, **21**, 4579–85.

17 Jeanpierre, C., Béroud, C., Niaudet, P. and Junien, C. (1998) *Nucleic Acids Research*, **26**, 271–4.

18 Reid, S., Renwick, A., Seal, S., Baskcomb, L., Barfoot, R. and Jayatilake, H., The Breast Cancer Suspectibility Collaboration (UK), Pritchard-Jones, K., Stratton, M.R., Ridolfi-Lüthy, A. and Rahman, N. for the Familial Wilms Tumour Collaboration (2005) *Journal of Medical Genetics*, **42**, 147–51.

19 Ahmed, H.U., AArya, M., Levitt, G., Duffy, P.G., Mushtaq, I. and Sebire, N.J. (2007) *Lancet Oncology*, **8**, 730–7.

20 Versteege, I., Sevenet, N., Lange, J., Rousseau-Merck, M., Ambros, P., Handgretinger, R., Aurias, A. and Delattre, O. (1998) *Nature*, **394**, 203–6.

21 Imbalzano, A.N. and Jones, S.N. (2005) *Cancer Cell*, **7**, 294–5.

22 Roberts, C.A., Leroux, M.M., Fleming, M.D. and Orkin, S.H. (2002) *Cancer Cell*, **2**, 415–25.

23 Rauch, A., Pfeiffer, R.A., Leipold, G., Singer, H., Tigges, M. and Hofbeck, M. (1999) *American Journal of Human Genetics*, **64**, 659–66.

24 Wieser, R., Fritz, B., Ullmann, R., Müller, I., Galhuber, M., Storlazzi, C.T., Ramaswamy, A., Christiansen, H., Shimizu, N. and Rehder, H. (2005) *Human Mutation*, **26**, 78–83.

25 Jackson, E.M., Shaikh, T.H., Gururangan, S., Jones, M.C., Malkin, D., Nikkel, S.M., Zuppan, C.W., Wainwright, L.M., Zhang, F. and Biegel, J.A. (2007) *Human Genetics*, **122**, 117–27.

26 Kalapurakal, J.A., Dome, J.S., Perlman, E.J., Malogolowkin, M., Haase, G.M., Grundy, P. and Coppes, M.J. (2004) *Lancet Oncology*, **5**, 37–46.

27 Tomlinson, G.E., Breslow, N.E., Dome, J., Guthries, K.A., Norkool, P., Li, S., Thomas, P.R.M., Perlman, J.E., Beckwith, B., D'Angio, G.J. and Green, D.M. (2005) *Journal of Clinical Oncology*, **23**, 7641–5.

15
Hereditary Renal Tumors of the Adult

Liesbeth Spruijt and Nicoline Hoogerbrugge

Summary

A hereditary predisposition to renal cell cancer (RCC) is suspected when a patient with RCC has a first-degree relative who has also been diagnosed with RCC, or in an individual patient presenting with bilateral and/or multiple tumors. The clinical diagnosis of hereditary RCC can be confirmed by germline DNA testing of the main predisposing genes (*VHL* for Von Hippel–Lindau disease, *MET* for hereditary papillary RCC (HPRC), *FH* for hereditary leiomyomatosis RCC, and *BHD* for Birt–Hogg–Dubé syndrome). In patients with clear cell RCC, *VHL* analysis is the first step and, if negative, should be followed by karyotyping for chromosome 3 translocations. Patients with papillary Type 1 RCC should be considered for *MET* analysis, and those with papillary Type 2 RCC for *FH* analysis. In patients with a chromophobe RCC or an oncocytoma, genetic analysis of the *BHD* gene is indicated.

Once a disease causing germline DNA mutation has been demonstrated in a family, genetic testing may be offered to at-risk relatives, and clinical follow-up has to be initiated for carriers of the familial germline mutation. A close surveillance of the kidneys is recommended in the index patient and in the first-degree relatives, and of all families with a high suspicion of a hereditary renal cancer syndrome, even if the genetic factor has not been genetically characterized. Treatment by nephron-sparing surgery should be considered in hereditary forms of RCC.

15.1
General Introduction [1–4]

Cancers of the kidney account for approximately 1.5% of all cancer related deaths. Less than 5% of these tumors are hereditary. Having a first-degree relative affected with renal cancer is a recognized risk factor for renal cell carcinoma (RCC). Familial or hereditary RCCs are characterized by: (i) early ages of onset compared to

Hereditary Tumors: From Genes to Clinical Consequences
Edited by Heike Allgayer, Helga Rehder and Simone Fulda
Copyright © 2009 WILEY-VCH Verlag GmbH & Co. KGaA, Weinheim
ISBN: 978-3-527-32028-8

sporadic cases; (ii) frequent bilateral occurrence; and (iii) multifocality. Renal cancer is not a single disease. It is made up of a number of different types of cancer occurring in the kidney. The different types of renal cancer have distinct histological characteristics, different clinical courses, and different underlying gene defects. Two main types of renal cancers are distinguished: RCC and transition cell cancers of the renal pelvis have specific hereditary causes and therefore will be discussed separately.

15.2
Renal Cell Carcinoma [5, 6]

15.2.1
Introduction

RCCs represent about 90% of all renal neoplasms. Based on their location within the nephron and the cell type from which the tumors originate, a classification system has previously been introduced in which epithelial cells of the proximal part of the renal tubule give rise to clear cell RCC (also referred to as conventional or non-papillary RCCs) (75%), and papillary RCCs (also referred to as chromophilic RCCs) (10–15%), whereas the collecting tubule of the nephron gives rise to chromophobe RCCs (5%) and renal oncocytomas (5%). At present, several genes related to these cancer syndromes have been identified, including the *VHL, MET, BHD,* and *FH* genes. The respective syndromes show dominant inheritance patterns. The identification of a predisposing gene offers the possibility for surveillance of mutation carriers with the possibility of earlier diagnosis and treatment.

15.2.2
Familial Clear Cell RCC

15.2.2.1 Von Hippel–Lindau (VHL) Disease [7–14]
Although VHL is a rare autosomal dominant disorder with a birth incidence of 1 per 35 000, the disease is the main cause of inherited RCC. The RCCs in VHL are mostly multiple and bilateral [7, 9]. Although RCC is the presenting feature in only 10% of the patients with VHL disease, the risk of developing a RCC rises to 70% by the age of 60 years. The mean age of a RCC in VHL at diagnosis is 40 to 44 years, and is very rare below age 20 [8]. VHL disease should therefore be suspected in all cases with young onset, familial clustering, or multiple renal clear cell carcinomas.

VHL is a tumor predisposition syndrome that is characterized by a wide variety of tumors, the most frequent being retinal angioma (60% of patients), cerebellar (60% of patients), spinal (13–44%) and brainstem haemangioblastomas (18%), clear cell RCC (28%), and phaeochromocytomas (7–20%). Renal cysts, pancreatic cysts, and endolymphatic sac tumors (ELST) are also relatively common findings

[7]. Less frequent is the occurrence of non-secretory endocrine pancreatic tumors and broad ligament cystadenoma. The clinical diagnostic criteria for VHL disease are:

- In isolated cases:
  - two or more hemangioblastomas (retinal or CNS),
  - a single hemangioblastoma in association with a visceral tumour or ELST.
- In familial cases:
  - a family history of retinal or CNS hemangioblastoma,
  - one hemangioblastoma, ELST or visceral tumour.

The VHL gene is a tumor suppressor gene located on 3p25-26, and has a function in the oxygen-sensing pathway [10–12]. There is evidence that there are VHL modifier genes that might explain the existence of phenotypical subtypes. Somatic inactivation of the VHL gene by mutation or hypermethylation is found in up to 70% of sporadic clear cell RCCs [14].

RCC may arise from the wall of renal cysts, and complex cysts require careful follow-up. Early detection of renal tumors can be established by ultrasound, CT, or magnetic resonance imaging (MRI). The screening recommendations for VHL are:

- Yearly eye examinations and blood pressure monitoring, starting by age 5;
- Yearly 24-hour urine collection test for elevated catacholamines, starting at age 10;
- Yearly abdominal ultrasounds, MRI, and/or CT scan, starting at age 15.

15.2.2.2 Constitutional Chromosome 3 Translocations [14–20]

Chromosome 3 anomalies are the explicit hallmark of sporadic clear cell RCCs. Until now, 8 RCC families with constitutional chromosome 3 translocations have been reported: t(1;3)(q32;q13), t(2;3)(q33;q21), t(2;3)(q35;q21), t(3;4)(p13;p16), t(3;6)(p13;q25), t(3;6)(q12;q15), t(3;8)(p13;q24), and t(3;8)(p14;q24). In addition, 2 sporadic RCC cases with constitutional translocations t(3;11)(p14;q15) and t(3;12)(q13;q24), respectively, have been described [14–20].

RCCs caused by a chromosome 3 anomaly are mainly multifocal and bilateral. Both loss of heterozygosity and VHL mutations were identified in tumors from such patients, and a three-step model for the development of RCC was proposed. Inheritance of a germline chromosome 3 balanced translocation would be followed by a non-disjunctional loss of the derivative chromosome that carries the 3p segment, and a somatic inactivation by mutation or hypermethylation of the remaining VHL gene. Other genes disrupted by translocation breakpoints could also be involved in renal tumorigenesis (*FHIT, TRC8, DIRC2, DIRC3, LSAMP,* and *NORE1A*). Some of these genes have been shown to act as tumor suppressors.

In 100 Dutch RCC families, a screening program aimed at early detection has been initiated, including yearly ultrasound examinations of the kidneys, and analysis of urine sediments [18, 19]. As a result of this program, several novel tumors were detected and removed surgically. In addition, they were subjected to

cytogenetic and molecular analyses, thereby substantiating the previously proposed multi-step RCC model. Although the positions of the translocation breakpoints clearly varied between the different families reported so far, they all mapped
in the proximal p- and q-arms of chromosome 3. This notion is in full agreement
with observations made in sporadic RCC cases, as listed in the Mitelman catalog
of chromosome aberrations in cancer (http://cgap.nci.nih.gov/chromosomes/
mitelman). Such a breakpoint distribution may be related to the location of putative RCC-causing genes within these regions and/or a lack of compatibility with
cell survival, when major parts of chromosome 3 are lost during subsequent RCC
development.

15.2.2.3 Familial Clear Cell Renal Cell Cancer (FCRC) [21, 22]

Families with renal carcinoma in multiple family members, who do not have one
of the known inherited forms of renal carcinoma, are considered to have FCRC.
A sibling of a patient with RCC is 2.5 times more likely to have RCC than a
member of the general population. A few families have been reported worldwide
with 2 to 5 affected members. In contrast to other familial renal carcinomas, the
diagnosis of RCC is made relatively late in life (>50 years) in these cases and
tumors occur in general unilaterally and solitary. Very likely, FCRC is a heterogeneous entity, but it is not yet excluded that it might also represent a single
entity.

15.2.2.4 SDHB-Associated Heritable Paraganglioma [23]

Autosomal inherited multiple paragangliomas are characterized by the occurrence
of paragangliomas in the head and neck (31%), and pheochromocytomas, either
adrenal (28%) or extraadrenal (48%). Multiple tumors occur in 28% of the patients.
The onset is on average at 30 years of age, and it has a penetrance of 77% by 50
years of age. The cause is a germline mutation in one of the genes encoding the
different subunits of the mitochondrial enzyme succinate dehydrogenase (*SDHB*,
SDHC, and *SDHD*). Three cases of clear cell RCC occurring at a young age have
been reported recently in patients with germline mutations in the *SDHB* gene
(located on chromosome 1p36), but generally appear less common in this disorder.
No corresponding somatic mutation has been found in sporadic RCC.

15.2.2.5 Tuberous Sclerosis Complex (TSC) [24, 25]

Tuberous sclerosis (TS) is an autosomal dominant hamartomatous disorder with
an incidence of 1 per 6000 to 25 000 live births. It is a multi-system disorder affecting skin, eyes, CNS, teeth, bones, heart, lungs, and kidney. The skin features such
as facial angiofibroma, white ash leaf-shaped macules, shagreen patch, and subungual fibromata, are characteristic and will raise the suspicion for this syndrome.
TS is well-known by nephrologists because of the occurrence of multiple renal
angiomyolipomas (~45%) and cysts (~30%). Clear cell RCCs have only been
observed in 1 to 2% of cases.

Two genes have been identified that are causative for TSC. The *TSC1* gene,
located on chromosome 16p13.3, encoding the protein hamartin, and the *TSC2*

gene, located on chromosome 9q34.3, encoding tuberin. Both genes acting as tumor suppressors are critical regulators of cell growth and proliferation, and are physically interactive. In approximately two-thirds of the patients there is no family history of TSC, and these patients apparently have a *de novo* mutation. In about 70 to 80% of the individuals that fulfil the definite diagnostic criteria, a *TSC1* or *TSC2* mutation can be detected. The remaining patients rather have mutations in unanalyzed noncoding regions or somatic mosaic mutations, than that an additional TSC locus is suspected. In familial cases there is an equal distribution in *TSC1*- and *TSC2*-gene mutations, but in the *de novo* cases the majority (~80%) have a mutation in the *TSC2* gene. *TSC2* is located adjacent to the autosomal dominant polycystic kidney locus (APKD1). The presence of severe renal cystic disease is strongly correlated with deletions in both *TSC2* and *APKD1* genes. Patients with the *TSC2* mutations tend to have a more severe phenotype with an increased prevalence of mental retardation, autistic disorders, and infantile spasm, and multiple clinical findings are more frequent in this group.

15.2.3
Familial Papillary RCC

15.2.3.1 Hereditary Papillary RCC (HPRC) [26]
Papillary renal cell carcinomas and clear cell renal cell carcinoma are both thought to originate from the proximal renal tube, even though they are caused by a different gene defect. HPRC appears less aggressive stage-for-stage than FCRC. Type I HPRC causes less aggressive basophilic tumors that have a favorable prognosis. Type 2 causes eosinophilic tumors with a worse prognosis. HPRC is caused by activating missense mutations in the *MET* proto-oncogene located in 7q31, encoding a receptor tyrosine kinase that is normally activated by hepatocyte growth factor (HGF). The disease is highly penetrant, that is, in gene carriers there is a high life-time risk of papillary kidney cancer. The renal cancer in HPRC, in general, has a late onset in the fourth to sixth decade of life.

The MET–HGF signaling pathway is important for cell proliferation, epithelial–mesenchymal transition, branching morphogenesis, differentiation, and regulation of cell migration in many tissues. The renal tumors in HPRC often show trisomy 7, including two of the chromosomes that harbor the *MET* gene mutations. This suggests that the duplication of chromosome 7 provides the second activating event in renal cells that is important in tumorigenesis [27]. Somatic mutations of MET are encountered in 13% of sporadic papillary Type 1 RCC.

15.2.3.2 Hereditary Leiomyomatosis Renal Cell Cancer (HLRCC) [28, 29]
HLRCC is a hereditary cancer syndrome in which affected individuals are at risk of developing multiple cutaneous and uterine leiomyomas, bladder cancers, and solitary papillary Type 2 RCCs. The RCCs are the most aggressive of the familial types, metastasize early, and in this way show a very different clinical course than the renal tumors in patients with VHL, HPRC, and BHD. HLRCC is caused by germline mutations in the tumor suppressor gene *FH* located at 1q42-43, encoding

the mitochondrial Krebs cycle enzyme fumarate hydratase (FH). About 40 different *FH* mutations have been identified and are distributed throughout the entire gene without evidence of a genotype–phenotype correlation [29]. Somatic mutations of *FH* are very rare in sporadic tumors. Because of the increased risk for RCC and the aggressive nature of the tumors, screening for kidney cancer is advised in HLRCC families.

15.2.3.3 Hyperparathyroidism–Jaw Tumor (HPT-JT) [30]

HPT-JT predisposes to multiple parathyroid adenomas, fibro-osseous tumors of the jaw, and a variety of renal lesions including cystic kidney disease, hamartomas, mesoblastic nephromas, and late-onset Wilms tumors. A papillary RCC was described in only one patient. The HRPT2 gene is mapped to chromosome 1q24-32. It acts as a tumor suppressor gene and encodes a new protein with unknown function, named parafibromin. Cloning efforts are currently continuing to isolate the gene, which may play a general role in the renal tumorigenesis.

15.2.3.4 Papillary Thyroid Carcinoma with Associated Renal Neoplasia (FPTC-PRN) [31]

In 5% of cases, papillary thyroid carcinomas occur in a familial context in association with benign nodular thyroid disease. A large three-generation family has been reported, with two affected members having associated multifocal papillary RCC or adenomas, and another member with renal oncocytomas. A link between renal involvement by PRCC and the germline abnormalities that are related to familial papillary thyroid carcinoma is suspected, but has not been determined. The gene responsible for familial papillary thyroid neoplasia is to be identified.

15.2.4
Familial Chromophobe RCC and Oncocytomas

15.2.4.1 Birt–Hogg–Dubé syndrome (BHD) [32–36]

BHD is an autosomal dominant genodermatosis that predisposes individuals to the triad of benign cutaneous lesions of the face, neck, and upper torso (fibrofolliculomas (84%), trichodiscomas and acrochordons), spontaneous recurrent pneumothorax (11–32%) and/or lung cysts (85%), and renal tumors. The skin lesions usually develop in the third or fourth decade of life. RCC may develop in 6 to 30% of gene carriers, with a mean age of diagnosis of 43 years [35]. The tumors are often bilateral and multifocal. A unique feature among the hereditary renal cancers is the variety of histologic types of renal tumors in BHD, including chromophobe (35%) and chromophobe–oncocytic hybrid RCCs (50%), but clear cell RCC (5%), oncocytomas (5%) and rarely papillary RCCs (5%) have also been observed. Colorectal polyps and tumors have been reported in some BHD families [32], but not in a risk-assessment study [34]. The disease is caused by germline mutations in the *FLCN* gene, a gene with a tumor suppressor role located on chromosome 17p11.2. In approximately half of the BHD patients, there are no known affected relatives [36]. Mutation detection is high (69–84%) in patients with skin manifestation of BDH [35, 36]. Due to the increased risk of kidney cancer, yearly screening with ultrasound, MRI, or CT scan should be considered starting at age 25.

15.2.5
Medullary Renal Carcinoma (MRC) [37–39]

Medullary carcinomas of the kidney are very rare, highly aggressive tumors that occur in young, often black patients with the sickle cell trait. The mean age of onset is between 11 and 39 years, and males predominate in this age group by 3 to 1. However, beyond age 24, the tumors occur equally in men and women. Hematuria is the most frequent initial symptom (60%). Medullary tumors are usually large and centrally located with adjacent lymphadenopathy, and as a rule already have metastasized when first discovered. The mean survival is only 15 weeks. These tumors most likely arise in the collecting ducts in or near the renal papillae. With ultrasound and CT-scan, an infiltrative and indefinite mass arising in the central region of the kidney, and invasion into the renal sinus can be detected. Characteristically, small multifocal nodules are seen in the medullary portion of the kidney.

The gene for sickle anemia trait is located on the short arm of chromosome 11. In one patient, a monosomy of chromosome 11 was reported [38], but in all other cases no specific genetic abnormality has been associated with renal medullary carcinoma. The genes associated with medullary carcinoma do not cluster with those of clear cell or papillary renal cell carcinoma; however, there was close clustering with transition cell carcinoma [39].

15.3
Transition Cell Cancers of the Renal Pelvis

15.3.1
Lynch Syndrome [40–45]

Urothelial cell carcinoma of the upper urinary tract, also called transitional cell carcinoma, are relatively uncommon tumors representing about 5% of the upper urinary tract tumors. Although familial occurrence has been reported, most cases are acquired and not inherited.

First-degree relatives with urothelial carcinoma have a two-fold increased risk [40]. Some families with Lynch syndrome demonstrate a predisposition to transitional cell carcinoma of the ureter and renal pelvis, but not to renal parenchymal tumors. Lynch syndrome or the hereditary nonpolyposis colorectal cancer syndrome (HNPCC) is an autosomal dominant inherited disorder caused by a germline mutation in one of the mismatch repair genes *MLH1*, *MSH2*, *MSH6*, or *PMS2* (see Chapter 17 on Lynch syndrome (HNPCC)). Carriers of such a mutation are at high risk of developing colon cancer, in particular the proximal colon. Most patients with Lynch syndrome develop tumors at a young age, often before the age of 45 to 50. In addition, there is increased risk of extracolonic cancer, such as cancer of the endometrium, ovary, stomach, small bowel, hepatobiliary tract, urether, and renal pelvis. Although the overall increased risk is more than 20-fold the risk of the normal population, possibly somewhat higher for urethral urothelial carcinoma than for renal pelvic urothelial carcinoma, the absolute life-time risk for mutation carriers is 4 to 10% [41–45].

15.3.2
Diagnostic Recommendations [46–49]

A hereditary predisposition to RCC should be suspected when a patient with RCC has a first-degree relative who has also been diagnosed with RCC. An inherited syndrome is also suspected in patients presenting with an apparent sporadic RCC, when the tumor is bilateral and/or multiple, or appears at a young age because of the high and life-long risk of recurrence [2, 3, 46]. When the diagnosis of familial RCC has been made, first-degree relatives at risk should be identified and advised to have genetic counseling. A detailed pedigree with family history should be obtained, and a thorough examination carried out since VHL, BHD, and HLRCC have extrarenal manifestations, and physical examination, ophthalmologic, neurological, dermatological examinations, and radiology may be helpful. Although a careful medical and family history in combination with physical examination can identify VHL, BHD, and HLRCC affected patients, other syndromes can only be detected when renal tumors have been diagnosed. The effective clinical management of patients with an inherited predisposition to RCC requires an early diagnosis of the syndrome, close kidney surveillance, and specific treatment of renal tumors, in addition to other potential manifestations specific to each condition.

The clinical diagnosis can be confirmed by genetic testing in most cases, since analysis of the main predisposing genes (*VHL, MET, BHD*, and *FH*) is now available [2]. The required genetic investigations depend on the histological type of renal tumor, and the associated features present in some of the hereditary renal cancer syndromes [2]. In patients with clear cell RCC, VHL analysis is the first step and, if negative, should be followed by karyotyping to look for potential chromosome three translocations. Patients with papillary Type 1 RCC should be considered for MET analysis, and those with papillary Type 2 RCC for FH analysis. In patients with chromophobe RCC or oncocytomas, genetic analysis of the *BHD* gene is indicated. Once a specific genetic anomaly has been demonstrated in the proband, genetic testing may be offered to at-risk relatives, and clinical follow-up has to be initiated for carriers of the familial germline mutation [2].

A close surveillance of the kidneys is recommended in the index patient and in the first-degree relatives, of all families with high suspicion of a hereditary renal cancer syndrome, even if the genetic factor has not been genetically characterized.

The available guidelines for the follow-up of patients with hereditary RCC are scarce. The standard evaluation of patients with suspected renal cell tumor includes an ultrasound and/or CT scan of the abdomen and pelvis, urine analysis, and urine cytology. Screening for microscopic hematuria in individuals with an increased risk for urinary tract malignancies is not invasive; however, it is not clear if microscopic hematuria is an appropriate and useful screening marker for these malignancies [47]. Ultrasound evaluation for the surveillance of renal masses can demonstrate such masses, as small as 1.5 cm with 80% accuracy [48]. This technique is therefore insensitive to small renal masses and can lead to a false-negative diagnosis [46]. CT-scan with contrast is the best single choice for surveillance. Gadolinium-enhanced MR imaging is the second choice for this purpose. It is supplementary to CT imaging, but the overall accuracy in the differentiation of tumors is higher with MRI than with CT imaging.

Clearly, not all reported hereditary forms of renal cancer have the same risk and the same tumor phenotype. Patients with an aggressive phenotype, such as HLRCC and MRC, should undergo imaging relatively frequently, every 3 to 6 months, whereas patients with a mild phenotype and lower risk for RCC, such as SDHB-associated heritable paraganglioma, TSC, and HPT-JT, may undergo imaging at 2- to 3-year intervals. [46]

The recommendation of surveillance for upper urethelial tract carcinoma in patients with Lynch syndrome is strongly disputed. Surveillance is only recommended in Lynch syndrome families with a documented urothelial tumor of the upper tract in a first-degree relative, and there are even some that believe that surveillance is these cases is not indicated [49]. There is no well-established screening test available, but the usually followed management is urinalysis, urine cytology, and periodic upper tract imaging by ultrasound every 1 to 2 years starting at the age of 25 to 30.

15.3.3
Therapeutic Recommendations [50–53]

In hereditary forms of RCC, nephron-sparing treatment regimens should be considered. These regimens include observation for clear cell RCC less than 3 cm in diameter in families with VHL, percutaneous ablation by radiofrequency or cryotherapy, or nephron sparing surgery. Promising results have been obtained, but close follow-up with imaging studies of treated lesions and long-term experience is still lacking [50, 51]. Nephron-sparing surgery is the standard method of treatment for patients with inherited RCC who tend to have multiple tumors, often requiring recurrent operations, but nephrectomy may be necessary in the course of the disease or because of the diagnosis of locally advanced RCC [52]. Observation of patients with hereditary forms of RCC until their tumors grow 3 cm or larger, followed by the enucleation or removal of all lesions once they reach this size threshold, has led to extremely few deaths from metastatic RCC in families with VHL, and has improved the quality of life for patients affected by multiple bilateral and recurring renal tumors [53]. Whether small renal tumors by virtue of size alone differ dramatically from larger tumors of similar histology is unclear, but size correlates well to prognosis.

Acknowledgment

We thank Prof. Dr. A. Geurts van Kessel for careful comment on this chapter.

References

1 Godley, P. and Kim, S.W. (2002) Renal cell carcinoma. *Current Opinion in Oncology*, **14**, 280–5.

2 Pavlovich, C.P. and Schmidt, L.S. (2004) Searching for the hereditary causes of renal-cell carcinoma. *Nature Reviews Cancer*, **4**, 381–93.

3 Zbar, B., Klausner, R. and Linehan, W.M. (2003) Studying cancer families to identify kidney cancer genes. *Annual Review of Medicine*, **54**, 217–33.

4 Zimmer, M. and Iliopoulos, O. (2003) Molecular genetics of kidney cancer. *Cancer Treatment and Research*, **116**, 3–27.

5 Linehan, W.M. and Zbar, B. (2004) Focus on kidney cancer. *Cancer Cell*, **6**, 223–8.

6 Thoenes, W., Storkel, S. and Rumpelt, H.J. (1986) Histopathology and classification of renal cell tumors (adenomas, oncocytomas and carcinomas). The basic cytological and histopathological elements and their use for diagnostics. *Pathology, Research and Practice*, **181**, 125–43.

7 Lonser, R.R., Glenn, G.M., Walther, M. et al. (2003) von Hippel–Lindau disease. *Lancet*, **361**, 2059–67.

8 Richard, S., Graff, J., Lindau, J. and Resche, F. (2004) von Hippel–Lindau disease. *Lancet*, **363**, 1231–4.

9 Chauveau, D., Duvic, C., Chretien, Y. et al. (1996) Renal involvement in von Hippel–Lindau disease. *Kidney International*, **50**, 944–51.

10 Latif, F., Tory, K., Gnarra, J. et al. (1993) Identification of the von Hippel–Lindau disease tumor suppressor gene. *Science*, **260**, 1317–20.

11 Kaelin, W.G. Jr (2002) Molecular basis of the VHL hereditary cancer syndrome. *Nature Reviews Cancer*, **2**, 673–82.

12 Maxwell, P.H., Wiesener, M.S., Chang, G.W. et al. (1999) The tumour suppressor protein VHL targets hypoxia-inducible factors for oxygen-dependent proteolysis. *Nature*, **399**, 271–5.

13 Ang, S.O., Chen, H., Hirota, K. et al. (2002) Disruption of oxygen homeostasis underlies congenital Chuvash poly-cythemia. *Nature Genetics*, **32**, 614–21.

14 Gnarra, J.R., Tory, K., Weng, Y. et al. (1994) Mutations of the VHL tumour suppressor gene in renal carcinoma. *Nature Genetics*, **7**, 85–90.

15 Cohen, A.J., Li, F.P., Berg, S. et al. (1979) Hereditary renal-cell carcinoma associated with a chromosomal translocation. *New England Journal of Medicine*, **301**, 592–5.

16 Bodmer, D., van den Hurk, W., van Groningen, J.J. et al. (2002) Understanding familial and non-familial renal cell cancer. *Human Molecular Genetics*, **11**, 2489–98.

17 Bodmer, D., Schepens, M., Eleveld, M.J., Schoenmakers, E.F. and Geurts van Kessel, A. (2003) Disruption of a novel gene, DIRC3, and expression of DIRC3-HSPBAP1 fusion transcripts in a case of familial renal cell cancer and t(2;3)(q35;q21). *Genes Chromosomes Cancer*, **38**, 107–16.

18 Bonne, A.C., Bodmer, D., Schoenmakers, E.F. et al. (2004) Chromosome 3 translocations and familial renal cell cancer. *Current Molecular Medicine*, **4**, 849–54.

19 Van Erp, F., Van Ravenswaaij, C., Bodmer, D. et al. (2003) Chromosome 3

translocations and the risk to develop renal cell cancer: a Dutch intergroup study. *Genetic Counseling*, **14**, 149–54.

20 Chen, J., Lui, W.O., Vos, M.D. *et al.* (2003) The t(1;3) breakpoint-spanning genes LSAMP and NORE1 are involved in clear cell renal cell carcinomas. *Cancer Cell*, **4**, 405–13.

21 Woodward, E.R., Clifford, S.C., Astuti, D., Affara, N.A. and Maher, E.R. (2000) Familial clear cell renal cell carcinoma (FCRC): clinical features and mutation analysis of the VHL, MET, and CUL2 candidate genes. *Journal of Medical Genetics*, **37**, 348–53.

22 Teh, B.T., Giraud, S., Sari, N.F. *et al.* (1997) Familial non-VHL non-papillary clear-cell renal cancer. *Lancet*, **349**, 848–9.

23 Vanharanta, S., Buchta, M., McWhinney, S.R. *et al.* (2004) Early-onset renal cell carcinoma as a novel extraparaganglial component of SDHB-associated heritable paraganglioma. *American Journal of Human Genetics*, **74**, 153–9.

24 Lendvay, T.S. and Marshall, F.F. (2003) The tuberous sclerosis complex and its highly variable manifestations. *The Journal of Urology*, **169**, 1635–42.

25 Au, K.S., Williams, A.T., Roach, E.S. *et al.* (2007) Genotype/phenotype correlation in 325 individuals referred for a diagnosis of tuberous sclerosis complex in the United States. *Genetics in Medicine*, **9**, 88–100.

26 Schmidt, L., Duh, F.M., Chen, F. *et al.* (1997) Germline and somatic mutations in the tyrosine kinase domain of the MET proto-oncogene in papillary renal carcinomas. *Nature Genetics*, **16**, 68–73.

27 Zhuang, Z., Park, W.S., Pack, S. *et al.* (1998) Trisomy 7-harbouring non-random duplication of the mutant MET allele in hereditary papillary renal carcinomas. *Nature Genetics*, **20**, 66–9.

28 Tomlinson, I.P., Alam, N.A., Rowan, A.J. *et al.* (2002) Germline mutations in FH predispose to dominantly inherited uterine fibroids, skin leiomyomata and papillary renal cell cancer. *Nature Genetics*, **30**, 406–10.

29 Alam, N.A., Rowan, A.J., Wortham, N.C. *et al.* (2003) Genetic and functional analyses of FH mutations in multiple cutaneous and uterine leiomyomatosis, hereditary leiomyomatosis and renal cancer, and fumarate hydratase deficiency. *Human Molecular Genetics*, **12**, 1241–52.

30 Carpten, J.D., Robbins, C.M., Villablanca, A. *et al.* (2002) HRPT2, encoding parafibromin, is mutated in hyperpara-thyroidism-jaw tumor syndrome. *Nature Genetics*, **32**, 676–80.

31 Malchoff, C.D., Sarfarazi, M., Tendler, B. *et al.* (2000) Papillary thyroid carcinoma associated with papillary renal neoplasia: genetic linkage analysis of a distinct heritable tumor syndrome. *The Journal of Clinical Endocrinology and Metabolism*, **85**, 1758–64.

32 Khoo, S.K., Giraud, S., Kahnoski, K. *et al.* (2002) Clinical and genetic studies of Birt–Hogg–Dube syndrome. *Journal of Medical Genetics*, **39**, 906–12.

33 Khoo, S.K., Kahnoski, K., Sugimura, J. *et al.* (2003) Inactivation of BHD in sporadic renal tumors. *Cancer Research*, **63**, 4583–7.

34 Zbar, B., Alvord, W.G., Glenn, G. *et al.* (2002) Risk of renal and colonic neoplasms and spontaneous pneumothorax in the Birt–Hogg–Dube syndrome. *Cancer Epidemiology, Biomarkers and Prevention*, **11**, 393–400.

35 Leter, E.M., Koopmans, A.K., Gille, J.J. *et al.* (2008) Birt–Hogg–Dube Syndrome: clinical and genetic studies of 20 families. *The Journal of Investigative Dermatology*, **128**, 45–9.

36 Schmidt, L.S., Nickerson, M.L., Warren, M.B. *et al.* (2005) Germline BHD-mutation spectrum and phenotype analysis of a large cohort of families with Birt–Hogg–Dube syndrome. *American Journal of Human Genetics*, **76**, 1023–33.

37 Davis, C.J. Jr, Mostofi, F.K. and Sesterhenn, I.A. (1995) Renal medullary carcinoma. The seventh sickle cell nephropathy. *The American Journal of Surgical Pathology*, **19**, 1–11.

38 Avery, R.A., Harris, J.E., Davis, C.J. Jr *et al.* (1996) Renal medullary carcinoma: clinical and therapeutic aspects of a newly described tumor. *Cancer*, **78**, 128–32.

39 Yang, X.J., Sugimura, J., Tretiakova, M.S. *et al.* (2004) Gene expression profiling of renal medullary carcinoma: potential clinical relevance. *Cancer*, **100**, 976–85.

40 Aben, K.K., Witjes, J.A., Schoenberg, M.P. *et al.* (2002) Familial aggregation of urothelial cell carcinoma. *International Journal of Cancer*, **98**, 274–8.

41 Vasen, H.F., Offerhaus, G.J., den Hartog Jager, F.C. *et al.* (1990) The tumour spectrum in hereditary non-polyposis colorectal cancer: a study of 24 kindreds in the Netherlands. *International Journal of Cancer*, **46**, 31–4.

42 Lenz, D.L. and Harpster, L.E. (2003) Urothelial carcinoma in a man with hereditary nonpolyposis colon cancer. *Reviews in Urology*, **5**, 49–53.

43 Sijmons, R.H., Kiemeney, L.A., Witjes, J.A. and Vasen, H.F. (1998) Urinary tract cancer and hereditary nonpolyposis colorectal cancer: risks and screening options. *The Journal of Urology*, **160**, 466–70.

44 Amira, N., Rivet, J., Soliman, H. *et al.* (2003) Microsatellite instability in urothelial carcinoma of the upper urinary tract. *The Journal of Urology*, **170**, 1151–4.

45 Ericson, K.M., Isinger, A.P., Isfoss, B.L. and Nilbert, M.C. (2005) Low frequency of defective mismatch repair in a population-based series of upper urothelial carcinoma. *BMC Cancer*, **5**, 23.

46 Choyke, P.L., Glenn, G.M., Walther, M.M., Zbar, B. and Linehan, W.M. (2003) Hereditary renal cancers. *Radiology*, **226**, 33–46.

47 Sugimura, K., Ikemoto, S.I., Kawashima, H., Nishisaka, N. and Kishimoto, T. (2001) Microscopic hematuria as a screening marker for urinary tract malignancies. *International Journal of Urology*, **8**, 1–5.

48 Baxter, G. and Sidhu, P. (2006) *Ultrasound of the Urogenital System*, Thieme Medical Publishers, Stuttgart.

49 Aarnio, M., Sankila, R., Pukkala, E. *et al.* (1999) Cancer risk in mutation carriers of DNA-mismatch-repair genes. *International Journal of Cancer*, **81**, 214–18.

50 Pavlovich, C.P., Walther, M.M., Choyke, P.L. *et al.* (2002) Percutaneous radio frequency ablation of small renal tumors: initial results. *The Journal of Urology*, **167**, 10–15.

51 Shingleton, W.B. and Sewell, P.E. Jr (2002) Percutaneous renal cryoablation of renal tumors in patients with von Hippel–Lindau disease. *The Journal of Urology*, **167**, 1268–70.

52 Herring, J.C., Enquist, E.G., Chernoff, A. *et al.* (2001) Parenchymal sparing surgery in patients with hereditary renal cell carcinoma: 10-year experience. *The Journal of Urology*, **165**, 777–81.

53 Neumann, H.P., Bender, B.U., Berger, D.P. *et al.* (1998) Prevalence, morphology and biology of renal cell carcinoma in von Hippel–Lindau disease compared to sporadic renal cell carcinoma. *The Journal of Urology*, **160**, 1248–54.

16
Gastrointestinal Polyposis Syndromes

Waltraut Friedl and Stefanie Vogt

Summary

The diagnosis of a colorectal polyposis syndrome is based on clinical findings of multiple gastrointestinal polyps on endoscopy. Histologic evaluation of polyps is required to allow differentiation between the different types of polyposis: adenomatous polyposis syndromes, juvenile polyposis syndrome, or Peutz–Jeghers syndrome (PJS). These polyposis syndromes have a different molecular genetic basis and a characteristic predisposition to different tumors. Therefore, specific surveillance programs are developed for patients with each of the polyposis syndromes.

Careful clinical diagnosis, including histology of the polyps is a prerequisite for appropriate molecular genetic testing. It should be kept in mind that the genetic defect underlying the disease cannot be identified in some of the patients. Therefore, a molecular genetic test in an affected individual can confirm but never exclude a suspected disease. This implies that clinical management of a patient diagnosed with one of the clinically defined polyposis syndromes should be based on the actual clinical findings in the patient and not on results of molecular tests.

Identification of a germline mutation in one of the genes involved in the etiology of polyposis syndromes in an affected individual is of importance for his family. It allows accurate predictive genetic testing of the family members, which identifies those persons who have inherited the mutation and thus the predisposition to the disease. As a consequence, clinical surveillance can be limited to the actual persons at risk within the family. Moreover, identification of the genetic defect in adenomatous polyposis syndromes is of relevance to differentiate between *APC*-associated autosomal-dominant familial adenomatous polyposis (FAP), and the MUTYH-associated autosomal-recessive polyposis (MAP); this differentiation is of high importance in genetic counselling and risk prediction in the families.

Hereditary Tumors: From Genes to Clinical Consequences
Edited by Heike Allgayer, Helga Rehder and Simone Fulda
Copyright © 2009 WILEY-VCH Verlag GmbH & Co. KGaA, Weinheim
ISBN: 978-3-527-32028-8

16.1
Introduction

Up to 5% of colorectal cancer (CRC) cases are caused by a monogenic predisposition. Among these, hereditary non-polyposis colorectal cancer (HNPCC, Lynch syndrome, see Chapter 17) accounts for 2 to 3% of cases, adenomatous polyposis syndromes for about 1%, and other polyposis syndromes together for less than 1% of CRC cases.

Unlike HNPCC, where the clinical diagnosis can be established only in the context of family history or molecular testing, the different gastrointestinal polyposis syndromes usually can be diagnosed clinically in an individual patient. Gastrointestinal polyposis syndromes encompass a heterogeneous group of hereditary tumor disposition entities. For clinical differentiation, histologic examination of polyps is essential (Figure 16.1). Based on polyp histology, polyposis disorders are divided into *adenomatous* polyposis syndromes including *APC*-associated familial adenomatous polyposis (FAP) and MUTYH-associated polyposis (MAP), *hamartomatous* polyposis syndromes (Peutz–Jeghers syndrome (PJS), juvenile polyposis

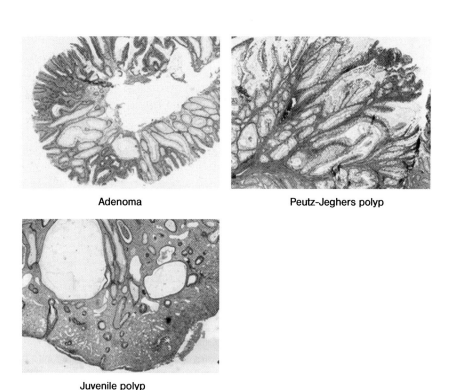

Adenoma   Peutz–Jeghers polyp

Juvenile polyp

Figure 16.1 Histopathologic differentiation of gastrointestinal polyps
(Images: N. Friedrichs, Pathological Institute, University Hospital Bonn).

syndrome, *PTEN* hamartoma tumor syndrome), and *hyperplastic* polyposis. These entities differ not only by type of polyps, but also by the clinical course, tumor spectrum, and genetic background (Table 16.1).

16.2
Adenomatous Polyposis Syndromes

Adenomatous polyposis syndromes encompass heterogeneous disorders that differ by clinical course, genetic background, and mode of inheritance. The first cases of FAP were described more than 120 years ago (for a review on history, see [1]). In 1991, the identification of the *APC* gene and mutations therein as the genetic cause of the disease has consistently promoted research in this field. Although presenting with variable phenotypes, FAP was considered as a monogenic, autosomal-dominantly inherited disease until 2002 when the recessively inherited MAP was discovered. Since then, the term familial adenomatous polyposis is used for the autosomal-dominant disorder caused by mutations in the *APC* gene, while the term *MUTYH*-associated polyposis is applied to the autosomal-recessive disorder caused by biallelic mutations in the *MUTYH* gene.

16.2.1
APC-Associated Familial Adenomatous Polyposis (FAP)

Polyposis conditions associated with germline mutations in the *APC* gene (OMIM #175100) include two main phenotypes that differ by the degree of colorectal polyposis: the classic (or typical) FAP, and the attenuated FAP (AFAP). Moreover, the two overlapping phenotypes (Gardner syndrome and Turcot syndrome) are currently considered phenotypic variants of classic FAP (Table 16.1).

   APC-associated FAP is present in about 1:10000 births worldwide. FAP follows an autosomal-dominant mode of inheritance, with a penetrance of almost 100%. Thus, offspring of FAP patients have a risk of 50% to inherit and develop the disease. About 15 to 20% of cases occur *de novo* [2–4]. Somatic mosaicism has been detected in about 15% of cases with *de novo* mutations [5].

16.2.1.1 Classic (Typical) FAP

Gastrointestinal Features By definition, classic FAP is characterized by the occurrence of more than a hundred and up to several thousands of *colorectal adenomas* (Figure 16.2). Polyps appear at a mean age of 16 years (range 7–36), and are distributed over the entire colorectum. First symptoms of typical FAP may be diarrhoea, constipation, rectal bleeding, and abdominal pain. If left untreated, some of the polyps will inevitably transform to CRC by a mean age of 39 years (review in [6, 7]).

   Gastric adenomas are relatively rare in the Western FAP population and are usually confined to the gastric antrum. At a higher frequency, fundic gland polyps

Table 16.1 Hereditary predispositions to gastrointestinal polyposis.

Disease	Abbreviation	Clinical characteristics	Mode of inheritance	Genes
Adenomatous polyposis syndromes				
Familial adenomatous polyposis	FAP		Autosomal-dominant	*APC*
• Classical FAP	FAP	>100 adenomatous polyps (at age <35 years)		
– Subtype: Gardner syndrome		Triad of polyposis, desmoids, and osteomas		
– Subtype: Turcot syndrome[a]		Association of polyposis and brain tumors (medulloblastoma)		
• Attenuated FAP	AFAP; AAPC	<100 adenomatous polyps		
MUTYH-associated polyposis	MAP	Adenomatous polyps (usually comparable to AAPC)	Autosomal-recessive	*MUTYH*
Hamartomatous polyposis syndromes				
Peutz–Jeghers syndrome	PJS	Peutz–Jeghers polyps; hyperpigmentation	Autosomal-dominant	*STK11*
Juvenile polyposis syndrome	JPS	Juvenile polyps	Autosomal-dominant	*SMAD4* *BMPR1A*
PTEN hamartoma tumor syndrome	PHTS		Autosomal-dominant	*PTEN*
Cowden syndrome	CS	Characteristic mucocutaneous lesions; macrocephaly; gastrointestinal hamartomatous polyps; benign breast, thyroid, and endometrial manifestations		
Bannayan–Riley–Ruvalcaba syndrome	BRRS	Multiple lipomas; macrocephaly; gastrointestinal hamartomatous polyps; pigmented macules on the glans penis (in males)		
Lhermitte–Duclos disease	LDD	Cerebellar gangliocytomatosis		

a Turcot syndrome, historically defined by the appearance of gastrointestinal polyps and brain tumors, is an allelic subtype of either FAP or Lynch syndrome.

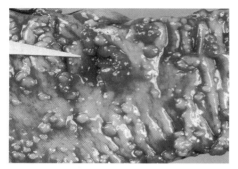

Figure 16.2 Fragment from a colectomy specimen in a patient with classic FAP (Image: K. Jäger, Marienhospital Brühl).

occur (in ~50% of patients); these polyps do not have an increased malignant potential and therefore do not need special management.

The prevalence of *duodenal adenomas* in FAP patients reported in the literature varies between 50 and 90% [7, 8] or even 20 to 100% [9]. Prevalence data vary, depending on age at endoscopy, but also on the diagnostic procedure used for surveillance.

Extraintestinal Features   FAP patients may develop benign tumors such as desmoids, osteoma, or epidermoid cysts.

- **Desmoid Tumors**   Desmoids are histologically benign tumors of the connective tissue; however, they can lead to life-threatening complications due to their locally invasive growth. In the general population, desmoids have an incidence of 2 to 5 per million. FAP patients have an 850-fold increased risk to develop desmoids, resulting in a prevalence of 10 to 25% in FAP. Desmoid tumors may occur sporadically or following surgical intervention, pregnancy, and oral contraceptive use.

- **Osteomas and Dental Anomalies**   Osteomas are osseous tumors located mainly in the facial skeleton and long bones. These tumors are benign and generally do not need therapeutic interventions except in cases where they create problems because of their local displacing growth. Osteomas were reported in 76 to 93% of FAP patients. Dental anomalies including unerupted, absent, or supernumerary teeth or odontomas are also reported in FAP; however, they occur less frequently as compared to osteoma.

- **Epidermoid Cysts and Fibromas**   These benign soft subcutaneous tumors are mainly located on the face, scalp, or extremities and have no clinical relevance.

- **Hypertrophy of the Retinal Pigment Epithelium (CHRPE)**   About 85% of FAP patients develop characteristic lesions of the retina referred to as congenital hypertrophy of the retinal pigment epithelium (CHRPE) [10]. CHRPE are multiple and mainly bilateral non-premalignent flat patches of the retina that do not affect visual abilities. CHRPE are detected by indirect ophthalmoscopy. Since CHRPE are present at birth, their detection in persons at risk can be used as a predictive marker for FAP in part of the families.

16.2.1.2 Attenuated FAP (AFAP, AAPC)

Leppert *et al.* [11] reported the first large family with an autosomal-dominant predisposition to an attenuated polyposis phenotype and CRC. The number of adenomas varied between 5 and 300. In AFAP, polyp growth starts roughly 10 to 15 years later than in classic FAP. Adenomas are localized predominantly in the proximal colon and have a flat shape, as illustrated by the term "hereditary flat adenoma syndrome" used in another family with a similar clinical picture [12]. In both families, the disease-causing gene was mapped to chromosomal region 5q containing the *APC* gene.

The term attenuated refers to the number and time of occurrence of colorectal polyps. Nevertheless, patients have an increased risk for CRC, and for cancer of the upper gastrointestinal tract. Extraintestinal manifestations of FAP (CHRPE, desmoids, osteomas) are rare in AFAP (see review on AFAP by [13, 14]).

16.2.1.3 Allelic Subtypes of Classic FAP

Gardner Syndrome The triade of colorectal adenomas, osteomas, and soft cyst-like surface tumors have been referred to as Gardner syndrome [15]. However, both Gardner syndrome and classic FAP are caused by mutations in the same gene. Moreover, most FAP patients have one or several extracolonic manifestations. Therefore, the term Gardner syndrome should no longer be used [16].

Turcot Syndrome The association of a central nervous tumor and multiple colorectal adenoma or carcinoma is defined as Turcot syndrome, an heterogeneous entity [17, 18]. Most cases are associated with germline mutations in the *APC* gene and are thus allelic to FAP; these patients usually develop a medulloblastoma. In a small number of cases, Turcot syndrome is associated with germline mutations in a DNA mismatch repair gene and is thus allelic to HNPCC; in these patients usually a glioblastoma is diagnosed as the central nervous tumor (see also Chapter 5 on hereditary brain tumors).

16.2.1.4 Genetics

Molecular Genetic Background FAP is caused by germline mutations in the tumor suppressor gene *APC* (Adenomatous Polyposis Coli). The detection of an interstitial deletion on the long arm of chromosome 5 in a patient with FAP was the first hint for mapping the involved gene to this chromosomal region [19]. The *APC* gene was mapped shortly thereafter [20, 21], and finally cloned in 1991 [22, 23].

The APC protein plays a regulatory role in the Wnt pathway by its interaction with β-catenin (Figure 16.3). The name Wnt is a combination of Wg (wingless), a

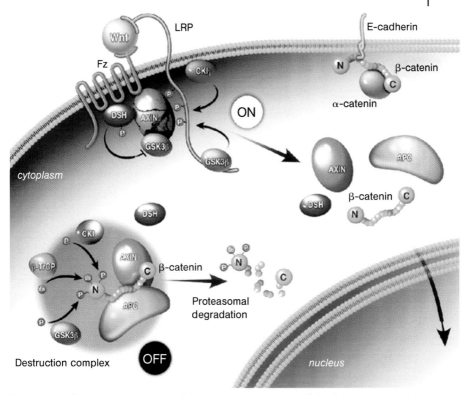

Figure 16.3 Schematic representation of the role of APC and β-catenin in the Wnt pathway. In the absence of Wnt (OFF), β-catenin is degraded by a destruction complex formed by APC, Axin, CKI, GSK3β, and β-TrPC. Wnt signaling (ON) mediates phosphorylation of LRP by CKIγ and GSK3β, which leads to recruiting Axin out of the destruction complex to the receptor complex. This mechanism is supported by Dsh, which binds Axin. Consequently, β-catenin is no longer degraded but enters the nucleus where it acts as a transcription cofactor. (Reprinted from Willert and Jones [24], with permission).

gene originally identified in *Drosophila melanogaster*, and *INT*, a gene that was originally identified in vertebrates, but was found to be homologous with the Wg gene. The Wnt signaling pathway is required at different stages of gut development and is mainly involved in cellular proliferation, survival, and motility (for review, see [24, 25]). The leading part of the Wnt cascade is the cytoplasmic protein β-catenin, a gene-specific transcription cofactor, which is involved both in cellular signaling and in cell adhesion. In the absence of Wnt signals, β-catenin interacts with E-cadherin and α-catenin to help mediate cell adhesion. The excess β-catenin is rapidly turned over by a destruction complex formed by APC, Axin, casein kinase I (CKI), glycogen synthase kinase 3β (GSK3β), and β-transducing repeat-containing protein (β-TrPC).

Binding of the Wnt ligand to the receptor induces formation of a receptor complex composed of the transmembrane proteins Frizzled (Fz), and LDL-

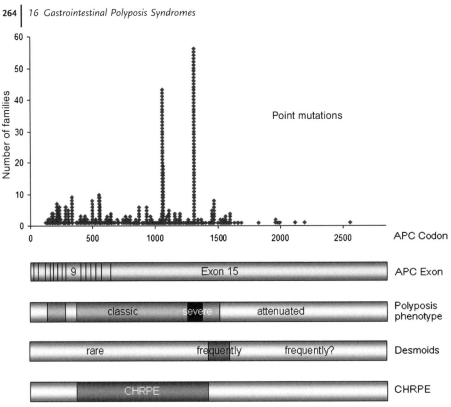

Figure 16.4 Distribution of 597 germline point mutations in the *APC* gene detected in 1166 unrelated FAP patients, and summary of genotype-phenotype correlations.

receptor-related protein (LRP), and triggers phosphorylation of LRP by GSK3β and CK1γ, a membrane-tethered kinase. This leads to a high affinity binding of LRP to Axin, thus disrupting the destruction complex and releasing β-catenin. The released β-catenin translocates to the nucleus, where it associates with the Tcf family of transcription factors to activate the transcription of target genes.

Mutant APC proteins are unable to bind Axin or to initiate the proteolytic degradation of β-catenin, which results in a sustained expression of Wnt target genes and a promotion of tumorigenesis [24, 25].

Molecular Diagnostics The *APC* gene contains 15 coding exons (in addition to a noncoding exon in the 5′-untranslated region and an alternatively spliced exon 10a), encoding a protein of 2843 amino acids (Figure 16.4). Currently, more than 1000 different germline mutations have been reported worldwide. Two mutational hot spots occur at codon 1309 (c.3927_3931delAAAGA;p.Glu1309AspfsX4) or codon 1061 (c.3183_3187delACAAA;p.Gln1062fsX) at frequencies of about 10 and 7%, respectively, in patients with classic FAP [26], while most families have their private mutations. The mutations are distributed mainly over the first half of the gene, and are predicted to result in a truncated APC protein. About 10% of patients with classic FAP have large deletions encompassing one or several exons or even the entire *APC* gene. The mutation detection rate is up to 80% in patients with classic FAP, but only about 30% in patients with AFAP.

Genotype–Phenotype Correlations   A consistent correlation between the site of mutation in the *APC* gene, and the clinical course of polyposis disease or extracolonic manifestations has been repeatedly reported (Figure 16.4). Patients with *APC* mutations around codon 1309 usually have a profuse phenotype with thousands of adenomas diagnosed in the early teens or even before 10 years of age [27–29], while patients with mutations at the very 5′ end of the gene (before codon 168), in the 3′ half of the gene (beyond codon 1580), or in the alternatively spliced region of exon 9, usually develop an attenuated colorectal phenotype [30–34].

Desmoids and osteomas are observed more frequently in patients with mutations distal to codon 1444 [29, 35–37].

A strong correlation has also been observed for the presence of CHRPE. With only a few exceptions, CHRPE were diagnosed in patients with mutations between exon 9, and the middle of exon 15 (codons 413–1444) [35, 38]. This observation is in line with the overall frequency of CHRPE of about 85% in patients with classic FAP, and the fact that about 85% of patients with classic FAP have a mutation within this region (Figure 16.4).

16.2.1.5 Clinical Management

Early detection of colorectal adenomas in persons at risk results in a reduction of colorectal cancer. Based on the difference of clinical phenotypes regarding age at onset, the number and distribution of colorectal adenomas in families with classic and AFAP distinct guidelines have been developed for their surveillance and therapy.

Recently, the current recommendations for clinical management of FAP have been re-evaluated by a European panel of experts, and guidelines regarding timing, type of investigation, and surveillance intervals for persons at risk, as well as the management of colorectal and duodenal polyposis, desmoids, and other manifestations in affected persons, have been worked out (Table 16.2) [8].

Surveillance Recommendations in Persons at Risk   In families with classic FAP, endoscopic surveillance for persons at risk can start with flexible sigmoidoscopy, as adenomas will always be present in the rectum. The risk of CRC is low below the age of 15 years, therefore starting sigmoidoscopy by the age of 15 would be appropriate. However, beginning endoscopic surveillance at the age of 10 to 12 years in asymptomatic children is recommended in order to accommodate children with this procedure before puberty. This implies that predictive genetic tests, to clarify the carrier status of children at risk, is also recommended at this age. Of course, for symptomatic children (e.g. children with bowel symptoms at a younger age), predictive genetic testing and endoscopic surveillance will be performed earlier.

Table 16.2 Surveillance protocol recommended for FAP patients and persons at risk (modified from Vasen *et al.* [8]).

	Typical FAP	**Attenuated FAP**
Surveillance in persons at risk		
Predictive molecular diagnostics	Age 10–12 years	18–20 years
Type of colorectal endoscopy	Rectosigmoidoscopy	Colonoscopy
Start of endoscopy[a]	Age 10–12 years	18–20 years
Interval of endoscopies	2 years[b]	2 years[b]
Upper limit of surveillance		
• in mutation carriers	Lifelong	Lifelong
• in persons where the disease-causing mutation in the affected relatives has not been identified	50 years	60 years
Surveillance in polyposis patients		
Endoscopy of the rectum (after IRA)	At intervals of 3–6 months	
Pouchoscopy (after IPAA)	At intervals of 6–12 months	
Start of esophago-gastro-duodenoscopy	Age 25–30 years, or at time of colectomy	
Interval of EGD[c]	1–5 years	

a Surveillance is limited to persons at risk who are mutation carriers (in families in whom a mutation was identified), and is recommended for all persons at risk from families in whom the disease-causing mutation was not identified.
b Once adenomas are detected, annual colonoscopy should be performed until prophylactic colectomy is planned.
c Intervals for esophago-gastro-duodenoscopy (EGD) depend on the Spigelman stage (see text).

Mutation carriers are recommended to undergo sigmoidoscopy every 2 years. When rectal adenomas are diagnosed by this procedure, a complete colonoscopy should be performed annually until prophylactic colectomy is planned. Surveillance for mutation carriers should be performed throughout life. Persons at risk in whose families no mutation was identified should continue the endoscopies until aged 50.

Persons at risk from families with AFAP should start surveillance at age 18 to 20, as polyp growth starts later in life. Due to the preferential location of adenomas in the proximal colon, a total colonoscopy is recommended.

Surgical Procedures for Colectomy So far, surgical removal of the polyp-containing large bowel is the only safe therapeutic procedure in patients with classic FAP. The time of surgery and type of colectomy depend on polyp development and distribution. To date, there are two main surgical options, both of them sphincter-preserving: subtotal colectomy with ileorectal anastomosis (IRA), and subtotal proctocolectomy with ileal pouch-anal anastomosis (IPAA). A third option is the total proctocolectomy with a permanent end ileostomy. This procedure is applied only in exceptional cases; it is the only choice for patients with very low rectal or anal cancer.

In IRA, about 10 to 15 cm of the sigmoid are preserved. The advantage of IRA is that it is a relatively simple operation procedure with relatively low complication rates, and results in an almost normal stool frequency. The major disadvantage is that colonic epithelium in the rectal stump is still a source of polyp growth and therefore regular endoscopic examination of the sigmoid is required.

In IPAA, the complete colon and rectum is surgically removed, and a pouch formed from the terminal ileum is directly attached to the sphincter. The advantage of this procedure is a lower risk of adenoma and cancer development; however, pouchoscopies are still required since adenomas can also develop in the pouch. The major disadvantages of IPAA are a higher complication rate during surgery, in general a higher stool frequency, and a higher risk of incontinence.

Factors influencing the choice of surgery are outlined in detail by Church [39]: IRA is the method of choice when less than 20 adenomas are contained in the rectum, while IPAA is recommended when polyp growth in the rectum is more aggressive.

Should the genotype influence decision making? This question is controversially discussed in the literature. Based on the statistically strong correlation between the site of mutation and severity of polyp growth, some clinicians aim at basing the decision making on the genotype. However, there are many reports on an intrafamilial variation of the polyposis phenotype; moreover, with the exception of the two hotspot mutations, almost each family has her own mutation, and the functional relevance of a mutation depends not only on the rough localization in the gene, but also on the exact type of a mutation [40, 41]. Basing decision making on genotype would create a lot of uncertainty among clinicians and families as to timing and type of surgery.

The observation of a higher incidence of desmoids in patients with an *APC* mutation localized 3′ to codon 1444 and the fact that surgical trauma may aggravate desmoid development, led to the recommendation to postpone prophylactic colectomy in patients with such germline mutations as long as possible. As patients with mutations in the 3′ half of the *APC* gene tend to have an attenuated colorectal polyposis phenotype, this recommendation can safely be applied. However, severe desmoids may also develop in patients with mutations in the first half of the gene. For those patients usually having a typical FAP, a delay in colorectal surgery may be more difficult [39]. Therefore, usually the degree of colorectal polyposis should determine time and type of surgery, and not the genotype.

Duodenal Polyposis Duodenal and periampullary cancer constitutes, together with desmoids, the second-most common cause of death in FAP patients who are under surveillance for colonic polyposis. The risk of duodenal cancer in FAP patients is about 5% and occurs at an average age of 52 years (range 18–78). Detailed reviews of literature data regarding incidence, surveillance, and clinical management in polyposis of the upper gastrointestinal tract are published [9, 42].

Most polyps are located in the second or third parts of the duodenum, and cluster around the ampulla of Vater. Severity of duodenal polyposis is classified according to the Spigelman system into stages 0 to IV; in this system, points are allocated for number, size, histology, and degree of dysplasia [9, 43]. Approximately 10 to 20% of FAP patients have the severe stage IV of the disease, with an increased risk to develop duodenal carcinoma.

In order to control for the adenomas in the duodenum, regular esophago-gastroduodenoscopies (EGD) are recommended. A side-viewing video-endoscopy is the optimal method for surveillance of the upper gastrointestinal tract. Since duodenal carcinomas are diagnosed rarely before the age of 30, surveillance should start at 25 to 30 years (or at time of surgery). The recommended intervals for EGD depend on the severity of the disease, with a 5-year interval in Spigelman stages 0 and I, 3 years in Spigelman stage II, and 1 to 2 years in stage III, while in stage IV surgery should be considered [8].

Among the drugs used for pharmacological treatment in FAP, it has been shown that sulindac has no effect in upper gastrointestinal polyposis, while the selective Cox-II inhibitor Celecoxib at a dose of 400 mg/day over a period of 6 months produced a 31% decrease in patients who had a severe stage of duodenal polyposis at the outset.

Desmoids An actual detailed review on etiology, pathology, and treatment of FAP-associated desmoids is given by Sturt and Clark [44]. Diagnosis of desmoids should always be considered as the first differential in the case of an FAP patient presenting with an abdominal or abdominal wall mass. Desmoids can be best diagnosed by CT scanning or MRI.

The method of choice for the treatment of desmoids to date is pharmacological treatment with sulindac, in combination with tamoxifen or toremifene [44–46]. Patients not responding to this treatment are recommended to undergo chemotherapy or radiotherapy. Surgical excision of desmoids is in general not recommended as a primary treatment because most of the tumors cannot be resected and have a high recurrence rate. However, the role of surgical treatment, especially in cases of mesenteric desmoids, is controversially discussed.

Other Tumors The risk for other tumors (thyroid, hepatoblastoma, medulloblastoma) is increased in FAP patients as compared to the general population [47–49]; however, the absolute incidence of these tumors remains low. Therefore, surveillance programs to control these tumors are controversially discussed; to date it is not clear whether the possible gain in life expectancy justifies the substantial psychosocial impact resulting from an excessive surveillance program for extraintestinal tumors [8].

Pharmacological Treatment   The history and current state of chemoprevention trials in FAP has been recently reviewed by Lynch [50]. A first therapeutic effect on colorectal polyp growth was reported following treatment with the nonsteroidal anti-inflammatory drug (NSAID) sulindac [51–53]. This drug cannot replace prophylactic surgery, but it was considered helpful in postponing the time of surgery in children, and it may be applied in patients who have undergone prophylactic surgery with IRA to control polyp growth in the rectosigmoid. Sulindac has several detrimental side effects, and is not efficient in duodenal polyposis. A more specific COX II inhibitor (Celecoxib) was shown to also decrease polyp growth in the duodenum [54, 55]. However, another COX II inhibitor (Rofecoxib) was found to have cardiovascular side effects [56]. Therefore, treatment with COX II inhibitors should be confined to patients with severe duodenal polyposis.

16.2.2
MUTYH-Associated Polyposis (MAP)

The presence of an autosomal-recessively inherited adenomatous polyposis syndrome was first reported in 2002. Al-Tassan *et al.* [57] described a family with three affected sibs who exhibited biallelic *MUTYH* mutations.

16.2.2.1   Clinical Features
Clinically, MAP, OMIM #608 456 is comparable to *APC*-associated AFAP. Extraintestinal manifestations are rare in this disorder. Due to the autosomal-recessive mode of inheritance, MAP usually occurs in isolated patients or in sibships having healthy parents. MAP has been diagnosed in 15 to 20% of patients with the AFAP phenotype.

16.2.2.2   Genetics
MAP is caused by biallelic germline mutations in *MUTYH*, a gene encoding a protein involved in base excision repair (BER). MUTYH is responsible for the excision of adenosine mismatched with 8-oxo-7,8-dihydroxy-2′-deoxyguanosine (8-oxoG), the most stable product of DNA damage caused by reactive oxygen species. Biallelic mutations in this highly conserved protein result in an increase in 8-oxoG–induced somatic $G:C > T:A$ transversions in other genes, including *APC* [58, 59].

   MUTYH is located on chromosome 1p35, and consists of 16 exons. In Caucasians, the two missense mutations *Y176C* and *G393D* (formerly referred to as *Y165C* and *G382D*) are found in a homozygous or compound-heterozygous state in about 70% of MAP patients [60–64].

16.2.2.3   Clinical Management
The surveillance program and therapeutic interventions are the same as in *APC*-mediated AFAP. However, the autosomal-recessive mode of inheritance implies a different risk for sibs and children of a patient to inherit the disease. Sibs of a patient may have a risk of 25% to develop the disease. Parents and children are

obligatory heterozygous. Tumor risk in heterozygotes is still not well evaluated. Farrington *et al.* [65] report an increase of tumor risk of 1.68 as compared to the general population. To date, it is not clear whether this low tumor risk justifies a regular surveillance program.

16.3
Hamartomatous Polyposis Syndromes

While adenomatous polyps are considered as neoplastic tissues with a high tendency to transform to cancer, hamartomatous polyps have a lower tendency to become cancerous. Nevertheless, neoplasia may develop inside the hamartomas, and a hamartoma–carcinoma sequence is also discussed [66, 67].

16.3.1
Peutz–Jeghers Syndrome (PJS)

16.3.1.1 Clinical Diagnosis

PJS (OMIM #175 200) is characterized by the occurrence of gastrointestinal polyposis, mucocutaneous pigmentation, and an increased risk of cancer of the gastrointestinal tract and at other sites (reviewed in [68, 69]). According to the clinical criteria for PJS, as defined by Tomlinson and Houlston [69], a definite diagnosis of PJS can be made if a person fulfils the following criteria:

- two or more characteristic PJS polyps in the gastrointestinal tract; or
- one PJS polyp in the gastrointestinal tract, together with either a characteristic PJS pigmentation or a family history of PJS.

The diagnosis of PJS can be assumed in individuals with a positive family history and florid, typical freckling.

Histopathology of gastrointestinal polyps is essential for the clinical diagnosis of PJS. The PJS polyps are characterized by the presence of smooth muscle bundles with a characteristic branching tree appearance (Figure 16.1). Polyps develop preferentially in the jejunum and ileum, but they can also occur elsewhere in the gastrointestinal tract, including the stomach and large bowel. Some PJS patients are diagnosed in the first decade of life as surgical emergencies, with attacks of pain or even intestinal obstruction, due to intussusception of the small bowel. Other symptoms may be bleeding with secondary anemia.

Mucocutaneous pigmentation presents as florid freckling of lips, buccal mucosa, vulva, fingers, and toes. It is rarely present at birth, but may develop during the first decade of life, frequently prior to the appearance of polyps. Pigmentation usually fades from the third decade onwards. It should be noted that some PJS patients never present the characteristic pigmentation, while some individuals have multiple dark lentigines as a normal variant [69].

Another characteristic feature of PJS is the occurrence of sex cord tumors with annular tubules (SCTAT) in females, a benign neoplasm of the ovaries. Males occasionally develop calcifying Sertoli cell tumors of the testes, which secrete estrogen and can lead to gynecomastia.

There are only rough estimates for the prevalence at birth, ranging from 1 : 25 000 to 1 : 280 000; however, these figures have not been epidemiologically assessed [68].

16.3.1.2 Genetics

Molecular Genetic Background PJS is an autosomal-dominant disorder. About 10 to 20% of PJS cases are apparently sporadic.

PJS is caused by germline mutations in the serin-threonin-kinase gene *STK11* (alias *LKB1*), localized on chromosomal region 19p13.3 [70, 71]. The *STK11* gene is essential for cell viability. The function has been linked with the control of the cellular energy balance, polarity, cell cycle, and proliferation [72, 73].

The formation of hamartomas may be caused by a dysregulation of the *mTOR* (mammalian target of rapamycin) pathway, a regulator of cell growth. *STK11* suppresses *mTOR* via several mediators. Mutant *STK11* fails to suppress *mTOR*, leading to a lapse of cell growth [73].

Molecular Diagnostics The *STK11* gene consists of 9 coding exons. A germline mutation was detected in about 90% of patients meeting the clinical criteria of PJS. Of them, two-thirds are point mutations distributed over the entire gene, except exon 9; one-third of the identified mutations are large deletions, most of them encompassing the entire gene, or the promoter region and exon 1 [74].

Evidence for a second PJS locus on chromosomal region 19q13.4 was suggested by results of linkage analysis in a PJS family [75]. However, the high detection rate of *STK11* mutations in PJS patients strongly questions the existence of a notable locus heterogeneity.

16.3.1.3 Tumor Risk

PJS patients have an increased risk of developing tumors at different sites. First studies estimated an about a 15-fold increased overall tumor risk [76], whereas a recent large collaborative study in Western Europe revealed lower relative risk figures [77]. In this study, the risk among PJS patients for developing any first cancer by age 70 years was 85%, while the risk for all cancers in the general population by age 70 years is approximately 18%; thus, the risk in PJS patients is increased about four-fold. However, when age-adjusted risk figures were considered, a considerably higher tumor risk at younger ages becomes evident (Table 16.3).

Among gastrointestinal tumors, CRC is the most frequent. The relative risk for pancreatic cancer is largely increased; however, the absolute risk is much lower than for other cancers in PJS. Among the extra-intestinal cancers, breast cancer represents the major risk in females, approaching the risk associated with mutations in *BRCA1* and *BRCA2* [77].

No correlation between the site of mutation or type of mutation (missense vs. chain-terminating mutations), and the clinical manifestation in PJS was found in

Table 16.3 Cumulative site-specific cancer risk by age in PJS patients (data from Headle *et al.*, 2006 [77], modified).

Type of cancer	Cancer risk by age (%)					
	20 y	30 y	40 y	50 y	60 y	70 y
All cancers	2 (0.3)[a]	5 (0.6)	17 (1.4)	31 (3.4)	60 (8.2)	85 (17.7)
Gastrointestinal[b]	– (<0.1)	1 (<0.1)	9 (0.1)	15 (0.3)	33 (1.3)	57 (3.9)
Breast (females)	– (<0.1)	– (<0.1)	8 (0.5)	13 (1.8)	31 (4.3)	45 (7.0)
Gynecologic[c]	– (<0.1)	1 (0.1)	3 (0.4)	8 (0.7)	18 (1.3)	18 (2.1)
Pancreas	– (<0.1)	– (<0.1)	3 (<0.1)	5 (<1.0)	7 (0.2)	11 (0.5)
Lung (male)	– (<0.1)	– (<0.1)	1 (<0.1)	4 (0.2)	13 (1.3)	17 (4.7)
(female)	(<0.1)	(<0.1)	(<0.1)	(0.1)	– (0.6)	– (2.0)

a The numbers in parantheses represent the frequencies of tumors in the general population.
b Gastroesophagal, small bowel, pancreatic, and colorectal cancers.
c Uterine, ovarian, and cervical cancers.

a large European collaborative study; moreover, no phenotypic difference between mutation-positive and mutation-negative patients was observed [77].

16.3.1.4 Clinical Management

The main problem during early childhood may be acute ileus due to intussusception in the vicinity of the polyps. This complication needs surgical removal of the part of the bowel carrying the polyps. Routine endoscopy and intra-operative enteroscopy with polypectomy is recommended in order to decrease the frequency of emergency laparotomy and bowel loss due to intussusception. As polyps preferentially develop in the small bowel, capsule or double-balloon endoscopy (every 2–3 years) is recommended. Polyps larger than 1.5 cm should be removed surgically, while sparing as much of the ileum as possible.

For female patients, the surveillance program recommended to *BRCA1/BRCA2* mutation carriers should be offered.

16.3.2
Juvenile Polyposis Syndrome (JPS)

16.3.2.1 Clinical Diagnosis

Isolated juvenile polyps are the most frequent bowel polyps in childhood and do not require special treatment. The diagnosis of familial juvenile polyposis (OMIM #174900) is clinically established when the following criteria are met [78]:

- at least five juvenile gastrointestinal polyps in a patient; or
- at least one typical juvenile polyp in the presence of a family history of JPS.

A detailed overview on JPS is given by Haidle and Howe [79]. The term juvenile polyposis does not refer to the young age of the patients, but rather reflects the presence of polyps with histology that is characteristic for juvenile polyps (Figure 16.1). Juvenile polyps vary in size, shape, and number. They may present as sessile or pedunculated, with a smooth or inflammatory eroded surface. Histology reveals cystic dilated crypts and proliferating filamentous stroma. Some patients may have only four to five juvenile polyps during their life, while other members of the same families may have more than a hundred polyps. Juvenile polyps are preferentially diagnosed in the distal large bowel. Some patients develop a severe gastric polyposis, with a tendency to transform to gastric cancer [80, 81]. Patients are frequently diagnosed due to chronic gastrointestinal bleeding associated with anemia.

The incidence of JPS at birth ranges between 1:16000 to 1:100000 and may account for about 10% of all gastrointestinal polyposis cases [79].

16.3.2.2 Genetics

Molecular Genetic Background Germline mutations in the genes *SMAD4* and *BMPR1A* (bone morphogenetic protein receptor, Type 1A) have been identified in JPS patients [82, 83]. Concerning nomenclature, *SMAD* is merged from the denomination of related genes in *C. elegans* (*Sma* genes), and *D. melanogaster* (*mad*, for "mothers against decapentaplegic"). The genes are implicated in signal transduction by members of the TGF-β family in these two organisms and also in vertebrates. Given that the human gene designated *DPC4* (deleted in pancreatic carcinoma, locus 4, on chromosome 18q) is highly similar to the *mad*- and *sma-2*, *-3*, and *-4* genes [84], *DPC4* was later termed *SMAD4*.

The proteins encoded by *SMAD4* and *BMPR1A* participate in the transforming growth factor-β (TGF-β)/SMAD signaling pathway. *SMAD* pathway target genes are involved in development, cell differentiation, and regulation of the cell cycle. TGF-β is the prototype of about 30 extra cellular ligands that form the TGF-β superfamily. Here, *SMAD4* plays an important role as a critical signal transducer that translocates all activated *SMADs* to the nucleus to activate target genes directly or indirectly [85]. BMPR1A is a ligand-specific receptor of the TGF-β/BMP signaling pathway. Its intracellular mediation is conducted by *SMADs* [86].

In JPS, mutant *SMAD4* or *BMPR1A* disequilibrate the control cycle, trigger polyposis, and consequently result in tumorigenesis.

Molecular Diagnostics About 20% of JPS patients have a germline point mutation in the *SMAD4* gene (other symbols: *MADH4, DPC4*). Another 20% have a germline mutation in the *BMPR1A* gene. Recently, large genomic deletions mainly in *SMAD4* (and to a lesser extent in *BMPR1A*) were detected in about 10% of patients meeting the clinical criteria of JPS [81]. It is likely that at least one other gene may be involved in the etiology of JPS.

Genotype-Phenotype Correlations The first observation of an over-representation of gastric polyposis in patients with *SMAD4* germline mutations as compared to *BMPR1A* mutation carriers [87] has been confirmed in additional investigations

[81, 88]. Moreover, some patients with *SMAD4* mutations may exhibit traits of hemorrhagic telangiectasia [81, 89].

16.3.2.3 Tumor Risk

JPS patients have an increased tumor risk that is confined mainly to the gastrointestinal tract. A recent study revealed a 34-fold increased risk of CRC, and a cumulative life-time risk of CRC of 38.7%. The mean age at diagnosis of CRC was 44 years [90]. In some studies, an increased risk of other gastrointestinal cancers, including stomach, small bowel, and pancreatic cancers has been reported [80, 81, 91, 92].

16.3.2.4 Clinical Management

Early clinical diagnostic surveillance and therapy is needed to prevent cancer development. Clear and appropriate recommendations for surveillance in JPS are reviewed by Zbuk and Eng [67]. Affected individuals should be endoscopically investigated when bowel symptoms such as rectal bleeding, anemia, abdominal pain, constipation, diarrhoea, or other changes in stool characteristics are observed. Complete blood count, colonoscopy, and upper endoscopy should be performed starting at the age of 15 years. When no polyps are observed, screening should be repeated at intervals of 3 years. If only a few polyps are detected, they should be removed, and screening should be performed annually until no additional polyps are observed; then 3-yearly intervals can resume. An excessive polyp burden may require colectomy or gastrectomy.

16.3.3
PTEN Hamartoma Tumor Syndrome (PHTS)

By definition, the PTEN hamartoma tumor syndrome (PHTS, OMIM #601728) is characterized by hamartomatous tumors at different sites and a germline mutation in the *PTEN* gene. It includes Cowden syndrome (CS), Bannayan–Riley–Ruvalcaba syndrome (BRRS), Proteus syndrome (PS), and Proteus-like syndrome. Of these, gastrointestinal polyps are found in CS and BRRS.

16.3.3.1 Clinical Diagnosis

CS is a multiple hamartomatous syndrome with a high risk of benign and malignant tumors of the thyroid (non-medullary), breast, and endometrium. Operational diagnostic criteria are published by Eng [93, 94]. Patients usually have macrocephaly and mucocutaneous lesions (facial trichilemmomas, acral keratoses, and papillomatous papules). Intestinal hamartomatous polyposis is a minor feature of CS.

The diagnosis of BRRS is based on the presence of macrocephaly, hamartomatous intestinal polyposis (in 45% of cases), lipomas and, in males, a speckled penis.

Unlike polyps in adenomatous or juvenile polyposis, the hamartomatous gastrointestinal polyps in CS are usually tiny and cause few symptoms. In BRRS, gastrointestinal hamartomatous polyps may occasionally cause intussusception or rectal bleeding. Both in CS and BRRS, the polyps seem not to increase the risk of CRC.

16.3.3.2 Genetics

PHTS is caused by germline mutations of *PTEN* (phosphatase and tensin homolog, deleted on chromosome 10). PTEN is a dual-specificity phosphatase within the protein-tyrosine-phosphatase superfamily. It counteracts the phosphatidylinositol 3-kinase (PI3K)/protein kinase B [PKB or Akt-Kinase (AKT)] pathway, which plays a role in nearly all aspects of tumor biology: cell transformation, growth, proliferation, migration, protection from apoptosis, genomic instability, angiogenesis, and metastasis. Activated PI3K induces PKB and stimulates subsequent signaling via downstream effectors.

PTEN, as an antagonist of this pathway, leads to a down-regulation of PKB activation. Thus, mutant PTEN fails to regulate cell homeostasis, ultimately causing tumorigenesis [95]. Besides, PTEN also interacts with other pathways (e.g. integrin signaling pathway, mitogen-activated kinase pathway, mTOR pathway) which, when malfunctioning, for example, due to mutant PTEN, may contribute to the tumorigenesis.

A germline mutation in the *PTEN* gene is detected in approximately 80% of patients with the clinical diagnosis of CS and in 60% of patients with BRRS [94, 96, 97].

16.3.3.3 Cancer Risk and Clinical Management

Patients with CS have a life-time risk of 50% of developing breast cancer, and a 5 to 10% risk of developing endometrial cancer. Moreover, about 10% of patients develop follicular thyroid cancer. Renal cell carcinoma and malignant melanoma may be minor components of neoplasia in CS. Currently it is not definitely evaluated whether patients with CS have an increased risk of developing CRC [67, 93].

Patients with *PTEN* mutations should follow the surveillance recommendations that are governed by the tumors mentioned above, especially breast cancer, endometrial cancer, and non-medullary thyroid cancer [67, 93].

References

1 Bülow, S., Berk, T. and Neale, K. (2006) The history of familial adenomatous polyposis. *Familial Cancer*, **5** (*3*), 213–20.

2 Bisgaard, M.L., Fenger, K., Bulow, S., Niebuhr, E. and Mohr, J. (1994) Familial adenomatous polyposis (FAP): frequency, penetrance, and mutation rate. *Human Mutation*, **3** (*2*), 121–5.

3 Aretz, S., Uhlhaas, S., Caspari, R., Mangold, E., Pagenstecher, C., Propping, P. *et al.* (2004) Frequency and parental origin of *de novo* APC mutations in familial adenomatous polyposis. *European Journal of Human Genetics*, **12** (*1*), 52–8.

4 Ripa, R., Bisgaard, M.L., Bulow, S. and Nielsen, F.C. (2002) *De novo* mutations in familial adenomatous polyposis (FAP). *European Journal of Human Genetics*, **10** (*10*), 631–7.

5 Aretz, S., Stienen, D., Friedrichs, N., Stemmler, S., Uhlhaas, S., Rahner, N. *et al.* (2007) Somatic APC mosaicism: a frequent cause of familial adenomatous polyposis (FAP). *Human Mutation*, **28** (*10*), 985–92.

6 Bülow, S. (1986) Clinical features in familial polyposis coli. Results of the Danish Polyposis Register. *Diseases of the Colon and Rectum*, **29** (*2*), 102–7.

7 Solomon, C. and Burt, R. (2005) APC-Associated Polyposis Conditions. www. genetests.org.

8 Vasen, H.F., Möslein, G., Alonso, A., Aretz, S., Bernstein, I., Bertario, L. *et al.* (2008) Guidelines for the clinical management of familial adenomatous polyposis (FAP). *Gut*, **57** (*5*), 704–13.

9 Gallagher, M.C., Phillips, R.K. and Bulow, S. (2006) Surveillance and management of upper gastrointestinal disease in Familial Adenomatous Polyposis. *Familial Cancer*, **5** (*3*), 263–73.

10 Traboulsi, E.I., Maumenee, I.H., Krush, A.J., Giardiello, F.M., Levin, L.S. and Hamilton, S.R. (1988) Pigmented ocular fundus lesions in the inherited gastrointestinal polyposis syndromes and in hereditary nonpolyposis colorectal cancer. *Ophthalmology*, **95** (*7*), 964–9.

11 Leppert, M., Burt, R., Hughes, J.P., Samowitz, W., Nakamura, Y., Woodward, S. *et al.* (1990) Genetic analysis of an inherited predisposition to colon cancer in a family with a variable number of adenomatous polyps. *The New England Journal of Medicine*, **322** (*13*), 904–8.

12 Lynch, H.T., Smyrk, T.C., Watson, P., Lanspa, S.J., Lynch, P.M., Jenkins, J.X. *et al.* (1992) Hereditary flat adenoma syndrome: a variant of familial adenomatous polyposis?. *Diseases of the Colon and Rectum*, **35** (*5*), 411–21.

13 Knudsen, A.L., Bisgaard, M.L. and Bulow, S. (2003) Attenuated familial adenomatous polyposis (AFAP). A review of the literature. *Familial Cancer*, **2** (*1*), 43–55.

14 Burt, R.W., Leppert, M.F., Slattery, M.L., Samowitz, W.S., Spirio, L.N., Kerber, R.A. *et al.* (2004) Genetic testing and

phenotype in a large kindred with attenuated familial adenomatous polyposis. *Gastroenterology*, **127** (*2*), 444–51.

15 Gardner, E.J. and Richards, R.C. (1953) Multiple cutaneous and subcutaneous lesions occurring simultaneously with hereditary polyposis and osteomatosis. *American Journal of Human Genetics*, **5** (*2*), 139–47.

16 Bülow, S. (1989) Familial adenomatous polyposis. *Annals of Medicine*, **21** (*4*), 299–307.

17 Turcot, J., Despres, J.P. and St Pierre, F. (1959) Malignant tumors of the central nervous system associated with familial polyposis of the colon: report of two cases. *Diseases of the Colon and Rectum*, **2**, 465–8.

18 Hamilton, S.R., Liu, B., Parsons, R.E., Papadopoulos, N., Jen, J., Powell, S.M. *et al.* (1995) The molecular basis of Turcot's syndrome. *The New England Journal of Medicine*, **332** (*13*), 839–47.

19 Herrera, L., Kakati, S., Gibas, L., Pietrzak, E. and Sandberg, A.A. (1986) Gardner syndrome in a man with an interstitial deletion of 5q. *American Journal of Medical Genetics*, **25** (*3*), 473–6.

20 Bodmer, W.F., Bailey, C.J., Bodmer, J., Bussey, H.J., Ellis, A., Gorman, P. *et al.* (1987) Localization of the gene for familial adenomatous polyposis on chromosome 5. *Nature*, **328** (*6131*), 614–16.

21 Leppert, M., Dobbs, M., Scambler, P., O'Connell, P., Nakamura, Y., Stauffer, D. *et al.* (1987) The gene for familial polyposis coli maps to the long arm of chromosome 5. *Science*, **238** (*4832*), 1411–13.

22 Groden, J., Thliveris, A., Samowitz, W., Carlson, M., Gelbert, L., Albertsen, H. *et al.* (1991) Identification and characterization of the familial adenomatous polyposis coli gene. *Cell*, **66** (*3*), 589–600.

23 Kinzler, K.W., Nilbert, M.C., Su, L.K., Vogelstein, B., Bryan, T.M., Levy, D.B. *et al.* (1991) Identification of FAP locus genes from chromosome 5q21. *Science*, **253** (*5020*), 661–5.

24 Willert, K. and Jones, K.A.R. (2006) Wnt signaling: is the party in the nucleus? *Genes and Development*, **20** (*11*), 1394–404.

25 Gregorieff, A. and Clevers, H. (2005) Wnt signaling in the intestinal epithelium:

from endoderm to cancer. *Genes and Development*, **19** (*8*), 877–90.

26 Friedl, W. and Aretz, S. (2005) Familial adenomatous polyposis–experience from a study on 1164 German unrelated polyposis patients. *Hereditary Cancer*, **3** (*3*), 95–114.

27 Nagase, H., Miyoshi, Y., Horii, A., Aoki, T., Ogawa, M., Utsunomiya, J. *et al.* (1992) Correlation between the location of germline mutations in the APC gene and the number of colorectal polyps in familial adenomatous polyposis patients. *Cancer Research*, **52** (*14*), 4055–7.

28 Caspari, R., Friedl, W., Mandl, M., Moslein, G., Kadmon, M., Knapp, M. *et al.* (1994) Familial adenomatous polyposis: mutation at codon 1309 and early onset of colon cancer. *Lancet*, **343** (*8898*), 629–32.

29 Davies, D.R., Armstrong, J.G., Thakker, N., Horner, K., Guy, S.P., Clancy, T. *et al.* (1995) Severe Gardner syndrome in families with mutations restricted to a specific region of the APC gene. *American Journal of Human Genetics*, **57**, 1151–8.

30 Heppner Goss, K., Trzepacz, C., Tuohy, T.M. and Groden, J. (2002) Attenuated APC alleles produce functional protein from internal translation initiation. *Proceedings of the National Academy of Sciences of the United States of America*, **99** (*12*), 8161–6.

31 Friedl, W., Meuschel, S., Caspari, R., Lamberti, C., Krieger, S., Sengteller, M. *et al.* (1996) Attenuated familial adenomatous polyposis due to a mutation in the 3' part of the APC gene. A clue for understanding the function of the APC protein. *Human Genetics*, **97** (*5*), 579–84.

32 Soravia, C., Berk, T., Madlensky, L., Mitri, A., Cheng, H., Gallinger, S. *et al.* (1998) Genotype-phenotype correlations in attenuated adenomatous polyposis coli. *American Journal of Human Genetics*, **62** (*6*), 1290–301.

33 van der Luijt, R.B., Meera Khan, P., Vasen, H.F., Breukel, C., Tops, C.M., Scott, R.J. *et al.* (1996) Germline mutations in the 3' part of APC exon 15 do not result in truncated proteins and are associated with attenuated adeno-

matous polyposis coli. *Human Genetics*, **98** (*6*), 727–34.

34 van der Luijt, R.B., Vasen, H.F., Tops, C.M., Breukel, C., Fodde, R. and Meera Khan, P. (1995) APC mutation in the alternatively spliced region of exon 9 associated with late onset familial adenomatous polyposis. *Human Genetics*, **96** (*6*), 705–10.

35 Caspari, R., Olschwang, S., Friedl, W., Mandl, M., Boisson, C., Boker, T. *et al.* (1995) Familial adenomatous polyposis: desmoid tumours and lack of ophthalmic lesions (CHRPE) associated with APC mutations beyond codon 1444. *Human Molecular Genetics*, **4** (*3*), 337–40.

36 Scott, R.J., Froggatt, N.J., Trembath, R.C., Evans, D.G., Hodgson, S.V. and E.R.M. (1996) Familial infiltrative fibromatosis (desmoid tumours) (MIM135290) caused by a recurrent 3' APC gene mutation. *Human Molecular Genetics*, **5**, 1921–4.

37 Eccles, D.M., van der Luijt, R., Breukel, C., Bullman, H., Bunyan, D., Fisher, A. *et al.* (1996) Hereditary desmoid disease due to a frameshift mutation at codon 1924 of the APC gene. *American Journal of Human Genetics*, **59**, 1193–201.

38 Olschwang, S., Tiret, A., Laurent-Puig, P., Muleris, M., Parc, R. and Thomas, G. (1993) Restriction of ocular fundus lesions to a specific subgroup of APC mutations in adenomatous polyposis coli patients. *Cell*, **75** (*5*), 959–68.

39 Church, J. (2006) In which patients do I perform IRA, and why?. *Familial Cancer*, **5** (*3*), 237–40; discussion 262-2.

40 Aretz, S., Uhlhaas, S., Sun, Y., Pagenstecher, C., Mangold, E., Caspari, R. *et al.* (2004) Familial adenomatous polyposis: aberrant splicing due to missense or silent mutations in the APC gene. *Human Mutation*, **24** (*5*), 370–80.

41 Friedl, W., Caspari, R., Sengteller, M., Uhlhaas, S., Lamberti, C., Jungck, M. *et al.* (2001) Can APC mutation analysis contribute to therapeutic decisions in familial adenomatous polyposis? Experience from 680 FAP families. *Gut*, **48** (*4*), 515–21.

42 Kadmon, M., Tandara, A. and Herfarth, C. (2001) Duodenal adenomatosis in familial adenomatous polyposis coli. A review of the literature and results from the

Heidelberg Polyposis Register. *International Journal of Colorectal Disease,* **16** (*2*), 63–75.

43 Spigelman, A.D., Williams, C.B., Talbot, I.C., Domizio, P. and Phillips, R.K. (1989) Upper gastrointestinal cancer in patients with familial adenomatous polyposis. *Lancet,* **2** (*8666*), 783–5.

44 Sturt, N.J. and Clark, S.K. (2006) Current ideas in desmoid tumours. *Familial Cancer,* **5** (*3*), 275–85.discussion 287–8.

45 Hansmann, A., Adolph, C., Vogel, T., Unger, A. and Moeslein, G. (2004) High-dose tamoxifen and sulindac as first-line treatment for desmoid tumors. *Cancer,* **100** (*3*), 612–20.

46 Moeslein, G. (2006) Invited commentary. *Familial Cancer,* **5**, 287–8.

47 Cetta, F., Toti, P., Petracci, M., Montalto, G., Disanto, A., Lore, F. *et al.* (1997) Thyroid carcinoma associated with familial adenomatous polyposis. *Histopathology,* **31** (*3*), 231–6.

48 Cetta, F., Montalto, G., Gori, M., Curia, M.C., Cama, A. and Olschwang, S. (2000) Germline mutations of the APC gene in patients with familial adenomatous polyposis-associated thyroid carcinoma: results from a European cooperative study. *The Journal of Clinical Endocrinology and Metabolism,* **85** (*1*), 286–92.

49 Aretz, S., Koch, A., Uhlhaas, S., Friedl, W., Propping, P., von Schweinitz, D. *et al.* (2006) Should children at risk for familial adenomatous polyposis be screened for hepatoblastoma and children with apparently sporadic hepatoblastoma be screened for APC germline mutations? *Pediatric Blood and Cancer,* **47** (*6*), 811–18.

50 Lynch, P.M. (2008) Chemoprevention with special reference to inherited colorectal cancer. *Familial Cancer,* **7** (*1*), 59–64.

51 Waddell, W.R. and Loughry, R.W. (1983) Sulindac for polyposis of the colon. *Journal of Surgical Oncology,* **24** (*1*), 83–7.

52 Winde, G., Gumbinger, H.G., Osswald, H., Kemper, F. and Bunte, H. (1993) The NSAID sulindac reverses rectal adenomas in colectomized patients with familial adenomatous polyposis: clinical results of a dose-finding study on rectal sulindac administration. *International Journal of Colorectal Disease,* **8** (*1*), 13–17.

53 Giardiello, F.M., Hamilton, S.R., Krush, A.J., Piantadosi, S., Hylind, L.M., Celano, P. *et al.* (1993) Treatment of colonic and rectal adenomas with sulindac in familial adenomatous polyposis. *The New England Journal of Medicine,* **328** (*18*), 1313–16.

54 Steinbach, G., Lynch, P.M., Phillips, R.K., Wallace, M.H., Hawk, E., Gordon, G.B. *et al.* (2000) The effect of celecoxib, a cyclooxygenase-2 inhibitor, in familial adenomatous polyposis. *The New England Journal of Medicine,* **342** (*26*), 1946–52.

55 Phillips, R.K., Wallace, M.H., Lynch, P.M., Hawk, E., Gordon, G.B., Saunders, B.P. *et al.* (2002) A randomised, double blind, placebo controlled study of celecoxib, a selective cyclooxygenase 2 inhibitor, on duodenal polyposis in familial adenomatous polyposis. *Gut,* **50** (*6*), 857–60.

56 Topol, E.J. (2004) Failing the public health – rofecoxib, Merck, and the FDA. *The New England Journal of Medicine,* **351** (*17*), 1707–9.

57 Al-Tassan, N., Chmiel, N.H., Maynard, J., Fleming, N., Livingston, A.L., Williams, G.T. *et al.* (2002) Inherited variants of MYH associated with somatic G:C– > T:A mutations in colorectal tumors. *Nature Genetics,* **30** (*2*), 227–32.

58 Jones, S., Emmerson, P., Maynard, J., Best, J.M., Jordan, S., Williams, G.T. *et al.* (2002) Biallelic germline mutations in MYH predispose to multiple colorectal adenoma and somatic G:C– > T:A mutations. *Human Molecular Genetics,* **11** (*23*), 2961–7.

59 Sampson, J.R., Dolwani, S., Jones, S., Eccles, D., Ellis, A., Evans, D.G. *et al.* (2003) Autosomal recessive colorectal adenomatous polyposis due to inherited mutations of MYH. *Lancet,* **362** (*9377*), 39–41.

60 Fleischmann, C., Peto, J., Cheadle, J., Shah, B., Sampson, J. and Houlston, R.S. (2004) Comprehensive analysis of the contribution of germline MYH variation to early-onset colorectal cancer. *International Journal of Cancer,* **109** (*4*), 554–8.

61 Gismondi, V., Meta, M., Bonelli, L., Radice, P., Sala, P., Bertario, L. *et al.* (2004) Prevalence of the Y165C, G382D and

1395delGGA germline mutations of the MYH gene in Italian patients with adenomatous polyposis coli and colorectal adenomas. *International Journal of Cancer*, **109** (*5*), 680–4.

62 Wang, L., Baudhuin, L.M., Boardman, L.A., Steenblock, K.J., Petersen, G.M., Halling, K.C. *et al.* (2004) MYH mutations in patients with attenuated and classic polyposis and with young-onset colorectal cancer without polyps. *Gastroenterology*, **127** (*1*), 9–16.

63 Aretz, S., Uhlhaas, S., Goergens, H., Siberg, K., Vogel, M., Pagenstecher, C. *et al.* (2006) MUTYH-associated polyposis: 70 of 71 patients with biallelic mutations present with an attenuated or atypical phenotype. *International Journal of Cancer*, **119**, 807–14.

64 Sieber, O.M., Lipton, L., Crabtree, M., Heinimann, K., Fidalgo, P., Phillips, R.K. *et al.* (2003) Multiple colorectal adenomas, classic adenomatous polyposis, and germline mutations in MYH. *The New England Journal of Medicine*, **348** (*9*), 791–9.

65 Farrington, S.M., Tenesa, A., Barnetson, R., Wiltshire, A., Prendergast, J., Porteous, M. *et al.* (2005) Germline susceptibility to colorectal cancer due to base-excision repair gene defects. *American Journal of Human Genetics*, **77** (*1*), 112–19.

66 Wang, Z.J., Ellis, I., Zauber, P., Iwama, T., Marchese, C., Talbot, I. *et al.* (1999) Allelic imbalance at the LKB1 (STK11) locus in tumours from patients with Peutz–Jeghers' syndrome provides evidence for a hamartoma-(adenoma)-carcinoma sequence. *The Journal of Pathology*, **188** (*1*), 9–13.

67 Zbuk, K.M. and Eng, C. (2007) Hamartomatous polyposis syndromes. *Nat. Clin. Pract. Gastroenterol. Hepatol.*, **4** (*9*), 492–502.

68 Amos, C., Frazier, M. and McGarrity, T. (2007) Peutz–Jeghers Syndrome. www.genetests.org

69 Tomlinson, I.P. and Houlston, R.S. (1997) Peutz–Jeghers syndrome. *Journal of Medical Genetics*, **34** (*12*), 1007–11.

70 Hemminki, A., Markie, D., Tomlinson, I., Avizienyte, E., Roth, S., Loukola, A. *et al.* (1998) A serine/threonine kinase gene defective in Peutz–Jeghers syndrome. *Nature*, **391** (*6663*), 184–7.

71 Jenne, D.E., Reimann, H., Nezu, J., Friedel, W., Loff, S., Jeschke, R. *et al.* (1998) Peutz–Jeghers syndrome is caused by mutations in a novel serine threonine kinase. *Nature Genetics*, **18** (*1*), 38–43.

72 Forcet, C., Etienne-Manneville, S., Gaude, H., Fournier, L., Debilly, S., Salmi, M. *et al.* (2005) Functional analysis of Peutz–Jeghers mutations reveals that the LKB1 C-terminal region exerts a crucial role in regulating both the AMPK pathway and the cell polarity. *Human Molecular Genetics*, **14** (*10*), 1283–92.

73 Katajisto, P., Vallenius, T., Vaahtomeri, K., Ekman, N., Udd, L., Tiainen, M. *et al.* (2007) The LKB1 tumor suppressor kinase in human disease. *Biochimica et Biophysica Acta*, **1775** (*1*), 63–75.

74 Aretz, S., Stienen, D., Uhlhaas, S., Loff, S., Back, W., Pagenstecher, C. *et al.* (2005) High proportion of large genomic STK11 deletions in Peutz–Jeghers syndrome. *Human Mutation*, **26** (*6*), 513–19.

75 Mehenni, H., Gehrig, C., Nezu, J., Oku, A., Shimane, M., Rossier, C. *et al.* (1998) Loss of LKB1 kinase activity in Peutz–Jeghers syndrome, and evidence for allelic and locus heterogeneity. *American Journal of Human Genetics*, **63** (*6*), 1641–50.

76 Giardiello, F.M., Brensinger, J.D., Tersmette, A.C., Goodman, S.N., Petersen, G.M., Booker, S.V. *et al.* (2000) Very high risk of cancer in familial Peutz–Jeghers syndrome. *Gastroenterology*, **119** (*6*), 1447–53.

77 Hearle, N., Schumacher, V., Menko, F.H., Olschwang, S., Boardman, L.A., Gille, J.J. *et al.* (2006) Frequency and spectrum of cancers in the Peutz–Jeghers syndrome. *Clinical Cancer Research*, **12** (*10*), 3209–15.

78 Jass, J.R., Williams, C.B., Bussey, H.J. and Morson, B.C. (1988) Juvenile polyposis – a precancerous condition. *Histopathology*, **13** (*6*), 619–30.

79 Haidle, J.L. and Howe, J.R. (2007) Juvenile Polyposis Syndrome. www.genetests.org/

80 Hofting, I., Pott, G., Schrameyer, B. and Stolte, M. (1993) [Familial juvenile polyposis with predominant stomach involvement]. *Zeitschrift für Gastroenterologie*, **31** (*9*), 480–3.

81 Aretz, S., Stienen, D., Uhlhaas, S., Stolte, M., Entius, M.M., Loff, S. *et al.* (2007) High proportion of large genomic deletions and genotype-phenotype update in 80 unrelated families with Juvenile Polyposis Syndrome. *Journal of Medical Genetics*, **44** (*11*), 702–9.

82 Howe, J.R., Roth, S., Ringold, J.C., Summers, R.W., Jarvinen, H.J., Sistonen, P. *et al.* (1998) Mutations in the SMAD4/DPC4 gene in juvenile polyposis. *Science*, **280** (*5366*), 1086–8.

83 Howe, J.R., Bair, J.L., Sayed, M.G., Anderson, M.E., Mitros, F.A., Petersen, G.M. *et al.* (2001) Germline mutations of the gene encoding bone morphogenetic protein receptor 1A in juvenile polyposis. *Nature Genetics*, **28** (*2*), 184–7.

84 Hahn, S.A., Schutte, M., Hoque, A.T., Moskaluk, C.A., da Costa, L.T., Rozenblum, E. *et al.* (1996) DPC4, a candidate tumor suppressor gene at human chromosome 18q21.1. *Science*, **271** (*5247*), 350–3.

85 Javelaud, D. and Mauviel, A. (2005) Crosstalk mechanisms between the mitogen-activated protein kinase pathways and *Smad* signaling down-stream of TGF-beta: implications for carcinogenesis. *Oncogene*, **24** (*37*), 5742–50.

86 Pardali, K. and Moustakas, A. (2007) Actions of TGF-beta as tumor suppressor and pro-metastatic factor in human cancer. *Biochimica et Biophysica Acta*, **1775** (*1*), 21–62.

87 Friedl, W., Uhlhaas, S., Schulmann, K., Stolte, M., Loff, S., Back, W. *et al.* (2002) Juvenile polyposis: massive gastric polyposis is more common in *MADH4* mutation carriers than in *BMPR1A* mutation carriers. *Human Genetics*, **111** (*1*), 108–11.

88 Sayed, M.G., Ahmed, A.F., Ringold, J.R., Anderson, M.E., Bair, J.L., Mitros, F.A. *et al.* (2002) Germline *SMAD4* or *BMPR1A* mutations and phenotype of juvenile polyposis. *Annals of Surgical Oncology*, **9** (*9*), 901–6.

89 Gallione, C.J., Repetto, G.M., Legius, E., Rustgi, A.K., Schelley, S.L., Tejpar, S. *et al.* (2004) A combined syndrome of juvenile polyposis and hereditary haemorrhagic telangiectasia associated with mutations in *MADH4* (*SMAD4*). *Lancet*, **363** (*9412*), 852–9.

90 Brosens, L.A., van Hattem, A., Hylind, L.M., Iacobuzio-Donahue, C., Romans, K. E., Axilbund, J. *et al.* (2007) Risk of colorectal cancer in juvenile polyposis. *Gut*, **56** (*7*), 965–7.

91 Howe, J.R., Mitros, F.A. and Summers, R.W. (1998) The risk of gastrointestinal carcinoma in familial juvenile polyposis. *Annals of Surgical Oncology*, **5** (*8*), 751–6.

92 Rozen, P., Samuel, Z., Brazowski, E., Jakubowicz, M., Rattan, J. and Halpern, Z. (2003) An audit of familial juvenile polyposis at the Tel Aviv Medical Center: demographic, genetic and clinical features. *Familial Cancer*, **2** (*1*), 1–7.

93 Eng, C. (2000) Will the real Cowden syndrome please stand up: revised diagnostic criteria. *Journal of Medical Genetics*, **37** (*11*), 828–30.

94 Zbuk, K., Stein, J. and Eng, C. (2006) PTEN Hamartoma Tumor Syndrome (PHTS). www.genetests.org.

95 Sansal, I. and Sellers, W.R. (2004) The biology and clinical relevance of the PTEN tumor suppressor pathway. *Journal of Clinical Oncology*, **22** (*14*), 2954–63.

96 Marsh, D.J., Kum, J.B., Lunetta, K.L., Bennett, M.J., Gorlin, R.J., Ahmed, S.F. *et al.* (1999) PTEN mutation spectrum and genotype-phenotype correlations in Bannayan–Riley–Ruvalcaba syndrome suggest a single entity with Cowden syndrome. *Human Molecular Genetics*, **8** (*8*), 1461–72.

97 Zhou, X.P., Waite, K.A., Pilarski, R., Hampel, H., Fernandez, M.J., Bos, C. *et al.* (2003) Germline PTEN promoter mutations and deletions in Cowden/Bannayan–Riley–Ruvalcaba syndrome result in aberrant PTEN protein and dysregulation of the phosphoinositol-3-kinase/Akt pathway. *American Journal of Human Genetics*, **73** (*2*), 404–11.

17
Lynch Syndrome (HNPCC)

Gabriela Möslein

Summary

Lynch syndrome (synonymous for HNPCC = hereditary non-polyposis colorectal cancer) is characterized by the development of colorectal, endometrial, gastric, and various other cancers, and is caused by a mutation in one of the mismatch repair (MMR) genes. One of the main challenges in the clinical management of Lynch syndrome remains the broad spectrum and heterogeneity among and between affected families. To date, no clinically relevant genotype-phenotype correlation for the two main affected genes *hMSH2* and *hMLH1* has been established. Clinical management of familial colorectal cancer (CRC) remains a challenge for clinicians. The overlap of syndromes with different underlying genetic causes and the differentiated risk management of colorectal and associated malignancies require state-of-the-art management recommendations.

Regarding the identification of Lynch syndrome, the available criteria (revised Bethesda guidelines) appear to be effective for the selection of families for analysis of tumor MMR status. To date, the significant proportion of mutation carriers in Germany are still unknown and diagnosis still relies on patients with index cancers. Taking into account the tremendous importance the identification of MMR mutation carriers implies, future directives could include routine antibody staining for MMR genes in all CRCs. Increasing evidence suggests that microsatellite instability (MSI) and/or immunohistochemical (IHC) are an important prognostic factor and may predict the response to chemotherapy, therefore a broad application of these tools is envisaged in the near future.

17.1
Introduction

Environmental factors have been demonstrated to play an important role in the etiology of most colorectal cancers (CRC). However, in approximately 15 to 30% of patients, inherited genetic factors are clearly significant. In about 5% of all cases,

Hereditary Tumors: From Genes to Clinical Consequences
Edited by Heike Allgayer, Helga Rehder and Simone Fulda
Copyright © 2009 WILEY-VCH Verlag GmbH & Co. KGaA, Weinheim
ISBN: 978-3-527-32028-8

CRC is associated with a highly penetrant dominant or recessive inherited cancer syndrome. The most frequent of these is Lynch syndrome (hereditary non-polyposis CRC; HNPCC) [1]. It is characterized by the development of multiple CRCs, endometrial cancer, and is also associated with various other cancers. The underlying genetic mechanism is a mutation in one of the mismatch repair (MMR) genes: *MLH1, MSH2, MSH6,* or *PMS2.* Familial adenomatous polyposis (FAP) may be seen as a counterpart to Lynch syndrome and is another well-described inherited CRC syndrome, responsible for less than 1% of all CRC cases. It may easily be identified by the pathognomonic identification of hundreds to thousands of adenomas in the colorectum. FAP is transmitted as an autosomal dominant trait and is caused by truncating mutations in the *APC* gene. Recently, the *MUTYH* gene has been identified as a further polyposis gene. The associated disorder has been termed MUTYH-associated polyposis (MAP) and displays an autosomal recessive pattern of inheritance [2]. For further details, see Chapter 16 on gastrointestinal polyposis syndromes. Clinically, the differentiation between Lynch syndrome, attenuated FAP, and MAP is not clearly delineated. However, distinguishing between the underlying predispositions is important for risk assessment and surveillance recommendations. The increasingly available molecular genetic services imply the opportunity of testing for the underlying genetic mechanisms, and open the opportunity of predictive testing of at-risk relatives. This medical approach revolutionizes medicine and opens an entirely new field of surgical strategy–prophylactic surgery.

17.2
Characteristics of Lynch Syndrome

Carriers of an MMR-gene mutation have a high risk of developing CRC, endometrial cancer, and other associated cancers. Risk assessment plays a decisive role for the surveillance strategies. The various types of cancers and the reported risks are summarized in Table 17.1 [3–10].

Cancers observed in Lynch syndrome families are frequently diagnosed at an alerting young age and tend to be multiple. The MMR defect leads to instability

Table 17.1 Life-time cancer risk in Lynch syndrome.

Colorectal cancer (men)	28–75%
Colorectal cancer (women)	24–38%
Endometrial cancer	27–71%
Ovarian cancer	3–13%
Gastric cancer	2–13%
Urinary tract cancer	1–12%
Brain tumor	1–4%
Bile duct/gallbladder cancer	2%
Small bowel cancer	4–7%

at microsatellites of tumor-DNA (microsatellite instability (MSI)). This phenomenon may be found in more than 90% of tumors associated with Lynch syndrome, whereas in the sporadic setting, it is found in about 15% of cases. With immunohistochemical (IH) analysis using antibodies against the four MMR proteins, loss of protein expression of the causative gene can be shown. Therefore, this pre-screening, ubiquitous, and less costly approach may in the future be more widely applied for broad identification of Lynch syndrome, pinpointing towards an algorithm for mutation detection.

In 1989, the Amsterdam criteria were proposed in order to provide stratified family material required for international collaborative studies [11]. At that time, in analogy to the identification of FAP, the focus was clearly oriented towards identifying families with a predisposition for CRC. This strategy was successful, and after identification and molecular characterization of families with MMR mutations, it became clear that other cancer localizations were inherent to the syndrome. Consequently, in 1999 the criteria were revised and since then include various extra-colonic (EC) tumors [12] weighed differently. The basis for the inclusion or exclusion of EC cancers is thin, and leads to a bias in every regard. In 1997, the Bethesda guidelines were developed to identify individuals with CRC that

Table 17.2 Amsterdam criteria II and revised Bethesda criteria.

Amsterdam criteria II

There should be at least three relatives with colorectal cancer or with a Lynch syndrome–associated cancer: cancer of the endometrium, small bowel, ureter, or renal pelvis.

• Onerelative should be a first-degree relative of the other two.

• At least two successive generations should be affected.

• At least one tumor should be diagnosed before age 50.

• FAP should be excluded in the colorectal cancer case if any.

• Tumors should be verified by histopathological examination.

Revised Bethesda criteria

1. Colorectal cancer diagnosed in a patient <50 years of age.

2. Presence of synchronous, metachronous colorectal, or other Lynch syndrome-related tumours[a], regardless of age.

3. Colorectal cancer with MSI-H histology diagnosed in a patient <60 years of age.

4. Patient with colorectal cancer and a first-degree relative with a Lynch syndrome-related tumor, with one of the cancers diagnosed under age 50 years.

5. Patient with colorectal cancer with two or more first-degree or second-degree relatives with a Lynch syndrome-related tumor, regardless of age.

---

a   Lynch syndrome related tumours include colorectal, endometrial, stomach, ovarian, pancreas, ureter, renal pelvis, biliary tract, and brain tumors, sebaceous gland adenomas and keratoacanthomas, and carcinoma of the small bowel.

should be tested for MSI [13, 14]. These guidelines were revised in 2004 [15]. The revised Amsterdam criteria and Bethesda guidelines are shown in Table 17.2, and to date are valid identifiers.

17.3
Genetic Alteration

The identification of the underlying genetic cause in Lynch syndrome families about 15 years ago has been the decisive contribution for the medical community to accept the existence of the heterogeneous hereditary cancer syndrome in a setting other than the clear-cut phenotype in FAP. Before this time, there was an ongoing debate about chance clustering of frequent tumors in families or a genetic predisposition. Since then, large numbers of families worldwide have been ana-lyzed and related to this genetic background – the collaborative effort has led to the identification of large numbers of affected families.

17.4
Lynch Syndrome, HNPCC or Familial Cancer?

Some confusion exists regarding the terminology for variants of hereditary colorec-tal and/or familial cancer. Various names for Lynch syndrome have been used in the past century. Usually, the syndrome has been known as HNPCC, since this name historically clarified that the syndrome described an inherited form of CRC and was associated with a very low number of adenomas (non-polyposis vs. FAP). However, the term HNPCC does not insinuate the frequent involvement of EC cancers. It has therefore internationally been proposed to reintroduce the name Lynch syndrome – reserved for families with strong evidence of MMR deficiency, for example, by the presence of an MMR defect, or the presence of MSI in tumours [15]. The term, familial CRC, should be reserved for families that meet the Amster-dam criteria but do not have evidence for MMR deficiency.

17.5
Clinical Identification

Differentiation between mutation carriers and non-mutation carriers is clinically most beneficial – from a medical and resource perspective – since intensified sur-veillance may be restricted to the predisposed individuals, whereas those without a gene defect may be dismissed from the program. Mutation detection is costly, since as many as four genes may need to be analyzed. Moreover, direct sequencing of the genes is required since the mutational spectra are wide. Therefore, it is important to define which patients should be submitted to mutation analysis and if so, should they be subjected to a prescreening test?

Table 17.3 MMR-gene mutation analysis in relation to clinical criteria and results of MSI- and IH-analysis in population-based or consecutive series of unselected colorectal cancer.

Author/year	Primary test used		MMR-genes analyzed	Total no. of CRC	Pathogenic mutations identified	Proportion of mutation carriers that meet the clinical criteria	
	IH: antibodies	MSI: markers				Amsterdam II	(Revised) Bethesda criteria
Aaltonen 1998	–	7	MLH1, MSH2	509	10 (1.9%)	7/10	10/10[a]
Debniak 2000	2	10	MLH1, MSH2	68[b]	6 (3.5 %)	1/6	?
Solavaara 2000	–	7	MLH1, MSH2	535	18 (3.3%)	12/18	17/18[a]
Cunningham 2001	3	6	MLH1, MSH2	257	5 (1.95%)	3/5	?
Hampel 2005	4	5	MLH1, MSH2, MSH6, PMS2	1066	23 (2.1%)	3/23	18/23
Pinol 2005	2	1	MLH1, MSH2	1222	11 (0.9%)	4/11	10/11
Total				4627	111 (24%)	30/73 (41%)	55/62 (89%)

a Communicated with authors.
b The original number of consecutive CRCs was 168, including 143 sporadic cases and 25 suspected cases. A total of 43 of the sporadic cases and 25 suspected cases were analyzed.

Currently, the Amsterdam II or the revised Bethesda criteria are used to select patients with suspected familial CRC for molecular genetic and/or IH analysis of the tumor, and those with evidence of MSI or loss of MMR expression are offered mutation analysis. There are six studies in which either MSI- or IH-analysis or both tests were performed as the primary screening tool in prospective and unselected series of CRC patients (Table 17.3) [16–21].

Previous studies have shown that the yield of mutation analysis (positive predictive value) in families that meet the Amsterdam criteria is approximately 50% and the yield in families that meet the Bethesda criteria between 10 and 20% [22] These six studies showed that the sensitivity of the Amsterdam criteria for the detection of mutations was 40% and that of the Bethesda guidelines was about 90%. This means that if the revised Bethesda guidelines had been used, about 10% of the mutation carriers would have been missed, mostly patients with CRC diagnosed between ages 50 and 60.

Is performing both MSI and IH necessary as a prescreening tool, or is one of both sufficient, and if so, which one is more recommendable? Most studies addressing this issue have been retrospective and methodology applied varied greatly. For IH-analysis, mostly only two antibodies (MLH1, MSH2) were employed; other studies used three or four antibodies (MLH1, MSH2, MSH6, PMS2). In the studies in which both MSI analysis and IH analysis have been performed prospectively, the sensitivity of MSI analysis was slightly better than that of IH analysis [17, 19–21, 23–27]. In one large (German) study, the outcome of both methods was tested prospectively in families that meet the Amsterdam, Bethesda, or age-independent modified criteria. MSI analysis (using the Bethesda set of 5 markers) and IH analysis (2 antibodies) was performed in 1119 index patients [24]. Two hundred and thirty pathogenic MMR gene mutations were identified, the sensitivity of MSI analysis being 100% and that of IH analysis 94%. A Dutch study demonstrated increased detection by including an antibody against PMS2 [28].

IH is broadly available, less cost-intensive, and pinpoints towards the specific underlying gene defect. Most authors prioritize the use of IH for these reasons, especially in families with a high probability for an MMR mutation (e.g. families that meet the Amsterdam criteria, or families with a high predicted probability based on calculations using the Wijnen [22] or Engel model). MSI may be recommended in addition, if IH is unconclusive.

17.6
Surveillance Colorectum

The term HNPCC is misleading, since the adenoma-carcinoma sequence applies to development of CRC in Lynch syndrome families. Due to the increased occurrence of CRC and the availability of a precursor lesion, colonoscopic surveillance has been recommended since the 1980s. The question to be raised is: does colonoscopic surveillance translate to a reduction in mortality?

Several studies address this issue [29–37]. All studies demonstrate a benefit of surveillance in detecting CRC at an earlier stage compared to historical controls. The only prospective controlled trial (Järvinen 1995/2000) showed that surveillance led to a 63% reduction in CRC. Two studies assessed the effect of surveillance on CRC-associated mortality. A Finnish study showed that colonoscopic surveillance significantly decreased the mortality associated with CRC [34, 38]. A study from The Netherlands evaluated the relative mortality in a large series of families over a period of 45 years and demonstrated a reduction in mortality [31]. The protocols that have been used in studies of surveillance have varied with respect to the surveillance intervals. Some studies advised a 3-yearly colonoscopy and others colonoscopy every year–the data available so far does not allow a clear-cut recommendation; however, the surveillance interval will lie between 1 and 3 years.

17.7
Familial Cancer

In a significant proportion (~30%) of families that meet the Amsterdam criteria, the results of MSI analysis and IH analysis of the colorectal tumor(s) are negative [40]. Clustering of CRC by chance or genetic defects other than those of MMR may be responsible for the disease in such families, and they do not have Lynch syndrome. These families are characterized by a more advanced age of onset of CRC than in Lynch syndrome families and the absence of endometrial cancer and multiple tumours. A recent study reported that the risk of developing CRC in such families is only increased by a factor of 2.3 [40]. Another study compared the results of surveillance in families with clustering of CRC with and without MSI [41]. The results showed that the yield of adenomas was the same in both types of families. However, CRC was only identified in the families with MSI tumors. In families without evidence for MMR deficiency, a less intensive colonoscopic surveillance program (e.g. colonoscopy: 1x/3–5 years, starting 5–10 years before the first diagnosis of CRC or >45 years) might be appropriate. In view of the absence of endometrial cancer in such families, surveillance of the endometrium is not indicated.

17.8
Surveillance of the Endometrium/Ovary

The international studies in Lynch syndrome families have shown that carriers of an MMR mutation have a high risk of developing endometrial cancer [7]. Though it is known that the majority of (sporadic) endometrial cancers are detected at an early stage, about 10 to 15% of patients with such tumors will ultimately die from metastatic disease. Due to this significant mortality and the high risk of developing endometrial cancer in Lynch syndrome families, specifically if the mutation is located on *MSH6*, surveillance is advised.

British and Dutch investigators evaluated the outcome of surveillance of 269 women from families suspected of having Lynch syndrome [42, 43]. The surveillance program consisted of ultrasound every 1 to 2 years. It did not lead to the detection of pre-malignant lesions or endometrial cancer. In another study from The Netherlands, 41 women from Lynch families underwent surveillance by transvaginal ultrasound (TVU) followed by aspiration biopsy in suspected cases. After a mean follow-up of 5 years, premalignant lesions, that is, complex atypia, were detected in three patients. There was one early stage interval cancer diagnosed 8 months after a normal ultrasound. A recent study of 175 subjects from Finland reported the results of surveillance by TVU and aspiration biopsy [44]. Complex atypia was found in 5 patients, endometrial cancer was found in 11, and there were two interval cancers. Six of the 11 screen-detected cancers were only identified by aspiration biopsy and not by TVU. American investigators reported on a retrospective cohort of 315 women, all mutation carriers, 61 of whom had prophylactic surgery and were then followed up for approximately 10 years. No endometrial cancer or ovarian cancer developed in those women who had prophylactic surgery, whereas 33% of the women who did not have surgery developed endometrial cancer and 5.5% developed ovarian cancer [45].

In conclusion, two of the three available studies suggested that surveillance may lead to the detection of pre-malignant lesions, and one study also to detection of endometrial cancer at an early stage. Due to the higher risk of developing endometrial cancer in carriers of a *MSH6* mutation, hysterectomy may be suggested for these women at the time of CRC surgery or after menopause. This surgery may also be considered for carriers of mutations in the other MMR genes, and for women who require surgery for a CRC. In view of the risk of ovarian cancer and the failure of early detection of such tumors by TVU and CA-125 estimation, bilateral salpingo-oophorectomy might be considered in mutation carriers after completion of family planning.

17.9
Surveillance for Other Related Cancers

Other cancers associated with Lynch syndrome include cancer of the stomach, ureter, renal pelvis (see Chapter 15 on hereditary renal tumors of the adult), small bowel, the bile ducts, and tumors of the brain. The life-time risk of developing one of these cancers is relatively low (<10%), and may be associated with the underlying MMR defect. The risk of developing gastric cancer may be higher in some countries, such as Germany. The International Society of Gastrointestinal Hereditary Tumours (InSiGHT) recommends surveillance for cancer of the stomach and urinary tract, if the specific type of cancer clusters in the family (more than one case) [46]. However, screening for urological cancers by cytology has not proven to have any benefit.

17.10
Surgical Management

Several studies showed that Lynch syndrome patients have an increased risk of developing multiple (synchronous and metachronous) CRCs. A Dutch study reported that the risk of developing a second colon tumor after treatment of a primary CRC in Lynch syndrome was 16% after 10 years of follow-up [37]. In view of this substantial risk, the question arises whether a subtotal colectomy instead of a segmental resection might be the preferred treatment in patients from Lynch syndrome families with a primary tumor. In a recent study, a decision analysis was performed to compare the life expectancy for patients undergoing subtotal colectomy or partial resection for a primary screen-detected CRC [47]. The results indicated that subtotal colectomy performed at a young age (<47 years) would lead to an increased life expectancy of up to 2.3 years. Unfortunately, the authors were not able to use quality of life (QOL) adjusted life expectance because studies on QOL that specifically consider Lynch syndrome patients are not available in the literature. Although for sporadic CRC, QOL after segmental resection has been reported to be better than after subtotal colectomy, in Lynch syndrome families QOL after segmental resection may be decreased by the need for colonoscopy (vs. sigmoidoscopy after subtotal colectomy) and increase of fear of a second primary.

Based on these findings and taking into account the substantial risk of developing a second tumor, subtotal colectomy with ileorectal anastomosis can be discussed if colon cancer is detected in a young patient participating in a surveillance program. A prospective study that also addresses QOL should evaluate which surgical option is the most appropriate in Lynch syndrome. Until the outcome of such studies is available, the Mallorca group recommends discussing the pros and cons of both options with a patient from a Lynch syndrome family who develops CRC.

17.11
Chemotherapy

Currently, at least three chemotherapeutic agents have been proven to be effective in the treatment of CRC, that is, 5FU with or without leucovorin, oxaliplatin, and irinotecan (CPT11). *In vitro* studies suggested that MMR-deficient colon cancer cells might not respond to 5FU-based chemotherapy [48]. On the other hand, CRC cell lines defective of MMR exhibit increased sensitivity to CPT11 (irinotecan) [49].

The effect of chemotherapy in patients with MSI-H or HNPCC tumors has been reported in only a few studies [50–54]. Most studies showed that there was no benefit of 5FU treatment in such patients. One small study on Stage IV CRC patients reported complete or partial responses to treatment with irinotecan in 4 out of 7 patients with MSI-H tumors compared to 7 out of 65 patients with MSI-L/MSS tumors [55].

Because most studies are retrospective, all authors urge caution in implementing these findings in clinical practice until they are confirmed by prospective studies. Because it may be unethical to withhold chemotherapy in a clinical trial for potentially curable advanced-stage colon cancer, the best format of such studies is to compare effective drugs such as CPT11 or oxalaplatin with 5FU. These approaches require validation in large patient cohorts before routine integration into clinical recommendations.

References

1 Lynch, H.T. and Chapelle de la, A. (2003) Hereditary colorectal cancer. *The New England Journal of Medicine*, **348**, 919–32.

2 Al Tassan, N., Chmiel, N.H., Maynard, J., Fleming, N., Livingston, A.L., Williams, G.T., Hodges, A.K., Davies, D. R., David, S.S., Sampson, J.R. and Cheadle, J.P. (2002) Inherited variants of MYH associated with somatic G:C → T:A mutations in colorectal tumors. *Nature Genetics*, **30**, 227–32.

3 Vasen, H.F., Wijnen, J.T., Menko, F.H., Kleibeuker, J.H., Taal, B.G., Griffioen, G., Nagengast, F.M., Meijers-Heijboer, E.H., Bertario, L., Varesco, L., Bisgaard, M.L., Mohr, J., Fodde, R. and Khan, P.M. (1996) Cancer risk in families with hereditary nonpolyposis colorectal cancer diagnosed by mutation analysis. *Gastroenterology*, **110**, 1020–7.

4 Dunlop, M.G., Farrington, S.M., Carothers, A.D., Wyllie, A.H., Sharp, L., Burn, J., Liu, B., Kinzler, K.W. and Vogelstein, B. (1997) Cancer risk associated with germline DNA mismatch repair gene mutations. *Human Molecular Genetics*, **6**, 105–10.

5 Aarnio, M., Sankila, R., Pukkala, E., Salovaara, R., Aaltonen, L.A., de la Chapelle, A., Peltomaki, P., Mecklin, J.P. and Jarvinen, H.J. (1999) Cancer risk in mutation carriers of DNA mismatch repair genes. *International Journal of Cancer*, **81**, 214–18.

6 Vasen, H.F., Stormorken, A., Menko, F.H., Nagengast, F.M., Kleibeuker, J.H., Griffioen, G., Taal, B.G., Moller, P. and Wijnen, J.T. (2001) *MSH2* mutation carriers are at higher risk of cancer than *MLH1* mutation carriers: a study of hereditary nonpolyposis colorectal cancer families. *Journal of Clinical Oncology*, **19**, 4074–80.

7 Hendriks, Y.M., Wagner, A., Morreau, H., Menko, F., Stormorken, A., Quehenberger, F., Sandkuijl, L., Moller, P., Genuardi, M., Van Houwelingen, H., Tops, C., van Puijenbroek, M., Verkuijlen, P., Kenter, G., Van Mil, A., Meijers-Heijboer, H., Tan, G.B., Breuning, M.H., Fodde, R., Wijnen, J.T., Brocker-Vriends, A.H. and Vasen, H. (2004) Cancer risk in hereditary nonpolyposis colorectal cancer due to *MSH6* mutations: impact on counseling and surveillance. *Gastroenterology*, **127**, 17–25.

8 Quehenberger, F., Vasen, H.F. and van Houwelingen, H.C. (2005) Risk of colorectal and endometrial cancer for carriers of mutations of the *hMLH1* and *hMSH2* gene: correction for ascertainment. *Journal of Medical Genetics*, **42**, 491–6.

9 Hampel, H., Stephens, J.A., Pukkala, E., Sankila, R., Aaltonen, L.A., Mecklin, J.P. and de la Chapelle, A. (2005) Cancer risk in hereditary nonpolyposis colorectal cancer syndrome: later age of onset. *Gastroenterology*, **129**, 415–21.

10 Jenkins, M.A., Baglietto, L., Dowty, J.G., Van Vliet, C.M., Smith, L., Mead, L.J., Macrae, F.A., St John, D.J., Jass, J.R., Giles, G.G., Hopper, J.L. and Southey, M. C. (2006) Cancer risks for mismatch repair gene mutation carriers: a population-based early onset case-family study. *Clinical Gastroenterology and Hepatology*, **4**, 489–98.

11 Vasen, H.F., Mecklin, J.P., Khan, P.M. and Lynch, H.T. (1991) The International Collaborative Group on Hereditary Non-Polyposis Colorectal Cancer (ICG-HNPCC). *Diseases of the Colon and Rectum*, **34**, 424–5.

12 Vasen, H.F., Watson, P., Mecklin, J.P. and Lynch, H.T. (1999) New clinical criteria for hereditary nonpolyposis colorectal cancer (HNPCC, Lynch syndrome) proposed by the International Collaborative group on HNPCC. *Gastroenterology*, **116**, 1453–6.

13 Rodriguez-Bigas, M.A., Boland, C.R., Hamilton, S.R., Henson, D.E., Jass, J.R., Khan, P.M., Lynch, H., Perucho, M., Smyrk, T., Sobin, L. and Srivastava, S. (1997) A National Cancer Institute Workshop on Hereditary Nonpolyposis Colorectal Cancer Syndrome: meeting highlights and Bethesda guidelines. *Journal of the National Cancer Institute*, **89**, 1758–62.

14 Boland, C.R., Thibodeau, S.N., Hamilton, S.R., Sidransky, D., Eshleman, J.R., Burt, R.W., Meltzer, S.J., Rodriguez-Bigas, M.A., Fodde, R., Ranzani, G.N. and Srivastava, S. (1998) A National Cancer Institute Workshop on Microsatellite Instability for cancer detection and familial predisposition: development of international criteria for the determination of microsatellite instability in colorectal cancer. *Cancer Research*, **58**, 5248–57.

15 Umar, A., Boland, C.R., Terdiman, J.P., Syngal, S., Ruschoff, C.A., Fishel, J., Lindor, R., Burgart, N.M., Hamelin, L.J., Hamilton, R., Hiatt, S.R., Jass, R.A., Lindblom, J., Lynch, A., Peltomaki, H.T., Ramsey, P., Rodriguez-Bigas, S.D., Vasen, M.A., Hawk, H.F., Barrett, E.T., Freedman, J.C. and Revised, A.N. and Srivastava, S. (2004) Bethesda Guidelines for hereditary nonpolyposis colorectal cancer (Lynch syndrome) and microsatellite instability. *Journal of the National Cancer Institute*, **96**, 261–8.

16 Aaltonen, L.A., Salovaara, R., Kristo, P., Canzian, F., Hemminki, A., Peltomaki, P., Chadwick, R.B., Kaariainen, H., Eskelinen, M., Jarvinen, H., Mecklin, J.P. and de la Chapelle, A. (1998) Incidence of hereditary nonpolyposis colorectal cancer and the feasibility of molecular screening for the disease. *The New England Journal of Medicine*, **338**, 1481–7.

17 Debniak, T., Kurzawski, G., Gorski, B., Kladny, J., Domagala, W. and Lubinski, J. (2000) Value of pedigree/clinical data, immunohistochemistry and micro-satellite instability analyses in reducing the cost of determining *hMLH1* and *hMSH2* gene mutations in patients with colorectal cancer. *European Journal of Cancer*, **36**, 49–54.

18 Salovaara, R., Loukola, A., Kristo, P., Kaariainen, H., Ahtola, H., Eskelinen, M., Harkonen, N., Julkunen, R., Kangas, E., Ojala, S., Tulikoura, J., Valkamo, E., Jarvinen, H., Mecklin, J.P., Aaltonen, L.A. and de la Chapelle, A. (2000) Population-based molecular detection of hereditary nonpolyposis colorectal cancer. *Journal of Clinical Oncology*, **18**, 2193–200.

19 Cunningham, J.M., Kim, C.Y., Christensen, E.R., Tester, D.J., Parc, Y., Burgart, L.J., Halling, K.C., McDonnell, S.K., Schaid, D.J., Walsh, V.C., Kubly, V., Nelson, H., Michels, V.V. and Thibodeau, S.N. (2001) The frequency of hereditary defective mismatch repair in a prospective series of unselected colorectal carcinomas. *American Journal of Human Genetics*, **69**, 780–90.

20 Hampel, H., Frankel, W.L., Martin, E., Arnold, M., Khanduja, K., Kuebler, P., Nakagawa, H., Sotamaa, K., Prior, T.W., Westman, J., Panescu, J., Fix, D., Lockman, J., Comeras, I. and de la Chapelle, A. (2005) Screening for the Lynch syndrome (hereditary nonpolyposis colorectal cancer). *The New England Journal of Medicine*, **352**, 1851–60.

21 Pinol, V., Castells, A., Andreu, M., Castellvi-Bel, S., Alenda, C., Llor, X., Xicola, R.M., Rodriguez-Moranta, F., Paya, A., Jover, R. and Bessa, X. (2005) Accuracy of revised Bethesda guidelines, microsatellite instability, and immuno-histochemistry for the identification of patients with hereditary nonpolyposis colorectal cancer. *The Journal of the American Medical Association*, **293**, 1986–94.

22 Wijnen, J.T., Vasen, H.F., Khan, P.M., Zwinderman, A.H., van der Klift, H., Mulder, A., Tops, C., Moller, P. and Fodde, R. (1998) Clinical findings with implications for genetic testing in families with clustering of colorectal cancer. *The New England Journal of Medicine*, **339**, 511–18.

23 Scartozzi, M., Bianchi, F., Rosati, S., Galizia, E., Antolini, A., Loretelli, C., Piga, A., Bearzi, I., Cellerino, R. and Porfiri, E. (2002) Mutations of *hMLH1* and *hMSH2* in patients with suspected hereditary nonpolyposis colorectal cancer: correlation with microsatellite instability and abnormalities of mismatch repair protein expression. *Journal of Clinical Oncology*, **20**, 1203–8.

24 Engel, C., Forberg, C., Holinski-Feder, E., Pagenstecher, C., Plaschke, J., Kloor, M., Poremba, C., Pox, C.R.J. *et al.* (2006) Novel strategy for optimal sequential application of clinical criteria, immunohistochemistry and microsatellite analysis in the diagnosis of hereditary nonpolyposis colorectal cancer. *International Journal of Cancer*, **118**, 115–22.

25 Southey, M.C., Jenkins, M.A., Mead, L., Whitty, J., Trivett, M., Tesoriero, A.A., Smith, L.D., Jennings, K., Grubb, G., Royce, S.G., Walsh, M.D., Barker, M.A., Young, J.P., Jass, J.R., St John, D.J., Macrae, F.A., Giles, G.G. and Hopper, J. L. (2005) Use of molecular tumor characteristics to prioritize mismatch repair gene testing in early-onset colorectal cancer. *Journal of Clinical Oncology*, **23**, 6524–32.

26 Barnetson, R.A., Tenesa, A., Farrington, S.M., Nicholl, I.D., Cetnarskyj, R., Porteous, M.E., Campbell, H. and Dunlop, M.G. (2006) Identification and survival of carriers of mutations in DNA mismatch repair genes in colon cancer. *The New England Journal of Medicine*, **354**, 2751–63.

27 Niessen, R.C., Berends, M.J., Wu, Y., Sijmons, R.H., Hollema, H., Ligtenberg, M.J., de Walle, H.E., de Vries, E.G., Karrenbeld, A., Buys, C.H., van der Zee, A.G., Hofstra, R.M. and Kleibeuker, J.H. (2006) Identification of mismatch repair gene mutations in young colorectal cancer patients and patients with multiple HNPCC-associated tumours. *Gut*, **55**, 1781–8.

28 de Jong, A.E., van Puijenbroek, M., Hendriks, Y., Tops, C., Wijnen, J., Ausems, M.G., Meijers-Heijboer, H., Wagner, A., van Os, T.A., Brocker-Vriends, A.H., Vasen, H.F. and Morreau, H. (2004) Microsatellite instability, immunohistochemistry, and additional PMS2 staining in suspected hereditary nonpolyposis colorectal cancer. *Clinical Cancer Research*, **10**, 972–80.

29 Love, R.R. and Morrissey, J.F. (1984) Colonoscopy in asymptomatic individuals with a family history of colorectal cancer. *Archives of Internal Medicine*, **144**, 2209–11.

30 Mecklin, J.P., Jarvinen, H.J., Aukee, S., Elomaa, I. and Karjalainen, K. (1987) Screening for colorectal carcinoma in cancer family syndrome kindreds. *Scand J Gastroenterol*, **22**, 449–53.

31 Vasen, H.F., Hartog Jager, F.C., Menko, F.H. and Nagengast, F.M. (1989) Screening for hereditary nonpolyposis colorectal cancer: a study of 22 kindreds in The Netherlands. *The American Journal of Medicine*, **86**, 278–81.

32 Vasen, H.F., Taal, B.G., Nagengast, F.M., Griffioen, G., Menko, F.H., Kleibeuker, J.H., Offerhaus, G.J. and Meera, K.P. (1995) Hereditary nonpolyposis colorectal cancer: results of long-term surveillance in 50 families. *European Journal of Cancer*, **31A**, 1145–8.

33 Jarvinen, H.J., Mecklin, J.P. and Sistonen, P. (1995) Screening reduces colorectal cancer rate in families with hereditary nonpolyposis colorectal cancer. *Gastroenterology*, **108**, 1405–11.

34 Jarvinen, H.J., Aarnio, M., Mustonen, H., Aktan-Collan, K., Aaltonen, L.A., Peltomaki, P., de la Chapelle, A. and Mecklin, J.P. (2000) Controlled 15-year trial on screening for colorectal cancer in families with hereditary nonpolyposis colorectal cancer. *Gastroenterology*, **118**, 829–34.

35 Renkonen-Sinisalo, L., Aarnio, M., Mecklin, J.P. and Jarvinen, H.J. (2000) Surveillance improves survival of colorectal cancer in patients with hereditary nonpolyposis colorectal cancer. *Cancer Detection and Prevention*, **24**, 137–42.

36 Arrigoni, A., Sprujevnik, T., Alvisi, V., Rossi, A., Ricci, G., Pennazio, M., Spandre, M., Cavallero, M., Bertone, A., Foco, A. and Rossini, F.P. (2005) Clinical identification and long-term surveillance of 22 hereditary non-polyposis colon cancer Italian families. *European Journal of Gastroenterology and Hepatology*, **17**, 213–19.

37 de Vos tot Nederveen Cappel, W.H., Nagengast, F.M., Griffioen, G., Menko, F.H., Taal, B.G., Kleibeuker, J.H. and Vasen, H.F. (2002) Surveillance for hereditary nonpolyposis colorectal cancer: a long-term study on 114 families. *Diseases of the Colon and Rectum*, **45**, 1588–94.

38 de Jong, A.E., Hendriks, Y.M., Kleibeuker, J.H., de Boer, S.Y., Cats, A., Griffioen, G., Nagengast, F.M., Nelis, F.G., Rookus, M.A., Vasen, H.F. (2006) Shift in mortality due to surveillance in the Lynch syndrome. *Gastroenterology*, **130**, 665–71.

39 de Jong, A.E., Nagengast, F.M., Kleibeuker, J.H., van de Meeberg, P.C., van Wijk, H.J., Cats, A., Griffioen, G. and Vasen, H.F. (2006) What is the appropriate screening protocol in Lynch syndrome?. *Familial Cancer*, **5**, 373–8.

40 Lindor, N.M., Rabe, K., Petersen, G.M., Haile, R., Casey, G., Baron, J., Gallinger, S., Bapat, B., Aronson, M., Hopper, J., Jass, J., LeMarchand, L., Grove, J., Potter, J., Newcomb, P., Terdiman, J.P., Conrad, P., Moslein, G., Goldberg, R., Ziogas, A., Anton-Culver, H., de Andrade, M., Siegmund, K., Thibodeau, S.N., Boardman, L.A. and Seminara, D. (2005) Lower cancer incidence in Amsterdam-I criteria families without mismatch repair deficiency: familial colorectal cancer type X. *The Journal of the American Medical Association*, **293**, 1979–85.

41 Dove-Edwin, I., de Jong, A.E., Adams, J., Mesher, D., Lipton, L., Sasieni, P., Vasen, H.F. and Thomas, H.J. (2006) Prospective results of surveillance colonoscopy in dominant familial colorectal cancer with and without Lynch syndrome. *Gastroenterology*, **130**, 1995–2000.

42 Dove-Edwin, I., Boks, D., Goff, S., Kenter, G.G., Carpenter, R., Vasen, H.F. and Thomas, H.J. (2002) The outcome of endometrial carcinoma surveillance by ultrasound scan in women at risk of hereditary nonpolyposis colorectal carcinoma and familial colorectal carcinoma. *Cancer*, **94**, 1708–12.

43 Rijcken, F.E., Mourits, M.J., Kleibeuker, J.H., Hollema, H. and van der Zee, A.G. (2003) Gynecologic screening in hereditary nonpolyposis colorectal cancer. *Gynecologic Oncology*, **91**, 74–80.

44 Renkonen-Sinisalo, L., Butzow, R., Leminen, A., Lehtovirta, P., Mecklin, J.P. and Jarvinen, H.J. (2006) Surveillance for endometrial cancer in hereditary nonpolyposis colorectal cancer syndrome. *International Journal of Cancer*, **120**, 821–4.

45 Schmeler, K.M., Lynch, H.T., Chen, L.M., Munsell, M.F., Soliman, P.T., Clark, M.B., Daniels, M.S., White, K.G., Boyd-Rogers, S.G., Conrad, P.G., Yang, K.Y., Rubin, M.M., Sun, C.C., Slomovitz, B.M., Gershenson, D.M. and Lu, K.H.

(2006) Prophylactic surgery to reduce the risk of gynecologic cancers in the Lynch syndrome. *The New England Journal of Medicine*, **354**, 261–9.

46 Weber, T. (2006) Clinical surveillance recommendation adopted for HNPCC. *Lancet*, **348**, 465.

47 de Vos tot Nederveen Cappel, W.H., Buskens, E., van Duijvendijk, P., Cats, A., Menko, F.H., Griffioen, G., Slors, J.F., Nagengast, F.M., Kleibeuker, J.H. and Vasen, H.F. (2003) Decision analysis in the surgical treatment of colorectal cancer due to a mismatch repair gene defect. *Gut*, **52**, 1752–5.

48 Carethers, J.M., Chauhan, D.P., Fink, D., Nebel, S., Bresalier, R.S., Howell, S.B. and Boland, C.R. (1999) Mismatch repair proficiency and *in vitro* response to 5-fluorouracil. *Gastroenterology*, **117**, 123–31.

49 Jacob, S., Aguado, M., Fallik, D. and Praz, F. (2001) The role of the DNA mismatch repair system in the cytotoxicity of the topoisomerase inhibitors camptothecin and etoposide to human colorectal cancer cells. *Cancer Research*, **61**, 6555–62.

50 Liang, J.T., Huang, K.C., Lai, H.S., Lee, P.H., Cheng, Y.M., Hsu, H.C., Cheng, A. L., Hsu, C.H., Yeh, K.H., Wang, S.M., Tang, C. and Chang, K.J. (2002) High-frequency microsatellite instability predicts better chemosensitivity to high-dose 5-fluorouracil plus leucovorin chemotherapy for stage IV sporadic colorectal cancer after palliative bowel resection. *International Journal of Cancer*, **101**, 519–25.

51 Ribic, C.M., Sargent, D.J., Moore, M.J., Thibodeau, S.N., French, A.J., Goldberg, R.M., Hamilton, S.R., Laurent-Puig, P., Gryfe, R., Shepherd, L.E., Tu, D., Redston, M. and Gallinger, S. (2003) Tumor microsatelliteinstability status as a predictor of benefit from fluorouracil-based adjuvant chemotherapy for colon cancer. *The New England Journal of Medicine*, **349**, 247–57.

52 Carethers, J.M., Smith, E.J., Behling, C.A., Nguyen, L., Tajima, A., Doctolero, R.T., Cabrera, B.L., Goel, A., Arnold, C.A., Miyai, K. and Boland, C.R. (2004) Use of 5-fluorouracil and survival in patients with microsatellite-unstable colorectal cancer. *Gastroenterology*, **126**, 394–401.

53 de Vos tot Nederveen Cappel, W.H., Meulenbeld, H.J., Kleibeuker, J.H., Nagengast, F.M., Menko, F.H., Griffioen, G., Cats, A., Morreau, H., Gelderblom, H. and Vasen, H.F. (2004) Survival after adjuvant 5-FU treatment for stage III colon cancer in hereditary nonpolyposis colorectal cancer. *International Journal of Cancer*, **109**, 468–71.

54 Fallik, D., Borrini, F., Boige, V., Viguier, J., Jacob, S., Miquel, C., Sabourin, J.C., Ducreux, M. and Praz, F. (2003) Microsatellite instability is a predictive factor of the tumor response to irinotecan in patients with advanced colorectal cancer. *Cancer Research*, **63**, 5738–44.

55 Hurlstone, D.P., Karajeh, M., Cross, S.S., McAlindon, M.E., Brown, S., Hunter, M.D. and Sanders, D.S. (2005) The role of high-magnification-chromoscopic colonoscopy in hereditary nonpolyposis colorectal cancer screening: a prospective "back-to-back" endoscopic study. *The American Journal of Gastroenterology*, **100**, 2167–73.

18
Gastrointestinal Stromal Tumors (GISTs)

Maria Debiec-Rychter

Summary

Gastrointestinal stromal tumors (GISTs), the most common mesenchymal tumors of the gastrointestinal tract (GI), evolve from a progenitor related to the interstitial cells of Cajal (ICC). Oncogenic mutations in the *KIT* or *PDGFRA* gene are detected in approximately 85% of sporadic GISTs.

Familial GIST syndrome is an autosomal dominant genetic disorder with germline mutations of the *KIT* or *PDFGRA* gene as an underlying cause of the disease. Familial GIST syndrome associated with a germline *KIT* mutation is characterized by multiple GISTs associated with hyperplasia of ICCs, and other clinicopathologic features, such as skin hyperpigmentation, GI motility dysfunctions, or mast cell abnormalities. Symptoms associated with GI bleeding are common, and may be the only manifestation of the disease. Germline *PDGFRA* mutations result in multiple GISTs, diffuse hyperplasia of ICCs, and GI dysmotility symptoms, but affected kindreds lack pigmentation or mast cells abnormalities.

Hereditary forms of the disease also arise in the settings of other hereditary syndromes, such as neurofibromatosis type 1 (NF1), the Carney–Stratakis syndrome, and the Carney triad. GIST development in patients with NF1 is caused by a somatic inactivation of the wildtype NF1 allele in the tumor and the absence of neurofibromin, resulting in hyperactivation of the signaling pathway downstream of *KIT*. Familial Carney–Stratakis syndrome is the dyad of multifocal, gastric GISTs and paragangliomas, transmitted as an autosomal-dominant trait with incomplete penetrance. The condition is caused by germline "loss-of-function" mutations in the succinate dehydrogenase subunit B (SDHB), C *(SDHC)*, or D *(SDHD)* genes. The association of gastric, multiple GISTs, with pulmonary chondromas and functional paragangliomas is known as the Carney triad. The genetic basis of the association is yet unknown.

Familial GISTs usually have a milder clinical course than sporadic cases. Imatinib mesylate may be effective in the prevention of development as well as in the treatment of hereditary GISTs.

18.1
Sporadic GISTs

18.1.1
Epidemiology and Clinicopathologic Features of GISTs

Gastrointestinal stromal tumors (GISTs) are the most common mesenchymal tumors and account for approximately 80% of gastrointestinal (GI) mesenchymal tumors, 0.1 to 3% of all GI tract malignancy, 5 to 6% of sarcomas, and 14% of all intestine malignancies [1]. An incidence of the entity is 14.5 cases per million people according to a retrospective evaluation of a series of intra-abdominal sarcomas [2]. African and Asian/Pacific Islander patients might have an increased risk of GIST compared with Caucasian patients [1, 3].

Mazur and Clark originally described these tumors in 1983 [4], noting that they contained smooth muscle and neural elements. Now recognized as a distinct clinicopathologic entity, previously GISTs were often classified as leiomyomas, leiomyosarcomas, or leiomyoblastomas [5, 6]. The peak incidence of GIST occurs late in life at a median age of 58 years; however, there are also reports of cases for GIST developing as early as in the first decade of life. The most common sites of origin for GIST are stomach (39–70%) and small intestine (31–45%). A small subset of GISTs arises outside the GI tract, and these tumors are known as extra-gastrointestinal GISTs. Histopathologically, GISTs are a heterogeneous group of tumors, featuring spindle cell, epithelioid, or mixed type morphology, and showing a wide clinical spectrum from benign to frankly malignant sarcomas. GISTs typically show expression of CD117/KIT (95%) and frequently CD34 (70%) antigens by immuno-staining, yet a small fraction of GISTs lack both diagnostic markers. Frequent clinical symptoms of GIST include bloating, GI bleeding, or fatigue related to anemia. GISTs are highly resistant to conventional radiation therapy and traditional chemotherapeutic agents. Surgery has been the basis of treatment for GISTs, but more than 50% of patients experience relapse within 5 years. The common metastatic sites for GIST include the liver and the omentum.

18.1.2
The KIT Gene

KIT is the normal cellular homolog of a viral oncogene (*v-KIT*, Hardy Zuckerman 4 feline sarcoma viral oncogene homologue), encoding a 145-kDa transmembrane glycoprotein. In humans, the *KIT* gene maps to chromosome 4q12, and is composed of 21 exons spanning 65 kb. *KIT* is a member of the receptor tyrosine kinase (TK) subclass III superfamily that also includes receptors for platelet-derived growth factors (PDGFRA and PDGFRB), macrophage colony-stimulating factor (CSF1R), and FLT3 (fms-related TK3). These TK receptors have an extracellular domain containing five immunoglobulin-like domains, a single transmembrane domain, and a cytoplasmic domain containing a split kinase domain [5].

Expression of the wildtype KIT receptor TK is essential in embryonic development. Binding of its ligand, stem cell factor (SCF), induces the dimerization of KIT and leads to an autophosphorylation of KIT on tyrosine residues, and to activation of downstream intracellular signal transduction proteins such as PI3K and AKT, signal transducers and activators of transcription (STATs), mitogen-activated protein kinases (MAPK), and JUN N-terminal kinase (JNK) [7]. The normal function of *KIT* is essential for hematopoiesis, melanogenesis, gametogenesis, development of interstitial cells of Cajal (ICCs), and mast cell growth and differentiation [8].

18.1.3
Pathogenesis and Molecular Features of GISTs

It is generally accepted that GISTs arise from a progenitor related to the ICCs, the innervated pacemaker cells that coordinate peristaltic activity throughout the gastrointestinal system, which also have the potential of giving rise to cells in the omentum and peritoneal surfaces [9, 10].

Expression of activated KIT receptor TK plays a critical role in ICCs differentiation and proliferation, and *KIT* expression is a characteristic feature of most GISTs [5, 6]. The characterization of GIST based on the expression of *KIT* was further complemented by the finding that in the majority of sporadic GISTs (70–85%), the KIT protein is constitutively activated through somatic "gain-of function" *KIT* mutations [11, 12]. Around one-third of GISTs (5–8%) that lack *KIT* mutations carry intragenic activating mutations in a related receptor TK, platelet-derived growth factor-receptor alpha *(PDGFRA)* [13]. Activating mutations in *KIT* and *PDGFRA* appear to be mutually exclusive oncogenic events, indicating that either one is sufficient to induce GIST tumorigenesis.

Oncogenic mutations in sporadic GISTs are of heterogeneous nature [5, 6]. The *KIT* mutations are found predominantly in the juxtamembrane domain of KIT receptor (70–80% of mutations), which is encoded by exon 11 of the gene, but mutations in the extracellular domain and the split kinase domains have been also described. The *KIT* exon 11 mutations are heterogeneous, encompassing mainly in-frame deletions of variable sizes, basic amino acid substitutions, or more complex deletions-insertions. The *KIT* mutations in the extracellular domain (encoded by exon 9) have been reported in 4 to 18% of all *KIT*-immunopositive primary GISTs. The vast majority of these mutations are a recurrent in-frame tandem duplication of six nucleotides, AY502-503dup. Interestingly, these GISTs are predominantly found in the small intestine, suggesting a genotype to phenotype correlation. *KIT* mutations in the split kinase domains (encoded by exon 13 and exon 17) have been uncommon, accounting for 0.6 to 1.4% of all mutations. In the case of exon 13, the predominant mutation identified is a missense mutation *K642E*. Mutations involving exon 17 are mainly *N822K* or *N822H* substitutions.

The mutations reported within *PDGFRA* involve exons 12, 14, and 18, being homologous to *KIT* exons 11, 13, and 17, respectively [14]. In more than 80% of cases, *PDGFRA* mutations target exon 18 at codons 842–849; the majority of them are point mutations leading to most common *D842V* substitution. Most of the *PDGFRA*-mutated GISTs are associated with a distinct clinicopathologic pheno-type, including gastric location, epithelioid morphology, and variable or absent *KIT* expression, with a predominantly indolent clinical course [15].

It is important to note that, even though *KIT* or *PDGFRA* mutations are detected in the majority of GISTs, there is still a significant subset of tumors that lack mutations in either gene [13, 14]. These tumors are referred to as wildtype GISTs. In adults, the wildtype GIST subset represents 10 to 15% of cases, and is a het-erogeneous group with no particular association with the anatomic site. In con-trast, pediatric GISTs predominantly express the wildtype *KIT/PDGFRA* genotype, and represent a distinct clinicopathologic and molecular group with predilection for females, multifocal manifestation at gastric sites, and a more indolent clinical course [16].

Consistent with this notion of a separate biological entity, a cDNA expression micro-array study of GISTs showed a uniform and non-complex gene expression profile, with homogenous unsupervized hierarchical clustering of a set of defined genes [5, 6]. Also, the cytogenetic profile in primary, low-risk GISTs features rela-tively simple karyotypic changes, with losses of chromosome 14q, 22q, and 1p being most common. During progression of the disease, losses in 9p and gains, or high-level amplification at 5p, 8q, 17q, and 20q are common and often coexisting.

18.1.4
Imatinib Mesylate in the Treatment of Advanced GISTs

Imatinib mesylate, originally referred to as STI571 (Glivec, Gleevec), is an oral 2-phenylaminopyrimidine derivative that acts as a selective inhibitor against onco-genic forms of Type III TKs such as KIT, *PDGFRA*, PDGFRB, and BCR-ABL, which is the causative chimeric fusion protein in chronic myelogenous leukemia. Malignant GISTs were found to be generally resistant to cancer chemotherapy and associated with poor outcome until 2000, when imatinib-mesylate was used to treat a near terminal patient on a compassionate basis [17]. Soon after, the encouraging results obtained in the first patients led to large clinical trials and prompt FDA approval of imatinib for the treatment of advanced GISTs. Of utmost importance, several clinical trials have proved that the response to imatinib correlates with the tumor genotype, with the best response observed in tumors with *KIT* exon 11 mutations. Moreover, a subset of GISTs, mainly wildtype and tumors harboring missense point mutations at *PDGFRA* codon 842 are primarily resistant to ima-tinib, underscoring the clinical value of the molecular classification of GISTs [5, 6, 14, 17].

18.2
Hereditary GISTs

Hereditary forms of the disease arise in the settings of primary familial GIST syndrome or other hereditary syndromes. Specifically, GIST has been found associated with neurofibromatosis type I (NF1) or von Recklinghausen's disease, the dyad of "paraganglioma and gastric stromal sarcoma" or Carney–Stratakis syndrome, and the Carney triad.

18.2.1
Familial GIST Syndrome

Familial GIST syndrome is an autosomal dominant genetic disorder, showing a high penentrance and representing a small subset of clinical GISTs [6]. Germline missense mutations or small in-frame deletions of the *KIT* or *PDFGRA* genes cause most familial cases of GIST: to date, 21 families have been identified (Table 18.1) [12, 18–39].

As in sporadic forms of the disease, all germline *KIT* mutations are gain-of-function, with mutations reported primarily in exon 11 and some in exons 13 and 17. The family described by Hartmann and co-workers [26] displayed a unique mutation in exon 8 of the *KIT* gene, an exon whose mutation has not previously been associated with sporadic GISTs.

Familial GIST syndrome, associated with germline *KIT* mutations, is characterized by certain clinicopathologic features, which are distinct from sporadic GISTs. Patients carrying this syndrome develop GISTs at a younger age (median – 46 years). The tumors are usually multiple in number (3 to >100 tumors), smaller in size, and occur in a background of polyclonal diffuse hyperplasia of ICCs within the myenteric plexus, both intimately and remote from the neoplastic lesions. The predominant site of tumor development is stomach and small intestine, but other GI locations are also reported. Additional abnormalities may be present, with a substantial clinical variability and no firm evidence of genotype-phenotype manifestation. In addition to GIST predisposition, germline *KIT* mutations result in other types of gastrointestinal pathology, particularly in disrupted bowel motility, such as dysphagia, constipation, or gastroesophageal reflux symptoms, suggesting that abnormalities of peristalsis and sphincter tone are clinically relevant. A significant number of familial GIST patients have cutaneous hyperpigmentation, particularly around the mouth, in the perineum, on the face, neck, digits, axillae, groin, and knees. Other features that are linked with the dysfunction of melanocytes, such as melanocytic navi, lentigines, café au lait spots, and vitiligo are also seen. Abnormalities of mast cells, mainly urticaria pigmentosa or systemic mastocytosis in infancy, are less frequently reported. Symptoms associated with GI bleeding (anemia and melanea) are common and may be the only manifestation of the disease. Some *KIT* mutant kindreds have increased incidences of other types of cancer, including melanoma, and esophageal, breast, and prostate carcinomas; however, it is not clear whether there is a direct link between the development of these cancers and inherited mutant *KIT*.

Mutation in the gene encoding PDGFRA has been reported in three families [37–39]. A germline *PDGFRA* D846Y substitution co-segregated with the GIST phenotype in a French family reported by Chompret and co-workers [36], in which five individuals revealed gastric nodules typical of GISTs. *PDGFR.A.* Asp846 is homologous to *KIT*. Asp820 located within the *KIT* TK II domain,

Table 18.1 Clinical features of reported families with germline *KIT* and *PDGFRA* mutations.

No	Mutation	GISTs location	Pigmentation anomalies	GI dysmotility symptoms	Mast cell anomalies	Ref.
1.	*KIT*: p.D417del	Sm. Intestine	No	No	Mastocytosis	[26]
2.	*KIT*: p.W557R	Sm. Intestine, Stomach	Cutaneous hyperpigmentation	Dysphagia	No	[24]
3.	*KIT*: p.W557R	Sm. Intestine,	No	No	No	[19]
4	*KIT*: p.W557R	Stomach	Generalized lentigines, melanocytic navi	No	No	[23]
4.	*KIT*: p.V559A	Stomach, Sm. Intestine,	No	No	Urticaria pigmentosa	[20]
5.	*KIT*: p.V559A	Stomach, Sm. Intestine	Cutaneous hyperpigmentation, melanocytic navi	No	No	[21]
6.	*KIT*: p.V559A	Stomach, Sm. Intestine	Lentigines, melanocytic nevi, café-au-lait spots, vitiligo	No	Urticaria pigmentosa	[27]
7.	*KIT*: p.V559A	Sm. Intestine	Nd	nd	nd	[28]
8.	*KIT*: p.V559A	Sm. Intestine	No	No	No	[34]
9.	*KIT*: p.V559del	nd	Yes	No	No	[31]
10.	*KIT*: p.V560G	Sm. Intestine	No	No	No	[34]
11.	*KIT*: p.Q575_P577delinsH	Rectum	No	Constipation	No	[35]
12.	*KIT*: p.L576_P577insQL	Stomach, Sm. Intestine	Cutaneous hyperpigmentation	No	No	[25]
13.	*KIT*: p.D579del	nd	Cutaneous hyperpigmantation	No	No	[18]
14.	*KIT*: p.D579del	Sm. Intestine	Nd	nd	nd	[32]
15.	*KIT*: p.K642E	Sm. Intestine	Nd	nd	nd	[12]

Table 18.1 *Continued*

No	Mutation	GISTs location	Pigmentation anomalies	GI dysmotility symptoms	Mast cell anomalies	Ref.
16.	*KIT*: p.K642E	Esophagus, Stomach, Sm. Intestine, Rectum	No		No	[33]
17.	*KIT*: p.D820Y	Stomach	No	Dysphagia	No	[22]
18.	*KIT*: p.D820Y	Stomach, Sm. Intestine	No	Small intestinal diverticulosis, dysphagia	No	[30]
19.	*PDGFRA*: p.D846Y	Stomach	Nd	nd	nd	[36]
20.	*PDGFRA*: p.Y555C	Sm. Intestine	No	No	No	[37]
21.	PDGFRA: p.D561A	Stomach, Sm. Intestine	No	Small intestinal diverticulosis	No	[39]

nd = no data.

and two families with germline *KIT* D820Y, have been described worldwide [22, 30].

The second family presented with a germline activating mutation in *PDGFRA* (p.Y555C), and the rare condition known as intestinal neurofibromatosis [37]. Intestinal neurofibromatosis (OMIM 162220), also called NF3b, is phenotypically described as multiple neurofibromas strictly limited to the intestine of adult onset with incomplete penetrance, autosomal dominant inheritance pattern, and absence of other features of NF1 or NF2 [39]. The tumors in the reported family were morphologically identical to intestinal neurofibromas, but immunohistochemically they did not express the S100 protein (a marker of neural differentiation) or any of the known GIST markers (such as KIT, CD34, or DOG1 proteins). We have proposed to classify these tumors as familial *KIT*-negative GISTs.

Recently, a 22-year-old patient with a germline *PDGFRA* D561V missense substitution, and a unique combination of multiple fibrous tumors and lipomas of the small intestine and several gastric GISTs, was described [38].

Notably, none of the additional components of familial GIST syndrome, such as hyperpigmentation, dysphagia, or mast cell abnormalities, previously described in germline KIT mutation kindreds, were present in the *PDGFRA* mutation carriers. Interestingly, in two families all affected family members displayed unusually large hands [36, 37] – a phenotype not described so far in families associated with germline *KIT* mutations, providing a clue in favor of a causal relationship between constitutive PDGFRA activation, and congenital malformation of the hands.

The clinical behavior of familial GIST is generally benign; however, despite the absence of metastases in most individuals, the symptoms associated with the development of GIST, particularly GI bleeding, may result in significant morbidity. Imatinib may be effective in the prevention of development as well as in the treatment of hereditary GISTs [33, 35]. The careful monitoring for the development of tumors is indicated, but the indolent clinical course in most of the reported families, and the multifocality of the disease, suggests that surgical intervention should be avoided in the absence of complications.

18.2.2
GISTs Associated with Neurofibromatosis Type I

Based on a single Swedish study, adults with NF1 have a 7% risk for GISTs [2]. GISTs in NF1 patients tend to be multiple and are located predominantly within the small intestine, though a few have been reported in other anatomic sites [40–43]. Abdominal pain, bowel obstruction, and massive gastrointestinal bleeding are the most common presenting clinical manifestations. Morphologically and immunohistochemically, GISTs occurring in NF1 patients stain positive for *KIT*, like most other GISTs. Compared to sporadic GISTs, NF1-GISTs are more likely to show S-100 reactivity, entrapped myenteric nerves within the tumor, and the presence of skeinoid fibers [40, 43]. Although they may fall into any GIST risk category, NF1-GISTs usually show low cell proliferation (growth) indicators, and they rarely metastasize. Andersson and co-workers [40] reported follow-up for 9 NF1 patients who had surgery for GIST; none of the patients died of GIST, and 6 of 9 were well up to 32 years later.

The vast majority of GISTs associated with NF1 do not have *KIT* or *PDGFRA* mutations [40–43]. We have recently demonstrated that GIST development in patients with NF1 is caused by a somatic inactivation of the wildtype NF1 allele in the tumor, resulting in the absence of neurofibromin as an alternative mechanism of hyperactive signaling events downstream of KIT [42]. Particularly, NF1-related GISTs show an increased signaling through the MAP-kinase pathway as compared with sporadic GIST. These findings clearly position GISTs in the range of clinical symptoms seen in NF1. There is only one published paper about response of NF1-GISTs to TK inhibitor drugs such as imatinib; Lee and co-authors [44] report a case of NF1-GIST that did respond to the treatment.

18.2.3
Carney–Stratakis Syndrome

In a subset of patients with gastric GISTs, the lesions are associated with paragangliomas (PGLs) [45]. The condition referred to as the dyad of paraganglioma and gastric stromal sarcoma or the Carney–Stratakis syndrome (OMIM 606864) is familial and transmitted as an autosomal-dominant trait with incomplete pene-trance. The patients present tumors at a young age (median age 19 years). They are multifocal and paragangliomas multicentric, supporting a genetic link between the two lesions [46]. PGLs are neuroendocrine tumors that may secrete catecholamines. They occur most frequently in the head (glomus tympanicum and jugulare), neck (carotid body and glomus vagale), adrenal medulla, and extra-adrenal sympathetic ganglia. Once the diagnosis is made, patients must be followed carefully in order to detect new lesions as early as possible, since both entities have malignant potential. A functioning paraganglioma may manifest itself by sympathetic effects such as hypertension, diaphoresis, and/or facial flush-ing. A ^{131}I-MIBG scan is useful for diagnosis, as this agent localizes to catechol-amine-producing tissues. If the lesion is unresectable, radiation and chemotherapy may be used.

GISTs in Carney–Stratakis syndrome patients do not carry the *KIT* or *PDGFRA* gene mutations. The underlying hereditary defect of the Carney–Stratakis syn-drome has been elucidated recently by identification of germline "loss-of function" mutations in the succinate dehydrogenase subunit B *(SDHB)*, C *(SDHC)*, or D *(SDHD)* genes in affected patients [46]. The identified mutations had been described before in sporadic or familial pheochromocytomas or extra-adrenal para-gangliomas, an autosomal dominant inherited cancer-susceptibility syndrome. Notably, the abdominal paragangliomas associated with GISTs are uniquely cor-related with *SDHC* mutations. The absence of *KIT* or *PDGFRA* somatic mutations and inactivation of one of the succinate dehydrogenase subunits in GISTs/PGLs from patients with the dyad, suggests that a deficient mitochondrial tumor sup-pressor gene pathway is responsible for tumor formation, rather than constitu-tively active TKs.

18.2.4
Carney Triad

In 1977, Carney described the triad of gastric epithelioid leiomyosarcoma, func-tioning extra-adrenal paraganglioma, and pulmonary chondroma (OMIM 604287) [47]. Nowadays, gastric leiomyosarcoma is re-classified as GIST. There is an approximately 10-fold female predominance. The genetic and pathologic basis of the association is currently unknown [48]. Due to the rarity of these tumors, the presence of any two of them is regarded as a sufficient basis for making the diag-nosis. The complete triad is present in about one-third of cases; gastric GISTs are most frequently present (~97%), followed by pulmonary chondroma (~83%), and paraganglioma (~53%). The tumors can appear in any order and in a wide frame of time. Two of these three entities have malignant potential, and the overall mortality of the triad is approximately 20%. Recently, esophageal leiomyoma has been described as an additional component occurring in some triad patients [49].

A number of tumors associated with this entity were tested for *KIT, PDGFRA, SDHA, SDHB, SDHC,* and *SDHD* mutations, but none was found [48–50]. These multifocal GISTs usually have a milder clinical course when present within the context of Carney's triad, than in sporadic cases. The lesion is typically treated by wide resection and omentectomy. Imatinib had no apparent effect on liver metastases in the case described by Diment *et al.* [50]. However, Delemarre and co-workers [51] did report a patient for whom imatinib was effective. Most paragangliomas are extra-adrenal (~85%) and nonfunctional. Pulmonary chondromas are benign hamartomas, and are multiple in about 63% of cases. They are frequently mistaken for metastases. The diagnosis is established by excision biopsy or, if the triad is already established, by needle biopsy. If the pulmonary lesions display characteristic diffuse popcorn calcification, a radiographic diagnosis is possible. If the pathology is unequivocally benign, the patient can be followed radiographically.

References

1 Demetri, G.D., Benjamin, R.S., Blanke, C.D., Blay, J.Y., Casali, P., Choi, H., Corless, C.L., Debiec-Rychter, M., DeMatteo, R.P., Ettinger, D.S., Fisher, G.A., Fletcher, C.D., Gronchi, A., Hohenberger, P., Hughes, M., Joensuu, H., Judson, I., Le Cesne, A, Maki, R.G., Morse, M., Pappo, A.S., Pisters, P.W., Raut, C.P., Reichardt, P., Tyler, D.S., Van den Abbeele, A.D., von Mehren, M., Wayne, J.D., Zalcberg, J. and NCCN Force Task (2007) NCCN Task Force report: management of patients with gastrointestinal stromal tumor (GIST) – update of the NCCN clinical practice guidelines. *Journal of the National Comprehensive Cancer Network*, **5**, S1–29.

2 Nilsson, B., Bumming, P., Meis-Kindblom, J.M., Oden, A., Dortok, A., Gustavsson, B., Sablinska, K. and Kindblom, L.G. (2005) Gastrointestinal stromal tumors: the incidence, prevalence, clinical course, and prognostication in the preimatinib mesylate era – a population-based study in western Sweden. *Cancer*, **103**, 821–9.

3 Chan, K.H., Chan, C.W., Chow, W.H., Kwan, W.K., Kong, C.K., Mak, K.F., Leung, M.Y. and Lau, L.K. (2006) Gastrointestinal stromal tumors in a cohort of Chinese patients in Hong Kong. *World Journal of Gastroenterology*, **12**, 2223–8.

4 Mazur, M.T. and Clark, H.B. (1983) Gastric stromal tumors. Reappraisal of histogenesis. *The American Journal of Surgical Pathology*, **7**, 507–19.

5 Corless, C.L., Fletcher, J.A. and Heinrich, M.C. (2004) Biology of gastrointestinal stromal tumors. *Journal of Clinical Oncology*, **22**, 3813–25.

6 Miettinen, M. and Lasota, J. (2006) Gastrointestinal stromal tumors: review on morphology, molecular pathology, prognosis, and differential diagnosis. *Archives of Pathology and Laboratory Medicine*, **130**, 1466–78.

7 Ullrich, A. and Schlessinger, J. (1990) Signal transduction by receptors with tyrosine kinase activity. *Cell*, **61**, 203–12.

8 Dolci, S., Williams, D.E., Ernst, M.K., Resnick, J.L., Brannan, C.I., Lock, L.F., Lyman, S.D., Boswell, H.S. and Donovan, P.J. (1991) Requirement for mast cell growth factor for primordial germ cell survival in culture. *Nature*, **352**, 809–11.

9 Kindblom, L.G., Remotti, H.E., Aldenborg, F. and Meis-Kindblom, J.M. (1998) Gastrointestinal pacemaker cell tumor (GIPACT): gastrointestinal stromal tumors show phenotypic characteristics of the interstitial cells of Cajal. *American Journal of Pathology*, **152**, 1259–69.

10 Sircar, K., Hewlett, B.R., Huizinga, J.D., Chorneyko, K., Berezin, I. and Riddell, R.H. (1999) Interstitial cells of Cajal as

precursors of gastrointestinal stromal tumors. *The American journal of Surgical Pathology*, **23**, 377–89.

11 Hirota, S., Isozaki, K., Moriyama, Y., Hashimoto, K., Nishida, T., Ishiguro, S., Kawano, K., Hanada, M., Kurata, A., Takeda, M., Muhammad, T.G., Matsuzawa, Y., Kanakura, K., Shinomura, Y. and Kitamura, Y. (1998) Gain-of-function mutations of *c-KIT* in human gastrointestinal stromal tumors. *Science*, **279**, 577–80.

12 Isozaki, K., Terris, B., Belghiti, J., Schiffmann, S., Hirota, S. and Vanderwinden, J.M. (2000) Germline-activating mutation in the kinase domain of *KIT* gene in familial gastrointestinal stromal tumors. *American Journal of Pathology*, **157**, 1581–5.

13 Heinrich, M.C., Corless, C.L., Duensing, A., McGreevey, L., Chen, C.J., Joseph, N., Singer, S., Griffith, D.J., Haley, A., Town, A., Demetri, G.D., Fletcher, C.D. and Fletcher, J.A. (2003) *PDGFRA* activating mutations in gastrointestinal stromal tumors. *Science*, **299**, 708–10.

14 Corless, C.L., Schroeder, A., Griffith, D., Town, A., McGreevey, L., Harrell, P., Shiraga, S., Bainbridge, T., Morich, J. and Heinrich, M.C. (2005) PDGFRA mutations in gastrointestinal stromal tumors: frequency, spectrum and *in vitro* sensitivity to imatinib. *Journal of Clinical Oncology*, **23**, 5357–64.

15 Lasota, J., Dansonka-Mieszkowska, A., Sobin, L.H. and Miettinen, M. (2004) A great majority of GISTs with PDGFRA mutations represent gastric tumors of low or no malignant potential. *Laboratory Investigation*, **84**, 874–83.

16 Prakash, S., Sarran, L., Socci, N., DeMatteo, R.P., Eisenstat, J., Greco, A. M., Maki, R.G., Wexler, L.H., LaQuaglia, M.P., Besmer, P. and Antonescu, C.R. (2005) Gastrointestinal stromal tumors in children and young adults: a clinico-pathologic, molecular, and genomic study of 15 cases and review of the literature. *Journal of Pediatric Hematology/Oncology*, **27**, 179–87.

17 Siddiqui, M.A. and Scott, L.J. (2007) Imatinib: a review of its use in the management of gastrointestinal stromal tumours. *Drugs*, **67**, 805–20.

18 Nishida, T., Hirota, S., Taniguchi, M., Hashimoto, K., Isozaki, K., Nakamura, H., Kanakura, Y., Tanaka, T., Takabayashi, A., Matsuda, H. and Kitamura, Y. (1998) Familial gastrointestinal stromal tumours with germline mutation of the *KIT* gene. *Nature Genetics*, **19**, 323–4.

19 Hirota, S., Okazaki, T., Kitamura, Y., O'Brien, P., Kapusta, L. and Dardick, I. (2000) Cause of familial and multiple gastrointestinal autonomic nerve tumors with hyperplasia of interstitial cells of Cajal is germline mutation of the *c-KIT* gene. *The American journal of Surgical Pathology*, **24**, 326–7.

20 Beghini, A., Tibiletti, M.G., Roversi, G., Chiaravalli, A.M., Serio, G., Capella, C. and Larizza, L. (2001) Germline mutation in the juxtamembrane domain of the kit gene in a family with gastrointestinal stromal tumors and urticaria pigmentosa. *Cancer*, **92**, 657–62.

21 Maeyama, H., Hidaka, E., Ota, H., Minami, S., Kajiyama, M., Kuraishi, A., Mori, H., Matsuda, Y., Wada, S., Sodeyama, H., Nakata, S., Kawamura, N., Hata, S., Watanabe, M., Iijima, Y. and Katsuyama, T. (2001) Familial gastrointestinal stromal tumor with hyperpigmentation: association with a germline mutation of the *c-KIT* gene. *Gastroenterology*, **120**, 210–15.

22 Hirota, S., Nishida, T., Isozaki, K., Taniguchi, M., Nishikawa, K., Ohashi, A., Takabayashi, A., Obayashi, T., Okuno, T., Kinoshita, K., Chen, H., Shinomura, Y. and Kitamura, Y. (2002) Familial gastrointestinal stromal tumors associated with dysphagia and novel type germline mutation of *KIT* gene. *Gastroenterology*, **122**, 1493–9.

23 Shibusawa, Y., Tamura, A., Mochiki, E., Kamisaka, K., Kimura, H. and Ishikawa, O. (2004) *c-KIT* mutation in generalized lentigines associated with gastrointestinal stromal tumor. *Dermatology*, **208**, 217–20.

24 Robson, M.E., Glogowski, E., Sommer, G., Antonescu, C.R., Nafa, K., Maki, R.G., Ellis, N., Besmer, P., Brennan, M. and Offit, K. (2004) Pleomorphic characteristics of a germ-line *KIT* mutation in a large kindred with gastrointestinal stromal tumors, hyperpigmentation, and

dysphagia. *Clinical Cancer Research*, **10**, 1250–4.

25 Carballo, M., Roig, I., Aguilar, F., Pol, M.A., Gamundi, M.J., Hernan, I. and Martinez-Gimeno, M. (2005) Novel *c-KIT* germline mutation in a family with gastrointestinal stromal tumors and cutaneous hyperpigmentation. *American Journal of Medical Genetics*, **132**, 361–4.

26 Hartmann, K., Wardelmann, E., Ma, Y., Merkelbach-Bruse, S., Preussner, L.M., Woolery, C., Baldus, S.E., Heinicke, T., Thiele, J., Buettner, R. and Longley, B.J. (2005) Novel germline mutation of *KIT* associated with familial gastrointestinal stromal tumors and mastocytosis. *Gastroenterology*, **129**, 1042–6.

27 Li, F.P., Fletcher, J.A., Heinrich, M.C., Garber, J.E., Sallan, S.E., Curiel-Lewandrowski, C., Duensing, A., van de Rijn, M., Schnipper, L.E. and Demetri, G.D. (2005) Familial gastrointestinal stromal tumor syndrome: phenotypic and molecular features in a kindred. *Journal of Clinical Oncology*, **23**, 2735–43.

28 Kim, H.J., Lim, S.J., Park, K., Yuh, Y.J., Jang, S.J. and Choi, J. (2005) Multiple gastrointestinal stromal tumors with a germline c-*KIT* mutation. *Pathology International*, **55**, 655–9.

29 Kinoshita, K., Hirota, S., Isozaki, K., Ohashi, A., Nishida, T., Kitamura, Y., Shinomura, Y. and Matsuzawa, Y. (2004) Absence of *c-KIT* gene mutations in gastrointestinal stromal tumours from neurofibromatosis type 1 patients. *The Journal of Pathology*, **202**, 80–5.

30 O'Riain, C., Corless, C.L., Heinrich, M.C., Keegan, D., Vioreanu, M., Maguire, D. and Sheahan, K. (2005) Gastrointestinal stromal tumors: insights from a new familial GIST kindred with unusual genetic and pathologic features. *The American Journal of Surgical Pathology*, **29**, 1680–3.

31 Tarn, C., Merkel, E., Canutescu, A.A., Shen, W., Skorobogatko, Y., Heslin, M.J., Eisenberg, B., Birbe, R., Patchefsky, A., Dunbrack, R., Arnoletti, J.P., von Mehren, M. and Godwin, A.K. (2005) Analysis of *KIT* mutations in sporadic and familial gastrointestinal stromal tumors: therapeutic implications through protein modeling. *Clinical Cancer Research*, **11**, 3668–77.

32 Lasota, J. and Miettinen, M. (2006) A new familial GIST identified. *The American Journal of Surgical Pathology*, **30**, 1342.

33 Graham, J., Debiec-Rychter, M., Corless, C.L., Reid, R., Davidson, R. and White, J.D. (2007) Imatinib in the management of multiple gastrointestinal stromal tumors associated with a germline KIT K642E mutation. *Archives of Pathology and Laboratory Medicine*, **131**, 1393–6.

34 Kang, D.J., Park, C.K., Choi, J.S., Jin, S.Y., Kim, H.J., Joo, M., Kang, M.S., Moon, W.S., Yun, K.J., Yu, E.S., Kang, H. and Kim, K.M. (2007) Multiple gastrointestinal stromal tumors: clinicopathologic and genetic analysis of 12 patients. *The American Journal of Surgical Pathology*, **31**, 224–32.

35 Wozniak, A., Rutkowski, P., Sciot, R., Ruka, W., Michej, W. and Debiec-Rychter, M. Rectal gastrointestinal stromal tumors associated with a novel germline *KIT* mutation. *International Journal of Cancer*, **122**, 2160–4.

36 Chompret, A., Kannengiesser, C., Barrois, M., Terrier, P., Dahan, P., Tursz, T., Lenoir, G.M. and Bressac-De Paillerets, B. (2004) PDGFRA germline mutation in a family with multiple cases of gastro-intestinal stromal tumor. *Gastroenterology*, **126**, 318–21.

37 de Raedt, T., Cools, J., Debiec-Rychter, M., Brems, H., Mentens, N., Sciot, R., Himpens, J., de Waver, I., Schoffski, P., Marynen, P. and Legius, E. (2006) Intestinal neurofibromatosis is a subtype of familial GIST and results from a dominant activating mutation in PDGFRA. *Gastroenterology*, **131**, 1907–12.

38 Heimann, R., Verhest, A., Verschraegen, J., Grosjean, W., Draps, J.P. and Hecht, F. (1988) Hereditary intestinal neurofibromatosis. I. A distinctive genetic disease. *Neurofibromatosis*, **1**, 26–32.

39 Pasini, B., Matyakhina, L., Bei, T., Muchow, M., Boikos, S., Ferrando, B., Carney, J.A. and Stratakis, C.A. (2007) Multiple gastrointestinal stromal and other tumors caused by platelet-derived growth factor receptor {alpha} gene mutations: a case associated with a germline V561D

defect. *Journal of Clinical Endocrinology and Metabolism*, **92**, 3728–32.

40 Andersson, J., Sihto, H., Meis-Kindblom, J.M., Joensuu, H., Nupponen, N. and Kindblom, L.G. (2005) NF1-associated gastrointestinal stromal tumors have unique clinical, phenotypic, and genotypic characteristics. *The American Journal of Surgical Pathology*, **29**, 1170–6.

41 Kinoshita, K., Hirota, S. and Isozaki, K. (2004) Absence of c-KIT gene mutations in gastrointestinal stromal tumors from neurofibromatosis type 1 patients. *Journal of Pathology*, **202**, 80–5.

42 Maertens, O., Prenen, H., Debiec-Rychter, M., Wozniak, A., Sciot, R., Pauwels, P., De Wever, I., Vermeesch, J. R., de Raedt, T., De Paepe, A., Speleman, F., van Oosterom, A., Messiaen, L. and Legius, E. (2006) Molecular pathogenesis of multiple gastrointestinal stromal tumors in NF1 patients. *Human Molecular Genetics*, **15**, 1015–23.

43 Miettinen, M., Fetsch, J.F., Sobin, L.H. and Lasota, J. (2006) Gastrointestinal stromal tumors in patients with neurofibromatosis 1: a clinicopathologic and molecular genetic study of 45 cases. *The American Journal of Surgical Pathology*, **30**, 90–6.

44 Lee, J.L., Kim, J.Y., Ryu, M.H., Kang, H.J., Chang, H.M., Kim, T.W., Lee, H., Park, J.H., Kim, H.C., Kim, J.S. and Kang, Y.K. (2006) Response to Imatinib in KIT- and PDGFRA-Wild Type Gastrointestinal Stromal Associated with Neurofibromatosis Type 1. *Digestive Diseases and Sciences*, **51**, 1043–6.

45 Carney, J.A. and Stratakis, C.A. (2002) Familial paraganglioma and gastric stromal sarcoma: a new syndrome distinct from the Carney triad. *American Journal of Medical Genetics*, **108**, 132–9.

46 Pasini, B., McWhinney, S.R., Bei, T., Matyakhina, L., Stergiopoulos, S.S., Muchow, M.M., Boikos, S.A., Ferrando, B., Pacak, K., Assie, G., Baudin, E.,

Chompret, A., Ellison, J.W., Briere, J.-J., Rustin, P., Gimenez-Roqueplo, A.-P., Eng, C., Carney, J.A. and Stratakis, C.A. (2007) Clinical and molecular genetics of patients with the Carney–Stratakis syndrome and germline mutations of the genes coding for the succinate dehydrogenase subunits SDHB, SDHC, and SDHD. *European Journal of Human Genetics*, **16**, 79–88.

47 Carney, J.A., Sheps, S.G., Go, V.L. and Gordon, H. (1977) The triad of gastric leiomyosarcoma, functioning extra-adrenal paraganglioma, and pulmonary chondroma. *The New England Journal of Medicine*, **296**, 1517–18.

48 Matyakhina, L., Bei, T.A., McWhinney, S.R., Pasini, B., Cameron, S., Gunawan, B., Stergiopoulos, S.G., Boikos, S., Muchow, M., Dutra, A., Pak, E., Campo, E., Cid, M.C., Gomez, F., Gaillard, R.C., Assie, G., Fuzesi, L., Baysal, B.E., Eng, C., Carney, J.A. and Stratakis, C.A. (2007) Genetics of Carney triad: recurrent losses at chromosome 1 but lack of germline mutations in genes associated with paragangliomas and gastrointestinal stromal tumors. *Journal of Clinical Endocrinology and Metabolism*, **92**, 2938–43.

49 Knop, S., Schupp, M., Wardelmann, E., Stueker, D., Horger, M.S., Kanz, L., Einsele, H. and Kroeber, S.M. (2006) A new case of Carney triad: gastrointestinal stromal tumours and leiomyoma of the oesophagus do not show activating mutations of KIT and platelet-derived growth factor receptor alpha. *Journal of Clinical Pathology*, **59**, 1097–9.

50 Diment, J., Tamborini, E., Casali, P., Gronchi, A., Carney, J.A. and Colecchia, M. (2005) Carney triad: case report and molecular analysis of gastric tumor. *Human Pathology*, **36**, 112–16.

51 Delemarre, L., Aronson, D., van Rijn, R., Bras, H., Arets, B. and Verschuur, A. (2006) Respiratory symptoms in a boy revealing Carney triad. *Pediatric Blood and Cancer*, **50**, 399–401.

19
Hereditary Gastric Cancer

Holger Vogelsang and Gisela Keller

Summary

Familial gastric cancer (FGC) aggregation with at least two first- or second-degree gastric cancer cases can be observed in 15 to 20% of the patients. Five percent of the families even show up with three or more gastric cancer cases. Finally, less than 2% of gastric cancer cases can be identified as mutation positive hereditary gastric cancer. Therefore strong FGC aggregation without identifiable mutational background represents the majority of families that have to be considered as potentially hereditary. This group cannot be dissected by genetic characteristics but by certain phenotypic characteristics, such as familial pattern, gastric cancer subtype, age of manifestation, and associated tumors. Germline mutation has been identified for three categories of hereditary gastric cancer: hereditary diffuse type gastric cancer (HDGC – E-cadherin gene), hereditary colorectal cancer (HNPCC – mismatch repair genes), and particularly rare syndromes (Li–Fraumeni–*p53* gene; polyposis syndromes–various genes). For all of these syndromes, at least some specific phenotypic-characteristics of single gastric cancer cases as well as the familial pattern can be described.

Mutation screening is stratified according to the number of gastric cancer cases, age of manifestation, histological subtype of gastric cancer observed, and associated family pattern of other tumor diseases. As the life-time risk for gastric cancer is particularly high in E-cadherin mutation carriers (HDGC) at 60 to 80%, and endoscopic surveillance for diffuse type gastric cancer instead of difficult prophylactic gastrectomy has been offered and performed. In all other syndromes there is no option of prophylactic therapy but only surveillance and extended radicality in cases of gastric cancer manifestation, as limited endoscopic or surgical therapy has to calculate the risk of synchronous multifocal or metachronous recurrent disease of the same organ. Predictive testing in first-degree relatives of germline mutation carriers can detect persons at risk for gastric cancer or other tumors and exclude non-mutation carriers from surveillance programs. In families with strong gastric cancer aggregation without identifiable germline mutation, at least all first-degree relatives have to be considered as persons at risk and surveillance has to

Hereditary Tumors: From Genes to Clinical Consequences
Edited by Heike Allgayer, Helga Rehder and Simone Fulda
Copyright © 2009 WILEY-VCH Verlag GmbH & Co. KGaA, Weinheim
ISBN: 978-3-527-32028-8

be offered according to the clinical phenotype observed (age of manifestation, gastric cancer subtype, and associated tumor disease). Additional macroscopic and histological potential risk factors (atrophic gastritis, metaplasia, neoplasia) assessed by endoscopy may help to stratify surveillance programs. The Munich Hereditary Gastric Cancer Registry at the University of Technology (www.tumorgen.de) collected data and performed mutation screening over a period of almost 15 years. Participants of an international interdisciplinary group working on hereditary and FGC, the International Gastric Cancer Linkage Consortium (IGCLC), have been performing studies on new candidate genes, establishing functional tests for missense mutations, analyzing mutation detection rates in cohorts of FGC cases, and publishing guidelines for the management of hereditary and FGC.

19.1
Introduction to Gastric Cancer

Gastric cancer is among the top five solid tumors worldwide, but incidence differs depending on countries. Korea, Japan, Chile, Portugal, and Tuscany (Italy) are regions with the highest incidence of gastric cancer compared to a low and altogether decreasing incidence in Europe and the United States (http://www-dep.iarc.fr/; http://www.who.int./healthinfo/paper13.pdf.). Cumulative incidence of the German population up to 74 years of age is 0.7% for females and 1.7% for males (http://www.krebsinfo.de/ki/daten/magen/mag_bas.html). The WHO classification describes four major histological subtypes of gastric cancer: tubular, papillary, mucinous, and signet cell [1]. Lauren classification has the most epidemiological and clinical impact by differentiating the intestinal, diffuse, mixed, and non-classifiable subtypes [2]. With regard to prognostic and clinical studies, only the intestinal and non-intestinal subtypes have been distinguished. Regarding localization, the gastric body has been subdivided into the proximal (including cardiac cancer), middle, and distal third, with some tumors affecting more than one third up to the whole stomach by the diffuse type gastric cancer (linitis plastica). The most well-known contribution to carcinogenesis is the impact of infection by Helicobacter pylori (HP). Its genotype, as well as the host genotype regarding cytokines, has been identified as important factors influencing oncogenesis [3, 4]. Moreover, genetic factors with major or minor impact to carcinogenesis have been supposed. Molecular aspects of gastric cancer carcinogenesis are summarized in Table 19.1.

Surveillance for gastric cancer, either by radiographic investigation or endoscopy, has been successfully implemented in Asian countries with a high incidence of gastric cancer. In Europe or the United States, with an intermediate or low incidence of gastric cancer, no surveillance strategies have been introduced. Because of gastric cancer causing no symptoms in the early stages, most tumors are diagnosed as locally advanced or even systemically metastasized. Endoscopic or conventional surgery offers curative treatment in the early stages. Complete

Table 19.1 Oncogenesis of gastric cancer.

	Subtypes		
	Diffuse	**Both**	**Intestinal**
Regular mucosa	E-cadherin	Germline mutation *MLH1, MSH2, MSH6* Polymorphism *H. pylori*	
Premalignant changes	Globoid dysplasia		Non-invasive neoplasia (low-grade) high-grade
Mutations/LOH		*p53* *APC* *MSI*-Pathway *TGF IIR* *BAX* *IGFRII* *MSH3/6* *E2F-4*	*k-Ras* *bcl-2*
Methylation	E-cadherin-promotor		
Amplification		*C-met*	
Expression		*Cyclin E* ↑ *EGF* ↑ *EGFR* ↑ *TGF-* ↑	
Early cancer			
Mutations/LOH			β-Catenin *DCC*
Expression		Transcription factors ↑	*VEGF* ↑
Advanced cancer			
Amplification			*C-erB2*
Expression			E-Cadherin ↓ SIP1 ↑

tumor resection, and moreover, long-term patient survival is less frequently achieved in locally advanced gastric cancer treated by surgery alone. Therefore, neoadjuvant and adjuvant strategies with chemo- or radio-chemotherapy have been implemented to improve the outcome [5–7]. Five-year survival of early gastric cancer of the mucosa or submucosa type is 95 and 85%, respectively. Prognosis of stage II and IIIA gastric cancer depends on the surgical experience related to the incidence. Whereas 5-year survival in the United States is between 15 and 30%, figures in Germany are somewhat better with 45 and 33%, and even better in Japan with 75 and 60% [8–10].

19.2
Criteria of Potential Heredity

Familial occurrence of the same tumor entity or somehow related tumor entities of other organs with at least two second-degree family members is a minimal requirement for potential heredity of a rather rare tumor disease, suggesting a possibly autosomal dominant pedigree, in most cases with penetrance lower than 100%. Early onset tumor manifestation suggests potentially hereditary factors. As the mean age of gastric cancer patients is between 63 and 65 years, and the age-related highest incidence is in the group of patients over 70 years of age, gastric cancer manifestation before 50 years or even younger than 40 years is remarkably young. Synchronous or metachronous tumor manifestation of the same organ or in other organs somehow potentially related might hint at hereditary disease.

19.3
Hereditary Gastric Cancer

There are two hereditary gastric cancer entities going along with familial occurrence of gastric cancer, suggesting an autosomal dominant pedigree with a penetrance below 100%: hereditary diffuse type gastric cancer (HDGC), and familial gastric cancer (FGC) with a so far unknown mutational background. Within hereditary non-polyposis colorectal cancer (HNPCC), gastric cancer is the third most common following colorectal and endometrial cancer. Nevertheless, most HNPCC families do not present with gastric cancer, some with single gastric cancer cases, and just a few with a familial type manifestation. Finally, there are some rare hereditary tumor or polyposis syndromes with an identified mutational background, along with an increased incidence of gastric cancer compared to the main population, but in most families not showing up with a familial type of gastric cancer manifestation (Table 19.2).

Table 19.2 Types of hereditary gastric cancer.

Entity	Gene	Familial clustering	Mean age (years)	Characteristics
HDGC	E-cadherin	Yes	40	Diffuse subtype, lobular breast cancer
HNPCC	Mismatch repair	Exceptionally	56–58	Colorectal cancer
FGC of unknown origin	Unknown heterogenous	Yes	Early/late onset families	
Li Fraumeni syndrome	*p53*	Exceptionally	35	Sarcomas, breast cancer, early onset tumors
Polyposis syndromes	Various (see Table 19.6)	No	No data	Gastrointestinal polyps (specific, hamartomatous, adenomatous)

19.4
Hereditary Diffuse Type Gastric Cancer (HDGC)

19.4.1
Clinical Presentation

This very rare FGC syndrome is caused by a germline mutation in the adhesion molecule E-cadherin with an autosomal-dominant pedigree pattern. First described in 1998, in New Zealand Maori families, European families had been presented in 1999 [11–15]. Since then, at least 68 families with E-cadherin germline mutations have been identified worldwide, with at least 8 families in Germany and Austria [16–27]. The leading tumor entity is gastric cancer of the diffuse subtype according to Lauren. In addition, the incidence of breast cancer of the lobular subtype is increased, and perhaps there might also be a slightly increased incidence of colorectal and questionably of prostatic cancer. The mean age of gastric cancer manifestation is about 40 years, with some very young patients aged 14 and 15 years. Life-time risk for gastric cancer has been calculated as 83% for female and 67% for male mutation carriers. A very rough calculation of the life-time risk for breast cancer is about 38% in female mutation carriers [17, 22, 28–30]. There are no data regarding the prevalence of HDGC to date.

Criteria for E-cadherin screening accepted internationally are presented in Table 19.3, with examples of pedigrees in Figure 19.1. Because of gastric cancer having

Table 19.3 Screening criteria for E-cadherin germline mutation.

1. At least two first- or second-degree family members with gastric cancer, non-intestinal, or unknown Lauren subtype. 1 younger than 50 years.

2. At least three first- or second-degree family members with gastric cancer, non-intestinal, or unknown Lauren subtype.

3. At least two first- or second-degree family members with gastric and breast cancer, non-intestinal, or unknown Lauren subtype and/or lobular subtype breast cancer. 1 younger than 50 years.

4. At least one family member with gastric or breast cancer, non-intestinal, or unknown Lauren subtype and/or lobular subtype breast cancer, and another first- or second-degree family member with abdominal tumour of unknown origin. 1 younger than 50 years.

5. One family member with early onset gastric cancer (<35–40 years) and otherwise negative family history for gastric and breast cancer.

Table 19.4 Probability of E-cadherin germline mutation detection depending on number and age of onset of gastric cancer.

Gastric cancer	<50 years	Diffuse subtype	*N*	Mutations *n* (%)
1 < 45 J	1	1	18	[1]
≥2	2	1	10	5 (50)
≥2	1	1	26	6 (23)
≥2	1	2	2	1
≥2	0	1	7	0
≥3	2	1	7	5 (71)
≥3	1	1	14	6 (43)
≥3	0	1	3	0
Overall			51	7 (14)

a bad prognosis in most families, just one gastric cancer case can be identified as being the diffuse subtype according to Lauren. In two or more gastric cancer cases, one of the diffuse subtype and one gastric cancer with an onset at an age of younger than 50 years, the probability of detecting an E-cadherin germline mutation is about 20%. Having two gastric cancer cases younger than 50 years, the probability increases to 50%. In families with three or more gastric cancer cases, two younger than 50 years and one of the diffuse subtype, the probability of an E-cadherin germline mutation increases to 70% (Table 19.4). In families with at least two gastric cancer cases and one diffuse subtype tumor and one younger than 50 years, the probability for an E-cadherin germline mutation is about 14%, with two verified diffuse subtype tumors increasing to 30%. Other criteria listed in Table 19.3 help to identify single families [16, 17, 20, 27, 28].

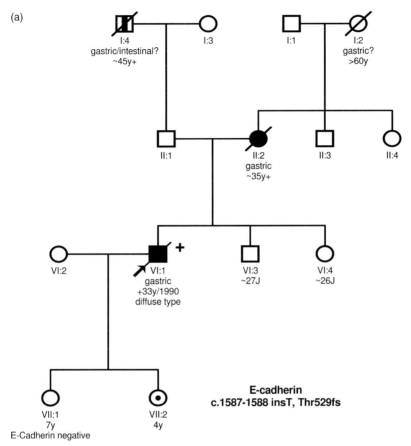

Figure 19.1 Pedigrees with HDGC and E-cadherin germline mutation fulfilling criteria 1 and possibly 2 (a) and criteria 3 and 4 (b). Third pedigree with very early onset gastric cancer (14 years) and lobular breast cancer (c). MSS: microsatellite stability; JHC: immunohistochemistry.

19.4.2
Molecular Genetics

E-cadherin (CDH1) is a calcium dependent cell adhesion molecule, which plays a key role in the structural integrity of epithelial tissues. The *E-cadherin* gene comprises 16 exons and is located on the long arm of chromosome 16. Somatic mutations of this gene are typically found in a substantial proportion of diffuse type gastric cancer and lobular breast carcinomas [31, 32]. E-cadherin germline mutations have been reported in several studies, and until today, at least 68 germline mutations in 273 families tested have been identified. Among these, 78% are

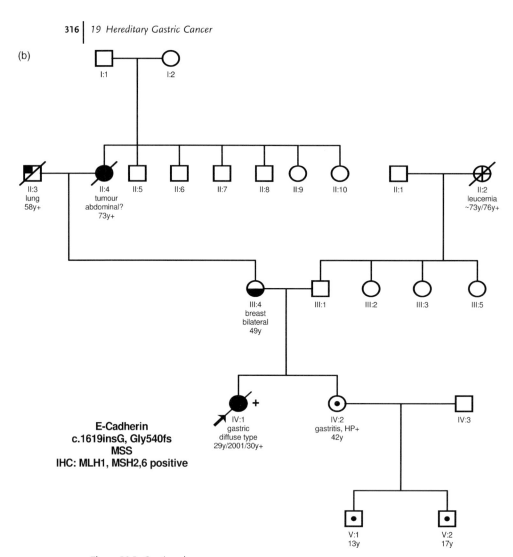

(b)

E-Cadherin
c.1619insG, Gly540fs
MSS
IHC: MLH1, MSH2,6 positive

Figure 19.1 *Continued*

truncating mutations, thus representing clear pathogenic mutations, and 22% are missense mutations. The mutations are distributed over the whole gene and no mutation hotspots were identified [27].

For some of the missense mutations, *in vitro* analysis revealed a functional decrease in cell adhesion and an increase of cell invasion, indicating a pathogenic significance of these mutations [33–35]. Intragenic deletion of one or more exons have been described as the second-hit mechanism of inactivation of the second allele, but not as a basis for germline mutations [36].

(c)

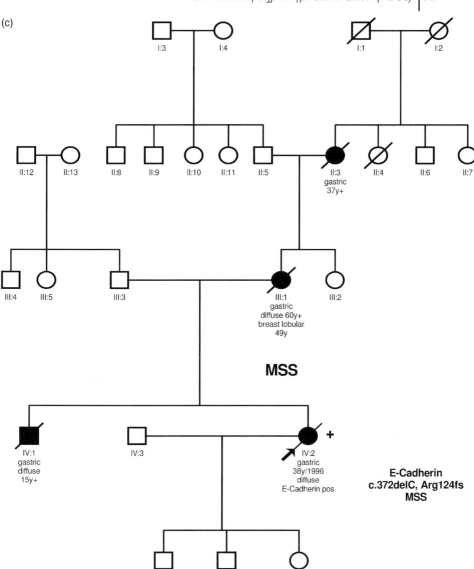

Figure 19.1 *Continued*

19.4.3
Histology

There have been no intestinal type gastric cancer cases identified in E-cadherin germline mutation carriers. As sporadic E-cadherin mutations have been described in about 50% of gastric cancer cases of the diffuse subtype according to Lauren, but not in pure intestinal subtype cases, it was unlikely to identify intestinal type gastric cancer in germline mutation carriers. Nevertheless, there might be rare cases of sporadic gastric cancers in germline carriers who did not develop fatal manifestations of the germline associated diffuse type gastric cancer. Very few cases indicate a manifestation of the mixed type gastric cancer, according to Lauren, in E-cadherin germline mutation carriers [17, 33]. A thorough investigation of prophylactically resected stomach specimens of mutation carriers without endoscopic evidence of gastric cancer helped to identify the premalignant lesion or *in situ* carcinoma of diffuse type gastric cancer. This so-called globoid dysplasia has been found in 7 out of 10 prophylactically resected gastric cancer specimens of germline mutation carriers [37, 38]. Nevertheless, all specimens showed between 1 and 161 early gastric cancer manifestations. Although their definite biological significance is not clear, since there is no 100% penetrance of gastric cancer manifestation in mutation carriers, at least 70 to 80% of mutation carriers definitely develop gastric cancer via these premalignant and early malignant lesions.

19.4.4
Surveillance, Predictive Testing, and Therapy

The International Gastric Cancer Linkage Consortium (IGCLC), an interdisciplinary group of scientists working on hereditary gastric cancer worldwide, published guidelines on clinical and genetic counseling in 1999, which had been supported by published results in the years following [28, 39]. Mutation carriers and persons at risk, not being genetically tested, are offered annual endoscopic surveillance with a special pre-endoscopic preparation of the stomach, mucosal, staining and random biopsies systematically taken out of the various gastric regions without using endoscopic ultrasound, and additional magnifying endoscopic techniques whenever possible. Because of the option of endoscopic surveillance, predictive testing for E-cadherin germline mutations has been offered to all persons at risk beyond the age 10 years, because of the youngest tumor manifestations at 14 and 15 years (Figure 19.1c).

Experienced clinicians expected a high risk of missing the early diagnosis of diffuse type gastric cancer in mutation carriers because of only minimal mucosal changes, early intramural spread, high life-time risk of developing gastric cancer, and little experience in the early detection of gastric cancer, particularly in Western compared to Asian countries. Therefore, the IGCLC established a concept of prophylactic gastrectomy as an alternative to endoscopic surveillance, offered to mutation carriers within a certain age range and fit for surgery following intensive clinical and genetic counselling, and stressing the benefit and risk of endoscopic surveillance as well as morbidity and mortality of prophylactic gastrectomy. Morbidity and mortality figures regarding high volume centers of gastric cancer surgery presented to the IGCLC suggested morbidity of around 10% and mortality less than 2% for non-tumor patients younger than 40 to 50 years of age (National University of Seoul, Korea; University of Siena, Italy; University of Technology Munich, Germany) [28].

The New Zealand group, initially describing E-cadherin germline mutations in Maori families, published their data on the surveillance program established in mutation carriers. Their at-risk persons did not accept the offer of prophylactic gastrectomy, but did accept surveillance endoscopy. Ten early gastric cancers have been diagnosed among 33 mutation carriers at risk, having had surveillance endoscopies over a period of 5 years. According to their data, they did not miss a gastric cancer as no advanced tumors beyond a T1-category had been detected, or any tumor-related death of persons at risk in the surveillance program [40, 41]. Besides endoscopic surveillance, E-cadherin germline mutation carriers in the United States and Canada accepted the option of prophylactic gastrectomy. Since 2000, more than 10 prophylactic gastrectomies have been published, one even performed with laparoscopic assistance [37, 38, 42, 43]. Preoperative endoscopy needs to be without evidence of gastric cancer in order not to perform lymphadenectomy along the hepatic and celiac artery. Complete removal of the gastric mucosa of the esophageal and duodenal resection line has to be ascertained by frozen section of the oral and distal resection margin. Since prophylactic resection demands low morbidity, a simple Roux Y reconstruction has been performed internationally. Nevertheless, a jejunal pouch with esophago-jejunoplication is our own reconstruction of choice, with low morbidity and some functional advantages [44, 45].

There have been no reports about mortality. Prophylactic gastrectomy should be performed in experienced oncological upper GI surgical centers, since this rare procedure demands low morbidity and mortality with a differentiated histopathological workup according to a standardized protocol [38]. The first ten prophylactically removed stomachs showed between 1 and 164 early gastric cancer manifestations and a suggested preneoplastic or carcinoma *in situ* lesion leading to diffuse type gastric cancer, called globoid dysplasia [37, 38]. Counselling for prophylactic gastrectomy should take into account the individual development of a mutation carrier (college, university or job training, wish for pregnancy, etc.) and the age (beyond 18 years, reasonable remaining life expectancy), and considering co-morbidity and life-long cancer risk [28].

Surveillance generally and following prophylactic gastrectomy has to include increased risk for breast cancer manifestation, not only in female mutation carriers. In addition, a potentially higher risk for colorectal and prostatic cancer should be kept in mind. Psycho-oncologic counselling and therapy should be offered with clinical and genetic counselling to potential or newly detected mutation carriers with or without gastric cancer, and parallel to the offer of prophylactic gastrectomy. In addition, nutritional counselling with surgery is mandatory.

Following prophylactic or curative gastrectomy, at least annual esophago-jejunos-copies should be performed to judge for gastric mucosal islets in the esophagus or at the anastomotic site. The gastric mucosal islets have been observed macro-scopically in about 6% of cases, but microscopically even more often [46, 47]. Whether there is an increased risk of adenocarcinoma due to these islets has not yet been reported. Theoretically, there is even an increased risk by gastric mucosa in Meckel's diverticula.

19.5
HNPCC Associated Gastric Cancer

19.5.1
Clinical Presentation

Gastric cancer has been considered of minor importance regarding the detection and definition of the HNPCC syndrome (see Chapter 17 on Lynch syndrome (HNPCC)). Though identified as the third most common on the list of HNPCC tumors with 4 to 5% close to small bowel cancer, it ranges far behind colorectal cancer with 70 to 80% and endometrial cancer with 10% [48, 49]. Gastric cancer has not been defined in the tumor list by the Amsterdam II criteria, but by the Bethesda criteria [50, 51]. As the majority of HNPCC families do not present with any gastric cancer manifestation, most families with gastric cancer present with just single cases. There is an undefined probability of non-HNPCC related spo-radic gastric cancer cases of germline positive as well as germline negative family members. Some families present with two or more gastric cancer cases, also showing associated rather young colorectal cancer manifestations (Figure 19.2). The mean age of patients with HNPCC-related gastric cancer is 56 to 58 years, and therefore 10 to 15 years older than colorectal cancer manifestation [48, 52, 53].

19.5.2
Molecular Genetics

Germline mutations in the DNA mismatch repair genes *MSH2, MLH1, MSH6,* and *PMS2* are the molecular genetic cause for the HNPCC syndrome [54–56]. A typical feature of the tumors of HNPCC patients is the occurrence of a high degree of microsatellite instability (MSI-H), which can be found in around 80% of the tumors in these patients. Microsatellites are short repetitive DNA sequences, which occur throughout the genome, mainly in non-coding regions. Microsatellite sequences are prone to errors during DNA replication, which are normally recog-nized and corrected by the DNA mismatch repair system. If the function of this repair system is impaired by mutations in one of the mismatch repair genes in the tumor, it leads to the occurrence of additional microsatellite alleles, called microsatellite instability. Defects in the DNA mismatch repair system not only

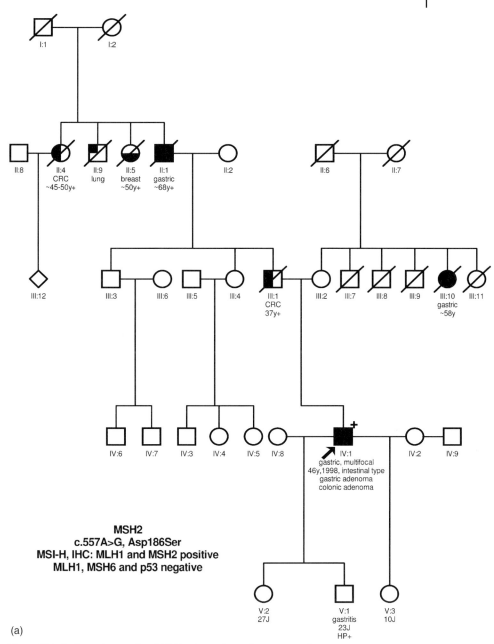

MSH2
c.557A>G, Asp186Ser
MSI-H, IHC: MLH1 and MSH2 positive
MLH1, MSH6 and p53 negative

(a)

Figure 19.2 Pathogenic germline MSH2 mismatch repair gene mutation in two families with multiple positive Bethesda but negative Amsterdam II criteria with 2 (a) and 4 gastric cancer (b) and early onset colorectal cancer. Negative mutation screening for MLH1, MSH6 and p 53. MSI-H: high rate microsatellite instability; IHC: immunohistochemistry.

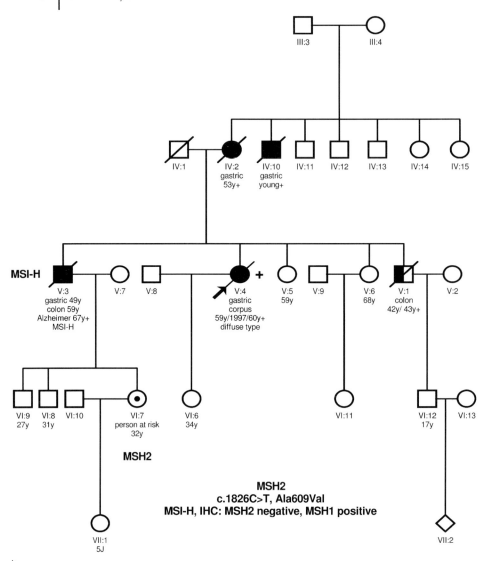

Figure 19.2 *Continued*

lead to microsatellite instability, but may also affect repetitive sequences in the coding region of genes, which are important for normal cell function and proliferation, thus contributing to tumor development.

The molecular diagnostics of an HNPCC syndrome is performed by analyzing a standardized panel of five microsatellite markers and/or by performing immunohistochemical analysis of the expression of the DNA mismatch repair genes in the tumor [57–59]. If at least two of the five markers demonstrate microsatellite instability, and/or loss of the expression of one of the mismatch repair gene is

Table 19.5 HNPCC associated gastric cancer. High rate microsatellite instability (*MSI-H*) and mutation analysis (*Mut*) for mismatch repair genes.

	MSI-H/tests	Mut/tests
Amsterdam positive, any age	4/21	1/4
≥3 gastric cancer	3/17	0/3
2 gastric cancer, 1 < 50 years	2/16	1/2
2 gastric cancer, first-degree	3/37	0/3
2 gastric cancer	3/12	1/3
≥1 gastric cancer + HNPCC tumor	3/14	2/3
1 gastric cancer ≤45 years	0/18	–
Overall (*n*)	18/113	5/18
Overall (%)	16%	28%

observed in the tumor, a germline mutation analysis is performed. Loss of the expression of a specific mismatch repair gene indicates which of the mismatch repair gene preferentially may harbor a germline mutation, and where mutation analysis should be started. In patients having been pre-selected by these criteria, pathogenic germline mutations have been found in 55 to 62% in *MSH2* or *MLH1* in German studies, and in 21% of the patients missense mutations with an unclear pathogenic function have been identified [59, 60]. In both genes, the majority of the pathogenic mutations are point mutations or small insertions or deletions, and the mutations are distributed over the whole genes. Larger genomic deletions encompassing one or several exons are found in 10 to 17% of the patients [60, 61]. Germline mutations in the *MSH6* gene are rare and have been reported in 4% of patients for whom the tumors have been first analyzed for microsatellite instability and/or by immunohistochemistry [62]. Overall, there is no genotype-phenotype correlation regarding gastric cancer manifestation. From the gastric cancer point of view, we tested microsatellite instability in 113 gastric cancer cases with familial or otherwise HNPCC-related background and detected high rate MSI (MSI-H) in 18%. Twenty-eight percent of MSI-H tumors turned out to be due to a germline mutation in one of the mismatch repair genes tested, which means an overall germline mutation rate of almost 5% (Table 19.5).

19.5.3
Histology

The Munich registry shows HNPCC related gastric cancer associated with the intestinal subtype without a predominant localization in the stomach. This is in accordance with most analyses regarding gastric cancer and microsatellite instability, regardless of an HNPCC relationship [63–66].

Though colorectal HNPCC related cancer shows certain histological characteristics, including low grading (G3) associated with high grade microsatellite instability, this has not been observed in the Munich registry or mentioned in the literature, with the exception of an article by dos Santos [66]. Low grading associated with high-grade microsatellite instability in gastric cancer has only been observed by Han [67].

19.5.4
Surveillance, Predictive Testing and Therapy

Originally, there had been no recommendation for surveillance endoscopies regarding gastric cancer in HNPCC families without gastric cancer manifestation. A Scandinavian study in HNPCC families including surveillance endoscopy for gastric cancer was not efficient, since gastric cancer cases were rare [68]. Pedigrees with gastric cancer cases should induce gastric cancer surveillance for persons at risk at about 2-year intervals. The recent data identifying gastric cancer as the third most common among HNPCC related tumors again stimulated the discussion about including upper GI endoscopy in the regular surveillance program, even in HNPCC families without a gastric cancer manifestation. Whereas the International Society of Gastrointestinal Hereditary Tumors recommends surveillance for cancer of the stomach if there is a clustering of more than one case in the family, the Mallorca group (European experts) recommends gastro-duodenoscopy starting at 30 to 35 years in 1- or 2-year intervals in countries with a high gastric cancer incidence [69]. Predictive testing is offered to persons at risk beyond 18 years of age, as tumor manifestation is not expected in adolescence. There is no indication for prophylactic surgery in HNPCC, neither for colorectal nor gastric cancer. Nevertheless, in cases of gastric pathology with high-grade neoplasia or early or distal cancer, an extended radicality is recommended as total gastrectomy is superior to endoscopic or distal gastric resection with regard to synchronic multifocal or metachronic gastric cancer disease. In HNPCC families, there is a strong indication for diagnostic endoscopy in cases of upper GI complaints or associated symptoms. Detection of HP infection should lead to eradication therapy, particularly in young persons at risk.

19.6
Familial Gastric Cancer of Unknown Origin

19.6.1
Clinical Presentation

Among gastric cancer patients, one or even two first- or second-degree relatives with gastric cancer have been observed in 18 and 5% of patients (Figure 19.3). Finally, less than 2%, that is about 10% of familial cases, have a detectable germline mutation, but nevertheless they all present with a FGC pattern. Presentation differs depending on two, three, or more family members with gastric cancer, the age of onset, Lauren subtype of the index patient, and possibly associated other

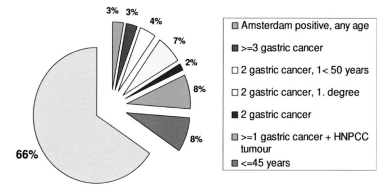

Figure 19.3 Family history of gastric cancer. Prospective analysis of clinical cases *n* = 177.

tumors within the family. They all have in common either negative screening criterias for HDGC and HNPCC, negative mutational screening for E-cadherin and microsatellite instability, or even mismatch repair genes.

There are different patterns of presentation for FGC. According to the Amsterdam I criteria in HNPCC, there are three or more family members with gastric cancer in at least two generations, one a first-degree relative to the others with at least one early onset gastric cancer before the age of 50 (Figure 19.4). In our own hereditary gastric cancer registry, there are twice as many diffuse subtype index cancer patients compared to the intestinal subtype, in parallel with a higher incidence of diffuse subtype gastric cancer among early onset gastric cancer patients without a positive family pattern. There are fewer families showing a wider relationship with early onset gastric cancer. Again, most index tumors are of the diffuse subtype. An Amsterdam-type relationship without early onset is less frequent with most index tumors classified as intestinal subtype (Figure 19.5). Finally, a wide relationship without early tumor onset has been observed more often with the same frequency of diffuse and intestinal subtype index tumors. There are single families with an association of gastric ulcer and gastritis (Figure 19.6) or type A gastritis to a strong familial pattern of gastric cancer. Finally, some families along with the FGC pattern, demonstrate some HNPCC associated tumors without early onset manifestation. In most cases, these tumors have to be identified preliminarily as sporadic tumors, at least not related to HNPCC. Nevertheless, it remains unclear whether these tumors have some syndromic characteristics or mark a phenotype associated to a so far unknown mutation.

19.6.2
Molecular Genetics

FGC with an early onset (<50 years) and diffuse subtype needs E-cadherin mutational screening. HNPCC-associated Bethesda criteria (see Chapter 17 on Lynch syndrome (HNPCC)) should be checked, and microsatellite analysis or immunohistochemistry for mismatch repair genes performed if necessary. A possible Li

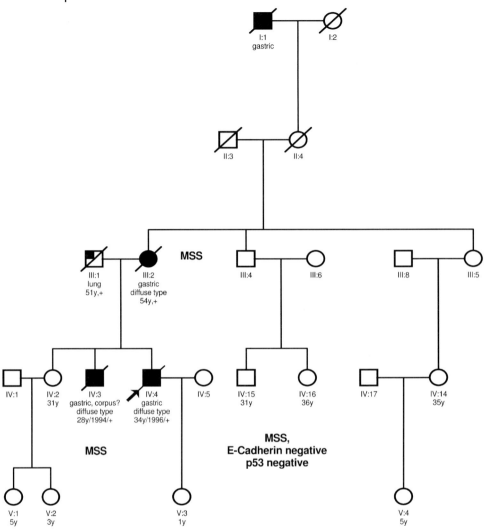

Figure 19.4 FGC fulfilling gastric cancer Amsterdam criteria with diffuse subtype and early onset. Negative testing for E-cadherin and microsatellite instability.

Fraumeni syndrome should be ruled out by pedigree presentation with associated tumor manifestations and *p53* mutational screening (see Chapter 3 on family cancer syndromes) [70]. Rare cases of familial breast and gastric cancer manifestation should lead to *BRCA2* mutation analysis (see Chapter 11 on herditary breast cancer) [71]. The association of gastric cancer and polyposis has to be kept in mind regarding various candidate genes. According to our clinical and molecular experience, we established an algorithm of molecular testing depending on the

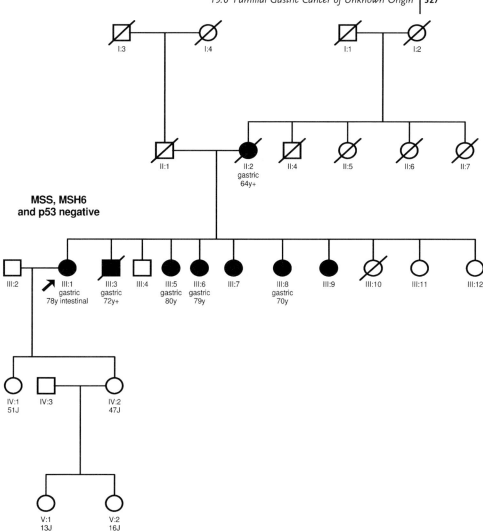

Figure 19.5 Amsterdam type relationship for gastric cancer with late onset and intestinal subtype with microsatellite stability and negative testing for *MSH6* and *p53*.

familial occurrence of gastric cancer, age of manifestation, histological subtype, other tumor diseases in the family or the patient, and a polyposis phenotype (Figure 19.7).

Neither catenins nor caspase-10, *SMAD4*, *RUNX3*, *HPP1*, or *Desmoglein 2*, worked on by different groups collaborating in the International Gastric Cancer Linkage Consortium, have turned out to be predisposing genes in FGC [17, 20, 72, 73].

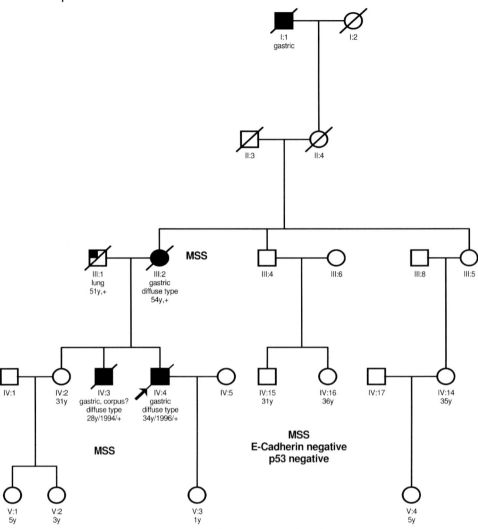

Figure 19.6 Familial occurrence of gastric cancer with early and late onset, gastric ulcer, and gastritis with negative mutational analysis.

19.6.3
Histology

Obviously, all different subtypes present in these families, according to Lauren, although the diffuse subtype occurs more often with early onset tumors. Verification of histology by obtaining the pathology report, and sometimes a second opinion by a reference pathologist, is extremely helpful. It also enables the clinician to establish some association to HP infection retrospectively. Some gastric

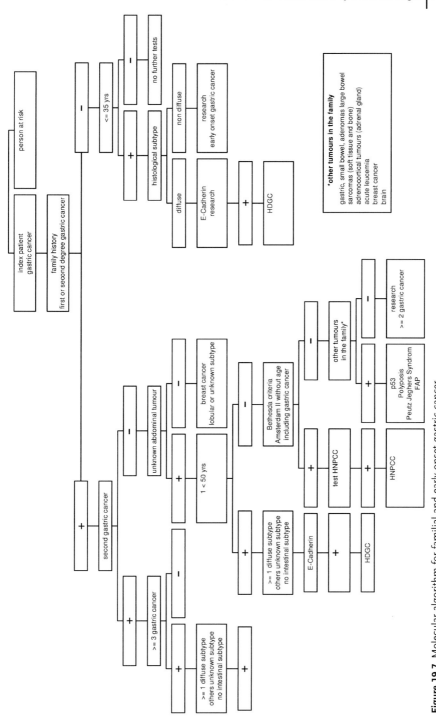

Figure 19.7 Molecular algorithm for familial and early onset gastric cancer.

cancer cases turn out to be gastric ulcer disease, and some as tumor diseases of other organs such as the esophagus. Particularly, the subtype classification according to Lauren differs among pathologists, and therefore a second opinion often changes the diagnosis and may induce E-cadherin mutational screening.

19.6.4
Surveillance and Therapy

As there are no established surveillance programs stratified according to FGC patterns, the individual recommendations are entirely based on expert opinion and related to statistical data and experience with familial colorectal cancer manifestation. On the background of their FGC occurrence, some persons at risk start surveillance endoscopies independently, as happened in the family demonstrated in Figure 19.8. The index patient had several surveillance endoscopies until the age of 55, when early diffuse type gastric cancer had been diagnosed and confirmed by a second pathologist as the gastric biopsy site could not be identified by re-endoscopy. The ideal age is 5, better 10 years before the youngest gastric cancer manifestation of the family so far. It should be recommended to first-degree relatives.

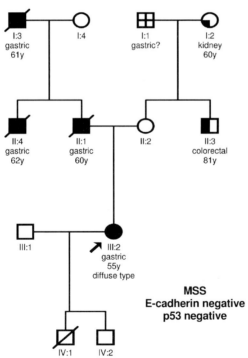

Figure 19.8 Mutation negative FGC without early onset manifestation. Index patient was diagnosed with early diffuse type gastric cancer by surveillance endoscopy.

If there is a leading Lauren subtype of gastric cancer, endoscopies should be performed annually for the diffuse type, and for the intestinal subtype, every 2 to 3 years should be reasonable. Additional gastric pathology such as atrophic gastritis, most likely caused by type B gastritis (HP associated) and rarely by type A gastritis (autoimmune, associated with pernicious anemia), and consecutive intestinal metaplasia should be diagnosed, which increases gastric cancer risk ten times. There are rare cases with even strong FGC manifestation. Particularly, a Type III incomplete intestinal metaplasia is associated with the highest cancer risk [74]. The potentially large extension of intestinal metaplasia along the lesser curvature might be an important predictive risk factor for cancer risk [75]. Detection of low-grade neoplasia, according to the Padua classification, can trigger surveillance intervals [76–79]. On the background of FGC, there is at least a theoretical benefit for HP eradication, particularly in young persons at risk. Longstanding low-grade neoplasia is supposed to be associated with a 10% gastric cancer risk, high-grade neoplasia confirmed by a second pathologist, even with a 60 to 70% gastric cancer risk in the course of many years [80]. The identification of a gastric cancer family should induce intensive clinical and additional genetic counseling, particularly for first-degree relatives.

Detection of high grade neoplasia or early gastric cancer in patients with a FGC background should consider a high risk for synchronous multifocal or metachronous gastric cancer. In the Munich hereditary gastric cancer registry, one-third of patients with multifocal gastric cancer and a positive family history eventually turned out to have a germline mutation. Also in Japan, a positive family history is associated with multifocality of gastric cancer [81]. Data on the metachronous risk for local recurrence or a second gastric cancer manifestation in gastric remnants following subtotal resection are contradictory, most series showing a metachronous risk of up to 20% [82–89]. Therefore, any limited therapy, such as endoscopic mucosal or submucosal resection, endoscopic or combined endoscopic-laparoscopic transmural resection, or even distal or subtotal gastric resection should be weighed against a total gastrectomy with extended prophylactic radicality, as performed with the index patient in Figure 19.8. Gastric pathology, age of onset, pedigree pattern, negative mutational screening, and co-morbidity should influence the surgical decision as well as intensive clinical and genetic counseling. The familial phenotype regarding other potentially associated tumor types should trigger surveillance and staging before surgery in case of gastric cancer occurrence. As far as we know, the familial background of gastric cancer should not influence the decision on neo-adjuvant chemotherapy in cases of a locally advanced gastric cancer manifestation.

19.7
Gastric Cancer as Part of Rare Hereditary Tumor Syndromes

There are some rare tumor syndromes connected with an increased risk for gastric cancer. As they will be described in other chapters (e.g. see Chapter 3 on family

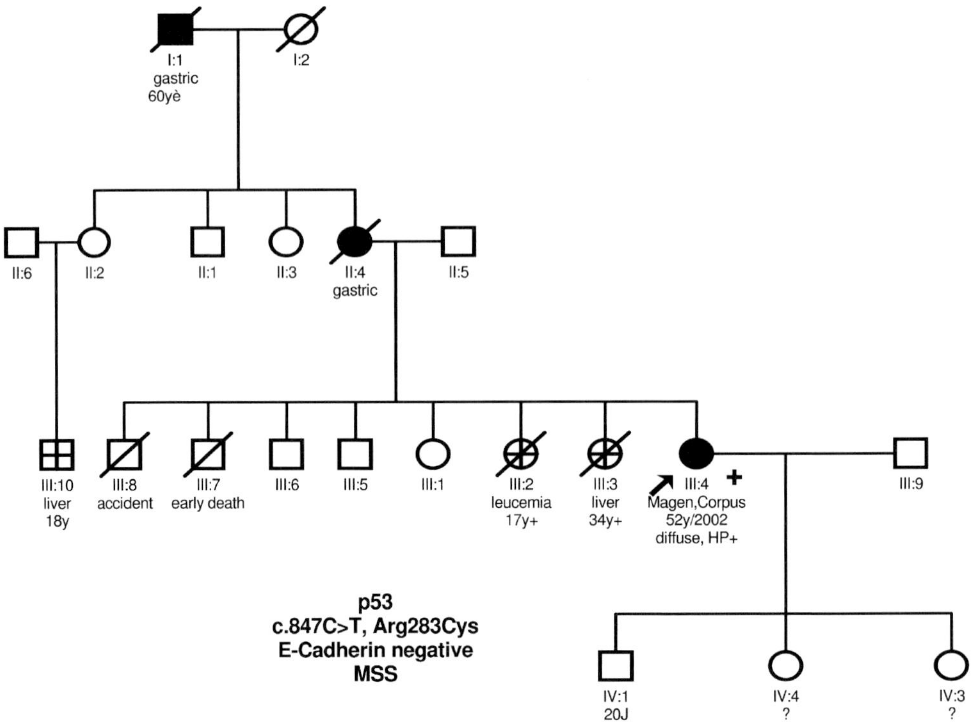

Figure 19.9 FGC within Li Fraumeni syndrome (*p53* germline mutation).

cancer syndromes), a gastric cancer association is mentioned briefly. Table 19.6 [70, 71, 90–100] summarizes information on these tumor syndromes.

In Li Fraumeni syndrome, gastric cancer is the second most common among the extra-syndromic malignancies following lung cancer, with typical early onset at about 35 years of age. Mostly single gastric cancer cases will be found within the pedigrees; however, some present with familial occurrence of gastric cancer (Figure 19.9). For example, most pedigrees show typical malignancies for Li Fraumeni syndrome as sarcomas, breast cancer, adrenocortical tumors, and leukemia. Within the group of FGC in Western countries, about 2 to 3% of cases might be attributable to a *p53* germline mutation [17, 20]. More single families have been identified in Korea and Japan [101, 102]. There is no general recommendation for Li Fraumeni carriers to have upper GI endoscopy, as long as there is no familial occurrence of gastric cancer.

Single breast cancer families have been observed with additional occurrence of gastric cancer and *BRCA2* mutations, although large series of *BRCA2* mutation carriers did not show an increased risk of gastric cancer [71, 90]. Pedigrees with breast and gastric cancer might also give a hint for an E-cadherin germline mutation in cases of diffuse type gastric and lobular type breast cancer. As surveillance programs should be adapted to additional organs being affected in selected fami-

Table 19.6 Rare tumor syndromes possibly or definitely associated with gastric cancer.

Entity	Gene	Chromosome	Characteristic tumours	Gastric cancer rsik	Gastric cancer surveillance	References
Li Fraumeni syndrome	*p53*	17p13	Sarcomas breast	Increased (number 2 extra-syndromic tumors following lung)	Depending on family pattern	Nichols *et al.* [70]
Hereditary breast cancer	*BRCA2*	13q12	Breast	Questionably increased	Depending on family pattern	Jakubowska *et al.* [71] van Asperen *et al.* [90]
Polyposis syndromes						
FAP	*APC*	5q21	Polyps colorectal	Increased in Asian Questionably increased in Western	Endoscopy for duodenal adenoms 25 years or earlier every 1–5 years according Spigelman score	Gallagher *et al.* [91] Hofgärtner *et al.* [92] Park *et al.* [93] Iwama *et al.* [94] Giardiello *et al.* [95]
Peutz–Jeghers	*STK11*	STK11	Polyps colorectal	RR213	Starting with 15 years every 3 years When polyps, every year	Zbuk and Eng [96] Latchford *et al.* [97] Giardiello *et al.* [98]
PTEN Hamartoma syndrome	*PTEN*	10q23	Polyps colorectal	not increased		Zbuk and Eng [96]
Juvenile polyposis	*BMR1A SMAD4/MADH4 PTEN*	10q22-23 18q21 10q23	Polyps colorectal	Questionably increased	Starting as teenager every 3 years	Howe *et al.* [99] Brosens *et al.* [100]

lies, upper GI endoscopy should be performed in these families at least 5 years before the youngest gastric cancer manifestation.

There are several reports about the increased gastric cancer risk in all polyposis syndromes (see Chapter 16 on gastrointestinal polyposis syndromes). For some very rare subtypes, data regarding gastric cancer risk are limited to the experience with small series. Although often stated, there are hardly any data on increased gastric cancer risk in familial polyposis coli (FAP) in Western countries compared to a slightly increased risk in Asia [91–95]. There is first evidence in Japanese patients that the incidence of gastric adenomas might be associated to chronic HP infection, which triggers gastric cancer risk [103]. Nevertheless, as there is a high risk for duodenal adenomas and consecutive carcinomas, surveillance includes upper GI endoscopy starting at about 25 years, having 1- to 5-year intervals, depending on duodenal adenoma appearance (Spigelman score). PTEN hamartoma syndrome is not connected with increased gastric cancer risk [96]. For juvenile polyposis, there are some contradictory results with gastric cancer being second most in one series [99] and no gastric cancer cases in another study cohort [100], but again upper GI endoscopy is part of the surveillance program starting in the teenage years with 3-year intervals. There have been large enough series with Peutz–Jeghers syndrome giving a relative risk for gastric cancer of 213. Surveillance includes upper GI endoscopies every 3 years without polyps and yearly when polyps have been detected [96–98].

19.8
Impact of Polymorphisms on Gastric Cancer Risk

Since gastric cancer incidence is particularly different between western and eastern populations, and proximal gastric cancer is increasing and distal cancer is deceasing in most countries of the Western world, polymorphism studies for gastric cancer have been critically looked at depending on the ethnic and regional background. Because of HP and the associated inflammation being the most important carcinogen for gastric cancer, it was not surprising that pro-inflammatory polymorphisms in IL-1B, IL1RN, and TNF-alpha, as well as special genotypes of HP, led to a gastric cancer risk with an odds ratio up to 87, taking into account the HP genotype and 9.7 for the 3 polymorphisms [4, 104]. These data could not be consistently confirmed in Japanese patients, but the interleukin-8 promoter polymorphism 251 was identified as a risk factor with an odds ratio of about 2, which again could not be confirmed in a Portuguese population [105–107]. Recently, the MDM2 promoter polymorphism (SNP309) has been associated with an increased gastric cancer risk in a Japanese population [108]. Although various enzymes with functionally relevant polymorphisms are involved in processes potentially associated with gastric cancer carcinogenesis (i.e. CYP2E1, GSTT1, GSTP1, GSTM1, ALDH2, and ODC), the majority do not individually influence gastric cancer risk, besides a possible association with dietary or smoking habits which might have secondary influence on gastric carcinogenesis [109].

19.9
Future Perspectives

Obviously, we are missing more potential candidate genes for FGC. As demonstrated, the clinical phenotype is very different, which is suggestive for not just one but several putative candidate genes. As most families are small and prognosis of gastric cancer is bad, linkage analysis for detecting new candidate genes is not feasible. Cooperating groups worldwide, such as the International Gastric Cancer Linkage Consortium, have initiated cooperative studies which might be a platform for finding new candidate genes. Stratified according to clinical, histological, and molecular criteria, pooled analyses of selected families and cases might offer new chances using constitutional and tumorous DNA finally paraffin derived, and array technology. In addition, genes involved in the oncogenesis of sporadic cancer are always potential candidate genes for hereditary gastric cancer as well.

Polymorphism studies depend on high-quality data assessment regarding patients and tumors, which can be achieved only by prospective multi-center case recruitment of high volume institutions.

Finally, differentiated animal models are missing, and a few settings can investigate gastric carcinogenesis, on the basis of TNF-alpha-dependent inflammation processes mediating COX2 and prostaglandins responsible for metaplasia and hyperplastic tumors [110].

Acknowledgments

The Munich Hereditary Gastric Cancer Registry is a cooperative initiative of the Interdisciplinary working group on hereditary cancer (www.tumorgen.de) at the Medical Faculty of the University of Technology, Munich, founded by G. Keller and. H. Vogelsang and supported by many contributions by clinicians, pathologists, geneticists and patients, initially funded by the German Cancer Aid (Deutsche Krebshilfe).

We thank Ms Susanne Brunnhölzl for her enormous technical assistance preparing the manuscript.

References

1 Hamilton, S.R. and Aaltonen, L. (2000) *World Health Organisation Classification of Tumours, Pathology and Genetics of Tumours of Digestive System*, IARC Press, Lyon.

2 Lauren, P. (1965) The two histological main types of gastric carcinoma: diffuse and so-called intestinal type carcinoma: an attempt at a histo-clinical classification. *Acta Pathologica et Microbiologica Scandinavica*, **64**, 31–43.

3 Machado, J.C., Pharoah, P., Sousa, S., Carvalho, R., Oliveira, C., Figueiredo, C., Amorim, A., Seruca, R., Caldas, C., Carneiro, F. and Sobrinho-Simoes, M. (2001) Interleukin 1B and interleukin 1RN polymorphisms are associated with

increased risk of gastric carcinoma. *Gastroenterology*, **121**, 823–9.

4 Machado, J.C., Figueiredo, C., Canedo, P., Pharoah, P., Carvalho, R., Nabais, S., Castro, A.C., Campos, M.L., Van Doorn, L.J., Caldas, C., Seruca, R., Carneiro, F. and Sobrinho-Simoes, M. (2003) A proinflammatory genetic profile increases the risk for chronic atrophic gastritis and gastric carcinoma. *Gastroenterology*, **125**, 364–71.

5 Ott, K., Sendler, A., Becker, K., Dittler, H.J., Helmberger, H., Busch, R., Kollmannsberger, C., Siewert, J.R. and Fink, U. (2003) Neoadjuvant chemotherapy with cisplatin, 5-FU, and leucovorin (PLF) in locally advanced gastric cancer: a prospective phase II study. *Gastric Cancer*, **6**, 159–67.

6 Lordick, F., Stein, H.J., Peschel, C. and Siewert, J.R. (2004) Neoadjuvant therapy for oesophagogastric cancer. *The British Journal of Surgery*, **91**, 540–51.

7 Macdonald, J.S., Smalley, S.R., Benedetti, J., Hundahl, S.A., Estes, N. C., Stemmermann, G.N., Haller, D.G., Ajani, J.A., Gunderson, L.L., Jessup, J.M. and Martenson, J.A. (2001) Chemoradiotherapy after surgery compared with surgery alone for adenocarcinoma of the stomach or gastroesophageal junction. *The New England Journal of Medicine*, **345**, 725–30.

8 Roder, J.D., Bottcher, K., Siewert, J.R., Busch, R., Hermanek, P. and Meyer, H.J. (1993) Prognostic factors in gastric carcinoma. Results of the German Gastric Carcinoma Study 1992. *Cancer*, **72**, 2089–97.

9 Maruyama, K., Sasako, M., Kinoshita, T., Sano, T. and Katai, H. (1996) Surgical treatment for gastric cancer: the Japanese approach. *Seminars in Oncology*, **23**, 360–8.

10 Wanebo, H.J., Kennedy, B.J., Chmiel, J., Steele, G. Jr, Winchester, D. and Osteen, R. (1993) Cancer of the stomach. A patient care study by the American College of Surgeons. *Annals of Surgery*, **218**, 583–92.

11 Gayther, S.A., Gorringe, K.L., Ramus, S.J., Huntsman, D., Roviello, F., Grehan, N., Machado, J.C., Pinto, E., Seruca, R., Halling, K., MacLeod, P., Powell, S.M., Jackson, C.E., Ponder, B.A. and Caldas, C. (1998) Identification of germline E-cadherin mutations in gastric cancer families of European origin. *Cancer Research*, **58**, 4086–9.

12 Guilford, P., Hopkins, J., Harraway, J., McLeod, M., McLeod, N., Harawira, P., Taite, H., Scoular, R., Miller, A. and Reeve, A.E. (1998) E-cadherin germline mutations in familial gastric cancer. *Nature*, **392**, 402–5.

13 Keller, G., Vogelsang, H., Becker, I., Hutter, J., Ott, K., Candidus, S., Grundei, T., Becker, K.F., Mueller, J., Siewert, J.R. and Hofler, H. (1999) Diffuse type gastric and lobular breast carcinoma in a familial gastric cancer patient with an E-cadherin germline mutation. *American Journal of Pathology*, **155**, 337–42.

14 Guilford, P.J., Hopkins, J.B., Grady, W.M., Markowitz, S.D., Willis, J., Lynch, H., Rajput, A., Wiesner, G.L., Lindor, N.M., Burgart, L.J., Toro, T.T., Lee, D., Limacher, J.M., Shaw, D.W., Findlay, M.P. and Reeve, A.E. (1999) E-cadherin germline mutations define an inherited cancer syndrome dominated by diffuse gastric cancer. *Human Mutation*, **14**, 249–55.

15 Richards, F.M., McKee, S.A., Rajpar, M.H., Cole, T.R., Evans, D.G., Jankowski, J.A., McKeown, C., Sanders, D.S. and Maher, E.R. (1999) Germline E-cadherin gene (*CDH1*) mutations predispose to familial gastric cancer and colorectal cancer. *Human Molecular Genetics*, **8**, 607–10.

16 Brooks-Wilson, A.R., Kaurah, P., Suriano, G., Leach, S., Senz, J., Grehan, N., Butterfield, Y.S., Jeyes, J., Schinas, J., Bacani, J., Kelsey, M., Ferreira, P., MacGillivray, B., MacLeod, P., Micek, M., Ford, J., Foulkes, W., Australie, K., Greenberg, C., LaPointe, M., Gilpin, C., Nikkel, S., Gilchrist, D., Hughes, R., Jackson, C.E., Monaghan, K.G., Oliveira, M.J., Seruca, R., Gallinger, S., Caldas, C. and Huntsman, D. (2004) Germline E-cadherin mutations in hereditary diffuse gastric cancer: assessment of 42 new families and review of genetic screening

criteria. *Journal of Medical Genetics*, **41**, 508–17.

17 Keller, G., Vogelsang, H., Becker, I., Plaschke, S., Ott, K., Suriano, G., Mateus, A.R., Seruca, R., Biedermann, K., Huntsman, D., Doring, C., Holinski-Feder, E., Neutzling, A., Siewert, J.R. and Hofler, H. (2004) Germline mutations of the E-cadherin (*CDH1*) and *TP53* genes, rather than of *RUNX3* and *HPP1*, contribute to genetic predisposition in German gastric cancer patients. *American Journal of Medical Genetics*, **41**, e89.

18 Dussaulx-Garin, L., Blayau, M., Pagenault, M., Le Berre-Heresbach, N., Raoul, J.L., Campion, J.P., David, V. and Bretagne, J.F. (2001) A new mutation of E-cadherin gene in familial gastric linitis plastica cancer with extra-digestive dissemination. *European Journal of Gastroenterology and Hepatology*, **13**, 711–15.

19 Oliveira, C., Bordin, M.C., Grehan, N., Huntsman, D., Suriano, G., Machado, J.C., Kiviluoto, T., Aaltonen, L., Jackson, C.E., Seruca, R. and Caldas, C. (2002) Screening E-cadherin in gastric cancer families reveals germline mutations only in hereditary diffuse gastric cancer kindred. *Human Mutation*, **19**, 510–17.

20 Oliveira, C., Ferreira, P., Nabais, S., Campos, L., Ferreira, A., Cirnes, L., Alves, C.C., Veiga, I., Fragoso, M., Regateiro, F., Dias, L.M., Moreira, H., Suriano, G., Machado, J.C., Lopes, C., Castedo, S., Carneiro, F. and Seruca, R. (2004) E-Cadherin (*CDH1*) and *p53* rather than *SMAD4* and Caspase-10 germline mutations contribute to genetic predisposition in Portuguese gastric cancer patients. *European Journal of Cancer*, **40**, 1897–903.

21 Humar, B., Toro, T., Graziano, F., Muller, H., Dobbie, Z., Kwang-Yang, H., Eng, C., Hampel, H., Gilbert, D., Winship, I., Parry, S., Ward, R., Findlay, M., Christian, A., Tucker, M., Tucker, K., Merriman, T. and Guilford, P. (2002) Novel germline *CDH1* mutations in hereditary diffuse gastric cancer families. *Human Mutation*, **19**, 518–25.

22 Kaurah, P., MacMillan, A., Boyd, N., De Senz, J.L.A., Chun, N., Suriano, G., Van Zaor, S.M.L., Gilpin, C., Nikkel, S., Connolly-Wilson, M., Weissman, S., Rubinstein, W.S., Sebold, C., Greenstein, R., Stroop, J., Yim, D., Panzini, B., McKinnon, W., Greenblatt, M., Wirtzfeld, D., Fontaine, D., Coit, D., Yoon, S., Chung, D., Lauwers, G., Pizzuti, A., Vaccaro, C., Redal, M.A., Oliveira, C., Tischkowitz, M., Olschwang, S., Gallinger, S., Lynch, H., Green, J., Ford, J., Pharoah, P., Fernandez, B. and Huntsman, D. (2007) Founder and recurrent *CDH1* mutations in families with hereditary diffuse gastric cancer. *The Journal of the American Medical Association*, **297**, 2360–72.

23 Roviello, F., Corso, G., Pedrazzani, C., De Marrelli, D.F.G., Berardi, A., Garosi, L., Suriano, G., De Vindigni, C.S.A., Leoncini, L., Seruca, R. and Pinto, E. (2007) Hereditary diffuse gastric cancer and E-cadherin: description of the first germline mutation in an Italian family. *European Journal of Surgical Oncology*, **33**, 448–51.

24 Rodriguez-Sanjuan, J.C., Fontalba, A., Mayorga, M., Bordin, M.C., Hyland, S.J., Trugeda, S., Garcia, R.A., Gomez-Fleitas, M., Fernandez, F., Caldas, C. and Fernandez-Luna, J.L. (2006) A novel mutation in the E-cadherin gene in the first family with hereditary diffuse gastric cancer reported in Spain. *European Journal of Surgical Oncology*, **32**, 1110–13.

25 Suriano, G., Yew, S., Ferreira, P., Senz, J., Kaurah, P., Ford, J.M., Longacre, T.A., Norton, J.A., Chun, N., Young, S., Oliveira, M.J., MacGillivray, B., Rao, A., Sears, D., Jackson, C.E., Boyd, J., Yee, C., Deters, C., Pai, G.S., Hammond, L.S., McGivern, B.J., Medgyesy, D., Sartz, D., Arun, B., Oelschlager, B.K., Upton, M.P., Neufeld-Kaiser, W., Silva, O.E., Donenberg, T.R., Kooby, D.A., Sharma, S., Jonsson, B.A., Gronberg, H., Gallinger, S., Seruca, R., Lynch, H. and Huntsman, D.G. (2005) Characterization of a recurrent germline mutation of the E-cadherin gene: implications for genetic testing and clinical management. *Clinical Cancer Research*, **11**, 5401–9.

26 More, H., Humar, B., Weber, W., Ward, R., Christian, A., Lintott, C., Graziano, F., Ruzzo, A.M., Acosta, E., Boman, B., Harlan, M., Ferreira, P., Seruca, R., Suriano, G. and Guilford, P. (2007) Identification of seven novel germline mutations in the human E-cadherin (*CDH1*) gene. *Human Mutation*, **28**, 203.

27 Carneiro, F., Oliveira, C., Suriano, G. and Seruca, R. (2008) Molecular pathology of familial gastric cancer, with an emphasis on hereditary diffuse gastric cancer. *Journal of Clinical Pathology*, **61**, 25–30.

28 Caldas, C., Carneiro, F., Lynch, H.T., Yokota, J., Wiesner, G.L., Powell, S.M., Lewis, F.R., Huntsman, D.G., Pharoah, P.D., Jankowski, J.A., MacLeod, P., Vogelsang, H., Keller, G., Park, K.G., Richards, F.M., Maher, E.R., Gayther, S.A., Oliveira, C., Grehan, N., Wight, D., Seruca, R., Roviello, F., Ponder, B.A. and Jackson, C.E. (1999) Familial gastric cancer: overview and guidelines for management. *Journal of Medical Genetics*, **36**, 873–80.

29 Pharoah, P.D., Guilford, P. and Caldas, C. (2001) Incidence of gastric cancer and breast cancer in *CDH1* (E-cadherin) mutation carriers from hereditary diffuse gastric cancer families. *Gastroenterology*, **121**, 1348–53.

30 Masciari, S., Larsson, N., Senz, J., Boyd, N., Kaurah, P., Kandel, M.J., Harris, L.N., Pinheiro, H.C., Troussard, A., Miron, P., Tung, N., Oliveira, C., Collins, L., Schnitt, S., Garber, J.E. and Huntsman, D. (2007) Germline E-cadherin mutations in familial lobular breast cancer. *Journal of Medical Genetics*, **44**, 726–31.

31 Becker, K.F., Atkinson, M.J., Reich, U., Becker, I., Nekarda, H., Siewert, J.R. and Hofler, H. (1994) E-cadherin gene mutations provide clues to diffuse type gastric carcinomas. *Cancer Research*, **54**, 3845–52.

32 Berx, G., Cleton-Jansen, A.M., Strumane, K., de Leeuw, W.J., Nollet, F., van Roy, F. and Cornelisse, C. (1996) E-cadherin is inactivated in a majority of invasive human lobular breast cancers by truncation mutations throughout its extracellular domain. *Oncogene*, **13**, 1919–25.

33 Suriano, G., Oliveira, C., Ferreira, P., Machado, J.C., Bordin, M.C., De Wever, O., Bruyneel, E.A., Moguilevsky, N., Grehan, N., Porter, T.R., Richards, F.M., Hruban, R.H., Roviello, F., Huntsman, D., Mareel, M., Carneiro, F., Caldas, C. and Seruca, R. (2003) Identification of *CDH1* germline missense mutations associated with functional inactivation of the E-cadherin protein in young gastric cancer probands. *Human Molecular Genetics*, **12**, 575–82.

34 Suriano, G., de Mulholland, D.W.O., Ferreira, P., Mateus, A.R., Bruyneel, E., Nelson, C.C., Mareel, M.M., Yokota, J., Huntsman, D. and Seruca, R. (2003) The intracellular E-cadherin germline mutation *V832M* lacks the ability to mediate cell-cell adhesion and to suppress invasion. *Oncogene*, **22**, 5716–19.

35 Suriano, G., Oliveira, M.J., Huntsman, D., Mateus, A.R., Ferreira, P., Casares, F., Oliveira, C., Carneiro, F., Machado, J.C., Mareel, M. and Seruca, R. (2003) E-cadherin germline missense mutations and cell phenotype: evidence for the independence of cell invasion on the motile capabilities of the cells. *Human Molecular Genetics*, **12**, 3007–16.

36 Oliveira, C., de Bruin, J., Nabais, S., Ligtenberg, M., Moutinho, C., Nagengast, F.M., Seruca, R., van Krieken, K.H. and Carneiro, F. (2004) Intragenic deletion of *CDH1* as the inactivating mechanism of the wildtype allele in an HDGC tumour. *Oncogene*, **23**, 2236–40.

37 Huntsman, D.G., Carneiro, F., Lewis, F.R., MacLeod, P.M., Hayashi, A., Monaghan, K.G., Maung, R., Seruca, R., Jackson, C.E. and Caldas, C. (2001) Early gastric cancer in young, asymptomatic carriers of germline E-cadherin mutations. *The New England Journal of Medicine*, **344**, 1904–9.

38 Carneiro, F., Huntsman, D.G., Smyrk, T.C., Owen, D.A., Seruca, R., Pharoah, P., Caldas, C. and Sobrinho-Simoes, M. (2004) Model of the early development of diffuse gastric cancer in E-cadherin mutation carriers and its implications for patient screening. *The Journal of Pathology*, **203**, 681–7.

39 Fitzgerald, R.C. and Caldas, C. (2006) Familial gastric cancer–clinical management. *Best Practice and Research Clinical Gastroenterology*, **20**, 735–43.

40 Charlton, A., Blair, V., Shaw, D., Parry, S., Guilford, P. and Martin, I.G. (2004) Hereditary diffuse gastric cancer: predominance of multiple foci of signet ring cell carcinoma in distal stomach and transitional zone. *Gut*, **53**, 814–20.

41 Shaw, D., Blair, V., Framp, A., Harawira, P., McLeod, M., Guilford, P., Parry, S., Charlton, A. and Martin, I. (2005) Chromoendoscopic surveillance in hereditary diffuse gastric cancer: an alternative to prophylactic gastrectomy? *Gut*, **54**, 461–8.

42 Lewis, F.R., Mellinger, J.D., Hayashi, A., Lorelli, D., Monaghan, K.G., Carneiro, F., Huntsman, D.G., Jackson, C.E. and Caldas, C. (2001) Prophylactic total gastrectomy for familial gastric cancer. *Surgery*, **130**, 612–17.

43 Francis, W.P., Rodrigues, D.M., Perez, N.E., Lonardo, F., Weaver, D. and Webber, J.D. (2007) Prophylactic laparoscopic-assisted total gastrectomy for hereditary diffuse gastric cancer. *Journal of the Society of Laparoendoscopic Surgeons*, **11**, 142–7.

44 Roder, J.D., Stein, H.J., Eckel, F., Herschbach, P., Henrich, G., Bottcher, K., Busch, R. and Siewert, J.R. (1996) [Comparison of the quality of life after subtotal and total gastrectomy for stomach carcinoma]. *Deutsche Medizinische Wochenschrift*, **121**, 543–9.

45 Roder, J.D., Herschbach, P., Henrich, G., Nagel, M., Bottcher, K. and Siewert, J.R. (1992) [The quality of life after total gastrectomy for stomach carcinoma. Esophagojejunal plication with pouch versus esophagojejunostomy without pouch]. *Deutsche Medizinische Wochenschrift*, **117**, 241–7.

46 Macha, S., Reddy, S., Rabah, R., Thomas, R. and Tolia, V. (2005) Inlet patch: heterotopic gastric mucosa– another contributor to supraesophageal symptoms? *Journal of Pediatrics*, **147**, 379–82.

47 von Rahden, B.H., Stein, H.J., Becker, K., Liebermann-Meffert, D. and Siewert, J.R. (2004) Heterotopic gastric mucosa of the esophagus: literature review and proposal of a clinicopathologic classification. *The American Journal of Gastroenterology*, **99**, 543–51.

48 Mueller-Koch, Y., Vogelsang, H., Kopp, R., Lohse, P., Keller, G., Aust, D., Muders, M., Gross, M., Daum, J., Schiemann, U., Grabowski, M., Scholz, M., Kerker, B., Becker, I., Henke, G. and Holinski-Feder, E. (2005) HNPCC– clinical and molecular evidence for a new entity of hereditary colorectal cancer. *Gut*, **54**, 1733–40.

49 Goecke, T., Schulmann, K., Engel, C., Holinski-Feder, E., Pagenstecher, C., Schackert, H.K., Kloor, M., Kunstmann, E., Vogelsang, H., Keller, G., Dietmaier, W., Mangold, E., Friedrichs, N., Propping, P., Krüger, S., Gebert, J., Schmiegel, W., Rueschoff, J., Loeffler, M., Moeslein, G. and the German HNPCC Consortium (2006) A genotype-phenotype comparison of 988 German *MLH1* and *MSH2* mutation carriers clinically affected with Lynch syndrome. *Journal of Clinical Oncology* **24**, 4285–92.

50 Rodriguez-Bigas, M.A., Boland, C.R., Hamilton, S.R., Henson, D.E., Jass, J.R., Khan, P.M., Lynch, H., Perucho, M., Smyrk, T., Sobin, L. and Srivastava, S. (1997) A National Cancer Institute Workshop on Hereditary Nonpolyposis Colorectal Cancer Syndrome: meeting highlights and Bethesda guidelines. *Journal of the National Cancer Institute*, **89**, 1758–62.

51 Umar, A., Boland, C.R., Terdiman, J.P., Syngal, S., de la, Chapelle, A., Ruschoff, J., Fishel, R., Lindor, N.M., Burgart, L.J., Hamelin, R., Hamilton, S.R., Hiatt, R.A., Jass, J., Lindblom, A., Lynch, H.T., Peltomaki, P., Ramsey, S.D., Rodriguez-Bigas, M.A., Vasen, H.F., Hawk, E.T., Barrett, J.C., Freedman, A.N. and Srivastava, S. (2004) Revised Bethesda Guidelines for hereditary nonpolyposis colorectal cancer (Lynch syndrome) and Microsatellite Instability 216. *Journal of the National Cancer Institute*, **96**, 261–8.

52 Aarnio, M., Salovaara, R., Aaltonen, L.A., Mecklin, J.P. and Jarvinen, H.J. (1997) Features of gastric cancer in hereditary non-polyposis colorectal cancer syndrome. *International Journal of Cancer*, **74**, 551–5.

53 Vasen, H.F., Wijnen, J.T., Menko, F.H., Kleibeuker, J.H., Taal, B.G., Griffioen, G., Nagengast, F.M., Meijers-Heijboer, E.H., Bertario, L., Varesco, L., Bisgaard, M.L., Mohr, J., Fodde, R. and Khan, P.M. (1996) Cancer risk in families with hereditary non-polyposis colorectal cancer diagnosed by mutation analysis. *Gastroenterology*, **110**, 1020–7.

54 Peltomaki, P. and Vasen, H.F. (1997) Mutations predisposing to hereditary non-polyposis colorectal cancer: database and results of a collaborative study. International Collaborative Group on Hereditary Non-polyposis Colorectal Cancer. *Gastroenterology*, **113**, 1146–58.

55 Peltomaki, P. (2005) Lynch syndrome genes. *Familial Cancer*, **4**, 227–32.

56 Liu, B., Parsons, R., Papadopoulos, N., Nicolaides, N.C., Lynch, H.T., Watson, P., Jass, J.R., Dunlop, M., Wyllie, A., Peltomaki, P., de la, Chapelle, A., Hamilton, S.R., Vogelstein, B. and Kinzler, K.W. (1996) Analysis of mismatch repair genes in hereditary non-polyposis colorectal cancer patients. *Nature Medicine*, **2**, 169–74.

57 Debniak, T., Kurzawski, G., Gorski, B., Kladny, J., Domagala, W. and Lubinski, J. (2000) Value of pedigree/clinical data, immunohistochemistry and microsatellite instability analyses in reducing the cost of determining *hMLH1* and *hMSH2* gene mutations in patients with colorectal cancer. *European Journal of Cancer*, **36**, 49–54.

58 Ponz, L.M., Di Benatti, P.G.C., Pedroni, M., Losi, L., Genuardi, M., Viel, A., Fornasarig, M., Lucci-Cordisco, E., Anti, M., Ponti, G., Borghi, F., Lamberti, I. and Roncucci, L. (2004) Genetic testing among high-risk individuals in families with hereditary non-polyposis colorectal cancer. *British Journal of Cancer*, **90**, 882–7.

59 Engel, C., Forberg, J., Holinski-Feder, E., Pagenstecher, C., Plaschke, J., Kloor, M., Poremba, C., Pox, C.P., Ruschoff, J., Keller, G., Dietmaier, W., Rummele, P., Friedrichs, N., Mangold, E., Buettner, R., Schackert, H.K., Kienle, P.,

Stemmler, S., Moeslein, G. and Loeffler, M. (2006) Novel strategy for optimal sequential application of clinical criteria, immunohistochemistry and microsatellite analysis in the diagnosis of hereditary non-polyposis colorectal cancer. *International Journal of Cancer*, **118**, 115–22.

60 Mangold, E., Pagenstecher, C., Friedl, W., Mathiak, M., Buettner, R., Engel, C., Loeffler, M., Holinski-Feder, E., Muller-Koch, Y., Keller, G., Schackert, H.K., Kruger, S., Goecke, T., Moeslein, G., Kloor, M., Gebert, J., Kunstmann, E., Schulmann, K., Ruschoff, J. and Propping, P. (2005) Spectrum and frequencies of mutations in *MSH2* and *MLH1* identified in 1721 German families suspected of hereditary non-polyposis colorectal cancer. *International Journal of Cancer*, **116**, 692–702.

61 Grabowski, M., Mueller-Koch, Y., Grasbon-Frodl, E., Koehler, U., Keller, G., Vogelsang, H., Dietmaier, W., Kopp, R., Siebers, U., Schmitt, W., Neitzel, B., Gruber, M., Doerner, C., Kerker, B., Ruemmele, P., Henke, G. and Holinski-Feder, E. (2005) Deletions account for 17% of pathogenic germline alterations in *MLH1* and *MSH2* in hereditary nonpolyposis colorectal cancer (HNPCC) families. *Genetic Testing*, **9**, 138–46.

62 Plaschke, J., Engel, C., Kruger, S., Holinski-Feder, E., Pagenstecher, C., Mangold, E., Moeslein, G., Schulmann, K., Gebert, J., von Knebel, D.M., Ruschoff, J., Loeffler, M. and Schackert, H.K. (2004) Lower incidence of colorectal cancer and later age of disease onset in 27 families with pathogenic *MSH6* germline mutations compared with families with *MLH1* or *MSH2* mutations: the German Hereditary Non-polyposis Colorectal Cancer Consortium. *Journal of Clinical Oncology*, **22**, 4486–94.

63 Bacani, J., Zwingerman, R., Di Nicola, N., Spencer, S., Wegrynowski, T., Mitchell, K., Hay, K., Redston, M., Holowaty, E., Huntsman, D., Pollett, A., Riddell, R. and Gallinger, S. (2005) Tumor microsatellite instability in early onset gastric cancer. *The Journal of Molecular Diagnostics*, **7**, 465–77.

64 Ottini, L., Palli, D., Falchetti, M., D'Amico, C., Amorosi, A., Saieva, C., Calzolari, A., Cimoli, F., Tatarelli, C., De Marchis, L., Masala, G., Mariani-Costantini, R. and Cama, A. (1997) Microsatellite instability in gastric cancer is associated with tumor location and family history in a high-risk population from Tuscany. *Cancer Research*, **57**, 4523–9.

65 Buonsanti, G., Calistri, D., Padovan, L., Luinetti, O., Fiocca, R., Solcia, E. and Ranzani, G.N. (1997) Microsatellite instability in intestinal- and diffuse-type. *The Journal of Pathology*, **182**, 167–73.

66 dos Santos, N.R., Seruca, R., Constancia, M., Seixas, M. and Sobrinho-Simoes, M. (1996) Microsatellite instability at multiple loci in gastric carcinoma: clinicopathologic implications and prognosis. *Gastroenterology*, **110**, 38–44.

67 Han, H.J., Yanagisawa, A., Kato, Y., Park, J.G. and Nakamura, Y. (1993) Genetic instability in pancreatic cancer and poorly differentiated type of gastric cancer. *Cancer Research*, **53**, 5087–9.

68 Renkonen-Sinisalo, L., Sipponen, P., Aarnio, M., Julkunen, R., Aaltonen, L.A., Sarna, S., Jarvinen, H.J. and Mecklin, J.P. (2002) No support for endoscopic surveillance for gastric cancer in hereditary non-polyposis colorectal cancer. *Scandinavian Journal of Gastroenterology*, **37**, 574–7.

69 Vasen, H.F., Moslein, G., Alonso, A., Bernstein, I., Bertario, L., Blanco, I., Burn, J., Capella, G., Engel, C., Frayling, I., Friedl, W., Hes, F.J., Hodgson, S., Mecklin, J.P., Moller, P., Nagengast, F., Parc, Y., Renkonen-Sinisalo, L., Sampson, J.R., Stormorken, A. and Wijnen, J. (2007) Guidelines for the clinical management of Lynch syndrome (hereditary non-polyposis cancer). *Journal of Medical Genetics*, **44**, 353–62.

70 Nichols, K.E., Malkin, D., Garber, J.E., Fraumeni, J.F. Jr and Li, F.P. (2001) Germline *p53* mutations predispose to a wide spectrum of early-onset cancers. *Cancer Epidemiology, Biomarkers and Prevention*, **10**, 83–7.

71 Jakubowska, A., Nej, K., Huzarski, T., Scott, R.J. and Lubinski, J. (2002) *BRCA2* gene mutations in families with aggregations of breast and stomach cancers. *British Journal of Cancer*, **87**, 888–91.

72 Lynch, H.T., Grady, W., Suriano, G. and Huntsman, D. (2005) Gastric cancer: new genetic developments. *Journal of Surgical Oncology*, **90**, 114–33.

73 Biedermann, K., Vogelsang, H., Becker, I., Plaschke, S., Siewert, J.R., Hofler, H. and Keller, G. (2005) Desmoglein 2 is expressed abnormally rather than mutated in familial and sporadic gastric cancer. *The Journal of Pathology*, **207**, 199–206.

74 Filipe, M.I., Munoz, N., Matko, I., Kato, I., Pompe-Kirn, V., Jutersek, A., Teuchmann, S., Benz, M. and Prijon, T. (1994) Intestinal metaplasia types and the risk of gastric cancer: a cohort study in Slovenia. *International Journal of Cancer*, **57**, 324–9.

75 Cassaro, M., Rugge, M., Gutierrez, O., Leandro, G., Graham, D.Y. and Genta, R.M. (2000) Topographic patterns of intestinal metaplasia and gastric cancer. *The American journal of Gastroenterology*, **95**, 1431–8.

76 Lauren, P. (1991) Histogenesis of intestinal and diffuse types of gastric carcinoma. *Scandinavian Journal of Gastroenterology Supplement*, **180**, 160–4.

77 Leung, W.K. and Sung, J.J. (2002) Review article: intestinal metaplasia and gastric carcinogenesis. *Alimentary Pharmacology and Therapeutics*, **16**, 1209–16.

78 Genta, R.M. and Rugge, M. (1999) Gastric precancerous lesions: heading for an international consensus. *Gut*, **45** (Suppl. 1), I5–8.

79 Rugge, M., Correa, P., Dixon, M.F., Hattori, T., Leandro, G., Lewin, K., Riddell, R.H., Sipponen, P. and Watanabe, H. (2000) Gastric dysplasia: the Padova international classification. *The American journal of Surgical Pathology*, **24**, 167–76.

80 Rugge, M., Cassaro, M., Di Mario, F., Leo, G., Leandro, G., Russo, V.M., Pennelli, G. and Farinati, F. (2003) The long-term outcome of gastric non-invasive neoplasia. *Gut*, **52**, 1111–16.

81 Ikeguchi, M., Fukuda, K., Oka, S., Hisamitsu, K., Katano, K., Tsujitani, S. and Kaibara, N. (2001) Clinicopathological findings in patients with gastric adenocarcinoma with familial aggregation. *Digestive Surgery*, **18**, 439–43.

82 Isozaki, H., Tanaka, N. and Okajima, K. (1999) General and specific prognostic factors of early gastric carcinoma treated with curative surgery. *Hepatogastroenterology*, **46**, 1800–8.

83 Moreaux, J. and Bougaran, J. (1993) Early gastric cancer. A 25-year surgical experience. *Annals of Surgery*, **217**, 347–55.

84 Newman, E., Brennan, M.F., Hochwald, S.N., Harrison, L.E. and Karpeh, M.S. Jr (1997) Gastric remnant carcinoma: just another proximal gastric cancer or a unique entity? *American Journal of Surgery*, **173**, 292–7.

85 Sano, T., Sasako, M., Kinoshita, T. and Maruyama, K. (1993) Recurrence of early gastric cancer. Follow-up of 1475 patients and review of the Japanese literature. *Cancer*, **72**, 3174–8.

86 Traynor, O.J., Lennon, J., Dervan, P. and Corrigan, T. (1987) Diagnostic and prognostic problems in early gastric cancer. *American Journal of Surgery*, **154**, 516–19.

87 Borie, F., Plaisant, N., Millat, B., Hay, J.M., Fagniez, P.L and De Saxce, B. (2003) Treatment and prognosis of early multiple gastric cancer. *European Journal of Surgical Oncology*, **29**, 511–14.

88 Moreaux, J. and Bougaran, J. (1993) Early gastric cancer. A 25-year surgical experience. *Annals of Surgery*, **217**, 347–55.

89 Pacelli, F., Doglietto, G.B., Alfieri, S., Carriero, C., Malerba, M., Crucitti, P.F., Caprino, P. and Crucitti, F. (1999) Survival in early gastric cancer: multivariate analysis on 72 consecutive cases. *Hepatogastroenterology*, **46**, 1223–8.

90 van Asperen, C.J., Brohet, R.M., Meijers-Heijboer, E.J., Hoogerbrugge, N., Verhoef, S., Vasen, H.F., Ausems, M.G., Menko, F.H., Gomez Garcia, E.B., Klijn, J.G., Hogervorst, F.B., van Houwelingen, J.C., Veer, L.J., Rookus, M.A. and van Leeuwen, F.E. (2005) Cancer risks in *BRCA2* families: estimates for sites other than breast and ovary. *Journal of Medical Genetics*, **42**, 711–19.

91 Gallagher, M.C., Phillips, R.K. and Bulow, S. (2006) Surveillance and management of upper gastrointestinal disease in Familial Adenomatous Polyposis. *Familial Cancer*, **5**, 263–73.

92 Hofgärtner, W.T., Thorp, M., Ramus, M.W., Delorefice, G., Chey, W.Y., Ryan, C.K., Takahashi, G.W. and Lobitz, J.R. (1999) Gastric adenocarcinoma associated with fundic gland polyps in a patient with attenuated familial adenomatous polyposis. *The American Journal of Gastroenterology*, **94**, 2275–81.

93 Park, J.G., Park, K.J., Ahn, Y.O., Song, I.S., Choi, K.W., Moon, H.Y., Choo, S.Y. and Kim, J.P. (1992) Risk of gastric cancer among Korean familial adenomatous polyposis patients. Report of three cases. *Diseases of the Colon and Rectum*, **35**, 996–8.

94 Iwama, T., Mishima, Y. and Utsunomiya, J. (1993) The impact of familial adenomatous polyposis on the tumorigenesis and mortality at the several organs. Its rational treatment. *Annals of Surgery*, **217**, 101–8.

95 Giardiello, F.M. and Offerhaus, J.G. (1995) Phenotype and cancer risk of various polyposis syndromes. *European Journal of Cancer*, **31A**, 1085–7.

96 Zbuk, K.M. and Eng, C. (2007) Hamartomatous polyposis syndromes. *Nature Clinical Practice Gastroenterology and Hepatology*, **4**, 492–502.

97 Latchford, A., Greenhalf, W., Vitone, L.J., Neoptolemos, J.P., Lancaster, G.A. and Phillips, R.K. (2006) Peutz–Jeghers syndrome and screening for pancreatic cancer. *The British Journal of Surgery*, **93**, 1446–55.

98 Giardiello, F.M., Brensinger, J.D., Tersmette, A.C., Goodman, S.N., Petersen, G.M., Booker, S.V., Cruz-Correa, M. and Offerhaus, J.A. (2000) Very high risk of cancer in familial Peutz–Jeghers syndrome. *Gastroenterology*, **119**, 1447–53.

99 Howe, J.R., Mitros, F.A. and Summers, R.W. (1998) The risk of gastrointestinal carcinoma in familial juvenile polyposis. *Annals of Surgical Oncology*, **5**, 751–6.

100 Brosens, L.A.H.A., Hylind, L.M., Iacobuzio-Donahue, C., Romans, K.E., Axilbund, J., Cruz-Correa, M., Tersmette, A.C., Offerhaus, G.J. and Giardiello, F.M. (2007) Risk of colorectal cancer in juvenile polyposis. *Gut*, **56**, 965–7.

101 Yamada, H., Shinmura, K., Okudela, K., Goto, M., Suzuki, M., Kuriki, K., Tsuneyoshi, T. and Sugimura, H. (2007) Identification and characterization of a novel germline *p53* mutation in familial gastric cancer in the Japanese population. *Carcinogenesis*, **28**, 2013–18.

102 Kim, I.J., Kang, H.C., Shin, Y., Park, H.W., Jang, S.G., Han, S.Y., Lim, S.K., Lee, M.R., Chang, H.J., Ku, J.L., Yang, H.K. and Park, J.G. (2004) A *TP53*-truncating germline mutation (*E287X*) in a family with characteristics of both hereditary diffuse gastric cancer and Li-Fraumeni syndrome. *Journal of Human Genetics*, **49**, 591–5.

103 Nakamura, S., Matsumoto, T., Kobori, Y. and Iida, M. (2002) Impact of *Helicobacter pylori* infection and mucosal atrophy on gastric lesions in patients with familial adenomatous polyposis. *Gut*, **51**, 485–9.

104 Figueiredo, C., Machado, J.C., Pharoah, P., Seruca, R., Sousa, S., Carvalho, R., Capelinha, A.F., Quint, W., Caldas, C., Van Doorn, L.J., Carneiro, F. and Sobrinho-Simoes, M. (2002) *Helicobacter pylori* and interleukin 1 genotyping: an opportunity to identify high-risk individuals for gastric carcinoma. *Journal of the National Cancer Institute*, **94**, 1680–7.

105 Taguchi, A., Ohmiya, N., Shirai, K., Mabuchi, N., Itoh, A., Hirooka, Y.,

Niwa, Y. and Goto, H. (2005) Interleukin-8 promoter polymorphism increases the risk of atrophic gastritis and gastric cancer in Japan. *Cancer Epidemiology, Biomarkers and Prevention*, **14**, 2487–93.

106 Shirai, K., Ohmiya, N., Taguchi, A., Mabuchi, N., Yatsuya, H., Itoh, A., Hirooka, Y., Niwa, Y., Mori, N. and Goto, H. (2006) Interleukin-8 gene polymorphism associated with susceptibility to non-cardia gastric carcinoma with microsatellite instability. *Journal of Gastroenterology and Hepatology*, **21**, 1129–35.

107 Canedo, P., Castanheira-Vale, A.J., Lunet, N., Pereira, F., Figueiredo, C., Gioia-Patricola, L., Canzian, F., Moreira, H., Suriano, G., Barros, H., Carneiro, F., Seruca, R. and Machado, J.C. (2008) The interleukin-8-251*T/*A polymorphism is not associated with risk for gastric carcinoma development in a Portuguese population. *European Journal of Cancer Prevention*, **17**, 28–32.

108 Ohmiya, N., Taguchi, A., Mabuchi, N., Itoh, A., Hirooka, Y., Niwa, Y. and Goto, H. (2006) *MDM2* promoter polymorphism is associated with both an increased susceptibility to gastric carcinoma and poor prognosis. *Journal of Clinical Oncology*, **24**, 4434–40.

109 You, W.C., Hong, J.Y., Zhang, L., Pan, K.F., Pee, D., Li, J.Y., Ma, J.L., Rothman, N., Caporaso, N., Fraumeni, J.F. Jr, Xu, G.W. and Gail, M.H. (2005) Genetic polymorphisms of *CYP2E1, GSTT1, GSTP1, GSTM1, ALDH2*, and *ODC* and the risk of advanced precancerous gastric lesions in a Chinese population. *Cancer Epidemiology, Biomarkers and Prevention*, **14**, 451–8.

110 Taketo, M.M. (2006) Mouse models of gastrointestinal tumors. *Cancer Science*, **97**, 355–61.

20
Pancreatic Cancer

Nils Habbe and Babette Simon

Summary

The fatality of pancreatic cancer (PC) is mostly caused by an advanced stage of diagnosis for the majority of patients. Nearly 5% of all PC patients exhibit a familial background of the disease. Inherited forms of PC occur in three distinct clinical settings: first, hereditary tumor syndromes revealing primarily a clinical phenotype other than PC with an increased risk of PC. Second, hereditary pancreatitis (HP) and cystic fibrosis (CF) predispose to the development of PC. The third setting is familial pancreatic cancer (FPC). High-risk individuals from these PC prone families need to be identified and enrolled in screening programs at expert centers, providing genetic counseling and further screening techniques. In case of identified suspicious lesions, surgery should be performed to avoid overtreatment and to keep the associated morbidity as low as possible.

20.1
Introduction

Pancreatic cancer (PC) has one of the worst prognoses among human cancers, and the mortality almost equals the incidence of this disease. Since a certain number of patients suffering from PC exhibit a familial background, several tumor registries have been founded to investigate the genetic basis of these FPC forms, and to provide a clinical screening program for persons from cancer prone families and therefore at risk, which is a crucial point for early detection.

20.2
History and Epidemiology of Familial Pancreatic Cancer

PC is the fifth leading cause of cancer-related deaths in the EU. As estimated by recent publications, around 59 000 patients were diagnosed with PC in 2006, and

Hereditary Tumors: From Genes to Clinical Consequences
Edited by Heike Allgayer, Helga Rehder and Simone Fulda
Copyright © 2009 WILEY-VCH Verlag GmbH & Co. KGaA, Weinheim
ISBN: 978-3-527-32028-8

approximately 64000 patients will die from this disease [1]. The poor 5-year survival rate of 5% is due to lack of accurate screening techniques to detect PC before the onset of symptoms, especially when compared to other malignancies such as colon cancer. Therefore, only a minority of patients harboring PC present with a local disease.

In the 1980s, several case reports indicated that PC accumulates in some families [2, 3]. The first thorough study investigating a cohort of families revealing an aggregation of PCs was published in 1989 [4]. In the aftermath of this study, several tumor registries were founded in the United States and Europe to further collect and analyze data on these cancer prone families, and to provide clinical screening as well as counseling to persons at risk.

Recent studies from Germany and Sweden demonstrated that hereditary pancreatic (HP) accounts for 2.7 and 1.9% of all PC cases, respectively [5, 6]. Overall, a familial predisposition to PC occurs in three different clinical settings. First, hereditary tumor syndromes that reveal primarily a clinical phenotype other than PC are known to be associated with an increased risk of PC. Second, HP and cystic fibrosis (CF) can predispose to the development of PC due to onset at an early age, and the concomitant changes and injuries in the pancreas. The third setting is the familial pancreatic cancer (FPC). This term is applied to families with at least two or more first-degree relatives with PC without fulfilling the criteria of other tumor predisposition syndromes.

20.3
Inherited Tumor Syndromes Associated with Pancreatic Cancer

20.3.1
Familial Atypical Multiple Mole Melanoma

Familial atypical multiple mole melanoma (FAMMM, see also Chapter 24 on Malignant Melanoma) is a disease characterized by 50 or more dysplastic nevi and melanoma in two or more first-degree relatives. About 25% of all FAMMM families are associated with the development of PC. In around 50% of these families, oncogenic mutations in the cyclin-dependent kinase 2A (CDKN2A) were identified. In contrast, melanoma prone kindreds not harboring a CDKN2A mutation revealed no PC, and the penetrance of the mutations varies considerably. Individuals of these FAMMM families carrying a CDKN2A mutation have a 13–22-fold increased risk of developing a PC [7]. Furthermore, carriers of a distinct CDKN2A mutation (p16-Leiden) have a cumulative 17% risk of developing PC by the age of 75 [8].

Interestingly, CDKN2A mutations also occur in kindreds with PC and melanoma which lack the FAMMM phenotype. Furthermore, mutations of the CDKN2A locus have not been described with FPC. Therefore, the occurrence of PC and melanoma seems to be another distinct tumor predisposition syndrome called melanoma-pancreatic cancer syndrome (MPCS) [9, 10].

20.3.2
Peutz–Jeghers Syndrome

Peutz–Jeghers syndrome (PJS) is an autosomal dominant tumor syndrome with an incidence of 1 in 25 000, defined by a clinical phenotype of multiple hamartomatous intestinal polyps in association with mucocutaneous pigmentations. This tumor syndrome is caused by germline mutations of the serine/threonine kinase 11 (STK11/LKB1). Patients suffering from PJS have a 132-fold increased risk of the development of PC, and a life-time risk of 36% [11, 12]

20.3.3
Hereditary Breast and Ovarian Cancer

Hereditary breast and ovarian cancer (HBOC) is mainly caused by mutations of the *BRCA1* and *BRCA2* genes (see Chapters 11 and 12). *BRCA1* mutation carriers from HBOC kindreds have a significantly increased risk of developing PC of 2.26 [13]. Larger studies for the development of PC of *BRCA2* mutation carriers in HBOC kindreds are still lacking, but an increased risk of 2.2 was estimated by a smaller study [14]. Furthermore, this study also revealed an elevated risk for colon, stomach, and prostate cancer, which was associated with mutations within the ovarian cancer cluster region (OCCR).

20.3.4
Hereditary Nonpolyposis Colon Cancer and Familial Adenomatous Polyposis

Hereditary nonpolyposis colon cancer (HPNCC) is caused by mutations in the mismatch repair gene (MMR) complex, including *hMSH2* and *hMLH1* [15] (see also Chapter 17 on Lynch syndrome (HNPCC)). As reported by a Finnish study, approximately 1% of MMR mutation carriers developed PC [16]. The estimated cumulated risk of HNPCC patients to develop PC is thought to be less than 5% [17].

Familial adenomatous polyposis is an autosomal dominant inherited disease leading to the development of hundreds of adenomatous polyps and is caused by a germline mutation in the *APC* gene (see Chapter 16 on gastrointestinal polyposis syndromes). Due to only occasional reports of FAP patients developing PC, a definitive link between these two tumor entities cannot be established to date [18].

20.3.5
Ataxia Telangiectasia

Ataxia telangiectasia (AT) is an autosomal recessive inherited disease. Its clinical presentation consists of cerebellar ataxia in combination with oculocutaneous telangiectasia, and cellular and humoral immune deficiencies. AT is caused by germline mutations in the *ATM* gene, and leads to a low risk of PC development [19].

20.3.6
Pancreatic Cancer and Basal Cell Carcinoma

The combined occurrence of PC and basal cell carcinoma of the skin in a subset of families has led to the suggestion that this might represent a rare new tumor syndrome, but further studies are needed to confirm this and the underlying gene defect [20].

20.4
Hereditary Pancreatitis and Cystic Fibrosis

HP is an autosomal dominant inherited disease characterized by recurrent episodes of acute pancreatitis with a progression to chronic pancreatitis and an early onset of the disease, often in childhood or adolescence. In approximately 70% of all cases, mutations in the protease serine 1 (PRSS1) were identified [21]. Mutations in this gene lead towards a disruption of the inactivation of trypsin, thus resulting in an intra-azinous activation of the zymogen cascade. The following autodigestion of the pancreas leads to episodes of acute and chronic pancreatitis, and embodies a long-term stimulus for the development of PC, due to persistent pancreatic injury.

Several families exhibited mutations in the serine protease inhibitor Kazal 1 gene (SPINK1) associated with HP, which serves only as a modifier gene [22].

Patients suffering from HP have a relative risk of 100% and a life-time risk of 44% to develop PC to the age of 70 years [23, 24]. Interestingly, inheritance of the disease from the paternal side and cigarette smoking further increase that risk [49].

CF is a common life-shortening inherited disorder, caused by mutations in the cystic fibrosis transmembrane regulator (CFTR) gene, leading to a disruption of the cyclic adenosine monophosphate (cAMP)-mediated chloride channel and thus leading to obstruction of ducts in several organs, including the pancreas, by mucous secretions. Several studies indicate an association of CF and PC, though these studies reveal significant differences in their results, ranging from a 2.6- to a 32-fold risk of the development of PC [25, 26].

20.5
Familial Pancreatic Cancer

As the previous section mainly focused on hereditary syndromes that also reveal a predisposition to PC, this section will address the heterogeneous group of families with at least two first-degree relatives with PC that do not fulfil the criteria of other tumor syndromes. The term FPC is not only used by most scientists and physicians when dealing with this distinct syndrome, but also by some groups for families with three or more members of any degree affected with PC [27].

The first larger systematic study was published by Lynch and colleagues in 1989. In the aftermath, international and national tumor registries (i.e. the North American National Familial Pancreatic Tumor Registry (NFPTR), the German National Case Collection of Familial Pancreatic Cancer (FaPaCa), and European Registry of Hereditary Pancreatitis and Familial Pancreatic Cancer (EUROPAC) were founded to collect a larger set of data on PC prone families, to characterize the clinical phenotype and the underlying genetic mechanisms [10, 28, 29]. The comprehensive and in-depth analysis of FPC families enrolled by these tumor registries led to a better understanding of this syndrome. As observed in FPC families, PC occurs in a vertical pattern, which is consistent with an autosomal dominant inheritance. The risk of developing a PC among first-degree relatives of a PC patient was determined to be 18-fold in families with two affected members, and 57-fold in kindreds with three or more affected family members [30, 31]. Furthermore, as estimated by a study performed by the EUROPAC and FaPaCa registries investigating 106 FPC families, FPC reveals an anticipation, as patients in younger generations died approximately 10 years earlier than their affected parents [32].

20.5.1
Genetic Background of Familial Pancreatic Cancer

The genetic basis of FPC remains largely unknown. In contrast to other inherited tumor syndromes, the progress in identifying the underlying genetic mutations (e.g. APC in FAP) and the efforts undertaken to identify the gene defect(s) leading to a familial aggregation of PC are still unrewarded.

In 2002, Eberle and colleagues reported that in one family with an early onset of pancreatic insufficiency, diabetes, and PC before the age of 40, the locus 4q32-34 appeared to be linked to this phenotype [33]. Furthermore, a germline mutation in the *palladin* gene, located on 4q32-34, was recently discovered in this unique Family X, but could not be confirmed in a larger cohort of FPC families [34, 35].

Studies investigating mutations of the major tumor suppressor genes known to be causing sporadic PC (i.e. *TP 53, CDKN2A, MADH4/DPC4*) also failed, and no inactivating mutations of these genes were found in FPC families [10, 36]. Furthermore, only a few or no germline mutations were found in other candidate genes such as *STK11/LKB1, RNASEL,* and *CHEK2* [5, 37, 38]. A subset of minor genes (*MAP2K4, ACVR1B/ALK4,* and *ACVR2*) exhibited no germline mutations in FPC kindreds, and the significance of the NOD23020insC remains to be elucidated, as it has been detected in 7% of 31 FPC families but also in 3% of controls [36, 39]. Recently, an investigation postulated an association between familial cancer, including a few cases of PC, and the polymorphism Trp149X of the *ARLTS1* gene, but could not be proven in FPC families [40].

The only exception to these disappointing analysis efforts is *BRCA2*. This gene was first considered to be a major tumor suppressor gene leading to the development of sporadic PC, as a homozygous deletion on locus 13q12.3 was observed in this tumor entity [41].

There are now three studies available addressing the potential link of *BRCA2* to FPC. First, Murphy and colleagues identified *BRCA2* germline mutations in 5 (17%) out of 29 families with 3 or more relatives harboring PC [36]. Noteworthy, 3 out of these 5 families were of Ashkenazi Jewish descent and revealed the 6174delT frameshift mutation previously found in sporadic PC in the Ashkenazi Jewish population. Hahn and colleagues discovered *BRCA2* germline mutations in 4 (15%) out of 26 European families with two or more first-degree relatives with confirmed PC. All families in this particular study were of non-Jewish descent and did not reveal the above-mentioned 6174delT frameshift [42]. Additionally, the BRCA2 K3326X alteration was significantly more prevalent in individuals with FPC (5.6%) than in controls (1.2%; $P < 0.01$) [43].

The latest study did not confirm the high prevalence of *BRCA2* mutations in FPC kindreds. Couch and colleagues identified *BRCA2* germline mutations in 10 (6%) out of 180 families in a multicentric approach [44].

Overall, *BRCA2* germline mutations are the most frequent inherited genetic alteration in FPC discovered to date.

20.5.2
Current Status of Surveillance and Treatment in FPC

As summarized above, the causative germline mutation leading towards FPC has not yet been identified. Therefore, high-risk persons cannot be detected by a single mutation analysis, as can be done for inherited tumor syndromes such as FAP, for which there are options for screening and prophylactic treatment.

The heterogeneity of inherited tumor syndromes associated with a high risk of PC requires an in-depth analysis of the family pedigree over at least three generations, and all cases of PC have to be confirmed by medical records and histology reports.

As confirmed by a consensus conference of experts, high-risk individuals should be enrolled in controlled, yearly-based screening programs performed in expert centers within multidisciplinary institutional review board–approved protocols [45]. The goal of screening programs is to detect pancreatic precursor lesions (PanIN, IPMN, MCN), with an emphasis on detecting carcinoma *in situ* (PanIN 3), as reliable tests and diagnostic markers are still lacking. High-risk persons (≥10-fold risk) for the development of PC should be screened, and screening should start at 40 years of age, or 10 years before the youngest manifestation of PC in the distinct family (Table 20.1).

A few published studies have evaluated surveillance programs in asymptomatic but high-risk groups of persons of FPC families. Canto and colleagues screened 38 high-risk persons from 17 FPC families by employing endoscopic ultrasound (EUS) and CT, followed by endoscopic retrograde cholangiopancreatography (ERCP) in case of a suspicious lesion. This study identified lesions in 6 patients, and limited pancreatic resections were performed, revealing PC in 1 patient, benign serous cystadenoma in 2 patients, one intraductal papillary mucinous tumor (IPMT), and non-neoplastic lesions in 2 patients [46]. A prospective con-

Table 20.1 Specific risk factors for inherited PC.

Low (<5-fold)	Moderate (5–10-fold)	High (≥10-fold)[a]
Hereditary non-polyposis colorectal cancer	History of PC in two first-degree relatives	FAMMM/ MPCS kindreds with p16 germline mutation and at least one case of PC in first-degree or second-degree relative
Familial adenomatous polyposis	Cystic fibrosis	Peutz–Jeghers syndrome
History of PC in one first-degree relative	Chronic pancreatitis	Hereditary pancreatitis
BRCA1 mutation carrier	*BRCA2* mutation carrier	>3 first-degree, second-degree, or third-degree relatives with PC
Ashkenazi Jewish descent		*BRCA2* mutation carrier with at least one first-degree or second-degree relative

a   Patients that should be enrolled in a surveillance program.

trolled study of screening EUS and CT followed by ERCP in 78 high-risk individuals from FPC kindreds, and 149 control subjects, was performed by the same group. Ten percent of the high-risk patients treated by limited pancreatectomy had precursor lesions for adenocarcinoma consisting of IPMNs (one with carcinoma *in situ*) [47]. The German FaPaCa registry also employs a EUS-based approach followed by two MRI with different dyes. To date, 4 patients underwent subtotal pancreatic resections, and histology revealed pancreatic lipoma in 1 patient, focal fibrosis with PanIN1b lesions in 2 patients, and a ductal epithelial cyst with PanIN1b lesion in 1 patient [48, 49].

It is obvious that surgery is recommended in cases where suspicious lesions or pancreatic masses were identified during the screening program. As revealed by the aforementioned data, false-positive results can occur in the EUS-based surveillance approaches, and therefore every surgical procedure has to be thoroughly planned to avoid overtreatment. The current surgical strategy employs the resection of the lesion bearing the relevant part of the pancreas, followed by frozen section. If examination of the frozen section leads to a diagnosis of PC or high-grade PanIN lesions, a total pancreatectomy will be performed, otherwise not. A prophylactic pancreatectomy in asymptomatic high-risk individuals cannot be recommended to date, especially with regard to the significant morbidity (e.g. Briddle's diabetes), and the unknown penetrance of the disease.

20.6
Conclusion

Since PC still remains a tumor entity with one of the worst prognoses and yet lacks distinct tests for early detection, it is crucial that high-risk persons from PC-prone families are enrolled in screening programs at expert centers in a setting of a national tumor registry. This, to date, is the only chance for these individuals to detect a potential pancreatic mass at an early stage.

References

1 Ferlay, J., Autier, P., Boniol, M. et al. (2007) Estimates of the cancer incidence and mortality in Europe in 2006. Annals of Oncology, 18, 581–92.

2 Ehrenthal, D., Haeger, L., Grin, T. et al. (1987) Familial pancreatic adenocarcinoma in three generations. A case report and a review of the literature. Cancer, 59 (9), 1661–4.

3 MacDermott, R.P. and Kramer, P. (1973) Adenocarcinoma of the pancreas in four siblings. Gastroenterology, 65 (1), 137–9.

4 Lynch, H.T., Lanspa, S.J., Fitzgibbons R.J. Jr, et al. (1989) Familial pancreatic cancer (part 1): genetic pathology review. The Nebraska Medical Journal, 74 (5), 109–12.

5 Bartsch, D.K., Kress, R., Sina-Frey, M. et al. (2004) Prevalence of familial pancreatic cancer in Germany. International Journal of Cancer, 110 (6), 902–6.

6 Hemminki, K. and Li, X. (2003) Familial and second primary pancreatic cancers: a nationwide epidemiologic study from Sweden. International Journal of Cancer, 103 (4), 525–30.

7 Goldstein, A.M., Fraser, M.C., Struewing, J.P. et al. (1995) Increased risk of pancreatic cancer inmelanoma-prone kindreds with p16INK4 mutations. The New England Journal of Medicine, 333 (15), 970–4.

8 Vasen, H.F., Gruis, N.A., Frants, R.R. et al. (2000) Risk of developing pancreatic cancer in families with familial atypical multiple mole melanoma associated with a specific 19 deletion of p16 (p16-Leiden). International Journal of Cancer, 87 (6), 809–11.

9 Whelan, A.J., Bartsch, D. and Goodfellow, P.J. (1995) Brief report: a familial syndrome of pancreatic cancer and melanoma with a mutation in the CDKN2 tumor-suppressor gene. The New England Journal of Medicine, 333 (15), 975–7.

10 Bartsch, D.K., Sina-Frey, M. and Lang, S. et al. (2002) CDKN2A germline mutations in familial pancreatic cancer. Annals of Surgery, 236 (6), 730–7.

11 Su, G.H., Hruban, R.H., Bansal, R.K. et al. (1999) Germline and somatic mutations of the STK11/LKB1 Peutz-Jeghers gene in pancreatic and biliary cancers. American Journal of Pathology, 154 (6), 1835–40.

12 Giardiello, F.M., Welsh, S.B., Hamilton, S.R. et al. (1987) Increased risk of cancer in the Peutz–Jeghers syndrome. The New England Journal of Medicine, 316 (24), 1511–14.

13 Thompson, D., Easton, D.F. and for the Breast Cancer Linkage Consortium (2002) Cancer incidence in BRCA1 mutation carriers. Journal of the National Cancer Institute, 94 (18), 1358–65.

14 Risch, H.A., McLaughlin, J.R., Cole, D.E. et al. (2001) Prevalence and penetrance of germline BRCA1 and BRCA2 mutations in a population series of 649 women with ovarian cancer. American Journal of Human Genetics, 68 (3), 700–10.

15 Fishel, R., Lescoe, M.K., Rao, M.R. et al. (1993) The human mutator gene homolog MSH2 and its association with hereditary nonpolyposis colon cancer. Cell, 75, 1027–8.

16 Aarnio, M., Sankila, R., Pukkala, E. *et al.* (1999) Cancer risk in mutation carriers of DNA-mismatch-repair genes. *International Journal of Cancer*, **81** (2), 214–18.

17 Lynch, H.T., Voorhees, G.J., Lanspa, S.J. *et al.* (1985) Pancreatic carcinoma and hereditary nonpolyposis colorectal cancer: a family study. *British Journal of Cancer*, **52**, 271–3.

18 Stewart, C.J., Imrie, C.W. and Foulis, A.K. (1994) Pancreatic islet cell tumour in a patient with familial adenomatous polyposis. *Journal of Clinical Pathology*, **47** (9), 860–1.

19 Lynch, H.T. (1994) Genetics and pancreatic cancer. *Archives of Surgery*, **129** (3), 266–8.

20 Sina-Frey, M., Bartsch, D.K., Grundei, T. *et al.* (2003) Pancreatic cancer and basal-cell carcinoma. *Lancet*, **361** (9352), 180.

21 Whitcomb, D.C., Gorry, M.C., Preston, R.A. *et al.* (1996) Hereditary pancreatitis is caused by a mutation in the cationic trypsinogen gene. *Nature Genetics*, **14** (2), 141–5.

22 Witt, H., Luck, W., Hennies, H.C. *et al.* (2000) Mutations in the gene encoding the serine proteaseinhibitor, Kazal type 1 are associated with chronic pancreatitis. *Nature Genetics*, **25** (2), 213–16.

23 Lowenfels, A.B., Maisonneuve, P. and Whitcomb, D.C. (2000) Risk factors for cancer in hereditary pancreatitis. International Hereditary Pancreatitis Study Group. *The Medical clinics of North America*, **84** (3), 565–73.

24 Lowenfels, A.B. and Maisonneuve, P. (2005) Risk factors for pancreatic cancer. *Journal of Cellular Biochemistry*, **95** (4), 649–56.

25 Maisonneuve, P., FitzSimmons, S.C., Neglia, J.P. *et al.* (2003) Cancer risk in nontransplanted and transplanted cystic fibrosis patients: a 10-year study. *Journal of the National Cancer Institute*, **95**, 381–7.

26 Neglia, J.P., Fitzsimmons, S.C., Maisonneuve, P. *et al.* (1995) The risk of cancer among patients with cystic fibrosis. Cystic Fibrosis and Cancer Study Group. *The New England Journal of Medicine*, **332**, 494–9.

27 Habbe, N., Langer, P., Sina-Frey, M. and Bartsch, D.K. (2006) Familial pancreatic cancer syndromes. *Endocrinology and Metabolism Clinics of North America*, **35** (2), 417–30. xi.

28 Hruban, R.H., Petersen, G.M., Ha, P.K. *et al.* (1998) Genetics of pancreatic cancer. From genes to families. *Surgical Oncology Clinics of North America*, **7** (1), 1–23.

29 Applebaum, S.E., Kant, J.A., Whitcomb, D.C. *et al.* (2000) Genetic testing. Counseling, laboratory, and regulatory issues and the EUROPAC protocol for ethical research in multicenter studies of inherited pancreatic diseases. *The Medical Clinics of North America*, **84** (3), 575–88.

30 Tersmette, A.C., Petersen, G.M., Overhaus, G.J. *et al.* (2001) Increased risk of incident pancreatic cancer among first-degree relatives of patients with familial pancreatic cancer. *Clinical Cancer Research*, **7**, 738–44.

31 Klein, A.P., Brune, K.A., Petersen, G.M. *et al.* (2004) Prospective risk of pancreatic cancer in familial pancreatic cancer kindreds. *Cancer Research*, **64** (7), 2634–8.

32 McFaul, C., Greenhalf, W., Earl, J. *et al.* (2006) Anticipation in familial pancreatic cancer. *Gut*, **55**, 252–8.

33 Eberle, M.A., Pfutzer, R., Pogue-Geile, K.L. *et al.* (2002) A new susceptibility locus for autosomal dominant pancreatic cancer maps to chromosome 4q32-34. *American Journal of Human Genetics*, **70** (4), 1044–8.

34 Pogue-Geile, K.L., Chen, R., Bronner, M.P. *et al.* (2006) Palladin mutation causes familial pancreatic cancer and suggests a new cancer mechanism. *PLOS Medicine*, **3**, e516.

35 Slater, E., Amrillaeva, V., Bartsch, D.K. *et al.* (2007) Palladin mutation causes familial pancreatic cancer: absence in European families. *PLoS Medicine*, **4** (4), e164.

36 Murphy, K.M., Brune, K.A., Griffin, C. *et al.* (2002) Evaluation of candidate genes MAP2K4, MADH4, ACVR1B and BRCA2 in familial pancreatic cancer: deleterious BRCA2 mutations in 17%. *Cancer Research*, **62**, 3789–93.

37 Gruetzmann, R., McFaul, C., Bartsch, D.K., *et al.* (2004) No evidence for germline mutations of the LKB1/STK11 gene in familial pancreatic carcinoma. *Cancer Letters*, **214**, 63–67.

38 Bartsch, D.K., Krysewski, K., Sina-Frey, M. *et al.* (2006) Low frequency of CHEK2 mutations in familial pancreatic cancer. *Familial Cancer*, **5** (4), 305–8.

39 Nej, K., Bartsch, D.K., Sina-Frey, M. *et al.* (2004) The NOD3020insC mutation and the risk of familial pancreatic cancer. *Hereditary Cancer in Clinical Practice*, **2**, 149–150.

40 Calin, G.A., Trapasso, F., Shimizu, M. *et al.* (2005) Familial cancer associated with a polymorphism in ARLTS1. *The New England Journal of Medicine*, **352** (16), 1667–76.

41 Schutte, M., da Costa, L.T., Hahn, S.A. *et al.* (1995) Identification by representational difference analysis of a homozygous deletion in pancreatic carcinoma that lies within the BRCA2 region. *Proceedings of the National Academy of Sciences USA*, **92**, 5950–4.

42 Hahn, S.A., Greenhalf, B., Ellis, I. *et al.* (2003) BRCA2 germline mutations of the LKB1/STK11 gene in familial pancreatic carcinoma. *Journal of the National Cancer Institute*, **95**, 214–21.

43 Martin, S.T., Matsubayashi, H., Rogers, C.D. *et al.* (2005) Increased prevalence of the BRCA2 polymorphic stop codon K3326X among individuals with familial pancreatic cancer. *Oncogene*, **24** (22), 3652–6.

44 Couch, F.J., Johnson, M.R., Rabe, K.G. *et al.* (2007) The prevalence of *BRCA2* mutations in familial pancreatic cancer. *Cancer Epidemiology Biomarkers and Prevention*, **16** (2), 342–6.

45 Brand, R.E., Lerch, M.M., Rubinstein, W.S. *et al.* (2007) Advances in counselling and surveillance of patients at risk for pancreatic cancer. *Gut*, **56**, 1460–9.

46 Canto, M.I., Goggins, M., Yeo, C.J. *et al.* (2004) Screening for pancreatic neoplasia in high-risk individuals: an EUS-based approach. *Clinical Gastroenterology and Hepatology*, **2**, 606–21.

47 Canto, M.I., Goggins, M., Hruban, R.H. *et al.* (2006) Screening for early pancreatic neoplasia in high-risk individuals: a prospective controlled study. *Clinical Gastroenterology and Hepatology*, **4**, 766–81.

48 Langer, P., Rothmund, M. and Bartsch, D.K. (2006) Prophylactic pancreas surgery. *Chirurg*, **77** (1), 25–32.

49 Lowenfels, A.B., Maisonneuve, P., Whitcomb, D.C. *et al.* (2001) Cigarette smoking as a risk factor for pancreatic cancer in patients with hereditary pancreatitis. *The Journal of the American Medical Association*, **286** (2), 169–70.

21
Liver Tumors

Sabine J. Presser

Summary

In contrast to other tumor entities, such as colon and mamma adenocarcinomas, hereditary aspects of malignant liver tumors have only been intensely studied within recent decades. Exogenous factors, such as viral hepatitis and food carcinogens, are traditionally regarded as hallmarks of liver carcinogenesis. However, the individual risk to develop liver cancer due to these factors also depends on a number of hereditary factors, such as susceptibility for viral infections and genetic variations in metabolizing liver enzymes, such as cytochrome P450 cyclooxogenases. Whereas hereditary aspects of carcinogen activation and detoxification are reviewed below, we would like to refer the interested reader to specific immunological literature with respect to the influence of host genetics on viral infections.

In addition, many inherited metabolic diseases significantly enhance the risk of liver cancer, and so are described in detail in this respect. They often follow a chronic progressive course and are linked to liver fibrosis. The molecular and cellular mechanisms responsible for malignant transformation of hepatocytes and biliary epithelial cells are not well understood. However, it appears that exogeneous factors also influence the cancer risk of inherited liver diseases.

Finally, a number of oncogenes and tumor suppressor genes are shown to be involved in the development and progression of liver cancer. Therefore, a brief description of the involved genes is included at the end of this chapter.

21.1
Introduction

Neoplasms of the liver may arise from any cell type within the liver parenchyma. Hepatocellular carcinoma (HCC) is by far the most common primary malignant tumor of the liver in adults (about 90% of all malignant liver tumors) and the fifth most common cancer worldwide, ranging third in cancer-related mortality.

Hereditary Tumors: From Genes to Clinical Consequences
Edited by Heike Allgayer, Helga Rehder and Simone Fulda
Copyright © 2009 WILEY-VCH Verlag GmbH & Co. KGaA, Weinheim
ISBN: 978-3-527-32028-8

However, the incidence of liver cancer shows striking geographic variations that can be explained by differences in the prevalence of viral hepatitis, in particular HBV and HCV. Almost any form of chronic liver disease that leads to cirrhosis may be complicated by liver cell carcinoma; therefore, cirrhosis should be considered a precancerous condition, independent of its origin.

Cholangiocellular carcinomas (CCC, 5–10%) exist in three main forms: intrahepatic, hilar, and extrahepatic. They are not associated with cirrhosis. Cholangio-carcinomas represent a rare but significant complication of long-standing ulcerative cholangitis, commonly preceded by sclerosing cholangitis. Mixed hepatocellular and bile duct carcinomas (combined HCC/CCC, 2%) are rarely seen. Hepatoblastoma accounts for approximately 5% of malignancies in childhood. Most hepatoblastomas are of the categories "epithelial" or "mixed epithelial" and "mesenchymal" [1]. Rare primary malignant nonepithelial tumors are angiosarcomas, leiomyosarcomas, and fibrosarcomas, arising from vascular or mesenchymal tissues within the liver, respectively.

Primary hereditary tumors of the liver are extremely rare. However, many genetic diseases, in particular metabolic disorders, lead to chronic liver disease that may in turn give rise to liver carcinoma. In addition, genetic variations have a significant influence on the incidence and progression of many liver tumors induced by exogenous factors such as viral infections (e.g. HBV, HCV) and toxic and carcinogenic agents (e.g. aflatoxins, benzopyrenes, vinyl chloride). Finally, a large number of somatic mutations in tumor suppressor genes and oncogenes have lately been associated with progression and metastasis of liver tumors.

21.2
Hereditary Diseases Affecting Liver Function and Carcinogenesis

21.2.1
Hemochromatosis

Hemochromatosis (HFE) is an autosomal recessive metabolic disease characterized by increased iron uptake that leads to iron overload and fibrosis, primarily of the liver but also of other organs, such as heart and skin. The disease has a prevalence of about 0.3 to 0.5% in Northern Europe and North America, and is caused by mutations of proteins involved in iron resorption and metabolism. Among affected homozygotes, primary HCC is responsible for up to one-third of deaths. Most common are homozygous defects in the HFE gene (HFE, chromosomal location 6p21.3), which encodes an MHC class I related protein (HLA-H) that associates with the transferrin receptor (TFR) and regulates the release of nutrient-resorbed iron from the enterocytes. Further autosomal recessive disorders are juvenile HFE (HFE2), caused by mutations in hemojuvelin (HJV, 19q13) and hepcidin (HAMP, 19q13) as well as HFE type 3 (HFE3), linked to TFR 2 mutations (TFR2, 7q22). In contrast, HFE type 4 (HFE4, 2q32) is an autosomal dominant disorder caused by mutations of ferroportin (SLC40A1, 2q32).

For successful treatment of HFE, an early diagnosis is important, relying on serum ferritin, transferrin saturation (TfSat) and genetic analysis. Due to its strong genetic linkage and high prevalence, HFE is even regarded as a candidate for population screening [2, 3]. Since HFE can easily be treated by iron depletion, this therapy constitutes an excellent form of cancer prevention. Iron is an essential transition metal that can adopt two different oxidation states (Fe^{3+}/Fe^{2+}). It constitutes a redox system with a high capacity to induce oxidative stress and lipid peroxidation, leading to membrane damage, organelle dysfunction and, as a result, to various degenerative diseases [4, 5]. Uncomplexed ionic iron is very toxic and is therefore bound to the iron binding proteins transferrin and lactoferrin with extremely high affinity. Iron homeostasis is primarily regulated by intestinal uptake and not by excretion. The liver, and to a much lesser extent the macrophages, serve as iron storage, enabling rapid iron delivery for erythropoiesis [6].

Clinical symptoms rarely occur before the total individuals burden of iron exceeds 15 g, as compared with a level below 5 g in healthy humans. This is usually the case in affected men during the third to sixth decade, in women several years later. Clinical manifestations include hepatomegaly, skin pigmentation, diabetes mellitus, hypopituitarism, hypogonadism, impotence, heart failure, liver cirrhosis, and HCC [7, 8]. The frequency of liver cirrhosis is up to 60% and of HCC up to 5%, as stated at a recent international consensus conference [9]. Most of the early symptoms are nonspecific, thus biochemical tests of iron status are important, using serum tests for TfSat, total iron binding capacity (TIBC), and ferritin [8, 9]. In patients with severe iron overload, serum transferrin may be completely saturated with iron. Primary HFE should be suspected in any cases where serum ferritin values exceed 200 µg/l at TfSat over 50%. In normal healthy subjects, serum TFR (sTfR) increased with decreasing TfSat values below 25%, while in HFE patients, increased levels occurred at TfSat levels as high as 50% [10].

Before the discovery of the HFE gene in 1996 [11], liver biopsy was often necessary to confirm the diagnosis. Since over 80% of all HFE patients are homozygous for the *C282Y* mutation [12], genetic testing has obviated the need for a liver biopsy in most cases [9]. At present, the only available non-invasive method is magnetic resonance imaging (MRI) for 3-D quantification of body iron deposition [13, 14]. However, it cannot replace liver biopsy with respect to assessing the cellular distribution pattern of iron.

There are a number of conditions in which TfSat should be measured to exclude a diagnosis of primary HFE. These include HCC and other chronic parenchymal liver diseases, cardiomyopathy and arrhythmias, diabetes mellitus, impotence, infertility, amenorrhoea, anterior pituitary failure, arthritis and arthralgia, increased skin pigmentation, and porphyria cutanea tarda [9].

The HFE gene on chromosome 6 encodes a protein of 343 amino acids that belongs to the major histocompatibility (MHC) class I family [11]. In populations of northern European origin, more than 80% of HFE patients have a point mutation at nucleotide 845, resulting in a cysteine-to-tyrosine substitution at position 282 (C282Y). It is estimated that 40 to 70% of C282Y homoyzogotes will develop clinical evidence of iron overload [15]. The allele frequency is about 3 to 5% in central Europe, up to 10% in Northern Europe, and less than 3% in the Mediterranean [16]. In Asian populations (Indian, Chinese), the *C282Y* mutation is rare or absent [17]. Another point mutation, leading to a histidine-to-aspartate substitution in position 63 (H63D), is more prevalent globally [18]. The average heterozygous carrier frequency of this mutation is 22% in European populations [15], but its penetrance is much lower than that for the *C282Y* mutation, leading to clinically apparent HFE in compound heterozygotes only (C282Y/H63D). The *C282Y* mutation appears to disrupt the association of the HFE protein with the TFR [19, 20]. Apparently, this interaction is essential for the physiological down-regulation of iron absorption when iron stores are full. The proposed mechanism is that mutated HFE protein is less able to bind to the TFR. This reduced binding increases the affinity of the TFR for iron-loaded transferrin, and thus more iron is transported into the cell [21]. HFE knockout mice develop an iron overload syndrome with clear similarities to human primary HFE, providing strong evidence that the HFE protein is directly involved in iron homeostasis [22]. Immunolocalization of the HFE protein in the small intestine is limited to cells in deep crypts, indicating that it is involved in the regulation of intestinal iron absorption [23].

Phlebotomy, the metal depletion treatment of choice in primary or secondary hemochromatosis [24], markedly improves survival and prevents most of the complications [7]. New approaches suggest removing 450 to 500 ml blood once a week until serum ferritin is reduced to about 50 mg/l, being followed by one venesection every 3 months. Patients with extensive iron deposits or acute liver cell damage and increased iron release into the circulation need combined treatment with the iron chelator desferrioxamine (Deferoxamine, Desferal, DFOA). The acute toxicity of this compound is rather low, and intravenous infusion should be given slowly to avoid hypotension. However, continued use induces a wide range of side-effects that include ophthalmic and auditory toxicity, changes in blood counts, allergic and skin reactions, and pulmonary, renal, and neurological effects [25]. Only 10 to 50 mg iron can be removed by one intravenous treatment, corresponding to about 4 g of iron within 1 year upon weekly in-clinic parenteral desferrioxamine administrations [26]. Due to the obvious need to find new effective chelators for peroral use, experimental and clinical studies are in progress [27, 28].

21.2.2
Wilson's Disease

Wilson's disease is an autosomal recessive disorder with chronic copper accumulation. The first symptoms become apparent in infancy, mainly in the liver, whereas other tissues, such as brain, cornea, and kidneys are affected later, partially owing to redistribution from the liver. The copper accumulation is related to impaired biliary excretion, which normally regulates the copper balance. The disease depends on the homozygous presence of a mutation in the *ATP7B* gene on the long arm of chromosome 13 [29–31], regulating the cellular trafficking of copper [32].

Wilson's disease is rare, with a prevalence estimated at about 1/30 000 to 1/50 000 [33]. However, many cases of atypical psychiatric or hepatic disorders may also be caused by undiagnosed Wilson's disease [34]. The carrier frequency is about 1% [33]. True Wilson's disease usually manifests between 5 and 30 years of age, with a variety of hepatic, neurologic, or psychiatric symptoms [35]. Liver cirrhosis and cardiac abnormalities [36] are common manifestations. Blocked biliary copper excretion, which characterizes the pathogenesis, also occurs in advanced cholestatic disease, for example, primary sclerosing cholangitis, but in the latter case the role of copper toxicity in disease progression is unclear [37].

The diagnosis is based on: (i) serum ceruloplasmin below the normal lower threshold of 200 mg/l; (ii) substantially increased urinary copper excretion (>100 µg/24 h, the best single screening test); and (iii) increased copper concentration in the liver (>250 µg/g dry weight), in the absence of signs of cholestatic liver disease [38]. Characteristic Kayser–Fleischer rings are often present due to copper deposits in the cornea [38]. Genetic screening is not done routinely, but all siblings of patients should be examined to identify presymptomatic homozygotes. Because Wilson's disease is autosomal recessive and rare, there is a very low probability that children of patients are homozygotes.

The mutated protein is a copper translocating ATPase located in hepatocytes at the *trans*-Golgi network and at the canalicular part of the cell membrane [30, 32, 39]. This enzyme (ATP7B) belongs to a large family of P-type ATPases that transport cations across cellular membranes. Malfunction of ATP7B is responsible for the defective biliary export of excess copper. Another role of ATP7B is to introduce copper into ceruloplasmin for export into the blood [32]. More than 250 different mutations have been described in the *ATP7B* gene, and it is highly likely that the large variability in clinical presentation seen in Wilson's disease is at least partly due to variability in the type and severity of gene disruption caused by the different mutations [40].

Strict low copper diets are no longer advised, but intake of liver and shellfish should be reduced. Drinking water may need to be tested for copper [38]. Successful treatment has been possible since 1956, when Walshe introduced the chelator D-penicillamine (DPA) to enhance copper excretion in affected patients [41]. The toxicity of oral and parenteral DPA is low, but its clinical use is limited because of side-effects such as hypersensitivity, bone marrow suppression, nephrotic syndrome, and various autoimmune reactions. The intestinal absorption of DPA is about 50%. The volume of distribution is close to that of extracellular water, and a major part of a systemic dose forms mixed disulfides with serum albumin. The metabolism is insignificant, and most of a systemic dose is rapidly excreted in the urine, as free DPA or the oxidized dimer [42, 43].

Since 1973, triethylene tetramine (trientine, trien, TETA) has been increasingly used clinically, and is now the drug of choice in the Western world [44, 45]. The normal administration route for TETA is oral, but the absorption is limited [46]. Only about 1% of an oral dose is recovered as free TETA in the urine, most of it being excreted as an acetylated conjugate identified as 1-acetyl-TETA. The rec-ommended dose for Wilson's disease patients is 0.75 to 2.0 g/day. Based on long-term experience, TETA is remarkably free of side-effects compared to DPA [47]. When given as the initial treatment, the TETA dose has been 250 mg, 4 to 6 times daily. The maintenance dose, 1 g daily to adults or 0.5 g to children, appears to be equivalent to penicillamine in halting the progression of the disease [34, 48].

In China, hundreds of patients have been treated with oral dimercaptosuccinic acid (DMSA) over the past 30 years, resulting in clinical improvement and increased urinary copper excretion [49].

Zinc is being strongly advocated by some groups as an alternative to chelation therapy [38, 50, 51]. Zinc acts by inducing hepatic metallothionein production, which sequesters copper into a nontoxic pool [52]. Compared to penicillamine, zinc has very low toxicity, and the only significant side-effect seems to be gastric discomfort in 10% of patients [35].

Wilson's disease depends on an *ATP7B* mutant on chromosome 13. Because successful treatment is available, early diagnosis is crucial using copper mea-surements in urine and liver biopsies. Treatment regimens involve chelation with TETA or penicillamine. Future research in these treatment regimens is justified.

21.2.3
Alpha 1-Antitrypsin Deficiency

Alpha-1-antitrypsin (AAT, PI1) is a serum protein encoded by the PI gene on chromosome 14q32.1. It is responsible for inhibiting trypsin and other proteases. Reduced AAT serum levels are associated with emphysema and liver disease. AAT is primarily produced by the liver and by macrophages [53], and released as a soluble protein into the blood stream. It is easily quantified by standard laboratory tests and serves as an acute phase marker. A large number of allelic variants have initially been described according to their differences in electrophoretic mobility [54].

The most common alleles and their frequency are: PI M1A: 0.20–0.23, PI M1V (A213V): 0.44–0.49, PI M2 (R101H): 0.10–0.11, PI M3 (E376D): 0.14–0.19, PI S (A213V & E264V): 0.02–0.04, and PI Z (E342K): 0.01–0.02. In addition, a number of null alleles result from frameshift mutations and large deletions. To date, 40 different alleles have been described in total. All M alleles are associated with a normal phenotype, and therefore usually not further differentiated. The Z allele is the major disease allele causing an accumulation of the protein in the endoplas-matic reticulum with only 15% released from the hepatocytes. The S allele results in a protein that is intracellularly degraded prior to secretion [55]. It is causing a mildly increased risk in combination with a Z or a null allele (with compound heterozygosity).

Already in the 1990s, it became clear that AAT deficiency may lead to severe medical problems. Complete absence of AAT was found to be associated with degenerative lung disease causing death at middle age [56], and identified as an inherited disease [57]. A little later, homozygous AAT deficiency (PI ZZ) was also described to cause familial infantile liver cirrhosis [58]. This was attributed by Udall *et al.* [59] to the obvious lack of protease inhibitors to counteract the effects of luminal proteases crossing the intestinal barrier in the neonate. The proposed mechanism was supported by the finding of Lake-Bakaar and Dooley [60] that AAT is also an important proteolytic inhibitor in the bile.

It is now accepted that the PI Z and the rare PI Malton mutation are associated with both emphysema and liver disease. In contrast, the PI S and some rare mutations are deficiency mutations that cause only an increased risk of emphysema. The same holds true for the null mutations [61].

It is assumed that liver injury and finally malignant transformation result from toxic effects of the mutant AAT molecule accumulating within the endoplasmic reticulum of hepatocytes. However, since only less than 15% of PI ZZ homozygous patients develop liver disease, it was proposed that other genetic and potentially exogenous factors, such as inflammation, are modulating the intracellular degradation of the abnormal AAT and thus its pathogenic effect. [62]. The underlying mechanism of AAT protein aggregation in the endoplasmic reticulum has been described in detail by Lomas *et al.* [63]. In 1987, Rakela reported that the mean age when liver disease became symptomatic, was 58 years for the ZZ phenotype, 66 years for the SZ phenotype, and 73 years for the MZ phenotype. Additional risk factors are male gender and obesity [64].

Heterozygosity of the PI Z allele was also found to be associated with liver disease in a large study based on 1055 liver biopsies. The prevalence of phenotype Pi MZ in the whole group was only 2.4%, but much higher in samples with liver cirrhosis (9%), and cryptogenic cirrhosis as well as chronic active hepatitis were 21%. The prognosis of the Pi MZ cirrhotic patients was poor; most died within one year [65]. The heterozygous phenotype is more prevalent in patients with hepatitis C, alcoholic liver disease, cryptogenic cirrhosis, and HCC [66, 67].

An association of non-M phenotypes with HCC was already described by Fargion *et al.* [68]. However, this risk and the risk of cirrhosis is only linked to the PI Z allele and not to PI null alleles, indicating that the intracellular accumulation of the mutated protein is responsible for this association. In a study with 317 patients with HCC, 6% had hepatic PI Z deposits (control group: 1.8%). In heterozygous AAT deficiency, HCC also develop in noncirrhotic livers and can be characterized by cholangiocellular differentiation. Bile duct lesions can frequently be found, which reflects a predisposition for the liver tissue for developing tumors with cholangiolar differentiation in AAT deficiency [69, 70].

An inherited deficiency of functional AAT in the plasma may be treated by weekly intravenous infusion of purified AAT, which can reverse the biochemical abnormalities in serum and lung fluid [71]. Since the combination of AAT deficiency and cigarette smoking increases significantly the risk to develop emphysema, the patients should be advised to avoid smoking throughout their life. However, the AAT supplementation therapy is expensive (30000–66000 US$ per year) and is not able to prevent the intracellular polymerization and accumulation of AAT in carrers of the Z-alleles [72]. The latter could potentially be treated with peptides that block the polymerization of the mutant protein [73, 74]. In addition, gene therapies have also been discussed to treat AAT deficiency [75–78]. The most definitive therapy is liver transplantation, which is used in end-stage liver disease and grants acquisition of the donor phenotype, a rise in serum levels of AAT, and prevention of associated diseases [79].

21.2.4
Cystic Fibrosis

Cystic fibrosis (CF, Mucoviscidosis) is one of the most common recessive human genetic diseases with an incidence between 1:2400 and 1:39000, depending on the ethnic origin [80]. It is caused by mutations in the CFTR gene (chromosomal location 7q31.3-q32), which encodes a chloride ion channel expressed in lung, pancreas, skin, and other tissues. The most common mutation is a deletion of phenylalanine 508 (delta-F508), which is found in about 75% of all CF patients [81]. In The Netherlands, the delta-F508 mutation has an allele frequency of about 1.6% [82]. The delta-F508 CFTR mutation results in the production of a misfolded CFTR protein that is retained in the endoplasmic reticulum and targeted for degradation.

Manifestations of CF relate not only to the disruption of the exocrine function of the pancreas but also to intestinal glands, the biliary tree, bronchial glands, and sweat glands. Gaskin *et al.* [83] found that 96% of patients with CF and evidence of liver disease had biliary tract obstruction, usually a stricture of the distal common bile duct. Bilton *et al.* [84] described a case of CF complicated by common bile duct stenosis.

Gabolde *et al.* [85] showed that the presence of cirrhosis in patients with CF is significantly associated with either homozygous or compound heterozygous mutations in the *MBL2* gene, which encodes mannose-binding lectin (MBL). Gabolde *et al.* compared 216 patients homozygous for the delta-F508 mutation and found that 5.4% of those homozygous or compound heterozygous for wildtype MBL had cirrhosis, while 30.8% of those homozygous or compound heterozygous for mutant alleles had cirrhosis ($p=0.008$).

21.2.5
Galactosemia

Patients suffering from galactosemia can present with hepatomegaly, icterus, cataracts, *E. coli* sepsis, failure to thrive, mental retardation, and urinary excretion of albumin and sugar [86]. Jaundice of intrinsic liver disease may be accentuated by severe hemolysis, and hemorrhagic diathesis may count for the onset of primary liver carcinoma [87].

Elsas [88] stated that more than 130 mutations in the *GALT* gene had been associated with GALT deficiency. Two common mutations, Q188R and K285N, accounted for more than 70% of galactosemia-producing alleles in the white population and were associated with classic galactosemia and impaired GALT function. Most patients are compound heterozygotes rather than true molecular homozygotes. Cramer *et al.* [89] hypothesized that women with galactosemia may be at increased risk of ovarian cancer, on the basis of a relationship between the N314D polymorphism and reduced GALT activity. Homozygosity for N314D is linked to a 4-fold increase in risk for all types of ovarian cancer and a 14-fold increase for endometrioid and clear cell ovarian cancer. Suzuki *et al.* [90] estimated that the birth incidence of classic galactosemia is 1 per 47 000 in the white population.

21.2.6
Fructosemia

Most cases of fructosemia are severely ill infants with recurrent hypoglycemia and vomiting, occurring at the time of weaning, when fructose or sucrose is added to the diet, resulting in marked malnutrition. Nordmann *et al.* [91] studied the immunologic and kinetic properties of the liver and suggested that a mutation of the structural gene is responsible for the abnormal fructose-1-phosphate aldolase activity in fructosemia. Since aldolase B is normally present in kidney and intestinal mucosa as well as in liver, Cox *et al.* [92] were able to detect heterozygotes by intestinal biopsy. Since children born by women with fructose intolerance may suffer from pulmonary edema, cirrhosis, and failure to thrive [93], a strict fructose-free diet is strongly advised during pregnancy.

21.2.7
Tyrosinemia

Lelong *et al.* [94] observed children with cirrhosis, renotubular syndrome, and increased plasma tyrosine. Malignant changes developed in the liver, and death from pulmonary metastases occurred. The disease was attributed to defects of FAH (fumaryl acetoacetate hydrolase), an enzyme involved with tyrosine metabolism.

In stage I of tyrosinemia, infants exhibit hepatic necrosis and hypermethioninemia. In stage II, nodular cirrhosis and chronic hepatic insufficiency are observed, and in stage III renal tubular damage. Low tyrosine diet arrests progression of the disease [95]. It had been postulated that the severe liver damage in tyrosinemia is the result of defective degradation of tyrosine. Hostetter *et al.* [96] showed, however, that liver damage is prenatal in onset, and that hypertyrosinemia developed only postnatally.

Holme *et al.* [97] demonstrated the feasibility of enzymatic diagnosis in chorionic villus material. They proposed enzyme determination in erythrocytes for rapid diagnosis and suggested that enzyme replacement by blood transfusion avoid acute metabolic crises [98, 99]. Dehner *et al.* [100] concluded that a liver replacement is necessary before the age of 2 years to preclude HCC. Liver transplantation is seen as the only definitive therapy for both the metabolic and the oncologic problem in this disorder [101], and should be performed at an early stage [102].

De Braekeleer and Larochelle [103] estimated the prevalence of hereditary tyrosinemia at birth to 1:1846 and a carrier rate of 5% in the Saguenay-Lac Saint Jean region. Grompe *et al.* [104] found that 100% of patients from the Saguenay-Lac St. Jean region of Quebec and 28% of patients from other regions of the world carry a splice donor site mutation in intron 12. As described by Russo and O'Regan [105], HCC was detected in 25% of the patients undergoing liver transplantation. Whereas more than 60% of the patients without liver transplantation died, 80% of the transplanted patients postoperatively had normal liver function, normal growth, and no recurrence of neurologic crises on a normal diet.

21.2.8
Glycogen Storage Disease

Glycogen storage disease (GSD) is caused by defects in the enzyme glucose-6-phosphatase. The liver and kidney are involved, and hypoglycemia is a major problem. Lipidemia also occurs and may lead to xanthoma formation. Survival to adulthood, previously rare, is now common. Hyperuricemia can be observed as well as gout. Liver adenomas are often present [106] and may undergo malignant transformation [107]. Stevenson *et al.* [108] and Burchell *et al.* [109] described HCC developing with GSD. Hepatoblastomas have been described in siblings [110–112], and have been found in association with Wilms tumor, polyposis coli, and the Beckwith–Wiedemann Syndrome (BWS) (see respective chapters in this book). Especially patients with BWS are at an increased risk of developing certain types of cancer. However, little is known about the cancer risk to a specific individual or how the genetic change are related. In over 95% of the cases, hepatomegaly and over 25% adenomas are detected, with elevated blood cholesterol concentration, triglycerides, and blood uric acid concentrations [113]. Bianchi [114] found 50 published cases of hepatocellular adenoma in GSD and 10 cases of HCC. In a multicenter study in the United States and Canada, Talente *et al.* [115] reviewed data from 42 adult patients with GSD. Clinical signs included short stature (90%), hepatomegaly (100%), hepatic adenomas (75%), increased alkaline phosphatase (61%) and gamma-glutamyltransferase (93%) activities, as well as increased serum cholesterol (76%) and triglyceride (100%) levels. Faivre *et al.* [116] reported 3 patients with GSD in whom liver transplantation was performed at 15, 17, and 23 years of age because of multiple hepatic adenomas with a fear of malignant transformation.

21.2.9
Beckwith–Wiedemann Syndrome

Patients with BWS are at increased risk of developing specific tumors, caused primarily by mutation in the chromosome 11p15.5 region (p57 (K1P2) and others). The cardinal features of this disorder are exomphalos, macroglossia, and gigantism in the neonate. Visceromegaly, adrenocortical cytomegaly, and dysplasia of the renal medulla are conspicuous features. Adrenal carcinoma, hepatoblastoma, and rhabdomyosarcoma occur with increased frequency [117].

Inheritance is autosomal dominant with variable expressivity, contiguous gene duplication at 11p15, and genomic imprinting resulting from a defective or absent copy of the maternally derived gene. Koufos *et al.* [118] discussed whether a pleiotropic mutation at 11p15.5 or a variety of allelic mutations at 11p15.5 underlie the pathogenesis of BWS and of the related tumors and whether these diseases may alternatively be due to defects at closely linked but separate loci. An unbalanced dosage of maternal and paternal alleles may be the common factor in the different etiologic forms of BWS and associated tumors [119].

Diagnosis is based on clinical findings. A careful cytogenetic analysis of the 11p15 region is recommended. Prenatal diagnosis by ultrasonography is possible [120–122]. Adrenal carcinoma, nephroblastoma, hepatoblastoma, and rhabdomyosarcoma occur with increased frequency, and justify biannual abdominal ultrasound examinations [123]. DeBaun and Tucker [124] studied 183 children with BWS. Thirteen children (7.1%) were identified with cancers before the fourth year of life, and the relative risk for hepatoblastoma was 2280.

21.2.10
FAP (Familial Adenomatous Polyposis)

Familial adenomatous polyposis (FAP) is an autosomal dominant disorder which typically presents with colorectal cancer in early adult life, secondary to extensive adenomatous polyps of the colon (see respective Chapter 16 on gastrointestinal polyposis syndromes). Polyps also develop in the upper gastrointestinal tract and malignancies may occur in other sites including the liver [125, 126]. Several groups noted the association of hepatoblastoma with polyposis coli [127–129]. An empiric risk of less than 1% for hepatoblastoma can be attributed to persons with FAP for their children [130]. Somatic mutations and loss of heterozygosity (LOH) were observed in over 50% of hepatoblastomas from patients without FAP [131].

21.2.11
Alagille Syndrome

Alagille syndrome is caused by mutations in the Jagged-1 gene (*JAG1*). In addition to neonatal jaundice caused by a reduction of intrahepatic bile ducts, several organs including the eyes, heart, bones, and nervous system, are affected [132].

HCC has been reported in children with Alagille syndrome [133–135] and in an adult with Alagille syndrome without cirrhosis [136]. Legius *et al.* [137] speculated that LOH for a cell cycle-regulating gene rather than underlying chronic liver disease may be the explanation of liver carcinoma. In a 19-year-old woman with Alagille syndrome, diagnosed at the age of 8 years, Kato *et al.* [138] described papillary thyroid carcinoma with multiple lung metastases. They reviewed 12 reported cases of HCC. Development of carcinoma was as early as at age 2 years and as late as at age 48 years.

Alagille syndrome is one of the major forms of chronic liver disease in childhood with severe morbidity and a mortality of 10 to 20%. Lykavieris *et al.* [139] reviewed the clinical outcome of 163 French children with Alagille syndrome. Overall, the prognosis was found to be worse in children presenting with neonatal cholestatic jaundice, nevertheless severe complications were possible, even after late-onset liver disease. Liver biopsy demonstrates multiple branches of the hepatic artery and portal vein in the portal tract without any accompanying bile ducts [140].

21.3
Liver Carcinogens

A number of chemicals such as aflatoxins, benzopyrenes, and PCBs, are known to induce liver carcinoma. Recently it has been found that polymorphisms in enzymes responsible for metabolizing these carcinogens in the liver modulate the risk of HCC in exposed patients.

The best studied hepatic carcinogen, aflatoxin B1 (AFB1), which is synthesized by certain *Aspergillus* strains, is metabolized in the liver by at least four different cytochrome P450 cyclooxogenases: 3A4, 1A2, 3A5, and 3A7 [141, 142]. Whereas P450 3A4 detoxifies AFB1 to AFQ_1, P450 1A2, P450 3A5, and P450 3A7 convert AFB1 to other toxic isoforms, AFM1 and AFBO, respectively [143, 144]. The hepatic expression of these cytochrome cyclooxogenases varies significantly inter-individually, due to common polymorphisms as well as enzyme induction by other compounds (e.g. drugs, chemicals, food compounds, etc.). In a recent analysis, Kamdem *et al.* [145] found a 12-fold interindividual variability in the production rate of the carcinogenic AFBO, and a 22-fold variability in the production rate of the detoxification product AFQ1. They attributed this variation predominantly to gene polymorphisms of cytochrome P450 3A5.

A polymorphism in the glutathione-S-transferase M1 (GSTM1-nul), which leads to a complete absence of the enzyme in the homozygous form, has been found to be significantly associated with the risk of HCC in chronic HBV carriers exposed to aflatoxin [146], and in liver transplanted patients when including XRCC1 (see below) in a multivariate analysis [147].

21.4
Cancer Genetics

Cancer research has revealed many key steps responsible on the molecular level for oncogenic cellular transformation. Many of the genes involved are participating in cell cycle control (Rb, E2F, etc.), intracellular signal transduction (tyrosine kinases, SOCS, β-catenin, APC, axin, etc.), transcriptional control (TCFs, HNFs, etc.), DNA methylation, and DNA repair. Oncogene activating or tumor suppressor gene inactivating mutations are usually acquired stepwise during malignant transformation but may also be present in the germline leading to an increased risk for certain malignancies (see Chapters 1, 2, 16, 30 and others). In addition to point mutations, also LOH and changes in methylation pattern are frequently observed in cancer cells.

In principle, similar genetic alterations are observed in HCC as in other malignancies. However, point mutations common to other carcinomas are often not as frequent in HCC. Mutations in the retinoblastoma (Rb) gene (see Chapter 7 on retinoblastoma), for example, have only been identified in a few cases of HCC [148], suggesting that this important tumor suppressor gene may be inactivated in HCC by other mechanisms, such as changes in methylation, or deletion of the chromosomal region (13q14) carrying this gene [149]. A complete loss of chromosome 13 has been found in about 30% of HCC (Laurent-Puig *et al.* [151], supporting this view. Similarly, inactivating mutations are also rare for p16INK4. [150]. On the other hand, LOH of the genomic region of p16INK4 on chromosome 9 is found in about 20% of HCC [151], and methylation of the p16INK4. promoter, abolishing protein expression, in up to 70% of HCC [150, 152]. Gankyrin, which accelerates the degradation of Rb, was overexpressed in all of 34 HCC, analyzed by [153], emphasizing the importance of Rb in HCC oncogenesis.

The tumor suppressor gene *p53*, which is essential for inducing apoptosis following chromosomal damage, was mutated in only 10 to 30% of HCC that had developed without any documented contact with aflatoxin. In contrast, the rate of the common inactivating R249S mutation alone rose to 50% of HCC resulting from exposure to this potent mutagenic carcinogen [154, 155].

In many adenocarcinomas, proteins involved in the mitogenic Wnt signaling pathway are mutated, in particular β-catenin (CTNNB1), adenomatous polyposis coli (APC), and Axin1 (AXIN1) (see also Chapter 16 on gastrointestinal polyposis syndromes). In over 40% of HCC, mutations of β-catenin were identified that lead to a decreased degradation and thus to an increased transcription of TCF/LEF dependent genes [151, 156–158]. For Axin, inactivation by point mutations, LOH or homozygous deletion was observed for only 5 to 8% of HCC [151, 159]. In contrast to other adenocarcinomas, no mutations have yet been observed for APC in HCC [160]. The transforming growth factor β (TGFβ) signaling pathway is also affected in HCC. Point mutations in the insulin growth factor 2 receptor (IGF2R) were identified in 10 to 20% of the cases, and some rare mutations in *Smad2* and *Smad4* genes. The promoter of the suppressor of cytokine signaling 1 (SOCS-1) was found to be silenced by an aberrant methylation in 65% of HCC [161]. Since SOCS-1 interact with Janus kinase (JAK), an antimitotic factor proliferation is induced.

A hallmark of HCC appears to be chromosomal instability, leading to common deletions of chromosomal fragments carrying tumor suppressor genes, thus causing LOH [151, 162, 163].

Yan *et al.* [164] recently described that common polymorphisms in the methylenetetrahydrofolate reductase (MTHFR) and thymidylate synthase (TYMS) genes influence the risk of HCC due to their modulation of uracil misincorporation into DNA. In addition, a polymorphism in the X-ray cross complementing group 1 (XRCC1) gene was linked to HCC, potentially due to its function in DNA repair [147] (see also Chapters 10 and 30 on lung tumors and molecular targeted therapy). Epigenetic effects induced by chronic iron overload due to hereditary HFE also appear to be involved in malignant transformation of liver cells [165].

References

1 Wittekind, Ch and Tannapfel, A. (1998) Pathologie der Lebertumore. *Chirurgische Gastroenterologie*, **14**, 175–83.

2 Asberg, A., Hveem, K., Thorstensen, K., Ellekjaer, E., Kannelonning, K., Fjosne, U. *et al.* (2001) Screening for hemo-chromatosis: high prevalence and low morbidity in an unselected population of 65 238 persons. *Scandinavian Journal of Gastroenterology*, **36**, 1108–15.

3 McCullen, M.A., Crawford, D.H.G. and Hickman, P.E. (2002) Screening for hemochromatosis. *Clinica Chimica Acta*, **315**, 169–86.

4 Halliwell, B. and Gutteridge, J. (1999) *Free Radicals in Biology and Medicine*, Oxford University Press, Oxford.

5 Valko, M., Morris, H. and Cronin, M.T.D. (2005) Metals, toxicity and oxidative stress. *Current Medicinal Chemistry*, **12**, 1161–208.

6 Canonne-Hergaux, F., Donovan, A., Delaby, C., Wang, H.J. and Gros, P. (2006) Comparative studies of duodenal and macrophage ferroportin proteins. *American Journal of Physiology. Gastrointestinal and Liver Physiology*, **290**, G156–63.

7 Niederau, C., Fischer, R., Pürschel, A., Stremmel, W., Häussinger, D. and Strohmeyer, G. (1996) Long-term survival in patients with hereditary hemochromatosis. *Gastroenterology*, **110**, 1107–19.

8 Brandhagen, D.J., Fairbanks, V.F. and Baldus, W. (2002) Recognition and management of hereditary hemochromatosis. *American Family Physician*, **65** (853–60), 65–6.

9 EASL International Consensus Conference on Haemochromatosis (2000) *Journal of Hepatology*, **33**, 485–504.

10 Brandao, M., Oliveira, J.C., Bravo, F., Reis, J., Garrido, I. and Porto, G. (2005) The soluble transferrin receptor as a marker of iron homeostasis in normal subjects and in HFE-related hemo-chromatosis. *Haematologica*, **90**, 31–7.

11 Feder, J.N., Gnirke, A., Thomas, W., Tsuchihashi, Z., Ruddy, D.A., Basava, A. *et al.* (1996) A novel MHC class I-like gene is mutated in patients with hereditary aemochromatosis. *Nature Genetics*, **13**, 399–408.

12 Rochette, J., Pointon, J.J., Fisher, C.A., Perera, G., Arambepola, M., Kodikara Arichchi, D.S., De Silva, S., Vandwalle, J.L., Monti, J.P., Old, J.M., Merryweather-Clarke, A.T., Weatherall, D.J. and Robson, K.J.H. (1999) Multicentric origin of hemochromatosis gene (*HFE*) mutations. *American Journal of Human Genetics*, **64**, 1056–62.

13 Brittenham, G.M. and Badman, D.G. (2003) Noninvasive measurement of iron. Report an NIDDK Workshop. *Blood*, **101**, 15–19.

14 Gandon, Y., Olivie, D., Guyader, D., Aube, C., Oberti, F., Sebille, V. *et al.* (2004) Non-invasive assessment of hepatic iron stores by MRI. *Lancet*, **363**, 357–62.

15 Hanson, E.H., Imperatore, G. and Burke, W. (2001) HFE gene and hereditary hemochromatosis: a HuGE review. *American Journal of Epidemiology*, **154**, 193–206.

16 Milman, N. and Pedersen, P. (2003) Evidence that the cys282-to-tyr mutation of the *HFE* gene originated from a population in southern Scandinavia and spread with the Vikings. *Clinical Genetics*, **64**, 36–47.

17 Beckman, L.E., Saha, N., Spitsyn, V., Van Landeghem, G. and Beckman, L. (1997) Ethnic differences in the HFE codon 282 (Cys/Tyr) polymorphism. *Human Heredity*, **47**, 263–7.

18 Merryweather-Clarke, A.T., Pointon, J.J., Shearman, J.D. and Robson, K.J. (1997) Global prevalence of putative haemo-chromatosis mutations. *Journal of Medical Genetics*, **34**, 275–8.

19 Ponka, P. (2000) Iron metabolism: physiology and pathophysiology. *The Journal of Trace Elements in Experimental Medicine*, **13**, 73–83.

20 Cullen, L.M., Anderson, G.J., Ramm, G.A., Jazwinska, E.C. and Powell, L.W. (1999) Genetics of hemochromatosis. *Annual Review of Medicine*, **50**, 87–98.

21 Feder, J.N., Penny, D.M., Irrinki, A., Lee, V.K., Lebron, J.A., Watson, N. *et al.* (1998) The hemochromatosis gene product complexes with the transferrin receptor and lowers its affinity for ligand binding. *Proceedings of the National Academy of Sciences of the United States of America*, **95**, 1472–7.

22 Zhou, X.Y., Tomatsu, S., Fleming, R.E., Parkkila, S., Waheed, A., Jiang, J. *et al.* (1998) HFE gene knockout produces mouse model of hereditary hemo-chromatosis. *Proceedings of the National Academy of Sciences of the United States of America*, **95**, 2492–7.

23 Parkkila, S., Waheed, A., Britton, R.S., Feder, J.N., Tsuchihashi, Z., Schatzman, R.C. *et al.* (1997) Immunohistochemistry of HLA-H, the protein defective in patients with hereditary hemochromatosis, reveals unique pattern of expression in gastrointestinal tract. *Proceedings of the National Academy of Sciences of the United States of America*, **94**, 2534–9.

24 Barton, J.C., McDonnell, S.M., Adams, P.C., Brissot, P., Powell, L.W., Edwards, C.Q. *et al.* (2001) Management of hemochromatosis. *Annals of Internal Medicine 1998*, **129**, 932–9.

25 Kontoghiorghes, G.J. (1995) Comparative efficacy and toxicity of desferrioxamine, deferiprone and other iron and aluminum chelating drugs. *Toxicology Letters*, **80**, 1–18.

26 Catsch, A. and Hartmuth-Hoene, A.-E. (1976) Pharmacology and therapeutic applications of agents used in heavy metal poisoning. *Pharmacology and Therapeutics. Part A*, **1**, 1–118.

27 Kontoghiorghes, G.J., Eracleous, E., Economides, C. and Kolnagou, A. (2005) Advances in iron overload therapies. Prospects for effective use of deferiprone (L1), deferoxamine, the new experimental chelators ICL670, GT56-252, L1NAII and their combinations. *Current Medicinal Chemistry*, **12**, 2663–81.

28 Neufeld, E.J. (2006) Oral chelators deferasirox and deferiprone for trans-fusional iron overload in thalassemia major: new data, new questions. *Blood*, **107**, 3436–41.

29 Bull, P.C., Thomas, G.R., Rommens, J.M., Forbes, J.R. and Cox, D.W. (1993) The Wilson's disease gene is a putative copper transporting P-type. ATPase similar to the Menkes gene. *Nature Genetics*, **5**, 327–37.

30 Tanzi, R.E., Petrukhin, K., Chernov, I., Pellequer, J.L., Wasco, W., Ross, B. *et al.* (1993) The Wilson's disease gene is a copper transporting. ATPase with homology to the Menkes disease gene. *Nature Genetics*, **5**, 344–50.

31 Yamaguchi, Y., Heiny, M.E. and Gitlin, J.D. (1993) Isolation and characterization of a human liver cDNA as a candidate gene for Wilson disease. *Biochemical and Biophysical Research Communications*, **197**, 271–7.

32 Horn, N. and Tüer, Z. (1999) Molecular genetics of intracellular copper transport. *The Journal of Trace Elements in Experimental Medicine*, **12**, 297–313.

33 Olivarez, L., Caggana, M., Pass, K.A., Ferguson, P. and Brewer, G.J. (2001) Estimate of the frequency of Wilson's disease in the US Caucasian population: a mutation analysis approach. *Annals of Human Genetics*, **65**, 459–63.

34 Brewer, G.J. and Yuzbasiyan-Gurkan, V. (1989) Wilson's disease: an update, with emphasis on new approaches to treat-ment. *Digestive Diseases*, **7**, 178–93.

35 Brewer, G. (2001) *Wilson's Disease: a Clinician's Guide to Recognition, Diagnosis and Management*, Kluwer Academic Publishers, Boston.

36 Kuan, P. (1987) Cardiac Wilson's disease. *Chest*, **91**, 579–83.

37 Aaseth, J. and Thomassen, Y. (1999) Trace elements in liver diseases: oxidative stress and antioxidative protectants, in *New Aspects of Trace Element Research* (eds M. Abdulla *et al*), Smith-Gordon, London, pp. 211–14.

38 Brewer, G.J. (2001) Zinc acetate for the treatment of Wilson's disease. *Expert Opinion on Pharmacotherapy*, **2**, 1473–7.

39 Shah, A.B., Chernov, I., Zhang, H.T., Ross, B.M., Das, K., Lutsenko, S. *et al.* (1997) Identification and analysis of mutations in the Wilson's disease gene (*ATP7B*): population frequencies, genotype-phenotype correlation, and

functional analyses. *American Journal of Human Genetics*, **61**, 317–28.

40 Mercer, J.F.B. (2001) The molecular basis of copper-transport diseases. *Trends in Molecular Medicine*, **7**, 64–9.

41 Walshe, J.M. (1956) Penicillamine, a new oral therapy for Wilson's disease. *American Journal of Medicine*, **21**, 487–95.

42 Planas-Bohne, F. (1981) Metabolism and pharmacokinetics of penicillamine in rats: an overview. *The Journal of Rheumatology*, **8** (Suppl. 7), 35–40.

43 Jellum, E., Munthe, E., Guldal, G. and Aaseth, J. (1979) Gold and thiol compounds in the treatment of rheumatoid arthritis. Excretory fate and tissue distribution of thiomalate in relation to gold after administration of myocrisin (auro-thiomalate). *Scandinavian Journal of Rheumatology. Supplement*, **28**, 28–36.

44 Walshe, J.M. (1973) Copper chelation in patients with Wilson's disease. A comparison of penicillamine and triethylene tetramine dihydrochloride. *The Quarterly Journal of Medicine*, **42**, 441–52.

45 Walshe, J.M. (1982) Treatment of Wilson's disease with trientine (triethylene tetramine) dihydrochloride. *Lancet*, **i**, 643–7.

46 Kodama, H., Murata, Y., Iitsuka, T. and Abe, T. (1997) Metabolism of administered triethylene tetramine dihydrochloride in humans. *Life Sciences*, **61**, 899–907.

47 Walshe, J.M. (1996) Treatment of Wilson's disease: the historical background. *The Quarterly Journal of Medicine*, **89**, 53–5.

48 Andersen, O. (1999) Principles and recent developments in chelation treatment of metal intoxication. *Chemical Reviews*, **99**, 2683–710.

49 Ren, M. and Yang, R. (1997) Clinical curative effects of dimercaptosuccinic acid on hepatolenticular degeneration and the impact of DMSA on biliary trace elements. *Chinese Medical Journal*, **110**, 694–7.

50 Hoogenraad, T.U., Van den Hamer, C.J.A., Koevoet, R. and De Ruyter Korver, E.G.W.M. (1978) Oral zinc in Wilson's disease. *Lancet*, **II**, 1262.

51 Hoogenraad, T.U. (2006) Paradigm shift in treatment of Wilson's disease: zinc therapy now treatment of choice. *Brain and Development*, **28**, 141–6.

52 Brewer, G.J., Dick, R.D., Yuzbasiyan-Gurkan, V., Johnson, V. and Wang, Y. (1994) Treatment of Wilson's disease with zinc XIII. therapy with zinc in presymptomatic patients from the time of diagnosis. *The Journal of Laboratory and Clinical Medicine*, **123**, 849–58.

53 Hafeez, W., Ciliberto, G. and Perlmutter, D.H. (1992) Constitutive and modulated expression of the human alpha-1 antitrypsin gene: different transcriptional initiation sites used in three different cell types. *Journal of Clinical Investigation*, **89**, 1214–22.

54 Hug, G., Chuck, G. and Fagerhol, MK. (1981) Pi (P-Clifton): a new alpha(1) antitrypsin allele in an American Negro family. *Journal of Medical Genetics*, **18**, 43–5.

55 Curiel, D.T., Holmes, M.D., Okayama, H., Brantly, M.L., Vogelmeier, C., Travis, W.D., Stier, L.E., Perks, W.H. and Crystal, R.G. (1989) Molecular basis of the liver and lung disease associated with the alpha-1-antitrypsin deficiency allele M (Malton). *Journal of Biological Chemistry*, **264**, 13938–45.

56 Laurell, C.-B. and Eriksson, S. (1963) The electrophoretic alpha-1-globulin pattern of serum in alpha-1-antitrypsin deficiency. *Scandinavian Journal of Clinical and Laboratory Investigation*, **15**, 132–40.

57 Eriksson, S. (1965) Studies in alpha 1-antitrypsin deficiency. *Acta Medica Scandinavica*, **177** (Suppl. 432), 1–85.

58 Gans, H., Sharp, H.L. and Tan, B.H. (1969) Antiprotease deficiency and familial infantile liver cirrhosis. *Surgery of Gynecology and Obstetrics*, **129**, 289–99.

59 Udall, J.N., Bloch, K.J. and Walker, W.A. (1982) Transport of proteases across neonatal intestine and development of liver disease in infants with alpha-1-antitrypsin deficiency. *Lancet*, **I**, 1441–3.

60 Lake-Bakaar, G. and Dooley, J.S. (1982) Alpha-1-antitrypsin deficiency and liver disease. *Lancet*, **II**, 159.

61 Crystal, R.G. (1990) Alpha-1-antitrypsin deficiency, emphysema, and liver disease:

genetic basis and strategies for therapy. *Journal of Clinical Investigation*, **85**, 1343–52.

62 Wu, Y., Whitman, I., Molmenti, E., Moore, K., Hippenmeyer, P. and Perlmutter, D.H. (1994) A lag in intracellular degradation of mutant alpha-1-antitrypsin correlates with the liver disease phenotype in homozygous PiZZ alpha-1-antitrypsin deficiency. *Proceedings of the National Academy of Sciences*, **91**, 9014–18.

63 Lomas, D.A., Evans, D.L., Finch, J.T. and Carrell, R.W. (1992) The mechanism of Z alpha-1-antitrypsin accumulation in the liver. *Nature*, **357**, 605–7.

64 Bowlus, C.L., Willner, I., Zern, M.A. *et al.* (2005) Factors associated with advanced liver disease in adults with alpha-1 antitrypsin deficiency. *Clinical Gastroenterology and Hepatology*, **3**, 390–6.

65 Hodges, R., Millward-Sadler, G.H., Path, M.R.C., Barbatis, C., Wright, R. and Phil, D. (1981) Heterozygous MZ alpha-1 antitrypsin deficiency in adults with chronic active hepatitis and cryptogenic cirrhosis. *New England Journal of Medicine*, **304**, 557–60.

66 Eigenbrodt, M.L., McCashland, T.M., Dy, R.M., Clark, J. and Galati, J. (1997) Heterozygous alpha-1 antitrypsin phenotypes in patients with end stage liver disease. *The American Journal of Gastroenterology*, **92**, 602–7.

67 Graziadei, I.W., Joseph, J.J., Wiesner, R.H., Therneau, T.M., Batts, K.P. and Porayko, M.K. (1998) Increased risk of chronic liver failurein adults with heterozygous alpha-1 antitrypsin deficiency. *Hepatology*, **28**, 1058–63.

68 Fargion, S., Klasen, E.C., Lalatta, F., Sangalli, G., Tommasini, M. and Fiorelli, G. (1981) Alpha-1-antitrypsin in patients with carcinoma and chronic active hepatitis. *Clinical Genetics*, **19**, 134–9.

69 Zhou, H. and Fischer, H.P. (1998) Liver carcinoma in PiZ alpha-1 antitrypsin deficiency. *American Journal of Pathology*, **22**, 742–8.

70 Zhou, H., Ortiz-Pallardo, M.E., Ko, Y. and Fischer, H.P. (2000) Is hetero-

zygous alpha-1 antitrypsin deficiency type PiZ a risk factor for primary liver cell carcinoma? *Cancer*, **88**, 2668–76.

71 Wewers, M.D., Casolaro, A., Sellers, S., Swayze, S.C., McPhaul, K.M., Wittes, J.T. and Crystal, R.G. (1987) Replacement therapy for alpha-1-antitrypsin deficiency associated with emphysema. *New England Journal of Medicine*, **316**, 1055–62.

72 Stoller, J.K. and Aboussouan, L.S. (2005) Alpha1-antitrypsin deficency. *Lancet*, **365**, 2225–36.

73 Burrows, J.A.J., Willis, L.K. and Permutter, D.H. (2000) Chemical chaperones mediate increased secretion of mutant alpha1-antitrypsin (AlAT) Z: a potential pharmacological strategy for prevention of liver injury and emphysema in AlAT deficiency. *Proceedings of the National Academy of Sciences of the United States of America*, **97**, 1796–801.

74 Lomas, D.A. and Mahadeva, R. (2002) Alpha 1-antitrypsin polymerization and serpinopathies: pathobiology and prospects for therapy. *Journal of Clinical Investigation*, **110**, 1585–90.

75 Garver, R.I. Jr, Chytil, A., Courtney, M. and Crystal, R.G. (1987) Clonal gene therapy: transplanted mouse fibroblast clones express human alpha-1-antitrypsin gene *in vivo*. *Science*, **237**, 762–4.

76 Kay, M.A., Baley, P., Rothenberg, S., Leland, F., Fleming, L., Ponder, K.P., Liu, T., Finegold, M., Darlington, G., Pokorny, W. and Woo, S.L.C. (1992) Expression of human alpha-1-antitrypsin in dogs after autologous transplantation of retroviral transduced hepatocytes. *Proceedings of the National Academy of Sciences*, **89**, 89–93.

77 Lemarchand, P., Jaffe, H.A., Danel, C., Cid, M.C., Kleinman, H.K., Stratford-Perricaudet, L.D., Perricaudet, M., Pavirani, A., Lecocq, J.-P. and Crystal, R.G. (1992) Adenovirus-mediated transfer of a recombinant human alpha-1-antitrypsin cDNA to human endothelial cells. *Proceedings of the National Academy of Sciences*, **89**, 6482–6.

78 Song, S., Morgan, M., Ellis, T., Poirier, A., Chesnut, K., Wang, J., Brantly, M., Muzyczka, N., Byrne, B.J., Atkinson, M. and Flotte, T.R. (1998) Sustained

secretion of human alpha-1-antitrypsin from murine muscle transduced with adeno-associated virus vectors. *Proceedings of the National Academy of Sciences*, **95**, 14384–8.

79 Vennarecci, G., Gunson, B.K., Ismail, T. *et al.* (1996) Transplantation for end stage liver disease related to alpha-1-antitrypsin. *Transplantation*, **61**, 1488–95.

80 Kerem, E., Kalman, Y.M., Yahav, Y., Shoshani, T., Abeliovich, D., Szeinberg, A., Rivlin, J., Blau, H., Tal, A., Ben-Tur, L., Springer, C., Augarten, A., Godfrey, S., Lerer, I., Branski, D., Friedman, M. and Kerem, B. (1995) Highly variable incidence of cystic fibrosis and different mutation distribution among different Jewish ethnic groups in Israel. *Human Genetics*, **96**, 193–7.

81 Lemna, W.K., Feldman, G.L., Kerem, B., Fernbach, S.D., Zevkovich, E.P., O'Brien, W.E., Riordan, J.R., Collins, F.S. and Tsui, L.-C., Beaud, A.L. (1990) Mutation analysis for heterozygote detection and the prenatal diagnosis of cystic fibrosis. *New England Journal of Medicine*, **322**, 291–6.

82 de Vries, H.G., Collee, J.M., de Walle, H.E.K., van Veldhuizen, M.H.R., Smit Sibinga, C.T., Scheffer, H. and ten Kate, L.P. (1997) Prevalence of delta-F508 cystic fibrosis carriers in The Netherlands: logistic regression on sex, age, region of residence and number of offspring. *Human Genetics*, **99**, 74–9.

83 Gaskin, K.J., Waters, D.L.M., Howman-Giles, R., de Silva, M., Earl, J.W., Martin, H.C.O., Kan, A.E., Brown, J.M. and Dorney, S.F.A. (1988) Liver disease and common-bile-duct stenosis in cystic fibrosis. *New England Journal of Medicine*, **318**, 340–6.

84 Bilton, D., Fox, R., Webb, A.K., Lawler, W., McMahon, R.F.T. and Howat, J.M.T. (1990) Pathology of common bile duct stenosis in cystic fibrosis. *Gut*, **31**, 236–8.

85 Gabolde, M., Hubert, D., Guilloud-Bataille, M., Lenaerts, C., Feingold, J. and Besmond, C. (2001) The mannose binding lectin gene influences the severity of chronic liver disease in cystic fibrosis. *Journal of Medical Genetics*, **38**, 310–11.

86 Goppert, F. (1917) Galaktosurie nach Milchzuckergabe bei angeborenem, familiaerem chronischem Leberleiden. *Klinische Wochenschrift*, **54**, 473–7.

87 Ruiz, M., Jover, S., Armas, M., Duque, M.R., Santana, C., Giros, M.L. and Boleda, M.D. (1999) Galactosaemia presenting as congenital pseudo-afibrinogenaemia. *Journal of Inherited Metabolic Disease*, **22**, 943–4.

88 Elsas, L.J.II and Lai, K. (1998) The molecular biology of galactosemia. *Genetics in Medicine*, **1**, 40–8.

89 Cramer, D.W., Greenberg, E.R., Titus-Ernstoff, L., Liberman, R.F., Welch, W.R., Li, E., Ng, W.G. (2000) Case-control study of galactose consumption and metabolism in relation to ovarian cancer. *Cancer Epidemiology, Biomarkers and Prevention*, **9** (1), 95–101.

90 Suzuki, M., West, C. and Beutler, E. (2001) Large-scale molecular screening for galactosemia alleles in a pan-ethnic population. *Human Genetics*, **109**, 210–15.

91 Nordmann, Y., Schapira, F. and Dreyfus, J.-C. (1968) A structurally modified liver aldolase in fructose intolerance: immunological and kinetic evidence. *Biochemical and Biophysical Research Communications*, **31**, 884–9.

92 Cox, T.M., Camilleri, M., O'Donnell, M.W. and Chadwick, V.S. (1982) Pseudodominant transmission of fructose intolerance in an adult and three offspring: heterozygote detection by intestinal biopsy. *New England Journal of Medicine*, **307**, 537–40.

93 Marks, F., Ordorica, S., Hoskins, I. and Young, B.K. (1989) Congenital hereditary fructose intolerance and pregnancy. *American Journal of Obstetrics and Gynecology*, **160**, 362–3.

94 Lelong, M., Alagille, D., Gentil, C.I., Colin, J., Le Tan, V. and Gabilan, J.C. (1963) Cirrhose congenitale et familiale avec diabete phospho-gluco-amine, rachitisme vitamin D-resistant et tyrosinurie massive. *Revue Francaise d'etudes Cliniques et Biologiques*, **8**, 37–50.

95 Scriver, C.R., Partington, M.W. and Sass-Kortsak, A. (1967) Conference on hereditary tyrosinemia held at the Hospital for Sick Children. *Canadian Medical Association Journal*, **97**, 1045–100.

96 Hostetter, M.K., Levy, H.L., Winter, H.S., Knight, G.J. and Haddow, J.E. (1983) Evidence for liver disease preceding amino acid abnormalities in hereditary tyrosinemia. *New England Journal of Medicine*, **308**, 1265–7.

97 Holme, E., Lindblad, B. and Lindstedt, S. (1985) Possibilities for treatment and for early prenatal diagnosis of hereditary tyrosinaemia. *Lancet*, I, 527 only.

98 Fisch, R.O., McCabe, E.R.B., Doeden, D., Koep, L.J., Kohlhoff, J.G., Silverman, A. and Starzl, T.E. (1978) Homotransplantation of the liver in a patient with hepatoma and hereditary tyrosinemia. *Journal of Pediatrics*, **93**, 592–6.

99 Gartner, J.C., Zitelli, B.J., Malatack, J.J., Shaw, B.W., Iwatsuki, S. and Starzl, T.E. (1984) Orthotopic liver transplantation in children: two-year experience with 47 patients. *Pediatrics*, **74**, 140–5.

100 Dehner, L.P., Snover, D.C., Sharp, H.L., Ascher, N., Nakhleh, R. and Day, D.L. (1989) Hereditary tyrosinemia type I (chronic form): pathologic findings in the liver. *Human Pathology*, **20**, 149–58.

101 van Spronsen, F.J., Berger, R., Smit, G.P.A., de Klerk, J.B.C., Duran, M., Bijleveld, C.M.A., van Faassen, H., Slooff, M.J.H. and Heymans, H.S.A. (1989) Tyrosinaemia type I. orthotopic liver transplantation as the only definitive answer to a metabolic as well as an oncological problem. *Journal of Inherited Metabolic Disease*, **12**, 339–42.

102 Sokal, E.M., Bustos, R., Van Hoof, F. and Otte, J.B. (1992) Liver transplantation for hereditary tyrosinemia – early transplantation following the patient's stabilization. *Transplantation*, **54**, 937–9.

103 De Braekeleer, M. and Larochelle, J. (1990) Genetic epidemiology of hereditary tyrosinemia in Quebec and in Saguenay-Lac-St-Jean. *American Journal of Human Genetics*, **47**, 302–7.

104 Grompe, M., St-Louis, M., Demers, S.I., Al-Dhalimy, M., Leclerc, B. and Tanguay, R.M. (1994) A single mutation of the fumarylacetoacetate hydrolase gene in French Canadians with hereditary tyrosinemia type I. *New England Journal of Medicine*, **331**, 353–7.

105 Russo, P. and O'Regan, S. (1990) Visceral pathology of hereditary tyrosinemia type I. *American Journal of Human Genetics*, **47**, 317–24.

106 Howell, R.R., Stevenson, R.E., Ben-Menachem, Y., Phyliky, R.L. and Berry, D.H. (1978) Hepatic adenomata with type I glycogen storage disease. *Journal of Nuclear Medicine*, **19**, 354–8.

107 Zangeneh, F., Limbeck, G.A., Brown, B.I., Emch, J.R., Arcasoy, M.M., Goldenberg, V.E. and Kelley, V.C. (1969) Hepatorenal glycogenosis (type I glycogenosis) and carcinoma of the liver. *Journal of Pediatrics*, **74**, 73–83.

108 Stevenson, R.E., Ben-Menachem, Y., Dudrick, S. and Howell, R.R. (1984) *Hepatocellular Carcinoma in Type 1 Glycogen Storage Disease*, Proc Greenwood Genet. Center 3, pp. 39–46.

109 Burchell, A., Jung, R.T., Lang, C.C., Bennet, W. and Shepherd, A.N. (1987) Diagnosis of type 1a and type 1c glycogen storage diseases in adults. *Lancet*, I. 1059–62.

110 Fraumeni, J.F., Rosen, P.J., Hull, E.W., Barth, R.F., Shapiro, S.R. and O'Connor, J.F. (1969) Hepatoblastoma in infant sisters. *Cancer*, **24**, 1086–90.

111 Napole, V.M. and Campbell, W.G. Jr (1977) Hepatoblastoma in infant sister and brother. *Cancer*, **39**, 2647–50.

112 Ito, E., Sato, Y., Kawauchi, K., Munakata, H., Kamata, Y., Yodono, H. and Yokoyama, M. (1987) Type 1a glycogen storage disease with hepatoblastoma in siblings. *Cancer*, **59**, 1776–80.

113 Smit, G.P.A. (1993) The long-term outcome of patients with glycogen storage disease type Ia. *European Journal of Pediatrics*, **152** (Suppl. 1), S52–5.

114 Bianchi, L. (1993) Glycogen storage disease I and hepatocellular tumours. *European Journal of Pediatrics*, **152** (Suppl. 1), S63–70.

115 Talente, G.M., Coleman, R.A., Alter, C., Baker, L., Brown, B.I., Cannon, R.A., Chen, Y.-T., Crigler, J.F. Jr, Ferreira, P., Haworth, J.C., Herman, G.E., Issenman, R.M., Keating, J.P., Linde, R., Roe, T.F., Senior, B. and Wolfsdorf, J.I. (1994) Glycogen storage disease in adults. *Annals of Internal Medicine*, **120**, 218–26.

116 Faivre, L., Houssin, D., Valayer, J., Brouard, J., Hadchouel, M. and Bernard, O. (1999) Long-term outcome of liver transplantation in patients with glycogen storage disease type Ia. *Journal of Inherited Metabolic Disease,* **22**, 723–32.

117 Wiedemann, H.-R. (1983) Tumours and hemihypertrophy associated with Wiedemann–Beckwith syndrome. *European Journal of Pediatrics,* **141**, 129.

118 Koufos, A., Grundy, P., Morgan, K., Aleck, K.A., Hadro, T., Lampkin, B.C., Kalbakji, A. and Cavenee, W.K. (1989) Familial Wiedemann–Beckwith syndrome and a second Wilms tumor locus both map to 11p15. 5. *American Journal of Human Genetics,* **44**, 711–19.

119 Brown, K.W., Williams, J.C., Maitland, N.J. and Mott, M.G. (1990) Genomic imprinting and the Beckwith–Wiedemann syndrome. *American Journal of Human Genetics,* **46**, 1000–1.

120 Nivelon-Chevallier, A., Mavel, A., Michiels, R. and Bethenod, M. (1983) Syndrome de Wiedemann-Beckwith familial: diagnostic antenatal echographique et confirmation histologique. *Journal de Genetique Humaine,* **31**, 397–402.

121 Winter, S.C., Curry, C.J.R., Smith, J.C., Kassel, S., Miller, L. and Andrea, J. (1986) Prenatal diagnosis of the Beckwith–Wiedemann syndrome. *American Journal of Medical Genetics,* **24**, 137–41.

122 Cobelis, G., Iannoto, P., Stabile, M., Lonardo, F., Della Bruna, M., Caliendo, E. and Ventruto, V. (1988) Prenatal ultrasound diagnosis of macroglossia in the Wiedemann–Beckwith syndrome. *Prenatal Diagnosis,* **8**, 79–81.

123 Azouz, E.M., Larson, E.J., Patel, J. and Gyepes, M.T. (1990) Beckwith–Wiedemann syndrome development of nephroblastoma during the surveillance period. *Pediatric Radiology,* **20**, 550–2.

124 DeBaun, M.R. and Tucker, M.A. (1998) Risk of cancer during the first four years of life in children from the Beckwith–Wiedemann Syndrome Registry. *Journal of Pediatrics,* **132**, 398–400.

125 Heimann, A., White, P.F., Riely, C.A., Ritchey, A.K., Flye, M.W. and Barwick, K.W. (1987) Hepatoblastoma presenting as isosexual precocity: the clinical importance of histologic and serologic parameters. *Journal of Clinical Gastroenterology,* **9**, 105–10.

126 Shneider, B.L., Haque, S., van Hoff, J., Touloukian, R.J. and West, A.B. (1992) Familial adenomatous polyposis following liver transplantation for a virilizing hepatoblastoma. *Journal of Pediatric Gastroenterology and Nutrition,* **15**, 198–201.

127 Kingston, J.E., Draper, G.J. and Mann, J.R. (1982) Hepatoblastoma and polyposis coli. *Lancet,* I, 457 only.

128 Li, F.P., Thurber, W.A., Seddon, J. and Holmes, G.E. (1987) Hepatoblastoma in families with polyposis coli. *The Journal of the American Medical Association,* **257**, 2475–7.

129 Krush, A.J., Traboulsi, E.I., Offerhaus, G.J.A., Maumenee, I.H., Yardley, J.H. and Levin, L.S. (1988) Hepatoblastoma, pigmented ocular fundus lesions and jaw lesions in Gardner syndrome. *American Journal of Medical Genetics,* **29**, 323–32.

130 Hughes, L.J. and Michels, V.V. (1992) Risk of hepatoblastoma in familial adenomatous polyposis. *American Journal of Medical Genetics,* **43**, 1023–5.

131 Oda, H., Imai, Y., Nakatsuru, Y., Hata, J. and Ishikawa, T. (1996) Somatic mutations of the APC gene in sporadic hepatoblastomas. *Cancer Reseach,* **56**, 3320–3.

132 Rosenfield, N.S., Kelley, M.J., Jensen, P.S., Cotlier, E., Rosenfield, A.T. and Riely, C.A. (1980) Arteriohepatic dysplasia: radiologic features of a new syndrome. *AJR. American Journal of Roentgenology,* **135**, 1217–23.

133 Ong, E., Williams, S.M., Anderson, J.C. and Kaplan, P.A. (1986) MR imaging of a hepatoma associated with Alagille syndrome. *Journal of Computer Assisted Tomography,* **10**, 1047–9.

134 Kaufman, S.S., Wood, R.P., Shaw, B.W. Jr, Markin, R.S., Gridelli, B. and Vanderhoff, J.A. (1987) Hepatocarcinoma in a child with the Alagille syndrome. *American Journal of Diseases of Children,* **141**, 698–700.

135 Rabinovitz, M., Imperial, J.C., Schade, R.R. and Van Thiel, D.H. (1989) Hepatocellular carcinoma in Alagille's syndrome: a family study. *Journal of Pediatric Gastroenterology and Nutrition*, 8, 26–30.

136 Adams, P.C. (1986) Hepatocellular carcinoma associated with arteriohepatic dysplasia. *Digestive Diseases and Sciences*, 31, 438–42.

137 Legius, E., Fryns, J.-P., Eyskens, B., Eggermont, E., Desmet, V., de Bethune, G. and Van den Berghe, H. (1990) Alagille syndrome (arteriohepatic dysplasia) and del(20)(p11.2). *American Journal of Medical Genetics*, 35, 532–5.

138 Kato, Z., Asano, J., Kato, T., Yamaguchi, S., Kondo, N. and Orii, T. (1994) Thyroid cancer in a case with the Alagille syndrome. *Clinical Genetics*, 45, 21–4.

139 Lykavieris, P., Hadchouel, M., Chardot, C. and Bernard, O. (2001) Outcome of liver disease in children with Alagille syndrome. a study of 163 patients. *Gut*, 49, 431–5.

140 Li, L., Krantz, I.D., Deng, Y., Genin, A., Banta, A.B., Collins, C.C., Qi, M., Trask, B.J., Kuo, W.L., Cochran, J., Costa, T., Pierpont, M.E.M., Rand, E.B., Piccoli, D.A., Hood, L. and Spinner, N.B. (1997) Alagille syndrome is caused by mutations in human Jagged1, which encodes a ligand for Notch1. *Nature Genetics*, 16, 243–51.

141 Forrester, L.M., *et al.* (1990) *Proceedings of the National Academy of Sciences*, 87, 8306–10.

142 Gallager, H.S., *et al.* (1994) *Cancer Research*, 54, 101–8.

143 Wild, C.P., Turner, P.C. (2002) The toxicology of aflatoxins as a basis for public health decisions. *Mutagenesis*, 17 (6), 471–81.

144 Wang, H., Dick, R., Yin, H., Licad-Coles, E., Kroetz, D.L., Szklarz, G., Harlow, G., Halpert, J.R., Correia, M.A (1998) Structure-function relationships of human liver cytochromes P450 3A: aflatoxin B1 metabolism as a probe. *Biochemistry*, 37, 12536–45.

145 Kamdem, L.K., Meineke, I., Götel-Armbrust, U., Brockmöler, J. and Wojnowski, L. (2006) Dominant contribution of P450 3A4 to the hepatic carcinogenic activation of aflatoxin B1. *Chemical Research in Toxicology*, 19, 577–86.

146 Chen, C.J., Yu, M.W., Liaw, Y.F., Wang, L.W., Chiamprasert, S., Matin, F., Hirvonen, A., Bell, D.A., Santella, R.M. (1996) Chronic hepatitis B carriers with null genotypes of glutathione S-transferase M1 and T1 polymorphisms who are exposed to aflatoxin are at increased risk of hepatocellular carcinoma. *American Journal of Human Genetics* 59, 128–34.

147 Borentain, P., Gérolami, V., Ananian, P., Garcia, S., Noundou, A., Botta-Fridlund, D., Le Treut, Y.P., Bergé-Lefranc, J.L., Gérolami, R. (2007) DNA-repair and carcinogen-metabolising enzymes genetic polymorphisms as an independent risk factor for hepatocellular carcinoma in Caucasian liver-transplanted patients. *European Journal of Cancer*, 43, 2479–86.

148 Lin, C.H. *et al.* (1996) *Annals of the Academy of Medicine, Singapore*, 25, 22–30.

149 Zhang, X., Xu, H.J., Murakani, Y., Sachse, R., Yashima, K., Hirohashi, S., Hu, S.X., Benedict, W.F., Sekiya, T. (1994) Deletions of chromosome 13q, mutations in retinoblastoma 1, and retinoblastoma protein state in human hepatocellular carcinoma. *Cancer Research*, 54, 4177–82.

150 Myung JinBaek, B.S., *et al.* (2000) p16 is a major inactivation target in hepatocellular carcinoma. *Cancer*, 89, 60–8.

151 Laurent-Puig, P., Legoix, P., Bluteau, O., Belghiti, J., Franco, D., Binot, F., Monges, G., Thomas, G., Bioulac-Sage, P., Zucman-Rossi, J. (2001) Genetic alterations associated with hepatocellular carcinomas define distinct pathways of hepatocarcinogenesis. *Gastroeneterology*, 120 (7), 1763–73.

152 Weihrauch, M., Benicke, M., Lehnert, G., Wittekind, C., Wrbitzky, R., Tannapfel, A. (2001) Frequent K-ras-2 mutations and p16 (INh 4A) methylation in hepatocellular carcinomas in workers exposed to vinyl chloride. *British Journal of Cancer*, 84, 982–9.

153 Higashitsuji, H., Itoh, K., Nagao, T., Dawson, S., Nonoguchi, K., Kido, T., Mayer, R.J., Ani, S., Fujita, J. (2000) Reduced stability of retinoblastoma protein by gankyrin, an oncogenic aukyrin-repeat protein overexpressed in hepatomas. *Nature Medicine*, **6**, 96–9.

154 Bressac, B., Kew, M., Wands, J., Ozturk, M. (1991) Selective G to T mutations of p53 gene in hepatocellular carcinoma from Southern Africa. *Nature*, **350**, 429–31.

155 Hsu, I.C., Metcalf, R.A., Sunt, Welsh, J.A., Wang, N.J., Harris, C.C. (1991) Mutational hot spot in the p53 gene in human hepatocellular carcinomas. *Nature*, **350**, 439–31.

156 de la Coste, A., Romagnolo, B., Billurat, P., Renard, C.A., Buendia, M.A., Soubrane, O., Fabre, M., Chelly, J., Beldjord, C., Kahn, A., Pacret, C. (1998) Somatic mutations of the beta-catenin gene are frequent in mouse and human hepatocellular carcinomas. *Proceedings of the National Academy of Sciences*, **95**, 8847–51.

157 Miyoshi, Y., Iwao, K., Nagasawa, Y., Aihara, T., Sasaki, Y., Imaoka, S., Murata, M., Shimano, T., Nakamura, Y. (1998) Activation of the beta-catenin gene in primary hepatocellular carcinomas by somatic alterations involving exon 3. *Cancer Research*, **58**, 2524–7.

158 Terris, B., Pineau, P., Bregeaud, L., Valla, D., Belghiti, J., Tiollais, P., Degott, C., Dejean, A. (1999) Close correlation between beta-catein gene alterations and nuclear accumulation of the protein in human hepatocellular carcinomas. *Oncogene*, **18**, 6583–8.

159 Satoh, T., Sasatumi, E., Wu, L., Tokunaga, O. (2000) Phlegmonous colitis – a specific and severe complication of chronic hepatic disease. *Virchows Arch*, **437** (6), 656–61.

160 Ishizaki, Y., Ikeda, S., Fujimori, M., Shimizu, Y., Kurihara, T., Itamoto, T., Kikuchi, A., Okajima, M., Asahra, T. (2004) Immunohistochemical analysis and mutational analyses of beta-catenin, axin family and APC genes in hepatocellular carcinomas. *International Journal of Oncology*, **24**, 1077–83.

161 Yoshikawa, H., Matsubara, K., Qiau, G.S., Jackson, P., Groopman, J.D., Manning, J.E., Harris, C.C., Herman, J.G. (2001) SOCS-1, a negative regulator of the JAK/STAT pathway, is silenced by methylation in human hepatocellular carcinoma and shows growth-suppression activity. *Nature Genetics*, **28**, 29–35.

162 Balsara, B.R., Pei, J., De Rienzo, A., Simon, D., Tosolini, A., Lu, Y.Y., Shen, F.M., Fan, X., Liu, W.Y., Buetow, K.H., London, W.T., Testa, J.R. (2001) Human hepatocellular carcinoma is characterized by a highly consistent pattern of genomic imbalances, including frequent loss of 16q23. 1-24.1. *Genes, Chromosome & Cancer*, **30**, 245–53.

163 Nishimura, T., Nishida, N., Itoh, T., Kuno, M., Minata, M., Komeda, T., Fukuda, Y., Ikai, I., Yamaoka, Y., Nakao, K. (2002) Comprehensive allelotyping of well-differentiated human hepatocellular carcinoma with semiquantitative determination of chromosomal gain or loss. *Genes, Chromosomes & Cancer*, **35**, 329–39.

164 Yuan, J.M., Lu, S.C., van den Berg, D., Govindarajan, S., Zhang, Z.G., Mato, J.M., Yu, M.C (2007) Genetic polymorphisms in the methylenete-trahydrofolate reductase and thymidylate synthase genes and risk of hepatocellular carcinoma. *Hepatology*, **46**, 749–58.

165 Lehmann, U., Wingen, L.U., Brakensiek, K., Wedemeyer, H., Becker, T., Heim, A., Metzig, K., Hasemeier, B., Kreipe, H., Flemming, P. (2007) Epigenetic defects of hepatocellular carcinoma are already found in non-neoplastic liver cells. *Human Molecular Genetics*, **16**, 1335–42.

22
DNA-Repair Deficiency and Cancer: Lessons from Lymphoma

Krystyna H. Chrzanowska, Martin Digweed, Karl Sperling, and Eva Seemanova

Summary

A peculiarity of the lymphatic system is its high rate of somatic recombination with associated hypermutability. In this process, DNA double-strand breaks (DSB) are generated and processed, whereby the genes responsible are often also involved in general DSB repair. Germline mutations in these genes are responsible for a particularly high risk for lymphoma. Genetic disorders such as ataxia-telangiectasia (A-T) and Nijmegen Breakage Syndrome (NBS), together with the characteristic somatic mutations discovered in sporadic lymphoma, have made major contributions to the understanding of DNA repair defects and carcinogenesis in general.

22.1
Introduction

Cells of the lymphatic system differ from all other cells in their hypermutability, due to the extreme degree of somatic recombination of the immunoglobulin and T-cell receptor genes necessary for the vast repertoire of antibodies and T-cell receptors. In the course of this somatic recombination, DNA-double-strand breaks (DSB) are induced and "repaired". The genes involved are also involved in general repair of DSBs, which leads to two significant facts: First, germline mutations in these DNA repair genes can be expected to be associated with a particularly high risk for lymphoma. The human genetic disorder, Nijmegen Breakage Syndrome (NBS), is an example of this. Approximately 30% of affected individuals develop lymphoma before 15 years of age. Second, the high rate of spontaneous mutations in lymphoid cells explains the high frequency of lymphoid malignancy, 6 to 10% of all neoplasia, with the tendency rising.

Furthermore, lymphoma serves as a model for the relationship of chromosome aberrations and cancer in general. It was a scientific breakthrough in the field of tumor genetics when, in October 1982, two research laboratories independently

Hereditary Tumors: From Genes to Clinical Consequences
Edited by Heike Allgayer, Helga Rehder and Simone Fulda
Copyright © 2009 WILEY-VCH Verlag GmbH & Co. KGaA, Weinheim
ISBN: 978-3-527-32028-8

demonstrated the nature of the characteristic translocations between chromosomes 8 and chromosome 2, 14 or 22, as seen in Burkitt lymphoma. It was found that the translocations always involved the same breakpoints and brought *c-myc*, a proto-oncogene at chromosome 8, into the vicinity of the particularly active genes for the heavy or light chains of the immunoglobulin genes on chromosomes 14, 2, and 22, respectively. The translocation leads to an elevated expression of the *c-myc* gene and so an early step towards tumor induction. For the first time in cancerogenesis, the relationship between a structural chromosome aberration and the expression of an affected gene could be established.

The natural hypermutability of lymphatic cells manifests as genomic instability in all cells from individuals with DNA repair defects, who all have a high cancer risk. In each case, the clinical phenotype and major cancer type reflect the particular repair process affected. In addition, many tumors are characterized by chromosome instability due to somatic mutations. In both cases, a large number of genetically unique cells are generated from which those capable of continual proliferation will be selected. Mutation and selection are the driving forces of cancerogenesis. In this review (based on an article published previously in German [1]), we consider the role of the DNA repair genes in this process, particularly as evidenced by the lymphomas.

22.2
DNA Repair

DNA is the only macromolecule which, when damaged, is repaired rather than replaced; indeed, this is a prerequisite for life itself. The enormous importance of DNA repair is made particularly clear by a consideration of how many different lesions occur every day in the cell nucleus (Figure 22.1). Not surprisingly, DNA repair processes are evolutionarily very old. The differences in DNA lesions are paralleled by variations in the repair processes. They can be grouped into five categories, although the delineation is less precise than often thought.

22.3
Base Excision Repair (BER)

This pathway is particularly involved in the repair of oxidative damage to DNA bases, but also plays a role in the replacement of defective nucleotides and repair of DNA single-strand breaks. In each case, the intact complementary strand serves as a template for DNA re-synthesis. Polymorphisms in genes involved in the BER pathway can have an influence on tumorigenesis. Pathological mutations have so far been found only in the glycosylase gene, *MYH* (Table 22.1).

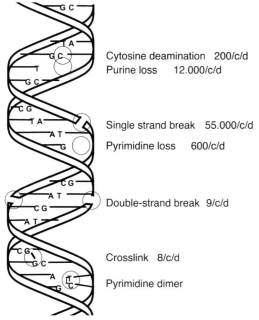

Cytosine deamination   200/c/d
Purine loss   12.000/c/d

Single strand break   55.000/c/d

Pyrimidine loss   600/c/d

Double-strand break 9/c/d

Crosslink   8/c/d

Pyrimidine dimer

Figure 22.1 Spontaneously occurring DNA lesions and their frequency per cell and day. Exogenous poisons can lead to immense increases in DNA lesions (after [1]).

22.4
Nucleotide Excision Repair (NER)

This is the pathway responsible for the repair of the majority of large lesions, which distort the DNA structure, for example, thymine dimers. Mutations in many of the involved genes lead to the disorder Xeroderma pigmentosum, in which patients have an extremely high skin tumor risk (Table 22.1). Mutations in the genes for transcription coupled repair are responsible for Cockayne syndrome and Trichothiodystrophy, which do not have an elevated cancer risk. Nevertheless, the expression of these genes (*XPD, ERCC1*) may be altered in tumors and thus influence their response to cytostatic therapy (see Chapter 30 on molecular targeted therapy).

22.5
Mismatch Repair (MMR)

Immediately after DNA replication, incorrectly incorporated bases are corrected by so-called mismatch repair. Germline mutations in the genes involved in

Table 22.1 DNA repair genes and genetic diseases with DNA repair defects and increased cancer risk.

Repair pathway	Number of genes involved	Mutations in DNA repair genes leading to increased cancer risk	Sensitivity towards mutagens
BER	~20	*MYH* (**colon cancer**); *ADPRT, APE1, OGG1, XRCC1* (so far only polymorphism)	Ionizing radiation; DNA mono-adducts
NER	~30	*ERCC1; XPA, XPB, XPC, XPD, XPE, XPF, XPG* (Xeroderma pigmentosum)	UV-light; DNA mono-adducts
MMR	11	*MSH2, MSH6, MLH1, PMS2* (Turcot S., HNPCC)	DNA mono-adducts; Crosslinker
RER	3	*MGMT* (so far only epigenetic modifications)	DNA mono-adducts
RR	~80	*BRCA1, BRCA2* (familial breast cancer); *ATM* (Ataxia-telangiectasia); *ATR* (Seckel S.); *NBS1* (Nijmegen Breakage S.); *MRE11* (AT-like S.); *RAD50* (RAD50 deficiency); *RECQL2* (Werner S.), *RECQL3* (Bloom S.); *RECQL4* (Rothmund-Thomson S.); *Lig4* (Ligase 4 deficiency); *Artemis* (RS-SCID); *FANCA, FANCB, FANCC, FANCD1/BRCA2, FANCD2, FANCE, FANCF, FANCG/ XRCC9, FANCJ/BRIP1, FANCL, FANCM, FANCN/PALB2* (Fanconi anemia)	Ionizing radiation, Bleomycin, Etoposid, Mitomycin C, cisPlatin

this pathway lead to an extremely increased risk for colon cancer in the disease, hereditary non-polyposis colorectal cancer (see Chapter 17 on Lynch syndrome (HNPCC)).

22.6
Reversion Repair (RER)

Modified bases are repaired by this pathway in a single reaction step. Mutations have not yet been described in any of the involved genes; however, methylation of the *MGMT* promoter is a predictive indicator for the response of gliomas to therapy with alkylating agents.

22.7
Recombination Repair (RR)

In contrast to all the lesions considered so far, which affected only one DNA strand, the lesions repaired by recombination are DSBs or interstrand crosslinks (ICLs). The eukaryotic cell has two main pathways for repair of DSBs (Figure 22.2). During homologous recombination (HR), a homologous sequence, in mammals usually the sister chromatid, is used as a template for repair. This process is practically error free but is restricted to the S- and G2-phase of the cell cycle. The alternative mechanism for repair of DSBs is non-homologous end joining (NHEJ), which is more universal but error prone. Since only a small portion of the mammalian genome has coding function, most of the deletions incurred during NHEJ will be tolerated by the cell. DSBs also arise as a consequence of base damage,

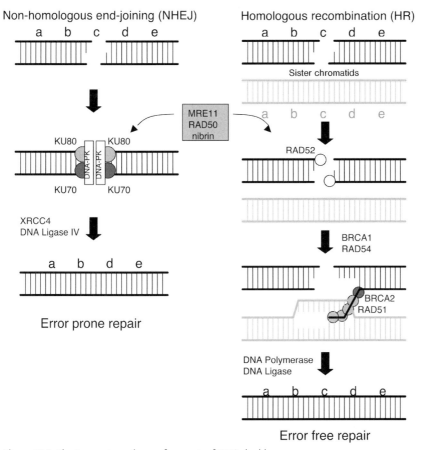

Figure 22.2 The two main pathways for repair of DNA double-strand breaks, and some of the proteins involved (after [1]).

single-strand breaks, or ICLs during DNA replication. Furthermore, DSBs are also intermediates in normal cellular processes such as meiotic recombination during meiosis, rearrangement of the immunoglobulin and T-cell receptor genes and, finally, maintenance of telomeres. Considering the frequency of DSBs, it is perhaps not surprising that so many genes are involved in their repair, and that these genes play an important role in carcinogenesis (Table 22.1). The consequences of unrepaired, or incorrectly repaired, DSBs are microscopically visible chromosome aberrations. Such aberrations are characteristic of the chromosome instability syndromes, all of which have an increased cancer risk.

However, the cellular response to DNA damage is more complex than the mere removal of a DNA lesion. When a DNA lesion occurs it must first be detected, for which sensor proteins are required. The sensors then transmit, via transducer proteins, a signal to the effector proteins, many of which are the actual DNA repair enzymes. A second group of effectors are those which, in proliferating cells, are responsible for arresting the cell cycle in order that DNA repair can be carried out. These two effector protein groups correspond to Kinzler und Vogelstein's "caretakers" and "gatekeepers". Loss or inactivation of both alleles of a caretaker gene leads to genomic instability, increased cancer risk, and reduced life expectancy. Interestingly, the two diseases, Cockayne Syndrome and Trichothiodystrophy, with an NER defect and premature aging but without increased cancer risk demonstrate that these phenomena can actually be separated from one another [2]. The gatekeeper group of genes is composed largely of the tumor suppressor genes, which in the case of severe damage initiate the self-destruction pathways of apoptosis.

As important and useful as these heuristic terms are, they remain abstractions, as individual genes can be involved in several discrete steps of a whole network. This network is in turn regulated by complex feedback control mechanisms, leading to a unique buffering capacity: the loss of one particular gene can be more or less compensated for by the other members of the network. The following will attempt to illustrate this complexity, using lymphoma as an example.

22.8
Genetic Diseases with a High Risk of Lymphoma: Ataxia-Telangiectasia and Nijmegen Breakage-Syndrome

Cardinal symptoms of ataxia-telangiectasia (A-T; OMIM 208900) are progressive cerebral ataxia, conjunctival telangiectasia, and immunodeficiency. About one-third of A-T patients develop malignancies, among children mostly lymphoma and leukemia. Older patients also develop solid tumors, such as breast cancer and colon carcinoma. Nijmegen Breakage-Syndrome (NBS; OMIM 251260) is clinically distinct from A-T through the characteristic facial features, microcephaly, and lack of ataxia. Again, both humoral and cellular immunodeficiency lead to frequent infections. Approximately 40% of NBS patients develop a lymphoma before the age of 20.

At the cellular level, A-T and NBS show many similarities. Cells from patients with both diseases have a high rate of spontaneous chromosome breakage. Characteristic of lymphocytes are clonal and non-clonal rearrangements involving the T-cell receptor and immunoglobulin genes. Occasionally, fusions of chromosome ends, so-called telomere fusions, are also observed. Cellular sensitivity towards ionizing radiation is remarkable, particularly the failure to arrest DNA synthesis after irradiation (radio resistant DNA synthesis).

Both genes are express ubiquitously. The *NBS* gene product, nibrin, is part of a trimeric complex together with *MRE11* and *RAD50* (the MRN complex). This complex is evolutionarily highly conserved, and in yeast consists of the proteins Mre11, Rad50, and Xrs2, whereby Xrs2 represents the functional ortholog of nibrin [3]. In yeast, and also in human cells, the MRN complex is involved in DSB repair by both HR and NHEJ. Only seconds after irradiation, the MRN complex relocates to the sites of DSBs where it holds the open DNA ends together. The protein product of the *AT* gene, ATM, is recruited to the DSBs and converted from an inactive dimer to an active, auto-phosphorylated monomer. The DNA-bound MRN complex is a prerequisite for the activation of ATM. This protein belongs to a highly conserved family of DNA-dependent protein kinases and, indeed, phosphorylates a large number of target proteins, including nibrin, p53, MDM2, CHK1, CHK2, BRCA1, and the histone, H2AX [4, 5]. However these proteins are also phosphorylated in ATM-deficient cells, albeit at much slower rates, by the related protein ATR. Particularly critical is the phosphorylation on the transcription factor and tumor suppressor *p53*, which regulates both cell cycle arrest and apoptosis.

As shown in Figure 22.3, the MRN complex is involved in the response to DNA damage upstream and downstream of ATM. Nibrin performs apparently as a *sensor*, since a complex of MRE11 and RAD50 alone does not relocate to DSBs after irradiation. In consequence, ATM is not activated, thus nibrin also clearly has a transducer function. Finally, nibrin is also an effector, since it is directly involved in DSB repair by HR and NHEJ, and in checkpoint control through its facilitating effect on ATM target phosphorylation.

In addition, ATM and nibrin are involved in the processing of DSBs, which occur during the maturation of immuno-competent cells. ATM is clearly involved in V(D)J recombination in T- and B-cells, whilst nibrin is never involved in this process: the sensor of DSBs and transducer to ATM during immune gene rearrangement is apparently a different protein. On the other hand, nibrin is clearly involved in immunoglobulin class switching, explaining the deficiencies in serum IgG and IgA observed in NBS patients. In both A-T and NBS patients, there is also a shift in the naive to memory T-cell ratio [6].

All these results can be assembled to obtain a greatly simplified pathophysiology of the diseases, A-T and NBS. Thus, because of the gene mutations, the mutation rate in rapidly proliferating lymphatic cells is particularly high with coincident deficiencies in cell cycle checkpoints and apoptosis induction. The development of T- and B-cell lymphoma during childhood is the almost inevitable outcome, particularly in immunodeficient patients. It remains to be explained why T-cell

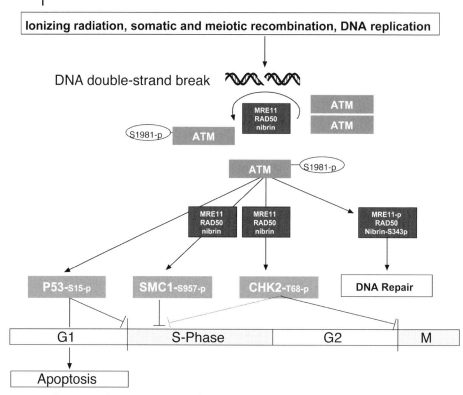

Figure 22.3 The MRE11/RAD50/nibrin complex and its role in the DNA double-strand break response. The diagram highlights the role of the MRN complex and ATM in DSB repair and checkpoint control. Some important critical phosphorylations are shown (-p). DSBs occur in mammalian cells not only after IR exposure, but also as a result of physiological processes, such as rearrangement of immunoglobulin genes and meiotic crossing over (after [1]). For details, see text.

lymphoma is four times more frequent than B-cell lymphoma among A-T patients. Under NBS patients, the B- and T-cell lymphomas occur equally often, but together much more frequently than in A-T patients.

The chromosome instability inherent in NBS and A-T affects all cells and, in both diseases, the risk for other haematological malignancies and for solid tumors is also increased. Patients with a deficiency in DNA repair are generally sensitive towards exogenous and endogenous mutagens. In this respect, free oxygen radicals generated during energy metabolism may pose a particular threat.

22.9
Lymphoma in Ataxia-Telangiectasia and Nijmegen Breakage Syndrome

Cancer is the most common cause of death in patients with NBS [7], and the second most common in A-T patients [8, 9]. The precise molecular classification of lympho-proliferative disease and lymphomas occurring in A-T and NBS is still incomplete, and it is often difficult to make a clear distinction between lympho-proliferation and overt lymphoma. Nevertheless, the calculated risk for developing lymphoma is clearly dramatically increased to over 1000-fold, and 252-fold for NBS and A-T patients, respectively (Boffetta *et al.*, personal communication and [8]).

The life-time cancer risk of developing malignancy among A-T patients has been estimated as about 38% [8], whilst in NBS it ranges from 40 to 65% in various reports [7, 10]. Roughly, 80 to 85% of all the malignancies in A-T patients, and 85 to 90% in NBS patients are either lymphoma or leukemia. The incidence of lymphoma, including non-Hodgkin lymphoma (NHL) and Hodgkin lymphoma (HL), is lower in A-T patients (50–60%) than in NBS patients (~80%) [8–10]. Median age of lymphoma development in A-T and NBS patients is about 8.5 and 9.5 years, respectively (Chrzanowska, unpublished materials and [11]).

In October 2007, an examination of the Polish NB.S. Registry, with 105 patients representing the largest national sample, revealed 51 lymphoid malignancies among 56 primary cancers. Among the 51 lymphoid malignancies, there were 46 lymphomas, including 44 cases of NHL and 2 of HL. A slight predominance of T-cell NHL (55%) over B-cell NHL (45%) was noted. Further analysis of the available data showed a high frequency of two morphological subtypes: T-cell lymphoblastic lymphoma (T-LBL) and diffuse large B-cell lymphoma (DLBCL), which were diagnosed in 13 of 23 patients (57%) and 10 of 19 patients (53%), respectively. Five Burkitt-like and one angio-immunobastic type T-cell lymphoma were also diagnosed; the histological subtypes of the remaining tumors were not specified.

The ratio of T- to B-cell lymphoid malignancies in A-T patients is more difficult to assess since many reports do not discriminate between the two. Some studies show a clear predominance of T-cell over B-cell tumors; however, when only lymphomas are considered, the proportions are almost equal [12, 13]. Other authors have pointed out that the histological origin of leukemia and lymphoma in A-T patients may be different, with the latter being predominantly of B-cell origin [14]. This situation will only be clarified by the publication of the characteristics of all tumors occurring in A-T patients in the future. Collectively, these data suggest the predominance of two phenotypes of lymphomas in NBS, those of precursor T-cell origin, and those representing mature large B-cell lymphomas.

In the general population, the majority of pediatric lymphomas stem from B-cells (B-NHL), and the most prevalent are Burkitt lymphoma (43%) and diffuse large B-cell lymphoma (13%) [15]. In comparison, in adults, DLBCL accounts for 30 to 40% of NHL [16]. Currently, DLBCL are grouped into three prognostically distinct types: the germinal center B-cell type (GCB), the activated B-cell type (ABC), and Type 3 or primary mediastinal DLBCL [17, 18]. A multicenter study of altogether 63 cases of DLBCL in pediatric patients revealed a striking predominance (83%) of the germinal center B-cell-like (GCB) type, indicating that pediatric DLBCL differs from adult DLBCL where this subtype makes up less than half of the cases [19]. In this connection it is interesting to note that sporadic childhood DLBCL has a generally more favorable prognosis than DLBCL in adulthood.

A thorough analysis of eight NBS-associated DLBCL tumors collected at one center (CMHI) revealed that all cases are of the BCL6$^-$/CD10$^-$ ABC type of DLBCL

(Gladkowska-Dura, personal communication). This tumor type exhibits a particularly aggressive biological behavior, and is associated with a much poorer prognosis. These findings are in line with an earlier report pointing out that the spectrum of lympho-proliferative disease in NBS patients appears to be more characteristic for adults than for children, and has an unfavorable clinical outcome [20, 21]. In addition, B-cell monoclonality was confirmed by gene rearrangement studies in all DLBCL tumors of these eight NBS patients, again showing a difference to other primary or secondary immuno-deficiencies in which around 60% of B-cell lympho-proliferations are oligoclonal and polymorphic in nature [22].

Patients with A-T and NBS are known to be at risk of developing secondary neoplasia; however, precise data have not been published. Earlier investigations of the additional risk for A-T patients already diagnosed with one type of neoplasm indicated that approximately 25% of patients with solid tumors subsequently developed NHL or leukemia. In contrast, when the primary tumor was lymphoid in origin, there was only a low risk of subsequent neoplasia [9]. In the Polish NBS Registry, nine patients with lymphoma developed a second malignancy. Among the secondary lympho-proliferations, there were seven lymphomas (6 B-cell and 1 T-cell) and two leukemias (T-ALL). It is striking that in all cases of lymphoma followed by a further lympho-proliferation, the primary lymphoma was Hodgkin lymphoma or NHL of B-cell origin; no subsequent neoplasia were observed in patients with NHL of T-cell origin. The median age at diagnosis of the second lympho-proliferation was 13 years.

In a further detailed analysis of six multiple lympho-proliferations in NBS patients, two types of secondary lymphomas could be defined. In four patients, the second tumor was a reoccurrence of the initial lymphoma, DLBCL. This could be a consequence of the relatively mild chemotherapy protocols employed due to their toxic complications in NBS patients: this is naturally of great concern. In two further patients, also with primary DLBCL, a true secondary lymphoma was found, including one peripheral T-cell lymphoma (Gladkowska-Dura, personal communication). These new malignancies reflect the higher mutation rate with its potential for cancer development in NBS patients.

Of the 35 Czech NBS patients born between 1960 and 2004, 15 have died from malignancies, 3 from infections, and 1 from congenital CNS malformation. Of the surviving patients, 5 have a malignancy, which they have survived for an average of 11 years (range 6–16) since diagnosis. Eleven patients are cancer-free at an average age of 11 years (range 1–33). The mean age at death from malignancy has increased to 12 years (range 1–29) since the introduction of modified treatment protocols.

In 2 of these patients, there were 2 or 3 secondary malignancies 3 to 4 years after diagnosis of the primary neoplasia. One boy had ALL at the age of 14, HL at the age of 17, and at 26, he developed a hepatic tumor. A girl who manifested with B-cell NHL at the relatively late age of 25 years, developed a T-cell NHL 3 years later. Three patients are living after successful treatment of their malignancy: the above-mentioned boy with three independent malignancies, a girl after malignant meningeoma, and a boy who had a rhabdomyosarcoma. Two patients, a boy and a girl, are alive at 20 years of age with NHL.

In conclusion, the spectrum of lymphoma NBS patients differs clearly not only from that of sporadic pediatric NHL, which are predominantly either Burkitt lymphoma or large cell anaplastic/diffuse lymphoma, but also from NHL in immunodeficient patients where oligoclonal B-cell proliferation predominates. Clearly, this reflects a different mechanism of lymphomagenesis in NBS patients.

22.10
Treatment of Malignancies in Nijmegen Breakage Syndrome

Twenty years ago, the oldest known Czech patient with NBS was 12 years of age; of 8 patients, 5 died, 4 from lymphoreticular malignancy. Survival ranged from a few days to weeks after diagnosis of malignancy. The former standard therapy for lymphoreticular malignancy including radiotherapy led to rapidly progressive organ insufficiency and death. Hyper-radiosensitivity of NBS patient cells was first reported in 1989 [23], and from that time, malignancy in children with NBS was treated by modified protocols completely avoiding ionizing radiation and radiomimetics. Initial doses of cytostatic drugs are considerably lower and are raised very slowly under careful clinical observation. Survival is now for several years after diagnosis and some patients have survived more than one malignancy (see Table 22.2).

Table 22.2 Treatment of malignancy in NBS

	1985	2005
Number of patients ascertained	8	35
Number of patients with malignancies	4	20
Total number of malignancies	4	23
Number of deceased patients	5	19
Death from malignancy	4	11 + 4
Death from infections	1	2 + 1
Death from congenital CNS malformation	0	1
Mean age at death from malignancy	5.5 y	12 y
Range	(1–10)	(1–29)
Mean survival after diagnosis of malignancy	0.1 y	3.3 y
Number of patients surviving after treatment of malignancy	0	5
Number of patients free from malignancy	3	11
Mean age	6 y	11 y
Range	(3–12)	(1–33)

A further major factor in the improvement of the clinical prognosis of NBS since 1998 is the possibility of very early and exact diagnosis by direct detection of the so-called Slavic mutation, 657del5, in exon 6 of the *NBS* gene [24]. Thus, confirmed homozygotes can be appropriately protected from mutagens, and particularly from ionizing radiation. Prior to identification of the *NBS* gene, the mean age at diagnosis was 7 years and was made solely on the basis of microcephaly, lymphoreticular malignancy, and toxic complications of standard tumor therapy. Since 1998, the mean age at diagnosis in the Czech Republic has dropped to 4 months (range 2–5 months) due to the routine analysis of the *NBS* gene in all infants with congenital microcephaly [25].

Needless to say, the prognosis for lympho-proliferative disease and malignant tumors in general has improved considerably over the past 20 years. For example, in the Czech Republic, the proportion of surviving patients has increased from 40% in 1985 to 80% in 2006, due to progress in combined therapy protocols. Thus, the successes in treating recurrent malignancies and modifications to chemotherapy have substantially improved the clinical prognosis for NBS patients.

22.11
Somatic Mutations in Sporadic Lymphoma

One of the most frequent deletions in lymphoid neoplasia is on the long arm of chromosome 11, leading to loss of the *ATM* gene at 11q22.3 [26]. More than 50% of mantel cell lymphomas (MCL) and 10 to 20% of chronic B-cell lymphocytic leukemia (B-CLL) have this deletion. Similarly, T-cell prolymphocytic leukemia (T-PLL) is often accompanied by a partial or complete loss of 11q. Inactivation of the second *ATM* allele could be demonstrated in all six T-PLLs, showing that *ATM* can behave as a typical "two-hit" tumor suppressor gene [27]. In the meantime, there is ample evidence that in many MCLs, B-CLLs, and T-PLLs, both ATM alleles are defective [26]. Inactivation of *ATM* clearly plays an important role in pathogenesis and tumor progression. Surprisingly, in NHL, which is common in A-T patients, mutation in both *ATM* alleles is only rarely observed. Similarly, mutations in the *NBS* gene play little or no role in sporadic lymphoma [28].

It is well documented that a large number of lymphoid neoplasias, particularly of the B-cell and myeloid lineages, are characterized by translocations of a more or less specific nature. In the case of Burkitt lymphoma, the translocation breakpoints are located in intron 1 of the proto-oncogene, *c-myc*, and in the Sμ switch region of the immunoglobulin heavy chain locus (IgH). In consequence, the *c-myc* gene is regulated by the promoter/enhancer of the *IgH* gene; a critical first step in the development of this lymphoma. Translocations can also lead to the generation of chimaeric proteins, such as the BCR-ABL tyrosine kinase in chronic myelogenous leukemia (CML).

Such specific translocations suggest that the chromosomes involved are topologically connected. Indeed, in B-cells, the *IgH* and *c-myc* loci are neighbors. In

CD34+ cells, the *ABL* gene and *BCR* region on chromosomes 9 and 22, respectively, are also in close proximity. However, it seems unlikely that this closeness is sufficient to explain the high specificity of such translocations in the development of some lymphomas.

Many of the breakpoints of chromosome translocations involve genes involved either in haematopoiesis, or in the regulation of the cell cycle [29]. A particularly instructive example is the translocation t(11;14)(q13;q32), which is highly characteristic for MCL. This translocation brings the cyclin *D1* gene, a central regulator of the G1-phase of the cell cycle on 11q13, under the control of the promoter of the immunoglobulin heavy chain gene on 14q32. Cyclin D1 is overexpressed in cells carrying this translocation, with predictable effects on cell proliferation.

Interestingly, haematological neoplasia often have two translocations, one affecting a gene involved in haematopoiesis whose disturbance blocks further differentiation, and one affecting a gene which leads to increased cell proliferation. In the case of MCL, the frequent inactivation of the *ATM* gene leads to loss of DNA repair processes and disturbances in cell cycle checkpoints, cumulating in the initiation of the malignancy [30].

22.12
Outlook and Perspectives

The relationship between increased mutation rates and carcinogenesis touches a central problem of tumor biology. Based on theoretical considerations of the spontaneous mutation rate, Loeb proposed that a cell accumulates less than three specific mutations within a normal lifetime: too few, considering the multistep nature of tumor initiation. He concluded that an increase in the mutation rate is a prerequisite for the malignant transformation of a cell [31]. Others were of a somewhat different opinion. Tomlinson and Bodmer stressed the importance of selection, leading to clonal expansion of those cells with a growth advantage. Just as selection is the driving force of evolution among organisms, so it is for the persistence of cells during tumorigenesis [32]. In this case, the normal spontaneous mutation rate is adequate, and an increased mutation rate can accelerate, but not cause, the emergence of a tumor. With respect to diseases with a defect in DNA repair, a constitutively increased mutation rate results in the early manifestation of cancer.

Knowledge of the molecular origin of hereditary and spontaneous lymphomas also has consequences for therapy. Before elucidation of the molecular defect, NBS and A-T patients with lymphoma were treated with radiotherapy, from which some of them died. Nowadays, these patients can be successfully treated with low dose chemotherapy.

In sporadic neoplasia, therapy sometimes depends on the particular chromosome translocation present. In case of the t(9;22) translocation in CML, the tyrosine kinase inhibitor Imatinib is the medication of choice since it inactivates the

BCR-AB.L. kinase. Patients with acute myeloid leukemia (AML) and a t(15;17) translocation are treated with all-trans retinoic acid, which is directed towards the chimaeric fusion receptor, PML-RAR. AML patients with inv(16) or t(8;21) respond better to treatment with high doses of Cytarabine than those patients without these chromosome rearrangements [29].

A great deal has been learned about cancerogenesis from the study of lymphoma, and the genes affected in haematological neoplasia. However, many questions still remain open – there is still much to be learned.

References

1 Digweed, M. and Sperling, K. (2007) DNA-Reparaturdefekte und Krebs. *Medgen*, **19**, 191–6.

2 Andressoo, J.O., Hoeijmakers, J.H. and Mitchell, J.R. (2006) Nucleotide excision repair disorders and the balance between cancer and aging. *Cell Cycle*, **5**, 2886–8.

3 Digweed, M. and Sperling, K. (2004) Nijmegen breakage syndrome: clinical manifestation of defective response to DNA double-strand breaks. *DNA Repair*, **3**, 1207–17.

4 Matei, I.R., Guidos, C.J. and Danska, J.S. (2006) ATM-dependent DNA damage surveillance in T-cell development and leukemogenesis: the DSB connection. *Immunological Reviews*, **209**, 142–58.

5 Matsuoka, S., Ballif, B.A., Smogorzewska, A., McDonald, E.R. 3rd, Hurov, K.E., Luo, J., Bakalarski, C.E., Zhao, Z. *et al.* (2007) ATM and ATR substrate analysis reveals extensive protein networks responsive to DNA damage. *Science*, **316**, 1160–6.

6 Marculescu, R., Vanura, K., Montpellier, B., Roulland, S., Le, T., Navarro, J.M., Jager, U., McBlane, F. *et al.* (2006) Recombinase, chromosomal translocations and lymphoid neoplasia: targeting mistakes and repair failures. *DNA Repair*, **5**, 1246–58.

7 The International Nijmegen Breakage Syndrome Study Group (2000) Nijmegen breakage syndrome. *Archives of Disease in Childhood*, **82**, 400–6.

8 Morrell, D., Cromartie, E. and Swift, M. (1986) Mortality and cancer incidence in 263 patients with ataxia-telangiectasia.

Journal of the National Cancer Institute, **77**, 89–92.

9 Hecht, F. and Hecht, B.K. (1990) Cancer in ataxia-telangiectasia patients. *Cancer Genet. Cytogenet*, **46**, 9–19.

10 Wegner, R.D., German, J.J., Chrzanowska, K.H., Digweed, M. and Stumm, M. (2007) Chromosomal Instability Syndromes other than ataxia-telangiectasia, in *Primary Immunodeficiency Diseases: A Molecular & Cellular Approach* (eds H.D. Ochs, C.I.E. Smith and J.M. Puck), Oxford University Press, New York, pp. 427–53.

11 Filipovich, A.H., Mathur, A., Kamat, D. and Shapiro, R.S. (1992) Primary immunodeficiencies: genetic risk factors for lymphoma. *Cancer Research*, **52**, 5465s–7s.

12 Stankovic, T., Kidd, A.M., Sutcliffe, A., McGuire, G.M., Robinson, P., Weber, P., Bedenham, T., Bradwell, A.R. *et al.* (1998) ATM mutations and phenotypes in ataxia-telangiectasia families in the British Isles: expression of mutant ATM and the risk of leukemia, lymphoma, and breast cancer. *American Journal of Human Genetics*, **62**, 334–45.

13 Taylor, A.M., Metcalfe, J.A., Thick, J. and Mak, Y.F. (1996) Leukemia and lymphoma in ataxia-telangiectasia. *Blood*, **87**, 423–38.

14 Gatti, R.A. (2002) Ataxia-telangiectasia, in *The Genetics Basis of Human Cancer* (eds B. Vogelstein and K.W. Kinzler), McGraw-Hill, New York, pp. 239–66.

15 Burkhardt, B., Zimmermann, M., Oschlies, I., Niggli, F., Mann, G., Parwaresch, R., Riehm, H., Schrappe, M. *et al.* (2005) The impact of age and gender on biology, clinical features and treatment

outcome of non-Hodgkin lymphoma in childhood and adolescence. *British Journal of Haematology*, **131**, 39–49.

16 Coiffier, B. (2001) Diffuse large cell lymphoma. *Current Opinion in Oncology*, **13**, 325–34.

17 Alizadeh, A.A., Eisen, M.B., Davis, R.E., Ma, C., Lossos, I.S., Rosenwald, A., Boldrick, J.C., Sabet, H. *et al.* (2000) Distinct types of diffuse large B-cell lymphoma identified by gene expression profiling. *Nature*, **403**, 503–11.

18 Rosenwald, A., Wright, G., Chan, W.C., Connors, J.M., Campo, E., Fisher, R.I., Gascoyne, R.D., Muller-Hermelink, H.K. *et al.* (2002) The use of molecular profiling to predict survival after chemotherapy for diffuse large-B-cell lymphoma. *New England Journal of Medicine*, **346**, 1937–47.

19 Oschlies, I., Klapper, W., Zimmer-mann, M., Krams, M., Wacker, H.H., Burkhardt, B., Harder, L., Siebert, R. *et al.* (2006) Diffuse large B-cell lymphoma in pediatric patients belongs predominantly to the germinal-center type B-cell lymphomas: a clinicopatho-logic analysis of cases included in the German BFM (Berlin–Frankfurt–Münster) Multicenter Trial. *Blood*, **107**, 4047–52.

20 Gladkowska-Dura, M.J., Dzierzanowska-Fangrat, K., Langerak, A.W. and Van Dongen, J.J.M. (2002) Immunopheno-typic and immunogenotypic profile of NHL in Nijmegen Breakage Syndrome (NBS) with special emphasis on DLBLC. *Journal of Clinical Pathology*, **55S**, A15.

21 Gladkowska-Dura, M.J., Chrzanowska, K.H. and Dura, W.T. (2000) Malignant lymphoma in Nijmegen Breakage Syndrome, *Annals of Diagnostic Pediatric Pathology*, **4**, 39–46.

22 Canioni, D., Jabado, N., MacIntyre, E., Patey, N., Emile, J.F. and Brousse, N. (2001) Lympho-proliferative disorders in children with primary immuno-deficiencies: immunological status may be more predictive of the outcome than other criteria. *Histopathology*, **38**, 146–59.

23 Taalman, R.D., Hustinx, T.W., Weemaes, C.M., Seemanova, E., Schmidt, A., Passarge, E. and Scheres, J.M. (1989) Further delineation of the Nijmegen breakage syndrome. *American Journal of Medical Genetics*, **32**, 425–31.

24 Varon, R., Vissinga, C., Platzer, M., Cerosaletti, K.M., Chrzanowska, K.H., Saar, K., Beckmann, G., Seemanova, E. *et al.* (1998) Nibrin, a novel DNA double-strand break repair protein, is mutated in Nijmegen breakage syndrome. *Cell*, **93**, 467–76.

25 Seeman, P., Gebertova, K., Paderova, K., Sperling, K. and Seemanova, E. (2004) Nijmegen breakage syndrome in 13% of age-matched Czech children with primary microcephaly. *Pediatric Neurology*, **30**, 195–200.

26 Boultwood, J. (2001) Ataxia-telangiectasia gene mutations in leukaemia and lymphoma. *Journal of Clinical Pathology*, **54**, 512–16.

27 Stilgenbauer, S., Schaffner, C., Litterst, A., Liebisch, P., Gilad, S., Bar-Shira, A., James, M.R., Lichter, P. *et al.* (1997) Biallelic mutations in the ATM gene in T-prolymphocytic leukemia. *Nature Medicine*, **3**, 1155–9.

28 Stumm, M., von Ruskowsky, A., Siebert, R., Harder, S., Varon, R., Wieacker, P. and Schlegelberger, B. (2001) No evidence for deletions of the NBS1 gene in lymphoma. *Cancer Genetics and Cytogenetics*, **126**, 60–2.

29 Aplan, P.D. (2006) Causes of oncogenic chromosomal translocation. *Trends in Genetics*, **22**, 46–55.

30 Fernandez, V., Hartmann, E., Ott, G., Campo, E. and Rosenwald, A. (2005) Pathogenesis of mantle-cell lymphoma: all oncogenic roads lead to dysregulation of cell cycle and DNA damage response pathways. *Journal of Clinical Oncology*, **23**, 6364–9.

31 Loeb, L.A. (1991) Mutator phenotype may be required for multistage carcinogenesis. *Cancer Research*, **51**, 3075–9.

32 Tomlinson, I. and Bodmer, W. (1999) Selection, the mutation rate and cancer: ensuring that the tail does not wag the dog. *Nature Medicine*, **5**, 11–12.

23
Familial Leukemias

Christa Fonatsch

Summary

Leukemias and other hematological neoplasias are frequently observed in association with different genetic disorders, as DNA repair deficiency syndromes, tumor predisposition syndromes, immunodeficiency syndromes, cancer family syndromes, and bone marrow failure syndromes, as well as in connection with several constitutional chromosome anomalies. Recently, in families with increased leukemia incidence, constitutional mutations have been identified in genes that are also affected by somatic mutations in sporadic leukemias. In addition to these high penetrance mutations, gene alterations with a low penetrance and polymorphisms seem to predispose to leukemia and/or modify the clinical course of the leukemia. Predisposing and modifying polymorphisms can be found in genes involved in cell proliferation, apoptosis, DNA repair, detoxification, and so on. A novel class of small RNA molecules, the so-called microRNAs, also play a role in cancer and presumably in leukemia pathogenesis. The findings on constitutional genetic alterations predisposing to leukemia start to close the gap between inborn and acquired genetic diseases.

23.1
Introduction

The frequent occurrence of leukemias and lymphomas in association with DNA repair deficiency syndromes (also called chromosome instability syndromes), and also with Down's syndrome represents a well established fact. But, most of the leukemias and lymphomas occur sporadically and only a small number of hematopoietic neoplasias are due to constitutional genetic diseases. Research has demonstrated that a number of monogenic diseases as well as syndromes caused by chromosome anomalies and also genetic polymorphisms, correlate with an increased risk to neoplasias of the hematopoietic system. These new findings create a bridge between leukemogenesis based on somatic (acquired) mutations

Hereditary Tumors: From Genes to Clinical Consequences
Edited by Heike Allgayer, Helga Rehder and Simone Fulda
Copyright © 2009 WILEY-VCH Verlag GmbH & Co. KGaA, Weinheim
ISBN: 978-3-527-32028-8

on the one hand, and on constitutional (inborn) genetic changes on the other. Familial leukemias as a part of syndromes, for example, of DNA repair deficiency, immunodeficiency, tumor predisposition, bone marrow failure, cancer family syndromes, and constitutional chromosome anomalies must be differentiated from non-syndromal familial leukemias. Affected members of these latter families develop hematopoietic neoplasias only, but do not show any malformations or pathological features. They constitute a special group of single gene, Mendelian disorders with pure familial leukemia.

23.2
Leukemias Associated with Genetic Syndromes

23.2.1
DNA Repair Deficiency Syndromes

DNA repair deficiency syndromes are autosomal recessive disorders, associated with an increased chromosomal instability. These disorders are described separately in this book. It has only to be mentioned that in patients with Bloom's syndrome that is due to a helicase gene defect (*BLM* gene), acute lymphoblastic leukemia (ALL) and acute myeloid leukemia (AML), as well as malignant lymphomas are observed. In connection with ataxia-telangiectasia (*ATM* gene), Hodgkin and non-Hodgkin lymphomas and ALL of the T-cell type occur. The Nijmegen Breakage Syndrome (*NBS* gene) is found to be associated with B-cell lymphomas. Fanconi's anemia *(*FA) can be induced by mutations of at least 13 genes. It is associated with a high risk of solid tumors, as well as aplastic anemia, myelodysplastic syndromes (MDS), and leukemia, and represents one of the bone marrow failure syndromes.

23.2.2
Bone Marrow Failure Syndromes

This heterogeneous group of diseases is characterized by bone marrow failure in association with somatic anomalies. The most common of these rare disorders include FA, Dyskeratosis congenita (DC), Shwachman-Diamond syndrome (SDS), severe congenital neutropenia (SCN), and Kostmann syndrome, as well as Diamond–Blackfan anemia (DBA) (Table 23.1).

23.2.2.1 Fanconi's Anemia
The most frequent clinical findings in patients with FA include short stature, hyper- and hypo-pigmentation, microcephaly, microphthalmia, and abnormal thumbs with or without hypoplastic radii. The cumulative incidence of haematologic malignancies (leukemia or MDS) was reported to be 40% [1]. The diagnosis of a malignant disease preceded the diagnosis of FA in more than 130 of the literature cases with cancer [2].

Table 23.1 Characteristics of the inherited bone marrow failure syndromes (after [12]).

	FA	DC	SDS	SCN (+Kostmann syndrome)	DBA
Mode of inheritance	AR, XR	XR, AR, AD	AR	AD, AR	AD
Somatic abnormalities	yes	yes	yes	rare	yes
Bone marrow failure	AA (>90%)	AA (~80%)	AA (20%)	Neut	RCA
Short telomeres	yes	yes	yes	?	yes
Cancer/leukemias	yes	yes	yes	yes	yes
Chromosome instability	yes	yes	yes	?	?
Genes identified	13	4	1	2	2

AA, aplastic anemia; AD, autosomal dominant; AR, autosomal recessive; DBA, Diamond-Blackfan anemia; DC, dyskeratosis congenita; FA, Fanconi's anemia; Neut, Neutropenia; RCA, red cell aplasia; SCN, severe congenital neutropenia; SDS, Shwachman-Diamond syndrome; XR, X-linked recessive.

Cells of FA patients are characterized by spontaneous chromosomal breakage and increased sensitivity to DNA cross-linking agents such as diepoxibutan (DEB) or mitomycin C (MMC). Interestingly, an accelerated shortening of telomeres, the ends of chromosomes, was found in FA cells by fluorescence-*in situ*-hybridization (FISH) [3]. This phenomenon is also observed in DC and in SDS, as described below.

In FA, a considerably heterogeneous disease, 13 subtypes/complementation groups are recognized: *FANCA, FANCB, FANCC, FANCD1/BRCA2, FANCD2, FANCE, FANCF, FANCG, FANCI, FANCJ/BACH1/BRIP1, FANCL, FANCM,* and *FANCN/PALBIX2* [2]. FA is usually an autosomal recessive disorder with the exception of the FANCB subgroup, which is X-linked.

Genotype-phenotype correlations have been reported for the genes *FANCD1/ BRCA2* and *FANCN/PALBIX2.* Mutations of these two genes have been described in patients with severe birth defects, brain tumors, Wilms tumor, and AML [2].

FA patients with MDS and/or AML frequently exhibit monosomy 7 in their bone marrow. FA-associated AML is often preceded by the occurrence of chromosome aberrations in bone marrow involving bands 3q26–29 [4, 5]. In association with a 3q26 abnormality in bone marrow and bone marrow- derived cell lines of an FA patient with AML and biallelic *FANCD1/BRCA2* disruption, an overexpression of the oncogenic transcription factor EVI1, located at 3q26, was observed [5].

23.2.2.2 Dyskeratosis Congenita

DC is characterized by abnormal skin pigmentation, nail dystrophy, mucosal leukoplakia, complications of the lung, and an elevated predisposition to cancer development. Mutations were found in the *DKC1* gene [6], encoding a nucleolar protein, dyskerin. Dyskerin plays a role in the biogenesis of ribosomes. Thus, it was suggested that DC is due to a disturbed ribosomal biogenesis. Dyskerin associates with the RNA component (TERC) of telomerase, the enzyme responsible for the stability of the telomeres. In patients with the X-linked form of DC, based on *DKC1* mutations, as well as in patients with the autosomal dominant form, induced by *TERC* mutations, significantly shortened telomeres were found [7].

Heterozygous mutations of the *TERT* gene, encoding the reverse transcriptase component of telomerase, were also found in several families with DC [8, 9].

Recently, a subtype of DC was found to be due to homozygous mutations of the gene *NOP10*, encoding a telomerase-associated protein [10].

In DC, the phenomenon anticipation can be observed, that means, the earlier occurrence of the disease in subsequent generations and a more severe expression of the disease. In DC, anticipation is associated with progressive telomere shortening. Decreased telomerase activity and reduced telomere lengths result in most cases from haploinsuffiency of the *TERC* or the *TERT* gene. Changes of the *TERC* sequence may also inhibit the wildtype copy in a dominant-negative fashion [11]. Therefore inherited telomerase gene mutations work by different mechanisms to decrease telomere lengths. DC represents the first disease that is significantly based on the constitutional disregulation of the telomere stability and is characterized by features of premature aging [12].

23.2.2.3 Shwachman-Diamond Syndrome

Clinical features of the rare autosomal recessive disorder SDS are exocrine pancreatic insufficiency and bone marrow failure. Patients with SDS are at an elevated risk to develop aplastic anemia, MDS, and AML. In SDS patients, defects of the hematopoietic stem cell as well as of the stroma are observed. Furthermore, an elevated rate of apoptosis and short telomeres do occur. Ninety percent of the patients show mutations in the *SBDS* gene, localized in 7q11 [13]. This gene has a function in ribosome formation. It is speculated that oncogenesis is correlated with an increased ribosomal biogenesis and translation, since the tumor suppressor gene *ARF* inhibits the production of ribosomal RNA, whereas the oncogene nucleophosmin promotes rRNA biosynthesis [12, 14]. Gene expression studies revealed that bone marrow cells of patients with SDS without transformation to AML exhibited an upregulation of several oncogenes and downregulation of several tumor suppressor genes, when compared to the gene expression patterns of healthy controls [15].

Many patients with SDS evolve to aplastic anemia, MDS, or AML. The age-dependent cumulative probability of leukemia is greater than 70% [2]. Several patients with SDS exhibit a specific chromosomal abnormality in bone marrow—an isochromosome of the long arms of chromosome 7–already before the development of MDS or AML [16, 17]. A study including 14 SDS patients with isochromosome 7q (i(7)(q10)) or other chromosome anomalies led to the conclusion that the *SBDS* mutation exerts a "mutator" effect, which may induce specific chromosome abnormalities such as an isochromosome i(7)(q10), and therefore is responsible for the development of MDS syndromes and AML [18].

23.2.2.4 Severe Congenital Neutropenia and Kostmann Syndrome

SCN includes a variety of hematologic disorders characterized by a severe neutropenia and associated with severe bacterial infections. The subtype Kostmann syndrome, an autosomal-recessive disorder, has been shown to be associated with mutations in the *HAX-1* gene encoding a mitochondria-targeted protein harboring so-called *BCL2*-homology domains [19]. HAX1 possesses anti-apoptotic properties and may suppress cell death [20]. In autosomal dominant neutropenia, heterozygous mutations in the *ELA-2* gene were discovered, which encodes the protein neutrophil elastase [21]. Interestingly, no individuals were identified with mutations in both *ELA-2* and *HAX-1* genes [20].

Malignant transformation into AML can occur in 10 to 15% of patients with SCN [22]. Several patients show an acquisition of additional genetic defects during the course of the disease, such as mutations of the granulocyte colony-stimulating factor (*G-CSF*) receptor gene and also chromosome aberrations. Patients with SCN are treated by recombinant human G-CSF and respond with an increase in absolute neutrophil count. But G-CSF treatment may accelerate the risk of leukemia [23]. Since, also in the pre-G-CSF era, leukemic transformation occurred in SCN patients, it remains unknown whether the increased survival due to G-CSF treatment leads to the manifestation of a higher rate of leukemia [20]. A study on 374 patients on long-term G-CSF therapy demonstrated an overall cumulative incidence of MDS/AML of 21% after 10 years [24]. It could be shown that patients less responsive to G-CSF had a cumulative incidence of MDS/AML of 40% after 10 years, compared to 11% of the more responsive patients [24].

The analysis of patterns of gene mutations in *de novo* AML compared to AML in patients with SCN revealed a high mutation rate of tyrosine kinase genes (*FLT3*, *KIT*, *JAK2*) in *de novo* AML, but no mutations in these genes were found in the SCN samples. Instead, somatic mutations of *CSF3R*, the gene encoding the G-CSF receptor, were detected in association with the development of AML or MDS in SCN patients [25, 26].

Leukemic transformation in SCN is associated with acquired chromosome aberrations, mostly the partial or complete loss of chromosome 7, abnormalities of chromosome 21, or activating *RAS* mutations [27, 28].

23.2.2.5 Diamond-Blackfan Anemia

The clinical picture of DBA includes hypoplastic anemia, macrocytic anemia, reticulocytopenia, erythroblastopenia, missing or reduced erythroid precursor cells, and a stop of differentiation of the erythroid lineage in the bone marrow. A short stature, craniofacial dysmorphies, and skeletal anomalies, as well as kidney and heart defects, have been found in DBA. The risk for hematopoietic neoplasias, mainly for AML, is moderately elevated [29]. Most cases of DBA are associated with autosomal dominant inheritance. In 20 to 25% of the patients, heterozygous mutations of the gene encoding the ribosomal protein *RPS19*, localized in 19q13.2, were described [14]. Mutations of the *RPS24* gene, localized in 10q22~23, are found in 2% of the DBA patients [2]. About 40% of the patients show a linkage to loci in 8p23.3~p22 [29].

The analysis of functional features of mutated *RPS19* led to the conclusion that some *RPS19* mutations alter the capacity of the protein to localize in the nucleolar structure, thus blocking maturation, or leading to an inadequate formation of 40s ribosomal subunits [30, 31].

Since several children with DBA and a cytogenetically proved deletion in 19q13.2 have been described, these cases are discussed as micro-deletion syndrome [32]. This fact leads to the well-established increased proneness to leukemia of specific constitutional chromosome anomalies.

23.2.3
Constitutional Chromosome Anomalies

23.2.3.1 Down's Syndrome (Trisomy 21)
About 10% of children with Down's syndrome manifest transient myeloproliferative diseases, but they also have a significantly increased risk to develop leukemia. During the first 5 years of life, this risk is 50-fold, during the next 10 years elevated to 10-fold [33]. A primary event predisposing to leukemia development may be the deficiency of haematopoietic precursor and stem cells as well as the rapid shortening of telomeres, detected in fetuses with Down's syndrome [34].

The most common cause of trisomy 21 is maternal meiosis I non-disjunction, which increases with advanced maternal age and, supposing one crossing over within the long arm of chromosome 21, leads to telomeric disomy (Figure 23.1). However, trisomy 21 in children with transient myeloproliferative diseases in most cases is due to non-disjunction of meiosis II, which is not related to maternal age and produces centromeric uniparental disomy (UPD) [35] (Figure 23.1). It could be discussed that a mutant allele, located in the chromosome 21 segment with UPD and therefore duplicated, may function in an autosomal-recessive mode and lead to the development of leukemia in children with Down's syndrome [36]. The gene *RUNX1/AML1*, which is located at 21q22 and thus in the middle of the long arm of chromosome 21, may represent such a key gene.

23.2.3.2 Trisomy 8
Patients with constitutional trisomy 8 in mosaic frequently suffer from MDS or AML. In sporadic myeloid leukemia, trisomy 8 as well as trisomy 21 represent very frequent somatic karyotype deviations. It is assumed that 15 to 20% of all

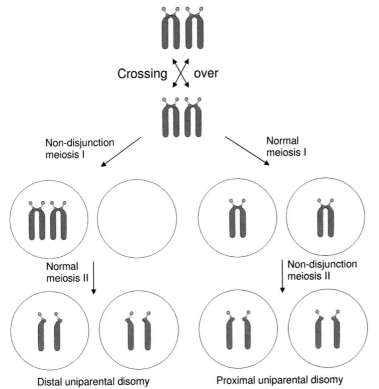

Figure 23.1 Scheme of meiosis of chromosomes 21 accomplishing one crossing over. Non-disjunction in M I results in disomy with duplication of a distal (telomeric) region, non-disjunction in M II leads to uniparental disomy for a proximal (centromeric) part of chromosome 21 (adapted from Benson and Horwitz [36]).

hematological dysplastic or neoplastic disorders with a supernumerary chromosome 8 are based on a constitutional trisomy 8 [37].

23.2.4
Hereditary Tumor Predisposition Syndromes

23.2.4.1 Li–Fraumeni Syndrome

The Li–Fraumeni syndrome (LFS) and its variant, the Li–Fraumeni-like (LFL) syndrome, are characterized by a specific spectrum of tumors (see Chapter 3 on family cancer syndromes). It includes breast cancer in juvenile age, osteosarcoma and soft tissue sarcoma, adrenocortical carcinoma, brain tumors and lung carcinomas, but also leukemias and lymphomas. About 75% of all patients with LFS show constitutional mutations of the *TP53* tumor suppressor gene (located in

17p13), whereas in families with LFL, *TP53* mutations as well as germline mutations of the *CHEK2* gene (located in 22q12) have been described [38].

23.2.4.2 Neurofibromatosis Type 1

Neurofibromatosis type 1, the presumably most frequent genetic disease with tumor predisposition, is described in this book by Wimmer, Kehrer-Sawatzki, and Legius.

23.2.4.3 Noonan Syndrome

Noonan syndrome, an autosomal dominant disorder, is characterized by short stature, distinct facial features, and heart defects. It is associated with a predisposition to a myeloproliferative disorder similar to the juvenile myelomonocytic leukemia (JMML), designated as NS/JMML, other MDS, and leukemias [39]. About 50% of all NS patients have germline mutations of the *PTPN11* gene [40, 41]. *PTPN11* encodes a tyrosine phosphatase, a positive regulator of RAS, and *PTPN11* mutations lead to an activation of the intracellular RAS signaling pathways. Most cases of NS result from one of several heterozygous gain-of-function mutations in genes of the RAS pathway, including *PTPN11, SOS1*, and *KRAS* [42, 43]. About 35% of all sporadic non-syndromal JMML patients show somatic *PTPN11* mutations [44].

An interesting observation concerns the acquisition of UPD in leukemic cells from patients with NS and constitutional mutation in one *PTPN11* allele. Loss of the wildtype allele of *PTPN11* with duplication of the mutant allele was an important "second hit", triggering the development of leukemia [45].

23.2.5
Hemochromatosis

Hereditary hemochromatosis, an autosomal recessive iron overload disease, is due to mutations of the *HFE* gene, localized in 6p21.3. *HFE* mutations have low penetrance, with a mild effect on serum iron levels. Elevated serum iron levels may increase the risk for oxidative damage to DNA, and thus may lead to an increased cancer risk. The most common mutations (variants) are *C282Y* and *H63D*. Childhood ALL has been shown to be associated with *C282Y*, with a significant gender effect in two British populations. An increase in *C282Y* mutation frequency was found in ALL patients compared to newborn controls, but in males only. The association mainly concerned heterozygosity for *C282Y* [46]. In contrast to these findings, a study from Finland did not confirm this gender-specific association [47]. Also, in Spanish patients with adult AML, the frequencies for *C282Y* and *H63D* were found to be from the same as controls [48]. A modification of susceptibility to leukemia conferred by *C282Y* by environmental and genetic factors is discussed to explain the geographically heterogeneous results [49].

H63D was found to be associated with adult acute leukemias in a study from Southern Italy [50]. The *H63D* mutation was significantly more frequent in adult ALL patients than in controls, whereas no difference was found between the incidences of this mutation in AML patients versus healthy controls [50]. However, this study shows limitations concerning a small size and imperfect matching between patient and control groups in age and sex distribution. In other examinations, *H63D* did not seem to be relevant for leukemia susceptibility [51, 52]. A significantly higher frequency of heterozygosity for the *C282Y* mutation was found in patients with refractory anemia with ringed sideroblasts compared with a matched control group, whereas the *H63D* genotype was not significantly increased [53].

It has to be mentioned that the *HFE* gene is an HLA class I-like gene and seems to be indirectly related to immune functions, since it plays a role in iron transport. Interestingly, the two missense alterations *C282Y* and *H63D* occur at a high frequency in hemochromatosis patients, but also in the normal population. The *H63D* variant has a relatively homogeneous global distribution and a frequency of 15 to 20%. *C282Y* frequency is lower and varies from 0.15% in the south to 4.7% in the north of Italy [54].

23.3
Hereditary Non-Syndromal Leukemia

23.3.1
Familial Thrombocytopenia with Leukemia Predisposition and Mutation of the *CBFA2/RUNX1/AML1* Gene

Familial platelet disorder with propensity to develop myeloid malignancy (FPD/ AML), an autosomal dominant disorder, has been described in at least 13 families to date. It is characterized by a disturbed megakaryopoiesis and thrombocytopoiesis. A consistent clinical feature is a mild to moderate bleeding tendency. FPD/ AML is induced by mutations of the *CBFA2* gene, localized in 21q22.1 [55]. *CBFA2* encodes a hematopoietic transcription factor. Most of the *CBFA2* mutations lead to haploinsuffiency, but also dominant-negative mutations have been described [56]. The incidence of MDS/AML in family members who inherited *CBFA2* mutations varies from 20 to 60% in different families, with a median of 35% [57]. In families with dominant-negative mutations, a higher incidence of leukemia has been observed compared to families with haploinsuffiency of the *CBFA2* gene [56–58].

A further gene predisposing to AML and MDS syndromes seems to be localized on 16q22 according to linkage analyses, but an involvement of the *CBFB* gene that resides in this chromosome band was excluded [59].

As secondary anomalies, monosomy 7, but also trisomies of chromosomes 8, 13, and 21 were observed [60]. In several families, anticipation occurred [61].

23.3.2
CEBPA Mutations and Familial AML

Recently, in a family with an increased incidence of AML, a constitutional mutation of the *CEBPA* gene was detected [62]. The *CEBPA* gene encodes the CCAAT/

enhancer-binding protein-alpha, a transcription factor, and is located in 19q13.1. The *CEBPA* gene plays a significant role in myeloid differentiation, and interacts with other proteins which are important for the regulation of myelopoiesis, as for example CBFA2. This second type of pure familial leukemia is characterized by a consistency of clinical and pathological phenotypes of patients [63]. As with patients with sporadic AML and *CEBPA* mutation, AML patients with constitutional *CEBPA* mutations suffer from AML of FAB subtypes M1 or M2, and clonal chromosome aberrations are rather uncommon. And they have a favorable prognosis. In spite of several relapses, the patients with familial leukemia due to *CEBPA* mutations show durable remissions [64, 65]. At present, 3 pedigrees with 10 affected members (9 males, 1 female) with germline *CEBPA* mutations have been described [63].

It has to be mentioned that *CBFA2* as well as *CEBPA* mutations also frequently occur as acquired gene defects in sporadic AML.

23.3.3
Familial Myelodysplasia of Childhood with Monosomy 7

Repeatedly, siblings with MDS and monosomy 7 have been reported, leading to the opinion that this type of MDS follows an autosomal recessive inheritance. Monosomy 7 also frequently occurs in children with MDS/juvenile myelomonocytic leukemia (JMML) and AML, within the scope of FA, SCN, Kostmann syndrome, SDS, as well as neurofibromatosis 1. About 20% of childhood MDS with monosomy 7 might be due to a genetic predisposing factor.

The so-called familial monosomy 7 that is not caused by the syndromes listed above, is in most cases associated with only myeloid leukemia; additional cerebellar ataxia does occur rarely [66, 67]. Since monosomy 7 is not a germline mutation in families with siblings with monosomy 7, a mutated (mutator) gene has been postulated which predisposes to the development of further genetic and chromosomal abnormalities [68].

23.3.4
Familial Chronic Lymphocytic Leukemia

B-cell chronic lymphocytic leukemia (CLL), the most common form of leukemia among older adults in Western countries, is characterized by the accumulation of lymphocytes in the blood, bone marrow, and lymphoid tissues. Epidemiological studies and case reports of families suggest that a subgroup of CLL is due to hereditary genetic predisposition. About 5 to 7% of all CLL cases may be based on a genetic component. However, a real predisposition gene for CLL has not yet been identified. CLL shows significant geographic variation, the highest rates occurring among whites in North America and Europe and the lowest in Asians [69].

Studies concerning the association of familial CLL with the HLA complex, as well as with the pseudoautosomal region (PAR) on X and Y chromosomes, demonstrated negative results [70, 71]. Both genes or gene complexes correlate with the familial Hodgkin's lymphoma. CLL and Hodgkin/Reed-Sternberg cells, the pathognomonic cell of Hodgkin lymphoma, have a common clonal origin, and therefore these investigations were obvious [70, 71]. Also, the analysis of the *ATM* gene in familial CLL did not reveal any association [72]; however, in a recent study [73] it could be shown that variants in the *ATM-BRCA2-CHEK2* DNA damage-response axis could be a cause of predisposition to CLL.

Approaches to elucidate the genetic background of familial CLL are linkage studies and association studies. By linkage studies, genes are localized using the co-inheritance of genetic markers and disease in families. Goldin *et al.* [74] performed a whole genome scan with 359 microsatellite markers in 18 families with CLL. One of the chromosome regions that showed increased sharing among affected relatives was the long arm of chromosome 13, which frequently exhibits deletions in patients with CLL. However, no germline mutations were found in the chromosome 13 region involved in deletions in CLL patients [75]. A single nucleotide polymorphism (SNP) genome-wide linkage scan of 206 families was performed by Sellick *et al.* [76], assembling families from the major European and American CLL consortia. A major susceptibility locus in chromosome band 2q21 that influences the risk of CLL was found. However, no significant evidence for a linkage to any of the regions of the genome, which are involved in specific chromosome aberrations (6q, 13q14, 17p, chromosome 12), was found [76]. In addition to a linkage to 2q21, evidence of a recessively acting locus for CLL in 6p22.1 and a dominantly acting locus mapping to 18q21.1 were described by Sellick *et al.* [76].

In association studies, frequencies of alleles of candidate genes are compared among cases and unrelated controls. In this way common genetic variants of modest risk can be detected. An alternative to studies of specific candidate genes represent large-scale genomic studies using SNPs of, for example, candidate cancer genes. In a large case-control study, Rudd *et al.* [73] analyzed 1467 coding non-synonymous SNPs from 865 candidate cancer genes in order to identify novel low-penetrance susceptibility alleles for CLL. As mentioned above, they found variants of genes in the *ATM-BRCA2-CHEK2* pathway to be associated with CLL.

An interesting new finding was reported by Calin *et al.* [77]. They studied the role of microRNAs in CLL. MicroRNAs (miRNAs) are involved in the regulation of different cell functions (see also the introductory Chapter 1 on tumor invasion, progression and metastasis). Calin *et al.* [77] detected that genes encoding the microRNA miR-15A and miR-16-1 located in the chromosome band 13q14, which is often deleted in CLL cells, may have somatic and germline changes in CLL patients. miR-16-1 and miR-15 seem to behave as tumor suppressors in CLL [78]. In two patients, a germline mutation in miR-16-1 was identified, accompanied by the deletion of the wildtype allele at 13q14 in their CLL cells. The combination of a loss of heterozygosity and a germline mutation corresponds to the Knudson model of inactivation of a tumor suppressor gene. Therefore, the authors discussed that these miRNA deletions and mutations may possibly predispose to additional mutations via regulatory changes involving oncogenes, and thus the deletion or mutation confers a selective advantage to B-cells [79]. However, as yet, germline mutations of miR genes were found only in two patients with CLL [77].

In several families with CLL, anticipation has been described [80]. In neurodegenerative disorders, anticipation is a consequence of an expansion of unstable trinucleotide repeat sequences. But it could be excluded that a CAG or CTG repeat amplification is the cause of anticipation in familial CLL [81].

Since, as yet, no specific mutation with a large effect–a high-penetrance gene mutation–could be identified, it is assumed that multiple genes with smaller effects–low-penetrance gene mutations or variants–cause much of the familial aggregation of CLL.

23.3.5
Genetic Susceptibility Factors for CLL and Other Leukemias

An elevated susceptibility to the development of leukemias could be produced by functionally active polymorphisms of genes involved in detoxification, DNA repair, cell cycle regulation, or apoptosis. Polymorphic genes with low penetrance implying a certain risk for tumor development are discussed as a cause for leukemias at an advanced age. Each of these predisposing alleles has a small effect, but in combination, they increase leukemia susceptibility [82].

A number of polymorphisms of candidate genes that could predispose to CLL or influence the clinical course have been evaluated. These are genes with a biological plausibility, because they are involved in apoptosis (*BAX:* [83]; *P2X7:* [84]) or xenobiotic metabolization (*GST:* [85, 86]; *N*-acetyltransferase 1 (*NAT1*) and 2 (*NAT2*): [86, 87]). Whereas Wiley *et al.* [84] initially identified an association between the *P2X7* receptor gene and risk of CLL, no association was found in follow-up studies [88]. Also for neither of the other genes mentioned above, an association with CLL was established [88].

Seedhouse *et al.* [89] demonstrated combined effects of specific genetic polymorphisms to the development of AML. Variants of the genes *RAD51* and *XRCC3* (see also Chapters 10 and 30 on lung tumors and molecular targeted therapy) coding for enzymes, which are involved in the DNA double-strand repair by homologous recombination, increase the risk for *de novo* and, more significantly for therapy-induced AML. If, in addition, a *GSTM1* deletion is present, causing the failure of an effect of this carcinogen detoxifying enzyme, the risk for AML is more increased. These data demonstrate that DNA double-strand breaks and their repair have an impact to pathogenesis of *de novo* as well as of therapy-induced AML. Also, polymorphisms of genes of mismatch repair, base excision repair, as well as of the homeobox gene *HLX1*, can influence the risk for the development of AML [90, 91].

The positive association between polymorphisms of genes involved in the protection of cells against double-strand breakage or toxic effects, and an elevated risk to develop AML, suggests the need to intensify the analysis of combined effects of genotypes that regulate specific cellular mechanisms. This could lead to new insights into the pathogenesis of sporadic leukemias, and perhaps to the discovery of their multifactorial genesis with a strong genetic component.

References

1 Kutler, D.I., Singh, B., Satagopan, J. *et al.* (2003) A 20-year perspective on the International Fanconi Anemia Registry (IFAR). *Blood,* **101,** 1249–56.

2 Alter, B.P. (2007) Diagnosis, genetics, and management of inherited bone marrow failure syndromes. *Hematology,* **2007,** 29–39.

3 Callén, E., Samper, E., Ramírez, M.J., Creus, A., Marcos, R., Ortega, J.J., Olivé, T., Badell, I., Blasco, M.A. and Surrallés, J. (2002) Breaks and telomeres and TRF2-independent end fusions in Fanconi anemia. *Human Molecular Genetics,* **11,** 439–44.

4 Tönnies, H., Huber, S., Kuhl, J.-S. *et al.* (2003) Clonal chromosome aberrations in bone marrow cells of Fanconi anemia patients: gains of the chromosomal segment 3q26q29 as an adverse risk factor. *Blood,* **101,** 3872–4.

5 Meyer, S., Fergusson, W.D., Whetton, A.D., Moreira-Leite, F., Pepper, S.D., Miller, C., Saunders, E.K., White, D.J., Will, A.M., Eden, T., Ikeda, H., Ullmann, R., Tuerkmen, S., Gerlach, A., Klopocki, E. and Tönnies, H. (2007) Amplification and translocation of 3q26 with overexpression of EVI1 in Fanconi anemia-derived childhood acute myeloid leukemia with biallelic *FANCD1/BRCA2* disruption. *Genes, Chromosomes and Cancer,* **46,** 359–72.

6 Heiss, N.S., Knight, S.W., Vulliamy, T.J. *et al.* (1998) X-linked dyskeratosis congenita is caused by mutations in a highly conserved gene with putative nucleolar functions. *Nature Genetics,* **19,** 32–8.

7 Vulliamy, T., Marrone, A., Goldman, F. *et al.* (2001) The RNA component of telomerase is mutated in autosomal dominant dyskeratosis congenita. *Nature,* **413,** 432–5.

8 Yamaguchi, H., Calado, R.T., Ly, H. *et al.* (2005) Mutations in *TERT,* the gene for telomerase reverse transcriptase, in aplastic anemia. *New England Journal of Medicine,* **352,** 1413–24.

9 Vulliamy, T. and Dokal, I. (2006) Dyskeratosis congenita. *Seminars in Hematology,* **43,** 157–66.

10 Walne, A.J., Vulliamy, T., Marrone, A. *et al.* (2007) Genetic heterogeneity in autosomal recessive dyskeratosis congenita with one subtype due to mutations in the telomerase-associated protein NOP10. *Human Molecular Genetics,* **16,** 1619–29.

11 Xin, Z.-T., Beauchamp, A.D., Calado, R.T., Bradford, J.W., Regal, J.A., Shenoy, A., Liang, Y., Lansdorp, P.M., Young, N.S. and Ly, H. (2007) Functional characterization of natural telomerase mutations found in patients with hematologic disorders. *Blood,* **109,** 524–32.

12 Dokal, I. (2006) Fanconi's anemia and related bone marrow failure syndromes. *British Medical Bulletin,* **77** and **78,** 37–53.

13 Bookcock, G.R., Morrison, J.A., Popovic, M. *et al.* (2003) Mutations in SBDS are associated with Shwachman-Diamond syndrome. *Nature Genetics,* **33,** 97–101.

14 Shimamura, A. (2006) Inherited bone marrow failure syndromes: molecular features. *Hematology,* **2006,** 63–71.

15 Rujkijyanont, P., Beyene, J., Wei, K., Khan, F. and Dror, Y. (2007) Leukemia-related gene expression in bone marrow cells from patients with the preleukemic disorder Shwachman-Diamond syndrome. *British Journal of Haematology,* **137,** 537–44.

16 Dror, Y. and Freedman, M.H. (1999) Shwachman-Diamond Syndrome: An inherited preleukemic bone marrow failure disorder with aberrant hematopoietic progenitors and faulty marrow microenvironment. *Blood,* **94,** 3048–54.

17 Göhring, G., Karow, A., Steinemann, D., Wilkens, L., Lichter, P., Zeidler, C., Niemeyer, C., Welte, K. and Schlegel-berger, B. (2007) Chromosomal aberrations in congenital bone marrow failure disorders – an early indicator of leukemogenesis? *Annals of Hematology*, **86**, 733–9.

18 Maserati, E., Minelli, A., Pressato, B., Valli, R., Crescenzi, B., Stefanelli, M., Menna, G., Sainati, L., Poli, F., Panarello, C., Zecca, M., Curto, F.L., Mecucci, C., Danesino, C. and Pasquali, F. (2006) Shwachman syndrome as mutator phenotype responsible for myeloid dysplasia/neoplasia through karyotype instability and chromosomes 7 and 20 anomalies. *Genes, Chromosomes and Cancer*, **45**, 375–82.

19 Klein, C., Grudzien, M., Appaswamy, G., Germeshausen, M., Sandrock, I., Schaffer, A.A. *et al.* (2007) HAX1 deficiency causes autosomal recessive severe congenital neutropenia (Kostmann disease). *Nature Genetics*, **39**, 86–92.

20 Carlsson, G., Melin, M., Dahl, N., Ramme, K.G., Nordenskjöld, M., Palmblad, J., Henter, J.I. and Fadeel, B. (2007) Kostmann syndrome or infantile genetic agranulocytosis, part two: understanding the underlying genetic defects in severe congenital neutropenia. *Acta Paediatrica*, **96**, 813–19.

21 Horwitz, M., Benson, K.F., Person, R.E., Aprikyan, A.G. and Dale, D.C. (1999) Mutations in ELA2, encoding neutrophil elastase, define a 21-day biological clock in cyclic haematopoiesis. *Nature Genetics*, **23**, 433–6.

22 Stein, R.A. (2007) Insights into the genetics of severe congenital neutropenia. *Clinical Genetics*, **72**, 308–10.

23 Kaushansky, K. (2006) Lineage-specific hematopoietic growth factors. *New England Journal of Medicine*, **354**, 2034–45.

24 Rosenberg, P.S., Alter, B.P., Bolyard, A.A., Bonilla, M.A., Boxer, L.A., Cham, B. *et al.* (2006) The incidence of leukemia and mortality from sepsis in patients with severe congenital neutropenia receiving long-term G-CSF therapy. *Blood*, **107**, 4628–35.

25 Dong, F., Brynes, R.K., Tidow, N., Welte, K., Lowenberg, B. and Touw, I.P. (1995) Mutations in the gene for the granulocyte colony-stimulating-factor receptor in patients with acute myeloid leukemia preceded by severe congenital neutropenia [see comments]. *New England Journal of Medicine*, **333**, 487–93.

26 Link, D.C., Kunter, G., Kasai, Y., Zhao, Y., Miner, T., McLellan, M.D., Ries, R.E., Kapur, D., Nagarajan, R., Dale, D.C., Bolyard, A.A., Boxer, L.A., Welte, K., Zeidler, C., Donadieu, J., Bellané-Chantelot, C., Vardiman, J.W., Caligiuri, M.A., Bloomfield, C.D., DiPersio, J.F., Tomasson, M.H., Graubert, T.A., Westervelt, P., Watson, M., Shannon, W., Baty, J., Mardis, E.R., Wilson, R.K. and Ley, T.J. (2007) Distinct patterns of mutations occurring in *de novo* AML versus AML arising in the setting of severe congenital neutropenia. *Blood*, **110**, 1648–55.

27 Freedman, M.H., Bonilla, M.A., Fier, C. *et al.* (2000) Myelodysplasia syndrome and acute myeloid leukemia in patients with congenital neutropenia receiving G-CSF therapy. *Blood*, **96**, 429–36.

28 Kalra, R., Dale, D., Freedman, M. *et al.* (1995) Monosomy 7 and activating RAS mutations accompany malignant trans-formation in patients with congenital neutropenia. *Blood*, **86**, 4579–86.

29 Gazda, H., Lipton, J.M., Willig, T.N., Ball, S., Niemeyer, C.M., Tchernia, G., Mohandas, N., Daly, M.J., Ploszynska, A., Orfali, K.A., Vlachos, A., Glader, B.E., Rokicka-Milewska, R., Ohara, A., Baker, D., Pospisilova, D., Webber, A., Viskochil, D.H., Nathan, D.G., Beggs, A.H. and Sieff, C.A. (2001) Evidence for linkage of familial Diamond-Blackfan anemia to chromosome 8p23.3-p22 and for non-19q non-8p disease. *Blood*, **97**, 2145–50.

30 Gregory, L.A., Aquissa-Touré, A.H., Pinaud, N., Legrand, P., Gleizes, P.E. and Fribourg, S. (2007) Molecular basis of Diamond-Blackfan anemia: structure and function analysis of RPS19. *Nucleic Acids Research*, **35**, 5913–21.

31 Flygare, J., Aspesi, A., Bailey, J.C., Miyake, K., Caffrey, J.M., Karlsson, S. and Ellis, S.R. (2007) Human *RPS19*, the gene mutated in Diamond-Blackfan anemia, encodes a ribosomal protein required for the maturation of 40S ribosomal subunits. *Blood*, **109**, 980–6.

32 Cario, H., Bode, H., Gustavsson, P., Dahl, N. and Kohne, E. (1999) A microdeletion syndrome due to a 3-Mb deletion on 19q13.2–Diamond-Blackfan anemia associated with macrocephaly, hypotonia, and psychomotor retardation. *Clinical Genetics*, **55**, 487–92.

33 Stiller, C.A. (2004) Epidemiology and genetics of childhood cancer. *Oncogene*, **23**, 6429–44.

34 Holmes, D.K., Bates, N., Murray, M., Ladusans, E.J., Morabito, A., Bolton-Maggs, P.H.B., Johnston, T.A., Walkenshaw, S., Wynn, R.F. and Bellantuono, I. (2006) Hematopoietic progenitor cell deficiency in fetuses and children affected by Down's syndrome. *Experimental Hematology*, **34**, 1611–15.

35 Iselius, L., Jacobs, P. and Morton, N. (1990) Leukemia and transient leukemia in Down's syndrome. *Human Genetics*, **85**, 477–85.

36 Benson, K.F. and Horwitz, M. (2006) Familial leukemia. *Best Practice and Research Clinical Haematology*, **19**, 269–79.

37 Maserati, E., Aprili, F., Vinante, F., Locatelli, F., Amendola, G., Zatterale, A., Milone, G., Minello, A., Bernardi, F., Lo Curto, F. and Pasquali, F. (2002) Trisomy 8 in myelodysplasia and acute leukemia is constitutional in 15–20% of cases. *Genes, Chromosomes and Cancer*, **33**, 93–7.

38 Siebert, R. (2003) Familiäre lymphatische und myeloische Neoplasien, in *Molekularmedizinische Grundlagen von hämatologischen Neoplasien* (ed. Ganten/ Ruckpaul), Springer, Berlin, Heidelberg, pp. 65–86.

39 Gelb, B.D. and Tartaglia, M. (2006) Noonan syndrome and related disorders: dysregulated RAS-mitogen activated protein kinase signal transduction. *Human Molecular Genetics*, **15** (Spec No. 2), R220–6.

40 Tartaglia, M., Mehler, E.L., Goldberg, R., Zampino, G., Brunner, H.G., Kremer, H., van der Burgt, I., Crosby, A.H., Ion, A., Jeffery, S., Kalidas, K., Patton, M.A.,

Kucherlapati, R.S. and Gelb, B.D. (2001) Mutations in *PTPN11*, encoding the protein tyrosine phosphatase SHP-2, cause Noonan syndrome. *Nature Genetics*, **29**, 465–8.

41 Van der Burgt, I. (2007) Noonan syndrome. *Orphanet Journal of Rare Diseases*, **2**, 4.

42 Kratz, C.P., Niemeyer, C.M. and Zenker, M. (2007) An unexpected new role of mutant Ras: perturbation of human embryonic development. *Journal of Molecular Medicine*, **85**, 223–31.

43 Roberts, A.E., Araki, T., Swanson, K.D., Montgomery, K.T., Schiripo, T.A., Joshi, V. A., Li, L., Yassin, Y., Tamburino, A.M., Neel, B.G. and Kucherlapati, R.S. (2007) Germline gain-of-function mutations in *SOS1* cause Noonan syndrome. *Nature Genetics*, **39**, 70–4.

44 Tartaglia, M., Niemeyer, C.M., Fragale, A., Song, X., Buechner, J., Jung, A., Hahnlen, K., Hasle, H., Licht, J.D. and Gelb, B.D. (2003) Somatic mutations in *PTPN11* in juvenile myelomonocytic leukemia, myelodysplastic syndromes and acute myeloid leukemia. *Nature Genetics*, **34**, 148–50.

45 Karow, A., Steinemann, D., Göhring, G., Hasle, H., Greiner, J., Harila-Saari, A., Flotho, C., Zenker, M., Schlegelberger, B., Niemeyer, C.M. and Kratz, C.P. (2007) Clonal duplication of a germline *PTPN11* mutation due to acquired uniparental disomy in acute lymphoblastic leukemia blasts from a patient with Noonan syndrome. *Leukemia*, **21**, 1303–5.

46 Dorak, M.T., Sproul, A.M., Gibson, B.E., Burnett, A.K. and Worwood, M. (1999) The *C282Y* mutation of HFE is another male-specific risk factor for childhood ALL [letter]. *Blood*, **94**, 3957–8.

47 Hannuksela, J., Savolainen, E.R., Koistinen, P. and Parkkila, S. (2002) Prevalence of *HFE* genotypes, *C282Y* and *H63D* in patients with hematologic disorders. *Haematologica*, **87**, 131–5.

48 Gimferrer, E., Nomdedeu, J., Gich, I., Barceló, M.J. and Baiget, M. (1999) Prevalence of hemochromatosis related *HFE* gene mutations in patients with acute myeloid leukemia. *Leukemia Research*, **23**, 597–8.

49 Dorak, M.T., Burnett, A.K. and Worwood, M. (2005) *HFE* gene mutations in

susceptibility to childhood leukemia: HuGE review. *Genetics in Medicine*, **7**, 159–68.

50 Viola, A., Pagano, L., Laudati, D., D'Elia, R., D'Amico, M.R., Ammirabile, M., Palmieri, S., Prossomariti, L. and Ferrara, F. (2006) *HFE* gene mutations in patients with acute leukemia. *Leukemia and Lymphoma*, **47**, 2331–4.

51 Dorak, M.T., Burnett, A.K. and Worwood, M. (2002) Hemochromatosis gene in leukemia and lymphoma. *Leukemia and Lymphoma*, **43**, 467–77.

52 Dorak, M.T. (2006) *HFE H63D* variant and leukemia susceptibility. *Leukemia and Lymphoma*, **47**, 2269–70.

53 Nearman, Z.P., Szpurka, H., Serio, B., Warshawsky, I., Theil, K., Lichtin, A., Sekeres, M.A. and Maciejewski, J.P. (2007) Hemochromatosis-associated gene mutations in patients with myelodysplastic syndromes with refractory anemia with ringed sideroblasts. *American Journal of Hematology*, **82**, 1076–9.

54 De Gobbi, M., D'Antico, S., Castagno, F., Testa, D., Merlini, R., Bondi, A. and Camaschella, C. (2004) Screening selected blood donors with biochemical iron overload for hemochromatosis: a regional experience. *Haematologica*, **89**, 1161–7.

55 Song, W.J., Sullivan, M.G., Legare, R.D., Hutchings, S., Tan, X., Kufrin, D., Ratajczak, J., Resende, I.C., Haworth, C., Hock, R., Loh, M., Felix, C., Roy, D.C., Busque, L., Kurnit, D., Willman, C., Gewirtz, A.M., Speck, N.A., Bushweller, J.H., Li, F.P., Gardiner, K., Poncz, M., Maris, J.M. and Gilliland, D.G. (1999) Haploinsufficency of *CBFA2* causes familial thrombocytopenia with propensity to develop acute myelogenous leukemia. *Nature Genetics*, **23**, 166–75.

56 Michaud, J., Osato, M., Cottles, G.M., Yanagida, M., Asou, N., Shigesada, K., Ito, Y., Benson, K.F., Raskind, W.H., Rossier, C., Antonarakis, S.E., Israels, S., McNicol, A., Weiss, H., Horwitz, M. and Scott, H.S. (2002) *In vitro* analyses of known and novel *RUNX1/AML1* mutations in dominant familial platelet disorder with predisposition to acute myelogenous leukaemia: implications for

mechanisms of pathogenesis. *Blood*, **99**, 1364–72.

57 Ganly, P., Walter, L.C. and Morris, C.M. (2004) Familial mutations of the transcription factor RUNX1 (AML1, CBFA2) predispose to acute myeloid leukaemia. *Leukaemia & Lymphoma*, **45**, 1–10.

58 Matheny, C.J., Speck, M.E., Cushing, P.R., Zhou, Y., Corpora, T., Regan, M., Newman, M., Roudaia, L., Speck, C.L., Gu, T.L., Griffey, S.M., Bushweller, J.H. and Speck, N.A. (2007) Disease mutations in RUNX1 and RUNX2 create nonfunctional, dominant-negative, or hypomorphic alleles. *EMBO Journal*, **26**, 1163–75.

59 Escher, R., Hagos, F., Michaud, J., Sveen, L., Horwitz, M., Olopade, O.I. *et al.* (2004) No evidence for core-binding factor CBFbeta as a leukemia predisposing factor in chromosome 16q22-linked familial AML. *Leukemia*, **18**, 881.

60 Osato, M. (2004) Point mutations in the RUNX1/AML1 gene: another actor in RUNX leukemia. *Oncogene*, **23**, 4284–96.

61 De Lord, C., Powles, R., Mehta, J., Wilson, K., Treleaven, J., Meller, S. and Catovsky, D. (1998) Familial acute myeloid leukaemia: four male members of a single family over three consecutive generations exhibiting anticipation. *British Journal of Haematology*, **100**, 557–60.

62 Smith, M.L., Cavenagh, J.D., Lister, T.A. and Fitzgibbon, J. (2004) Mutation of *CEBPA* in familial acute myeloid leukemia. *New England Journal of Medicine*, **351**, 2403–7.

63 Owen, C., Barnett, M. and Fitzgibbon, J. (2008) Familial myelodysplasia and acute myeloid leukaemia–a review. *British Journal of Haematology*, **140**, 123–32.

64 Sellick, G.S., Spendlove, H.E., Catovsky, D., Pritchard-Jones, K. and Houlston, R.S. (2005) Further evidence that germline CEBPA mutations cause dominant inheritance of acute myeloid leukemia. *Leukemia*, **19**, 1276–8.

65 Nanri, T., Uike, N., Kawakita, T., Iwanage, E., Hoshino, K., Mitsuya, H. and Asou, N. (2006) A pedigree harboring a germ-line N-terminal C/EBPBa mutation and development of acute myeloblastic leukemia with a somatic C-terminal

C/EBPa mutation [abstract]. *Blood*, **108**, 1916a.

66 Luna-Fineman, S., Shannon, K.M. and Lange, B.J. (1995) Childhood monosomy 7: Epidemiology, biology, and mechanistic implications. *Blood*, **85**, 1985–99.

67 Hasle, H., Arico, M., Basso, G., Biondi, A., Cantu Rajnoldi, A., Creutzig, U., Fenu, S., Fonatsch, C., Haas, O.A., Harbott, J., Kardos, G., Kerndrup, G., Mann, G., Niemeyer, C.M., Ptoszkova, H., Ritter, J., Slater, J., Stary, J., Stollmann-Gibbels, B., Testi, A.M., Van Wering, E.R. and Zimmermann, M. (1999) Myelodysplastic syndrome, juvenile myelomonocytic leukemia, and acute myeloid leukemia associated with complete or partial monosomy 7. European Working Group on MDS in Childhood (EWOG-MDS). *Leukemia*, **13**, 376–85.

68 Minelli, A., Maserati, E., Rossi, G., Bernardo, M.E., De Stefano, P., Cecchini, M.P., Valli, R., Albano, V., Pierani, P., Leszl, A., Sainati, L., Lo Curto, F., Danesino, C., Locatelli, F. and Pasquali, F. (2004) Familial platelet disorder with propensity to acute myelogenous leukemia: genetic heterogeneity and progression to leukemia via acquisition of clonal chromosome anomalies. *Genes, Chromosomes and Cancer*, **40**, 165–71.

69 Linet, M.S., Devesa, S.S. and Morgan, G.J. (2006) The leukemias, in *Cancer Epidemiology and Prevention*, 3rd edn (eds D. Schottenfeld and J.F. Fraumeni Jr), Oxford University Press, New York, pp. 841–71.

70 Bevan, S., Catovsky, D., Matutes, E., Antunovic, P., Auger, M.J., Ben-Bassat, I., Bell, A., Berrebi, A., Gaminara, E.J., Junior, M.E., Mauro, F.R., Quabeck, K., Rassam, S.M.B., Reid, C., Ribeiro, I., Stark, P., van Dongen, J.J.M., Wimperis, J., Wright, S., Marossy, A., Yuille, M.R. and Houlston, R.S. (2000) Linkage analysis for major histocompatibility complex-related genetic susceptibility in familial chronic lymphocytic leukaemia. *Blood*, **96**, 3982–4.

71 Houlston, R.S., Catovksy, D. and Yuille, M.R. (2000) Pseudoautosomal linkage in chronic lymphocytic leukaemia. *British Journal of Haematology*, **109**, 895–905.

72 Yuille, M., Condie, A., Hudson, C.D., Bradshaw, P.S., Stone, E.M., Matutes, E., Catovsky, D. and Houlston, R.S. (2002) ATM mutations are rare in familial chronic lymphocytic leukemia. *Blood*, **100**, 603–9.

73 Rudd, M.F., Sellick, G.S., Webb, E.L., Catovsky, D. and Houlston, R.S. (2006) Variants in the *ATM-BRCA2-CHEK2* axis predispose to chronic lymphocytic leukemia. *Blood*, **108**, 638–44.

74 Goldin, L.R., Ishibe, N., Sgambati, M., Marti, G.E., Fontaine, L., Lee, M.P., Kelley, J.M., Scherpbier, T., Buetow, K.H. and Caporaso, N.E. (2003) A genome scan of 18 families with chronic lymphocytic leukemia. *British Journal of Haematology*, **121**, 866–73.

75 Ng, D., Toure, O., Wei, M.H., Arthur, D.C., Abbasi, F., Fontaine, L., Marti, G.E., Fraumeni, J.F., Goldin, L.R., Caporaso, N. and Toro, J.R. (2007) Identification of a novel chromosome region, 13q21.33-q22.2, for susceptibility genes in familial chronic lymphocytic leukemia. *Blood*, **109**, 916–25.

76 Sellick, G.S., Goldin, L.R., Wild, R.W., Slager, S.L., Ressenti, L., Strom, S.S., Dyer, M.J.S., Mauro, F.R., Marti, G.E., Fuller, S., Lyttelton, M., Kipps, T.J., Keating, M.J., Call, T.G., Catovsky, D., Caporaso, N. and Houlston, R.S. (2007) A high-density SNP genome-wide linkage search of 206 families identifies susceptibility loci for chronic lymphocytic leukemia. *Blood*, **110**, 3326–33.

77 Calin, G.A., Ferracin, M., Cimmino, A., Di Leva, G., Shimizu, M., Wojcik, S.E., Iorio, M.V., Visone, R., Sever NI Fabbri, M., Iuliano, R., Palumbo, T., Pichiorri, F., Roldo, C., Garzon, R., Sevignani, C., Rassenti, L., Alder, H., Volinia, S., Liu, C.G., Kipps, T.J., Negrini, M. and Croce, C.M. (2005) A microRNA signature associated with prognosis and progression in chronic lymphocytic leukemia. *New England Journal of Medicine*, **353**, 1793–801.

78 Calin, G.A., Dumitru, C.D., Shimizu, M. *et al.* (2002) Frequent deletions and down-regulation of micro-RNA genes *miR15* and *miR16* at 13q14 in chronic lymphocytic

leukemia. *Proceedings of the National Academy of Sciences of the United States of America*, **99**, 15524–9.

79 Caporaso, N., Goldin, L., Plass, C., Calin, G., Marti, G., Bauer, S., Raveche, E., McMaster, M.L., Ng, D., Landgren, O. and Slager, S. (2007) Chronic lymphocytic leukemia genetics overview. *British Journal of Haematology*, **139**, 630–4.

80 Caporaso, N., Marti, G.E. and Goldin, L. (2004) Perspectives on familial chronic lymphocytic leukemia: genes and the environment. *Seminars in Hematology*, **41**, 201–6.

81 Auer, R.L., Dighiero, G., Goldin, L.R., Syndercombe-Court, D., Jones, C., McElwaine, S., Newland, A.C., Fegan, C.D., Caporaso, N. and Cotter, F.E. (2006) Trinucleotide repeat dynamic mutation identifying susceptibility in familial and sporadic chronic lymphocytic leukemia. *British Journal of Haematology*, **136**, 73–9.

82 Houlston, R.S., Sellick, G., Yuille, M., Matutes, E. and Catovsky, D. (2003) Causation of chronic lymphocytic leukaemia – insights from familial disease. *Leukemia Research*, **27**, 871–6.

83 Saxena, A., Moshynska, O., Sankaran, K., Viswanathan, S. and Sheridan, D.R. (2002) Association of a novel single nucleotide polymorphism, *G(-248)A*, in the 5′-UTR of *BAX* gene in chronic lymphocytic leukemia with disease progression and treatment resistance. *Cancer Letter*, **187**, 199–205.

84 Wiley, J.S., Dao-Ung, L.P. and Gu, B.J. (2002) A loss-of-function polymorphic mutation in the cytolytic *P2X7* receptor gene and chronic lymphocytic leukaemia: a molecular study. *Lancet*, **359**, 1114–19.

85 Yuille, M., Condie, A., Hudson, C., Kote-Jarai, Z., Stone, E., Eeles, R., Matutes, E., Catovsky, D. and Houlston,

R. (2002) Relationship between glutathione S-transferase M1, T1, and P1 polymorphisms and chronic lymphocytic leukemia. *Blood*, **99**, 4216–18.

86 Chiu, B.C., Kolar, C., Gapstur, S.M., Lawson, T., Anderson, J.R. and Weisenburger, D.D. (2005) Association of NAT and GST polymorphisms with non-Hodgkin's lymphoma: a population-based case-control study. *British Journal of Haematology*, **128**, 610–15.

87 Morton, L.M., Schenk, M., Hein, D.W., Davis, S., Zahm, S.H., Cozen, W., Cerhan, J.R., Hartge, P., Welch, R., Chanock, S.J., Rothman, N. and Wang, S.S. (2006) Genetic variation in *N*-acetyltransferase 1 (NAT1) and 2 (NAT2) and risk of non-Hodgkin lymphoma. *Pharmacogenetics and Genomis*, **16**, 537–45.

88 Slager, S.L., Kay, N.E., Fredericksen, Z.S., Wang, A.H., Liebow, M., Cunningham, J. M., Vachon, C.M., Call, T.G. and Cerhan, J.R. (2007) Susceptibility genes and B-chronic lymphocytic leukemia. *British Journal of Haematology*, **139**, 762–71.

89 Seedhouse, C., Faulkner, R., Ashraf, N., Das-Gupta, E. and Russell, N. (2004) Polymorphisms in genes involved in homologous recombination repair interact to increase the risk of developing acute myeloid leukemia. *Clinical Cancer Research*, **10**, 2675–80.

90 Seedhouse, C., Bainton, R., Lewis, M., Harding, A., Russell, N. and Das-Gupta, E. (2002) The genotype distribution of the *XRCC1* gene indicates a role for base excision repair in the development of therapy-related acute myeloblastic leukemia. *Blood*, **100**, 3761–6.

91 Jawad, M., Seedhouse, C., Russell, N. and Plumb, M. (2006) Polymorphisms in human homeobox *HLX1* and DNA repair *RAD51* genes increase the risk of therapy-related acute myeloid leukemia. *Blood*, **108**, 3916–18.

24

Malignant Melanoma

Carola Berking and Anja Katrin Bosserhoff

Summary

Familial melanoma represents approximately 10% of all melanomas. In patients with hereditary melanoma, the onset of the disease is at a young age (below 40), and the incidence of multiple melanomas is relatively high (30%). The most commonly mutated gene in familial melanoma is the *cdkn2a* gene (germline mutations in 30–50%), which encodes for two different proteins, P16^{INK4a} and P14^{ARF}, and is a key regulator of the cell cycle. Another high penetrance gene identified in melanoma is *cdk4*, which is involved in cell cycle progression. However, *cdk4* germline mutations are rare and play a minor role in hereditary melanoma.

Some low penetrance genes have been described in melanoma, including DNA repair genes such as *ercc1* or *xrcc3*, and pigmentation genes such as *mc1r*. While specific variants of the *mc1r* gene have been associated with an increased risk for melanoma, conflicting data exist on other potential low penetrance genes regarding their role in the susceptibility to melanoma. Genetic testing of familial melanoma patients is generally not recommended.

24.1
Introduction

24.1.1
Epidemiology

Cutaneous melanoma arises from the malignant transformation of melanocytes, the pigment-producing cells in the skin. The incidence and mortality rates have increased dramatically during the past decades among Caucasian populations. The current incidence rates of melanoma vary substantially throughout the world, ranging from 0.4 per 100 000 in Japan and 40 per 100 000 in Australia [1]. In the

A list of abbreviations is provided at the end of this chapter.

Hereditary Tumors: From Genes to Clinical Consequences
Edited by Heike Allgayer, Helga Rehder and Simone Fulda
Copyright © 2009 WILEY-VCH Verlag GmbH & Co. KGaA, Weinheim
ISBN: 978-3-527-32028-8

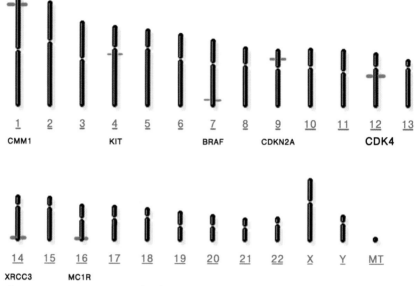

Figure 24.1 Genetic mapping of melanoma susceptibility genes.

United States, the incidence is between 9 (for females) and 13 (for males) per 100 000, with a current estimated life-time risk of approximately 1 in 68. Mortality rates are more than five-fold lower than incidence rates, but they also have increased.

The proportion of genetically conditioned familial melanoma is approximately 6 to 14%. Familial melanoma is usually defined as a cluster of two (some define three) or more first-degree relatives with melanoma. In these patients, the onset of melanoma is at a young age (median 36 vs. 57 years in males and 29 vs. 59 years in females), with 10% diagnosed before the age of 20 (sporadic: 2%). The rate of multiple primary melanomas is high with 30% versus 4% in sporadic melanoma, and the majority of patients have dysplastic nevi. Several studies aimed at determining the "melanoma susceptibility gene" affected in these patients, associated with the hope to find general mechanisms of sporadic melanoma development.

During the past years, linkage analysis, segregation analysis, and comparative genomic hybridization (CGH) were used to map the changes associated with hereditary melanoma (Figure 24.1). Here, we summarize the state-of-the-art knowledge on genomic regions and genes involved in hereditary melanoma with high penetrance or low penetrance [2].

24.1.1.1 High Penetrance Genes

cdkn2a (9p21) "Familial Atypical Multiple Mole Melanoma" (FAMMM) Syndrome
Among all known tumor suppressor genes involved in melanoma development, the *cdkn2a* (cyclin-dependent kinase inhibitor 2A) gene is probably the most

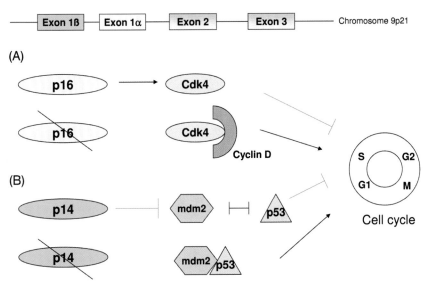

Figure 24.2 Composition and transcripts of the *cdkn2a* gene. Depending on alternative splicing, transcript P16^INK4A (Exon 1α, 2, and 3) binds and inhibits CDK4. If P16^INK4A is inactivated, CDK4 can form a complex with cyclin D, this leading to phosphorylation of the RB protein. This results in a release of transcription factors required for the transition from G1 to S phase, that is, cell cycle progression and growth (A). The alternative transcript P14^ARF (Exon 1β, 2, and 3) stabilizes P53 by preventing MDM2-induced P53 degradation. If P14^ARF is inactivated, MDM2 binds to P53 and promotes P53 ubiquitination. This prevents cells from undergoing apoptosis and facilitates cell cycle progression (B).

important. *Cdkn2a*, also known under the names *mts1*, *cmm2*, *cdk4i*, *ink4a/arf*, *tp16*, and *p16* gene, is unique among human genes, because it encodes two different proteins, P16^INK4a and P14^ARF [3, 4]. They are translated in different reading frames from two alternatively spliced transcripts (ARF stands for alternative reading frame). *Cdkn2a* is located on the short arm of chromosome 9 (9p21 region), and is composed of four exons: 1 α, 1 β, 2, and 3. The P16 transcript contains exon 1α, exon 2, and exon 3, while the P14 transcript consists of exon 1β, exon 2, and exon 3 (Figure 24.2).

Approximately half of all melanoma families show a linkage to chromosome 9p21-22. It is assumed that 30 to 50% of hereditary melanomas develop due to germline mutations in the *cdkn2a* gene. It has been shown that the number of affected individuals within a melanoma family correlates with the probability of germ line *cdkn2a* mutations within the family [5]. Carriers of these mutations also exhibit an increased risk for pancreatic carcinoma. The *cdkn2a* gene is an important negative regulator of the cell cycle. The transcript P16 binds and inhibits cyclin-dependent kinases CDK4 and CDK6, which in turn prevents complex formation of CDK4 with cyclin D1 (Figure 24.2). This complex normally phosphorylates and inactivates the retinoblastoma (RB) protein resulting in the transition from the G1 to S phase, that is, activation of cell division. Thus, P16 inhibits cell division at the G1/S restriction point in the cell cycle by inhibiting the kinase activity of CDK4, by inhibiting the CDK-activating kinase (CAK)-dependent phosphorylation of CDK4, and by inhibiting the assembly of the cyclin D/CDK4 complex. A more recently discovered additional function of P16 is the delay at the G2/M cell cycle checkpoint by accumulation of P16 in melanocytic cells exposed to ultraviolet radiation (UVR), probably in order to enable the repair of UVR-induced DNA damage [6]. Thus, if P16 is not present in a functional form or only available in very small concentrations, an essential control mechanism of cell division and cell cycle delay is missing, whereby a cell can acquire UVR-induced genetic defects, and transform into a tumor cell.

The transcript P14^{ARF} (P19^{ARF} in the mouse) can affect the P53/MDM2 pathway, although its exact function is not clear and may differ between mouse and man. It has been shown that, upon activation by hyperproliferative stimuli (e.g. RAS, MYC), P14^{ARF} can interact with MDM2 leading to stabilization of P53 by preventing MDM2 to inhibit P53 [7]. Thus, P14^{ARF} can induce cell cycle arrest in G1/S and G2/M phases. In this way, P14^{ARF} may support apoptosis or growth arrest of cancer cells. In addition, P14^{ARF} can inhibit cell growth independent of P53 and can interact with RB as well as possibly further unknown proteins. Ries *et al.* showed that hyper-proliferation and malignant transformation mediated by RAS only occur in cells lacking P19^{ARF} [8]. Therefore, P19^{ARF} seems to play a role as a tumor suppressor, hindering the effect of RAS-mediated growth factor signaling. Genetic analyses of two families, in which coincidence of cutaneous melanoma and glial tumors was observed, showed linkage to 9p21; however, without germline mutations in *p16*. These results suggest a role for P19^{ARF} in melanoma pathogenesis, which is also supported by the discovery of mutations in exon 1β [9].

Although these data indicate a tumor suppressive function of P14^{ARF}, several other studies could not yet demonstrate a decisive role of this protein in melanoma predisposition, as well as in sporadic melanoma development and progression.

cdk4 **(12q13)** Cyclin-dependent kinase 4 (cdk4) is the second highly penetrant susceptibility gene identified in melanoma. It is involved in cell cycle progression and inhibited by P16 protein. It has been shown that a point mutation in the *cdk4* gene with an arginine-to-cysteine substitution at codon 24 (R24C) encodes a mutated CDK4 protein, which corresponds to a tumor-specific antigen recognized by cytolytic T lymphocytes. The *R24C* mutation functionally disrupts the binding of P16 to CDK4, thereby disabling CDK4-inhibitory activities of P16.

Germline R24C mutations in the *cdk4* gene have been described in few melanoma families. This mutation is rarely found and seems to be relevant only for a very small subgroup of hereditary melanoma [10].

cmm1 **(1p36) "Dysplastic Nevus Syndrome"** Locus *cmm1* on chromosome 1p36 was the first melanoma susceptibility gene to be discovered [11]. Since then, no candidate gene has been identified from this chromosomal region. In addition, other groups could not confirm the locus [12, 13]. This discrepancy in the findings may be explained by the selection of subgroups analyzed. The first cohort consisted of patients with multiple dysplastic nevi, whereas in the other groups patients were included with melanoma only, or with dysplastic nevi without the history of melanoma. It can be speculated that different loci are affected in these kindred.

As more than 50% of melanoma-prone families do not show mutations in the three high penetrance genes, additional mutations, for example, in intronic, promoter, or enhancer regions, are expected. Furthermore, additional loci for high penetrance genes could be determined in the future such as the potential gene on 1p36.

24.1.1.2 Low Penetrance Genes

Xeroderma Pigmentosum (XP) Xeroderma pigmentosum (XP) is a rare, autosomal recessive and chronically progressive skin disease. In the literature, XP is summarized under the generic term of secondary photodermatosis. Photodermatoses are characterized by pathological changes of the skin due to the influence of visible light or UVR. The pathogenesis of XP is based upon defects in the repair of DNA damage. Genes of DNA repair enzymes are affected by mutations, for example, in *ercc1*, an enzyme participating in the so-called nucleotide excision repair. The damage of UVR-induced chromosomal DNA cannot be compensated in XP patients, leading to an increased photosensitivity with substantial skin damage, as well as the development of skin cancer including melanoma. Kraemer *et al.* reported that malignant skin neoplasms were present in 70% of XP patients at a median age of 8 years, which is approximately 50 years earlier than in the average white population in the United States [14]. Melanoma arises in 22% of the XP patients, who are at a 1000-fold increased risk to develop melanoma at an age younger than 20 years. Lynch *et al.* suggested that complementation group C XP patients may be particularly prone to melanoma [15].

***xrcc3* (14q32)** Winsey *et al.* revealed an association between polymorphisms in DNA repair genes and the development of melanoma [16]. The presence of a T allele at position 18067 in exon 7 of the *xrcc3* gene was significantly associated with melanoma development. However, follow-up studies excluded *xrcc3* from being associated with melanoma [17, 18].

***mc1r* (16q24)** The melanocortin 1 receptor gene *mc1r* codes for a seven-pass transmembrane receptor implicated in pigmentation. It is activated by ligands such as melanocyte-stimulating hormone (MSH; melanotropin), adrenocorticotropic hormone (ACTH), and by signals via heterotrimeric guanine nucleotide-binding proteins (G proteins) to activate adenylate cyclase. *Mc1r* belongs to the group of low penetrance genes. Valverde *et al.* reported that certain variants of the *mc1r* gene were more common in individuals with melanoma than in control subjects and that this association was greater than the association between melanoma and the skin type [19]. *Mc1r* variants in the second and seventh transmembrane domains were more common in melanoma cases than controls with a relative risk of 3.91 for carriers of variant alleles compared to normal homozygotes. In addition, it was noted that a particular allele, asp84 to glu (D84E), was present in 23% of the melanoma subjects, while it was absent in controls. The D84E allele accounted for most of the association with melanoma. The aspartate at codon 84 is highly conserved throughout the melanocortin receptor family, as well as in other G protein-coupled receptors. However, the functional significance of this mutation in the development of melanoma remains unclear.

Palmer *et al.* studied the relationship between melanoma risk and *mc1r* polymorphisms [20]. They reported the occurrence of 5 common *mc1r* variants in an Australian population-based sample of 460 individuals with familial and sporadic cutaneous malignant melanoma (CMM), and of 399 control individuals. *Mc1r* variants were found in 72% of patients with CMM, whereas only 56% of the control individuals carried at least one variant (P < 0.01). This finding was independent of the strength of family history of melanoma. Three "active" alleles previously associated with red hair (R151C, R160W, and D294H) doubled CMM risk for each additional allele carried. No such independent association could be demonstrated with the V60L and D84E variants. They concluded that the effect of *mc1r* variant alleles on CMM is partly mediated by the determination of the pigmentation phenotype. Comparison of melanoma patients without concomitant chronically sun-damaged skin with 171 healthy controls showed that the overall melanoma risk was higher by a factor of 3.3 in individuals with any *mc1r* variant allele as compared to individuals with no variant alleles, and that the risk increased with the number of variant *mc1r* alleles.

Interestingly, variation of the *mc1r* modulates the risk based on other melanoma susceptibility genes. A *cdkn2a* mutation in the presence of a homozygous consensus *mc1r* genotype had a raw penetrance of 50% with a mean age at onset of 58.1 years. Box *et al.* could show that the presence of one *mc1r* variant allele increased the raw penetrance of *cdkn2a* mutation to 84% with a mean age at onset of 37.8 years [21].

Van der Velden *et al.* found that the *mc1r* variant R151C modified melanoma risk in melanoma families with a *cdkn2a* mutation [22]. They suggested that the R151C variant may be involved in melanoma pathogenesis in two ways: both as a determinant of fair skin; and as a component of another independent pathway, since the variant contributed to increased melanoma risk even after statistical correction for its effect on skin type.

In addition, *mc1r* variants are strongly associated with *braf* mutations in melanomas on non-chronically sun-damaged skin [23]. It could be shown that *braf* mutations were more frequent in melanomas on non-chronically sun-damaged skin with germline *mc1r* variants than in those with 2 wildtype *mc1r* alleles.

24.2
More Melanoma-Susceptibility Genes

The v-raf murine sarcoma viral oncogene homolog BIX1 *braf* gene encodes a serine/threonine kinase, which is involved in the RAS-RAF-mitogen-activated protein kinase (MAPK) pathway [24]. This pathway can be stimulated by extracellular mitogenic signals such as diverse growth factors leading to cell proliferation. Somatic mutations in the *braf* gene have been demonstrated in 40 to 88% of melanoma and up to 74 to 82% of melanocytic nevi. In most cases, it is a V600E change leading to a constitutive activation of *braf*. Therefore, it has been speculated that *braf* may be a low-risk melanoma susceptibility gene. Whether certain polymorphic variants of the *braf* gene are associated with an increased melanoma risk is not yet clear. While some studies could show a significant risk of carriers of certain intronic *braf* variants or of germline single nucleotide polymorphisms (SNP) within the *braf* gene, others could not find similar associations.

Polymorphisms in the genes for epidermal growth factor receptor (EGFR) and for isozymes of glutathione-S-transferase (GST), *gstm1* and *gstt1*, were shown to be associated with melanoma risk, but these observations could not be confirmed by other groups [2].

Furthermore, an influence on melanoma susceptibility has been discussed for polymorphisms in the vitamin D receptor *(vdr)* gene, in the oculocutaneous albinism 2 (oca2) gene, the endothelin receptor B *(ednrb)* gene, and the *p53* gene, but these mostly single reports need to be confirmed in a larger series of patients by independent groups.

In addition, there were speculations on a linkage of malignant melanoma to chromosomes 6p, 2, 3, 10, and 11. However, no genes have been matched to these loci to date.

24.3
Sporadic Melanoma

In sporadic melanoma, innumerable cellular and molecular changes during melanocytes transformation and melanoma progression have been described. The most frequently mutated gene is *braf* (V600E), which leads to constitutive activation of the RAS/RAF/MAPK pathway (see above). Less commonly, but instead of mutated *braf*, *nras* mutations occur in 15 to 20% of melanoma with constitutive activation of the oncogene *ras*. In certain subgroups of melanoma, where mutations of *braf* or *nras* are infrequent, oncogenic mutations in *kit* were found by CGH: in 39% of melanomas on mucosal membranes, in 36% of melanomas on acral skin (soles, palms, nail bed), and in 28% of melanomas on chronically sun-damaged skin [25]. *Kit* encodes for c-KIT, which is the receptor for the growth factor SCF (stem cell factor) and regulates proliferation and maturation of melanocytes essentially during embryonic development.

Further genetic aberrations have been identified predominantly in the three major tumor suppressor pathways: The P16/RB pathway, the P14^{ARF}/P53 pathway, and the PI3kinase/PTEN/AKT pathway. However, it is noteworthy that typical tumor suppressor genes, such as *p53* (1–10%), or oncogenes, such as *c-myc* or *ß-catenin* (2%), are not, or only rarely, mutated in melanoma.

24.4
Conclusion

The vast majority of malignant melanomas occur sporadically. However, also in sporadic melanoma a familiar background with low penetrance has been speculated. Genetically determined phenotypic variability, such as skin color and activity of DNA repair mechanisms, have a major impact on melanoma development.

The identification of germline mutations in the *cdkn2a* gene in affected members of familial melanoma kindreds worldwide highlights the role of *cdkn2a* in melanoma predisposition. The potential benefit of genetic testing of this region in at-risk individuals has been controversially discussed, but eventually is not recommended. One reason is that the genotype does not necessarily predict the phenotype, another that the prevention and surveillance strategies would not be different compared to other patients with a history of sporadic or familial melanoma. Therefore, rather programs of prevention and surveillance irrespective of DNA status are recommended instead.

There is some evidence that besides a hereditary susceptibility for melanoma, environmental factors are involved in the development of melanoma. Among gene carriers of *cdkn2a* (*cmm2*) mutations, a history of sun exposure was more common in kindreds with melanoma than without melanoma. Likewise, the cumulative incidence of melanoma in families with 9p21 mutations was 21 times higher among members born after 1959, compared with those born before 1900. Due to changing habits regarding sun exposure over time, the increase in penetrance observed in these families was attributed to an environmental-genetic interaction between exposure to sun and mutations at the 9p21. This means that members of melanoma-prone families as well as individuals without familial but with constitutional risk factors for melanoma (e.g. skin type I and II, freckling) both may profit from strict sun protection measures. This is why the regular use of sunscreens with a high enough sun protection factor, the use of long-sleeved and long-legged clothes, hat and sunglasses, and the avoidance of direct sun exposure between 11 a.m. and 3 p.m. on sunny days should be propagated.

Abbreviations

ARF	alternative reading frame
CDK4	cyclin-dependent kinase 4
CDK8	cyclin-dependent kinase 8
CDKN2A	cyclin-dependent kinase inhibitor 2A
CGH	comparative genomic hybridization
CMM	cutaneous malignant melanoma
MAPK	mitogen-activated protein kinase
MC1R	melanocortin 1 receptor
RB	retinoblastoma
UVR	ultraviolet radiation
XP	Xeroderma pigmentosum

References

1 Berwick, M. and Weinstock, M.A. (2003) Epidemiology: Current trends, in *Cutaneous Melanoma* (eds C.M. Balch, A. Houghton, A. Sober and S.J. Soong), Quality Medical Publishing, St. Louis, pp. 16–23.

2 Fargnoli, M.C., Argenziano, G., Zalaudek, I. and Peris, K. (2006) High- and low-penetrance cutaneous melanoma susceptibility genes. *Expert Review of Anticancer Therapy*, **6**, 657–70.

3 Ortonne, J.P. (2002) Photobiology and genetics of malignant melanoma. *The British Journal of Dermatology*, **146**, 11–16.

4 Pollock, P.M., Weeraratna, A. and Trent, J.M. (2003) Genetics and molecular staging, in *Cutaneous Melanoma* (eds C.M. Balch, A. Houghton, A. Sober and S.J. Soong), Quality Medical Publishing, St. Louis, pp. 687–712.

5 Hayward, N. (2000) New developments in melanoma genetics. *Current Oncology Reports*, **2**, 300.

6 Piepkorn, M. (2000) The expression of *p16(INK4a)*, the product of a tumor suppressor gene for melanoma, is upregulated in human melanocytes by UVB irradiation. *Journal of the American Academy of Dermatology*, **42**, 741–5.

7 Quelle, D.E., Zindy, F., Ashmun, R.A. and Sherr, C.J. (1995) Alternative reading frames of the *INK4a* tumor suppressor gene encode two unrelated proteins capable of inducing cell cycle arrest. *Cell*, **83**, 993–1000.

8 Ries, S., Biederer, C., Woods, D., Shifman, O., Shirasawa, S., Sasazuki, T., McMahon, M., Oren, M. and McCormick, F. (2000) Opposing effects of Ras on p53: transcriptional activation of mdm2 and induction of p19ARF. *Cell*, **103**, 321–30.

9 Laud, K., Marian, C., Avril, M.F., Barrois, M., Chompret, A., Goldstein, A.M., Tucker, M.A., Clark, P.A., Peters, G., Chaudru, V., Demenais, F., Spatz, A., Smith, M.W., Lenoir, G.M., Bressac-de Paillerets, B. and French Hereditary Melanoma Study Group (2006) Comprehensive analysis of *CDKN2A* (p16INK4A/p14ARF) and *CDKN2B* genes in 53 melanoma index cases considered to be at heightened risk of melanoma. *Journal of Medical Genetics*, **43**, 39–47.

10 Goldstein, A.M., Chidambaram, A., Halpern, A., Holly, E.A., Guerry, I.V.D., Sagebiel, R., Elder, D.E. and Tucker, M.A. (2002) Rarity of *CDK4* germline mutations in familial melanoma. *Melanoma Research*, **12**, 51–5.

11 Bale, S.J., Dracopoli, N.C., Tucker, M.A., Clark, W.H. Jr , Fraser, M.C., Stanger, B.Z., Green, P., Donis-Keller, H., Housman, D.E. and Greene, M.H. (1989) Mapping the gene for hereditary

cutaneous malignant melanoma-dysplastic nevus to chromosome 1p. *New England Journal of Medicine*, **320**, 1367–72.

12 van Haeringen, A., Bergman, W., Nelen, M.R., van der Kooij-Meijs, E., Hendrikse, I., Wijnen, J.T., Khan, P.M., Klasen, E.C. and Frants, R.R. (1989) Exclusion of the dysplastic nevus syndrome (DNS) locus from the short arm of chromosome 1 by linkage studies in Dutch families. *Genomics*, **5**, 61–4.

13 Cannon-Albright, L.A., Goldgar, D.E., Wright, E.C., Turco, A., Jost, M., Meyer, L.J., Piepkorn, M., Zone, J.J. and Skolnick, M.H. (1990) Evidence against the reported linkage of the cutaneous melanoma-dysplastic nevus syndrome locus to chromosome Ip36. *American Journal of Human Genetics*, **46**, 912–18.

14 Kraemer, K.H., Lee, M.M., Andrews, A.D. and Lambert, W.C. (1994) The role of sunlight and DNA repair in melanoma and nonmelanoma skin cancer. The xeroderma pigmentosum paradigm. *Archives of Dermatology*, **130**, 1018–121.

15 Lynch, H.T., Fusaro, R.M. and Johnson, J.A. (1984) Xeroderma pigmentosum. Complementation group C and malignant melanoma. *Archives of Dermatology*, **120**, 175–9.

16 Winsey, S.L., Haldar, N.A., Marsh, H.P., Bunce, M., Marshall, S.E., Harris, A.L., Wojnarowska, F. and Welsh, K.I. (2000) A variant within the DNA repair gene *XRCC3* is associated with the development of melanoma skin cancer. *Cancer Research*, **60**, 5612–16.

17 Han, J., Colditz, G.A., Samson, L.D. and Hunter, D.J. (2004) Polymorphisms in DNA double-strand break repair genes and skin cancer risk. *Cancer Research*, **64**, 3009–13.

18 Bertram, C.G., Gaut, R.M., Barrett, J.H., Randerson-Moor, J., Whitaker, L., Turner, F., Bataille, V., Silva, I., Swerdlow, A.J., Bishop, D.T. and

Newton Bishop, J.A. (2004) An assessment of a variant of the DNA repair gene *XRCC3* as a possible nevus or melanoma susceptibility genotype. *The Journal of Investigative Dermatology*, **122**, 429–32.

19 Valverde, P., Healy, E., Sikkink, S., Haldane, F., Thody, A.J., Carothers, A., Jackson, I.J. and Rees, J.L. (1996) The Asp84Glu variant of the melanocortin 1 receptor (MC1R) is associated with melanoma. *Human Molecular Genetics*, **5**, 1663–6.

20 Palmer, J.S., Duffy, D.L., Box, N.F., Aitken, J.F., O'Gorman, L.E., Green, A.C., Hayward, N.K., Martin, N.G. and Sturm, R.A. (2000) Melanocortin-1 receptor polymorphisms and risk of melanoma: is the association explained solely by pigmentation phenotype? *American Journal of Human Genetics*, **6**, 176–86.

21 Box, N.F., Duffy, D.L., Chen, W., Stark, M., Martin, N.G., Sturm, R.A. and Hayward, N.K. (2001) MC1R genotype modifies risk of melanoma in families segregating *CDKN2A* mutations. *American Journal of Human Genetics*, **69**, 765–73.

22 van der Velden, P.A., Sandkuijl, L.A., Bergman, W., Pavel, S., van Mourik, L., Frants, R.R. and Gruis, N.A. (2001) Melanocortin-1 receptor variant R151C modifies melanoma risk in Dutch families with melanoma. *American Journal of Human Genetics*, **69**, 774–9.

23 Landi, M.T., Bauer, J., Pfeiffer, R.M., Elder, D.E., Hulley, B., Minghetti, P., Calista, D., Kanetsky, P.A., Pinkel, D. and Bastian, B.C. (2006) MC1R germline variants confer risk for *BRAF*-mutant melanoma. *Science*, **313**, 521–2.

24 Dhomen, N. and Marais, R. (2007) New insight into *BRAF* mutations in cancer. *Current Opinion in Genetics & Development*, **17**, 31–9.

25 Curtin, J.A., Busam, K., Pinkel, D. and Bastian, B.C. (2006) Somatic activation of KIT in distinct subtypes of melanoma. *Journal of Clinical Oncology*, **24**, 4340–6.

25
Xeroderma Pigmentosum, Cockayne Syndrome, Trichothiodystrophy – Defects in DNA Repair and Carcinogenesis

Steffen Emmert

Summary

The ultra-violet (UV) portion of sunlight is the most important exogenic factor in skin cancer development. If UV-induced DNA damage cannot be properly repaired by cells, patients are prone to skin cancer, including squamous cell carcinoma, basal cell carcinoma, as well as cutaneous melanoma. These skin cancers comprise the most common cancers in humans. The median age of such skin cancer development in the normal population is about 60 years. UV-induced DNA damage is repaired by the nucleotide excision repair (NER) system. The rare genetic diseases Xeroderma pigmentosum (XP), Cockayne syndrome (CS), and trichothiodystrophy (TTD) mirror the extreme clinical consequences of severely impaired NER. XP patients are very sun-sensitive, severely freckle in sun exposed skin areas, and also develop sun-induced skin cancers, at a median age of 8 years. CS and TTD patients are also sun-sensitive, but are not skin cancer prone. This demonstrates that functional NER can protect about 5 to 6 decades of life from UV-induced skin cancer development, and that some genetic defects in NER (CS and TTD) do not result in cancer proneness. In this chapter, the NER cascade, as well as the varieties of NER defective syndromes, is reviewed.

25.1
The Nucleotide Excision Repair (NER) – Defective Syndromes

A total of seven different autosomal-recessive inherited genetic diseases including xeroderma pigmentosum (XP), Cockayne syndrome (CS), and the photosensitive form of trichothiodystrophy (TTD) demonstrate the clinical consequences of defects in the NER pathway. All entities share an increased sun-sensitivity and freckling in the sun-exposed skin as clinical symptoms. However, XP patients are highly skin cancer prone, but CS and TTD patients are not [1–3].

Hereditary Tumors: From Genes to Clinical Consequences
Edited by Heike Allgayer, Helga Rehder and Simone Fulda
Copyright © 2009 WILEY-VCH Verlag GmbH & Co. KGaA, Weinheim
ISBN: 978-3-527-32028-8

25.1.1
Xeroderma Pigmentosum (XP)

The first patient with "dry skin (xeroderma) and hyperpigmentations" was described by Moritz Kaposi in 1863. In 1882, this entity was finally named XP [4]. Albert Neisser was the first to report neurological abnormalities associated with XP in 1883. In 1968, James Cleaver was the first to bridge the gap between the clinical picture XP and its underlying defect in NER.

XP is a rare autosomal-recessive inherited genetic disease occurring worldwide. The incidence of XP in Europe and the United States is about 1:1 million [1]. In northern Africa and Japan, the incidence is 10 times higher [5]. Both sexes are affected equally [6, 7]. In Europe and Northern America, mutations in the *XPD* and *XPC* genes are most common. In Japan, mutations in the *XPA* gene are most common, and due to the isolated location of Japan, only a few founder mutations in the *XPA* gene were identified that constitute most of the XP mutations [8, 9]. In about 30% of all cases, consanguinity of the parents is present. As an autosomal recessive disorder, there usually is no positive family history. The heterozygous parents are regarded as clinically healthy to date. However, the hypothesis exists that those heterozygous carriers of an XP mutation might have an increased skin cancer risk at an older age [10]. The frequency of such heterozygous carriers (1:500) is much higher than XP patients [9].

The median age of first XP symptoms is 1 to 2 years [6]. Three key cutaneous features exist: sun-sensitivity, freckling in sun-exposed areas, and skin cancer proneness. While babies are normal at birth, in the first years of life diffuse erythema, scaling, and pronounced freckle-like pigmentation develop (Figure 25.1a and b). In accordance with the increased sun sensitivity, changes are seen over sun-exposed skin areas, in particular the face, head, and neck, but will subsequently involve the lower legs and even the trunk in severe cases. Normally, the skin changes are sharply demarcated from sun-protected skin. One needs to become alert when babies present with severe solar dermatitis/sunburn, often associated with constant crying, for which no other explanation can be found. The sunburn will usually persist for extended periods of time, not uncommonly for several weeks, and may include blister formation upon minimal sun exposure, even behind window glass. Sometimes infants are misdiagnosed as being scalded, and investigations are initiated concerning child abuse.

Further on, pigmentary changes in sun-exposed skin develop in infancy. Telangiectasias and atrophic hyper- as well as hypo-pigmentations become apparent, which are normally signs of chronic sun exposure over decades. As the skin suffers actinic damage, the surface becomes atrophic and dry, which has led to the term "xeroderma" (dry skin) for this condition (Figure 25.1b and d).

Assessment of more than 830 XP patients revealed 8 years as the median age of first skin cancer development. In the normal Caucasian population, the median age of first skin cancer development is about 60 years [1, 11]. This indicates that NER normally protects over 5 to 6 decades from skin cancer development. The distribution and types of skin cancers are identical in XP patients and the normal

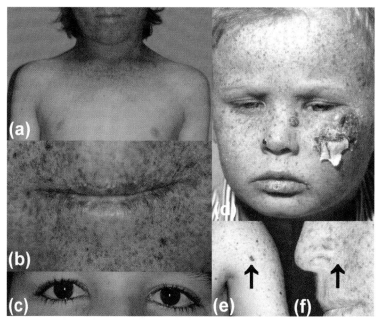

Figure 25.1 Clinical symptoms of XP. Skin changes sharply demarcated to sun-exposed skin (a) typical poikilodermic aspect of XP skin changes including the lips (atrophic dry skin with hyper- and hypo-pigmentations); (b) involvement of the anterior eyes (pterygium); (c) child with classical XP symptoms and large squamous cell carcinoma on the left cheek; (d) melanoma on XP skin ((e), arrow); basal cell carcinoma on XP skin ((f), arrow).

population, and include all classical UV-induced skin cancers such as basal cell carcinomas (Figure 25.1f), squamous cell carcinomas (Figure 25.1d), and melanomas (Figure 25.1e) [12]. The risk for the development of skin tumors is increased about 1000-fold, as compared with the normal population [12, 13].

In addition to their DNA damage repair deficiency, XP patients also show signs of immune deficiency. Although typical symptoms of immune deficiency, such as multiple infections, are not usually observed in XP patients, prominent depletion of Langerhans cells induced by UV radiation has been described [14]. Various other defects in cell-mediated immunity such as impaired cutaneous responses to recall antigens, impaired lymphocyte proliferative responses to mitogens, and decreased production of interferon, as well as reduced natural killer cell activity, have been detected in XP patients. Recently, impaired UVB-induced cytokine induction in XP fibroblasts was reported [15]. This, as well as the immunosuppressive effects of UV irradiation, is highly likely to contribute to skin tumor promotion in XP patients.

Besides the above-mentioned cancers, keratoakanthomas and sarcomas including fibrosarcomas and angiosarcomas have been described [16]. The incidence of tumors of the oral mucosa (inner lips, gingival, and tip of the tongue – presumably sun exposed), the anterior eye (usually nonmelanoma cancers of the conjunctiva or cornea), and other organs (brain cancer, lung cancer, and leukemia) is also increased. The frequency of internal tumors is elevated about 10-fold compared to normal individuals [12]. Tobacco smoke may be regarded as "internal sun" for XP patients, since benz-a-pyrene derivates induce DNA damage that is repaired by nucleotide excision [1]. Particularly, the occurrence of leukemias has been reported in XP [17]. The incidence of central nervous system tumors is about 10-fold higher than in normal individuals. The neurological tumors include astrocytoma, medulloblastoma, glioblastoma, and malignant schwannoma [18].

As the repair defect is present in all cells of the body, the sun-exposed portions of the eyes are also affected. Photophobia, conjunctivitis, keratitis, and neoplasias of the eye lids and conjunctivae may develop. Corneal abnormalities include corneal clouding, vascularization, and corneal ulcers, causing impaired vision in about 15%. These symptoms may progress to inflammatory lesions such as pingueculae (conjunctival growths limited to the bulbar conjunctiva) and pterygia (conjunctival growths that extend onto the corneal surface) (Figure 25.1c). In the general population, these lesions are rarely seen in children [19]. Blepharitis, ectropion, symblepharon, loss of eyelashes, atrophy, and scarring represent some less common ophthalmological features of XP [6, 7]. Interestingly, the posterior portions of the eye such as the retina are rarely affected, because UV-light is absorbed by anterior eye portions, and only visible light (400–800 nm) reaches the retina. The risk of ocular neoplasias is increased about 1000-fold, comparable to the XP skin cancer risk. These cancers occur in up to 15% of patients and are most often localized in the cornea and conjunctiva, while melanomas occur in about 5% [6, 20]. In addition, fibrovascular pannus of the cornea, pterygium, and epitheliomas of the lids and conjunctivae may occur.

Unfortunately, a causative therapy such as gene therapy is currently not available. Thus, the overall goal is to prevent the patient from sunlight to minimize the formation of DNA damage. This includes shifting the daily activities into the night as much as possible, which has led to the term "moon babies" or "children of the moon" for XP patients. In addition, protective clothing, hats, and appropriate eye care serve to minimize UV-induced damage. Special clothing suits are available with high UV protective but yet light fabrics. Sometimes, cooling systems are incorporated into the suit. Sunscreens should be regularly applied to all exposed surfaces, including the hands and the lower lids. Preferably, physical and chemical sunscreens are to be used simultaneously and around the entire year, even in winter months, and during evening as well as early morning hours. UV detectors may be helpful to measure the UV exposure outdoors as well as indoors.

This and the availability of dermatologists for establishing early clinical diagnosis and regular skin examination at 3 to 6 months intervals led to the situation that in general the skin problems of XP patients are manageable. Today, progressive neurological symptoms seem to be the most critical issue in XP patient care [21]. In addition, family support groups exist that offer assistance in XP patient management. Information as well as contact addresses can be found on their websites. For example, XP support groups in the United States (http://www.xps.

org/), the United Kingdom (http://xpsupportgroup.org.uk), France (http://asso.orpha.net/AXP/index.html), and in Germany (http://www.xerodermapigmentosum.de) also assist clinical and basic research efforts by raising funds, participating in patient registries, and donating samples for molecular research.

Some therapeutic approaches are under way. Prevention of skin cancer in XP patients has also been achieved to some degree with the use of oral isotretinoin [22]. In the last years, a delivery system has been developed consisting of packaging repair enzymes into liposomes that can be applied to the skin as a hydrogel lotion on a regular basis. This technique could deliver any repair enzyme at a defined concentration and frequency to epidermal skin cells. In 2001, the *Lancet* published a first successful and prospective pilot study that investigated the efficacy of T4 endonuclease liposomal therapy in 30 XP patients [23]. Twenty patients applied the repair enzyme-containing lotion to their skin and 10 patients a placebo containing lotion. After 1 year of treatment, a 68% reduction in the development of actinic keratoses, and a 30% reduction in basal cell cancer development could be detected compared to the placebo group. Stege *et al.* [24] investigated the efficacy of a second liposomal encapsulated repair enzyme, photolyase. Nineteen healthy volunteers were treated with a photolyase containing liposomal lotion. This treatment reduced the content of cyclobutane-pyrimidine dimers in UVB-irradiated skin of the probands up to 45%.

Until today, early diagnosis and consequent avoidance of sunlight, as well as regular dermatological screening have helped to increase life expectancy. The prognosis is significantly impaired, since fewer than 40% of patients survive beyond 20 years of age [6]. However, some individuals with milder disease may survive to about 40 years. The probability of a 40-year life expectancy is estimated at 70%. Overall, the life expectancy for XP patients is reduced by 30 years. Patients are likely to die from cancer (33%), infections (11%), and various other diseases [6].

Overall the life expectancy correlates with the severity of the disease. In a recent workshop, where researchers and clinicians interested in human diseases of DNA repair deficiency and premature aging met in September 2006 [21], suggestive trends emerged providing rational explanations for the relative severity of the disease in patients. The severity of the clinical phenotype may often correlate with the severity of the molecular defect. Molecular-genetic markers were identified that appear to retrospectively explain the patient's phenotype. In general, "null" mutations lead to severe phenotypes and the retention of some functional activity in at least one allele may result in milder phenotypes with better prognosis [25]. This implies that genetic testing may be beneficial in XP patients, even for prognostic purposes. The establishment of centers of excellence for that purpose may be very helpful in this regard.

25.1.2
XP Plus Neurologic Abnormalities

About 30% of all XP patients develop neurological abnormalities in addition to their XP skin problems [19, 26]. Usually, patients with defects in the *XPA, XPB,*

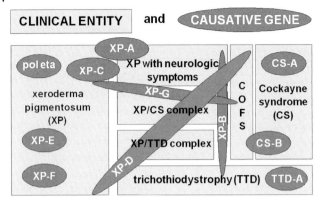

Figure 25.2 Seven clinical entities based on 11 defective genes (modified from Kraemer *et al.* [19]).

XPD, or *XPG* gene may present with additional neurological symptoms (Figure 25.2). The onset and severity of the neurological symptoms can be very variable, but all share a progressive character (Table 25.1). Commonly, around the fifth to tenth year of life, neurological symptoms may become evident. The earliest clinical signs of the presence of XP plus neurological symptoms are diminished or absent deep tendon reflexes, followed by progressive high-frequency hearing loss. This may necessitate the use of a hearing aid. Mental deterioration with disabilities in speaking, walking, and balance may follow (spasticity, ataxia). This may include abnormal gait and difficulty to walk, eventually leading to the use of a wheelchair. Swallowing difficulties may become problematic, leading to the aspiration of food, and necessitate the implantation of a gastric feeding tube [27–30]. For example, in 32 Japanese patients with XPA, mental retardation, microcephaly, nystagmus, dysarthria, ataxia, and short stature were described as the most prominent neurological symptoms [6, 31]. Often, these progressive neurological manifestations are more disabling than the cutaneous symptoms.

The corresponding histopathology of these symptoms is a primary neuronal degeneration with loss of neurons, without inflammation or abnormal depositions. The MRI shows diffuse atrophy of the cerebrum and cerebellum with sparing of the white matter. Enlarged ventricles may be seen in early childhood. The progressive nature of the neurological degeneration suggests that there might be ongoing damage that is not repaired. As neurons do not divide, this may occur due to an accumulation of endogenous, for example, oxidative, DNA damage. There are indications that some oxidative DNA damage is repaired via the NER system. In parallel, it was found that XP genes are also involved in base excision repair following oxidative DNA damage [19, 32]. However, there are many unanswered questions regarding the genesis of the neurological symptoms, for example, as to why only 30% of the XP patients develop neurological degeneration.

Table 25.1 Summary of the clinical features of NER-defective syndromes.

Clinical features	Phenotype				
	XP	**XP plus neurologic abnormalities**	**CS (±XP)**	**TTD (±XP)**	**COFS**[a]
sun-sensitivity	yes	yes, severe	yes	yes/no	
freckling	yes	yes			
skin cancer (NM[b] and M[c])	yes	yes			
photophobia	yes	yes	yes	yes/no	
conjunctival growths	yes	yes			
cancer (anterior eye portion)	yes	yes			
congenital cataracts			yes	yes	
pigmentary retinal degeneration			yes		
sensorineural deafness		yes	yes		
ataxia		yes, in some	yes		
progressive cognitive impairment		yes	yes	yes	yes
developmental delay		yes	yes	yes	
primary neuronal degeneration		yes			
loss of subcutaneous tissue			yes		
dwarfism		yes, in some	yes	yes	yes
brain calcification			yes	yes, in some	
demyelinating neuropathy			yes	yes, in some	
ichthyosis				yes	
brittle hair				yes	
brittle nails				yes	
tiger-tail hair				yes	
sulfur-deficient hair				yes	
hypertrichosis					yes
skeletal abnormalities					yes
microcephaly/craniofacial abnormalities					yes

a COFS: Cerebro-Oculo-Facio-Skeletal Syndrome.
b Non-melanoma skin cancer (basal and squamous cell carcinoma).
c Melanoma skin cancer.

25.1.3
Cockayne Syndrome (CS)

In 1936 a syndrome with the clinical hallmarks of cachectic dwarfism, hearing disability, and retinal atrophy was first described by Cockayne [1]. Patients suffering from the autosomal-recessive inherited genetic disease CS are sun-sensitive but, in contrast to XP patients, not prone to skin cancer [2]. A characteristic facies including a thin face, flat cheeks, and a prominent tapering nose (bird-like face), skin sensitivity to sunlight (with or without xerosis), neurologic and psychomotoric impairment with mental retardation, growth retardation (dwarfism), dental caries, deafness, and progressive ophthalmologic disorders including cataracts or retinitis pigmentosa, account for typical clinical symptoms (Table 25.1). Commonly, microcephaly and calcifications of the basal ganglia or other areas in the central nervous system occur. Cachectic dwarfism and neurologic disabilities are early diagnostic symptoms [1, 33]. Nance and Berry [33] suggested three clinical CS categories: i) CSI, a classic form including most of the CS patients; ii) CSII, a severe form with early onset and rapid progression; and iii) CSIII, a mild form with late onset and slow progression of symptoms. Pathologically, neurologic impairment correlates to a primary demyelinization of neurons. This contrasts the primary neuronal degeneration found in XP patients.

Defects in two genes, *CSA* and *CSB*, involved in the transcription-coupled repair sub-pathway of NER (Figures 25.2 and 25.3), are known to result in CS [34, 35]. However, the exact underlying functional and molecular mechanisms leading to CS symptoms, especially the absence of skin cancer proneness, are still to be investigated [36]. As the *CS* genes are involved in transcription-coupled repair of active genes, there may be a defect in transcription beyond bulky DNA damage. Other studies also indicate defective repair of endogenous oxidative DNA damage in actively transcribed genes in CS cells [2, 37].

25.1.4
XP/CS Complex

Thorough clinical studies in the 1970s revealed that there are patients showing symptoms of both XP and CS. Robbins *et al.* [28, 38] recognized these patients as an independent clinical entity, XP/CS complex. Sun-sensitivity, freckling, and skin cancer proneness (XP symptoms) as well as bird-like face, severe neurologic and psychomotoric disabilities, dwarfism, and defects in mental and physical development (CS symptoms) characterize XP/CS complex patients (Table 25.1) [25, 39, 40].

It was found that certain mutations in XP genes can lead to CS symptoms. A survey in 2002 revealed that 3 out of 12 XP/CS complex patients had a defect in the *XPB* gene, 2 patients had a defect in the *XPD* gene, and 7 XP/CS complex patients had *XPG* gene defects (Figure 25.2) [25]. Mutations in the *CSA* or *CSB* genes do not seem to result in XP symptoms. At least two different *XP* gene functions seem to be affected in XP/CS complex patients: One defect disturbs NER, the other affects repair of oxidative DNA damage in the global genome, or transcription-coupled repair of oxidative DNA damage [25, 41–46].

25.1.5
Trichothiodystrophy (TTD)

TTD is the third major NER-associated autosomal recessive inherited entity. Price introduced the term TTD in 1979 [47]. Sun-sensitivity is a clinical sign in about 50% of all TTD patients, which reflects the cellular repair defect of UV-induced photoproducts. Interestingly, as in CS patients this is not accompanied by skin

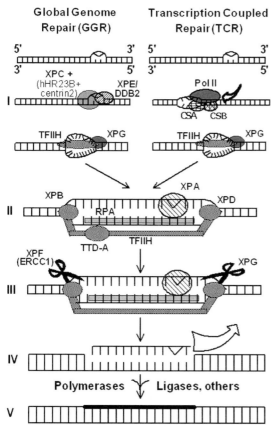

Global Genome Repair (GGR)

Transcription Coupled Repair (TCR)

Figure 25.3 The NER pathway. In the global genome *XPC* and *XPE* recognize the DNA damage and initiate the NER cascade. In actively transcribed genes, the stalled polymerase II in concert with *CSA* and *CSB* are thought to initiate the NER cascade. *XPB* and *XPD* are components of the 10 units containing multiprotein complex TFIIH (transcription factor II H), and demarcate the damage due to their helicase activity. TTD-A is also part of the TFIIH complex. *XPF* and *XPG* are endonucleases that cut the damage containing DNA strand. The resulting gap is filled using polymerases and ligases and the complementary DNA strand as a template. RPA: replication protein A.

cancer proneness [48]. Other prominent clinical symptoms include ichthyotic skin changes, nail changes, and erythemas (Table 25.1). Dystrophic, short, brittle hair, with reduced sulfur content, is a hallmark of TTD patients [2, 48]. Polarized microscopy reveals a typical tiger tail pattern of the hair due to a lack of sulfur-rich hair matrix proteins that results in changes of the amino acid content of the hair. The amount of cysteine is greatly reduced, as the amino acids proline, threonine, and serine. As a consequence, a relative increase in methionine, phenylalanine, alanine, leucine, lysine, and aspartic acid can be found [48, 49]. Sulfur-rich hair matrix proteins normally confer hair shaft stability [50].

Retrospectively, several syndromes are sub-summarized under TTD, including Pollitt syndrome, Tay syndrome, Sabinas syndrome, Marinesco–Sjögren syndrome, and ONMR (onychotrichodysplasia, neutropenia, mental retardation) as well as PIBIDS. The symptoms of PIBIDS include photosensitivity, ichthyosis, brittle hair and nails, intellectual impairment, decreased fertility, and short stature [2, 48]. PIBIDS patients have initially been studied to investigate the genetic basis of TTD [51].

Most of all photosensitive TTD cases (95%) are caused by mutations in the *XPD* gene [52]. *XPB* gene defects were identified in two TTD patients [53, 54]. Since a functional test is lacking for the non-photosensitive TTD patients, genetic testing was preferentially performed in photosensitive, NER defective TTD patient cells. Using such functional tests, one TTD patient was identified who obviously had a defect in transcription factor IIH (TFIIH) function, but no mutation in the *XPD* or *XPB* genes that are subunits of TFIIH [48, 55]. Complementation testing suggested a further putative TTD causing gene that was named *TTD-A*. This gene was identified in 2004 as a further tenth subunit of the TFIIH complex, and comprises the human TFBIX5 ortholog of yeast [56] (Figures 25.2 and 25.3).

25.1.6
XP/TTD Complex

A detailed characterization of *XPD* mutations revealed that they either lead to XP or TTD symptoms or are null mutations dependent on their location in the *XPD* gene [57, 58]. It was suggested that TTD results as a consequence of an *XPD*-triggered deficiency in basal transcription and that XP results from a defect in NER [59–61]. Therefore, individuals that carry compound heterozygous *XPD* mutations (one mutation leading to XP, the other to TTD) should present an XP/TTD complex phenotype comparable to the already identified XP/CS complex phenotype. Indeed, this hypothesis driven by genetics could be confirmed by the identification of two patients, XP189MA and XP38BR, who carry compound heterozygous *XPD* gene mutations, and exhibit a XP/TTD complex phenotype (Table 25.1 and Figure 25.2) [62].

25.1.7
COFS (Cerebro-Oculo-Facio-Skeletal Syndrome)

COFS syndrome was first reported by Lowry *et al.*, and delineated by Pena and Shokeir as an autosomal recessive brain and eye disorder in 1974, occurring in French-Indian families within the genetically isolated Manitoba Aboriginal population [63]. Typical clinical signs include microcephaly with cerebral atrophy, hypoplasia of the corpus callosum, hypotonia, severe mental retardation, cataracts, microcornea, optic atrophy, progressive joint contractures, and postnatal growth deficiency [64] (Table 25.1). Some symptoms, such as progressive demyelination with brain calcification or cataracts, are similar to CS. However, COFS syndrome eye defects (e.g. microcornea) appear to be more severe than those associated with CS, and in contrast to CS, cutaneous photosensitivity is not always noted in COFS patients [64] (Table 25.1). Recently, causative mutations in the *CSB, XPG,* and *XPD* genes have been identified in COFS patients [64, 65] (Figure 25.2).

25.2
The Nucleotide Excision Repair (NER) Pathway

All patients with the above-mentioned syndromes share defects in genes that are involved in the NER pathway (*XP, CS,* and *TTD* genes). However, there is one exception. Some patients suffering from XP have a normal NER. In 1999, these patients were identified as having a defect in polymerase eta, for example, they are defective in translesional synthesis (Figure 25.2). Polymerase eta can bypass cyclobutane pyrimidene dimers. XP patients belonging to this group of XP variant patients (XPV) do not accumulate DNA mutations due to the defective repair of UV-induced DNA damage but due to the alternative use of more error-prone polymerases for translesional bypassing [66–70].

All *XP* (*XPA-XPG*), *CS* (*CSA* and *CSB*), and *TTD* (*TTD-A*) genes participate in the multi-step process of NER (Figure 25.3) in a defined order [2, 71]: i) the DNA damage is recognized; ii) then demarcated; iii) followed by strand incision at both sides of the DNA lesion; iv) then the lesion containing oligonucleotide is removed; and v) the gap is filled with a newly synthesized oligonucleotide using the complementary strand as a template (Figure 25.3).

25.2.1
Damage Recognition (I)

There are two ways as to how cellular DNA damage can be sensed and located (Figure 25.3). The slower sub-pathway which, however, operates in a genome-wide manner, is called global genome repair (GGR). Here, the XPC protein binds to the damage and initiates the further repair steps. The XPC protein is part of a heterotrimeric complex with HHR23B and centrin, and acts as the damage sensor [2, 72–74]. Another damage sensor in GGR is the UV-damaged DNA-binding protein (UV-DDB) consisting of the DDBIX1 and DDBIX2 subunits. DDBIX2 corresponds to the *XPE* gene product [75]. DDB has a higher binding affinity and specificity for certain types of DNA damage than *XPC* and seems to assist *XPC* in detection of specific DNA damage such as cyclobutane pyrimidine dimers [72, 76–79]. Patients with *XPC* gene mutations usually develop a classical XP phenotype with skin cancer proneness but no neurological abnormalities. This may be due to the retained transcription coupled repair (TCR) activity in XPC patients (see below).

In actively transcribed genes, the damage recognition is mediated via the stalled RNA polymerase II [80–82]. This NER sub-pathway is called the TCR, and acts much faster than GGR (Figure 25.3). Here, *XPC* and *DDB* are dispensable [83]. XPC and XPE patients, therefore, have normal TCR capabilities. In contrast, CS patients (*CSA* or *CSB* defective) have normal GGR, but are deficient in TCR [84]. The CS proteins may support the polymerase II complex to allow its temporary removal, and may play a general role in the processing of stalled polymerases during transcription [41]. This may be one reason for the severe neurologic abnormalities in some CS patients and usually no neurological abnormalities in XPC or XPE patients.

25.2.2
Damage Demarcation (II)

To allow for excision repair, the DNA double helix has to be unraveled around the damage. This is accomplished by the multifunctional basal transcription factor IIH (TFIIH) complex, consisting of 10 subunits including the XPB, XPD, and TTD-A proteins [56]. The XPB protein possesses 3′-5′ helicase activity, and the XPD protein 5′-3′ helicase activity. TTD-A plays a role in regulating the level of the transcription factor IIH and leads to TTD, if mutated. This indicates that TTD results as a consequence of defective basal transcription, because TTD-A is not involved in NER. TFIIH is also needed by RNA polymerase II to initiate transcription at promoter sites [85]. Thus, TFIIH has at least two different functions, which are basal transcription and NER. This can explain the great phenotypic heterogeneity of defects in the *XPD* and *XPB* genes (Figure 25.2). Depending on the type and location of the mutation within the gene, either NER, basal transcription, or both may be disabled, leading to combinations of XP, TTD, or even CS symptoms (disabled TCR). The replication protein A (RPA) supports the activity of TFIIH and stabilizes the "DNA-bubble" around the damage (Figure 25.3). The XPA protein is recruited to the site of DNA damage later than TFIIH and complexes with RPA [86]. Although the exact role of the XPA-RPA complex is not well understood, XPA in conjunction with RPA may monitor DNA bending and unwinding, and verify the damage-specific localization of repair complexes rather than recognize DNA damage [87]. XPA patients usually are defective in GGR as well as in TCR, which can explain the preponderance of XP with neurological symptoms, if XPA is mutated (Figure 25.2).

25.2.3
Incision of the Damage Containing DNA Strand (III)

Two endonucleases, XPG and XPF (complexed with ERCC1), are recruited to incise the damage containing strand. ERCC1-XPF cleaves the DNA strand at the 5′ boundary, and XPG at the 3′ boundary of the bubble structure (Figure 25.3) [88]. XPG interacts with RPA and TFIIH, which may allow exact positioning of the first cut [25, 89]. XPG is also required non-enzymatically for subsequent 5′ incision by the XPF-ERCC1 heterodimer, which may define the strand excision 24 to 32 nucleotides upstream. XPG is another multifunctional protein, for example, also involved in base excision of oxidative DNA damage. This may indicate why XPG patients often show neurological abnormalities, because oxidative DNA damage may persist in non-dividing neurons.

25.2.4
Removal of the Damage Containing Oligonucleotide (IV)

The actions described above always result in an excised oligonucleotide between 24 and 32 nucleotides in length [90]. It may be that the excised oligonucleotide is not just degraded after transport into the cytoplasm, but may induce UV-protective cell functions. It has been shown that small oligonucleotides with specific sequences were capable of inducing DNA repair, as well as melanogenesis without UV-exposure of the cells [91].

25.2.5
Gap Filling (V)

The resulting single-strand gap is filled by a newly synthesized oligonucleotide using the complementary strand as a template (DNA repair synthesis). This involves DNA polymerase δ and/or polymerase ε activity, and depends on proliferating-cell nuclear antigen (PCNA) and replication factor C (RFC). Reconstitution of *in vitro* repair synthesis was successfully accomplished using purified PCNA, RFC, and either polymerase δ or polymerase ε [92, 93]. The very last step of NER consists of 3′ strand rejoining by DNA ligase I [26].

Acknowledgment

SE is supported by the Deutsche Forschungsgemeinschaft DFG (GRK 1034).

References

1 Bootsma, D., Kraemer, K.H., Cleaver, J.E. and Hoeijmakers, J.H. (2002) Nucleotide excision repair syndromes: xeroderma pigmentosum, Cockayne syndrome, and trichothiodystrophy, in *The Genetic Basis of Human Cancer* (eds B. Vogelstein and K.W. Kinzler), McGraw-Hill, New York, pp. 211–37.

2 de Boer, J. and Hoeijmakers, J.H. (2000) Nucleotide excision repair and human syndromes. *Carcinogenesis*, **21**, 453–60.

3 Leibeling, D., Laspe, P. and Emmert, S. (2006) Nucleotide excision repair and

cancer. *Journal of Molecular Histology*, **37**, 225–38.

4 von Hebra, F. and Kaposi, M. (1874) *On Diseases of the Skin, including the Exanthema* (ed. W. Tay), New Sydenham Society, London, p. 252.

5 Takebe, H., Nishigori, C. and Satoh, Y. (1987) Genetics and skin cancer of xeroderma pigmentosum in Japan. *Japanese Journal of Cancer Research: Gann*, **78**, 1135–43.

6 Kraemer, K.H., Lee, M.M. and Scotto, J. (1987) Xeroderma pigmentosum. Cutaneous, ocular, and neurologic abnormalities in 830 published cases. *Archives of Dermatology*, **123**, 241–50.

7 Goyal, J.L., Rao, V.A., Srinivasan, R. and Agrawal, K. (1994) Oculocutaneous manifestations in xeroderma pigmentosa. *British Journal of Ophthalmology*, **78**, 295–7.

8 Moriwaki, S. and Kraemer, K.H. (2001) Xeroderma pigmentosum–bridging a gap between clinic and laboratory. *Photodermatology, Photoimmunology & Photomedicine*, **17**, 47–54.

9 Hirai, Y., Kodama, Y., Moriwaki, S., Noda, A., Cullings, H.M., Macphee, D. G., Kodama, K., Mabuchi, K., Kraemer, K.H., Land, C.E. and Nakamura, N. (2006) Heterozygous individuals bearing a founder mutation in the XPA DNA repair gene comprise nearly 1% of the Japanese population. *Mutation Research*, **601**, 171–8.

10 Swift, M. and Chase, C. (1979) Cancer in families with xeroderma pigmentosum. *The Journal of the National Cancer Institute*, **62**, 1415–21.

11 Kraemer, K.H. and Slor, H. (1985) Xeroderma pigmentosum. *Clinics in Dermatology*, **3**, 33–69.

12 Kraemer, K.H., Lee, M.M., Andrews, A.D. and Lambert, W.C. (1994) The role of sunlight and DNA repair in melanoma and nonmelanoma skin cancer. The xeroderma pigmentosum paradigm. *Archives of Dermatology*, **130**, 1018–21.

13 English, J.S. and Swerdlow, A.J. (1987) The risk of malignant melanoma, internal malignancy and mortality in xeroderma pigmentosum patients. *The British Journal of Dermatology*, **117**, 457–61.

14 Jimbo, T., Ichihashi, M., Mishima, Y. and Fujiwara, Y. (1992) Role of excision repair in UVB-induced depletion and recovery of human epidermal Langerhans cells. *Archives of Dermatology*, **128**, 61–7.

15 Suzuki, H., Kalair, W., Shivji, G.M., Wang, B., Toto, P., Amerio, P., Kraemer, K.H. and Sauder, D.N. (2001) Impaired ultraviolet-B-induced cytokine induction in xeroderma pigmentosum fibroblasts. *The Journal of Investigative Dermatology*, **117**, 1151–5.

16 De Silva, B.D., Nawroz, I. and Doherty, V.R. (1999) Angiosarcoma of the head and neck associated with xeroderma pigmentosum variant. *The British Journal of Dermatology*, **141**, 166–7.

17 Schroeder, T.M. (1974) Relationship between chromosomal instability and leukemia. *Hamatologie und Bluttransfusion*, **14**, 94–6.

18 Nakamura, T., Ono, T., Yoshimura, K., Arao, T., Kondo, S., Ichihashi, M., Matsumoto, A. and Fujiwara, Y. (1991) Malignant schwannoma associated with xeroderma pigmentosum in a patient belonging to complementation group D. *Journal of the American Academy of Dermatology*, **25**, 349–53.

19 Kraemer, K.H., Patronas, N.J., Schiffmann, R., Brooks, B.P., Tamura, D. and DiGiovanna, J.J. (2007) Xeroderma pigmentosum, trichothiodystrophy and Cockayne syndrome: a complex genotype-phenotype relationship. *Neuroscience*, **145**, 1388–96.

20 Vivian, A.J., Ellison, D.W. and McGill, J.I. (1993) Ocular melanomas in xeroderma pigmentosum. *British Journal of Ophthalmology*, **77**, 597–8.

21 Kraemer, K.H., Sander, M. and Bohr, V.A. (2007) New areas of focus at workshop on human diseases involving DNA repair deficiency and premature aging. *Mechanisms of Aging and Development*, **128**, 229–35.

22 Kraemer, K.H., DiGiovanna, J.J., Moshell, A.N., Tarone, R.E. and Peck, G.L. (1988) Prevention of skin cancer in xeroderma pigmentosum with the use of oral isotretinoin. *New England Journal of Medicine*, **318**, 1633–7.

23 Yarosh, D., Klein, J., O'Connor, A., Hawk, J., Rafal, E. and Wolf, P. (2001) Effect of topically applied T4 endonuclease V in liposomes on skin cancer in xeroderma pigmentosum: a randomised study. Xeroderma Pigmentosum Study Group. *Lancet*, **357**, 926–9.

24 Stege, H., Roza, L., Vink, A.A., Grewe, M., Ruzicka, T., Grether-Beck, S. and Krutmann, J. (2000) Enzyme plus light therapy to repair DNA damage in ultraviolet-B- irradiated human skin. *Proceedings of the National Academy of*

Sciences of the United States of America, **97**, 1790–5.

25 Emmert, S., Slor, H., Busch, D.B., Batko, S., Albert, R.B., Coleman, D., Khan, S.G., Abu-Libdeh, B., DiGiovanna, J.J., Cunningham, B.B., Lee, M.M., Crollick, J., Inui, H., Ueda, T., Hedayati, M., Grossman, L., Shahlavi, T., Cleaver, J.E. and Kraemer, K.H. (2002) Relationship of neurologic degeneration to genotype in Three Xeroderma Pigmentosum Group G Patients. *The Journal of Investigative Dermatology*, **118**, 972–82.

26 Emmert, S., Leibeling, D. and Runger, T.M. (2006) Syndromes with genetic instability: model diseases for (skin) cancerogenesis. *Journal der Deutschen Dermatologischen Gesellschaft*, **4**, 721–33.

27 Hakamada, S., Watanabe, K., Sobue, G., Hara, K. and Miyazaki, S. (1982) Xeroderma pigmentosum: neurological, neurophysiological and morphological studies. *European Neurology*, **21**, 69–76.

28 Robbins, J.H. (1988) Xeroderma pigmentosum. Defective DNA repair causes skin cancer and neurodegeneration. *The Journal of the American Medical Association*, **260**, 384–8.

29 Robbins, J.H., Brumback, R.A. and Moshell, A.N. (1993) Clinically asymptomatic xeroderma pigmentosum neurological disease in an adult: evidence for a neurodegeneration in later life caused by defective DNA repair. *European Neurology*, **33**, 188–90.

30 Rolig, R.L. and McKinnon, P.J. (2000) Linking DNA damage and neurodegeneration. *Trends in Neurosciences*, **23**, 417–24.

31 Mimaki, T., Itoh, N., Abe, J., Tagawa, T., Sato, K., Yabuuchi, H. and Takebe, H. (1986) Neurological manifestations in xeroderma pigmentosum. *Annals of Neurology*, **20**, 70–5.

32 Thoms, K.M., Kuschal, C. and Emmert, S. (2007) Lessons learned from DNA repair defective syndromes. *Experimental Dermatology*, **16**, 532–44.

33 Nance, M.A. and Berry, S.A. (1992) Cockayne syndrome: review of 140 cases. *American Journal of Medical Genetics*, **42**, 68–84.

34 Lehmann, A.R. (1982) Three complementation groups in Cockayne

syndrome. *Mutation Research*, **106**, 347–56.

35 Miyauchi, H., Horio, T., Akaeda, T., Asada, Y., Chang, H.R., Ishizaki, K. and Ikenaga, M. (1994) Cockayne syndrome in two adult siblings. *Journal of the American Academy of Dermatology*, **30**, 329–35.

36 Stefanini, M., Fawcett, H., Botta, E., Nardo, T. and Lehmann, A.R. (1996) Genetic analysis of twenty-two patients with Cockayne syndrome. *Human Genetics*, **97**, 418–23.

37 Licht, C.L., Stevnsner, T. and Bohr, V.A. (2003) Cockayne syndrome group B cellular and biochemical functions. *American Journal of Human Genetics*, **73**, 1217–39.

38 Robbins, J.H., Kraemer, K.H., Lutzner, M.A., Festoff, B.W. and Coon, H.G. (1974) Xeroderma pigmentosum. An inherited diseases with sun sensitivity, multiple cutaneous neoplasms, and abnormal DNA repair. *Annals of Internal Medicine*, **80**, 221–48.

39 Moriwaki, S., Stefanini, M., Lehmann, A.R., Hoeijmakers, J.H., Robbins, J.H., Rapin, I., Botta, E., Tanganelli, B., Vermeulen, W., Broughton, B.C. and Kraemer, K.H. (1996) DNA repair and ultraviolet mutagenesis in cells from a new patient with xeroderma pigmentosum group G and cockayne syndrome resemble xeroderma pigmentosum cells. *The Journal of Investigative Dermatology*, **107**, 647–53.

40 Rapin, I., Lindenbaum, Y., Dickson, D.W., Kraemer, K.H. and Robbins, J.H. (2000) Cockayne syndrome and xeroderma pigmentosum. *Neurology*, **55**, 1442–9.

41 Cooper, P.K., Nouspikel, T., Clarkson, S.G. and Leadon, S.A. (1997) Defective transcription-coupled repair of oxidative base damage in Cockayne syndrome patients from XP group G. *Science*, **275**, 990–3.

42 Klungland, A., Hoss, M., Gunz, D., Constantinou, A., Clarkson, S.G., Doetsch, P.W., Bolton, P.H., Wood, R.D. and Lindahl, T. (1999) Base excision repair of oxidative DNA damage activated by XPG protein. *Molecular Cell*, **3**, 33–42.

43 Lalle, P., Nouspikel, T., Constantinou, A., Thorel, F. and Clarkson, S.G. (2002) The founding members of xeroderma pigmentosum group G produce XPG protein with severely impaired endonuclease activity. *The Journal of Investigative Dermatology*, **118**, 344–51.

44 Le Page, F., Kwoh, E.E., Avrutskaya, A., Gentil, A., Leadon, S.A., Sarasin, A. and Cooper, P.K. (2000) Transcription-coupled repair of 8-oxoguanine: requirement for XPG, TFIIH, and CSB and implications for Cockayne syndrome. *Cell*, **101**, 159–71.

45 Nouspikel, T. and Clarkson, S.G. (1994) Mutations that disable the DNA repair gene *XPG* in a xeroderma pigmentosum group G patient. *Human Molecular Genetics*, **3**, 963–7.

46 Nouspikel, T., Lalle, P., Leadon, S.A., Cooper, P.K. and Clarkson, S.G. (1997) A common mutational pattern in Cockayne syndrome patients from xeroderma pigmentosum group G: implications for a second XPG function. *Proceedings of the National Academy of Sciences of the United States of America*, **94**, 3116–21.

47 Price, V.H., Odom, R.B., Ward, W.H. and Jones, F.T. (1980) Trichothio-dystrophy: sulfur-deficient brittle hair as a marker for a neuroectodermal symptom complex. *Archives of Dermatology*, **116**, 1375–84.

48 Itin, P.H., Sarasin, A. and Pittelkow, M.R. (2001) Trichothiodystrophy: update on the sulfur-deficient brittle hair syndromes. *Journal of the American Academy of Dermatology*, **44**, 891–920.

49 Van Neste, D.J., Gillespie, J.M., Marshall, R.C., Taieb, A. and De Brouwer, B. (1993) Morphological and biochemical characteristics of trichothiodystrophy-variant hair are maintained after grafting of scalp specimens on to nude mice. *The British Journal of Dermatology*, **128**, 384–7.

50 Tsambaos, D., Nikiforidis, G., Balas, C. and Marinoni, S. (1994) Trichothio-dystrophic hair reveals an abnormal pattern of viscoelastic parameters. *Skin Pharmacology*, **7**, 257–61.

51 Stefanini, M., Lagomarsini, P., Arlett, C.F., Marinoni, S., Borrone, C., Crovato, F., Trevisan, G., Cordone, G. and Nuzzo, F. (1986) Xeroderma pigmentosum (complementation group D) mutation is present in patients affected by tricho-thiodystrophy with photosensitivity. *Human Genetics*, **74**, 107–12.

52 Nuzzo, F. and Stefanini, M. (1989) The association of xeroderma pigmentosum with trichothiodystrophy: a clue to a better understanding of XP-D? in *DNA Damage and Repair* (ed. A. Castellani), Plenum Press, New York, London, pp. 61–72.

53 Taieb, A., Van Neste, D., Lacombe, D., Mezzina, M. and Sarasin, A. (1994) Bébé collodion d' évolution favorable définissant un nouveau groupe génétique de trichothiodystrophie. *Annales de Dermatologie et de Venereologie*, S80.

54 Weeda, G., Eveno, E., Donker, I., Vermeulen, W., Chevallier-Lagente, O., Taieb, A., Stary, A., Hoeijmakers, J.H., Mezzina, M. and Sarasin, A. (1997) A mutation in the *XPB/ERCC3* DNA repair transcription gene, associated with trichothiodystrophy. *American Journal of Human Genetics*, **60**, 320–9.

55 Stefanini, M., Vermeulen, W., Weeda, G., Giliani, S., Nardo, T., Mezzina, M., Sarasin, A., Harper, J.I., Arlett, C.F. and Hoeijmakers, J.H. (1993) A new nucleotide-excision-repair gene associated with the disorder trichothiodystrophy. *American Journal of Human Genetics*, **53**, 817–21.

56 Giglia-Mari, G., Coin, F., Ranish, J.A., Hoogstraten, D., Theil, A., Wijgers, N., Jaspers, N.G., Raams, A., Argentini, M., van der Spek, P.J., Botta, E., Stefanini, M., Egly, J.M., Aebersold, R., Hoeijmakers, J. H. and Vermeulen, W. (2004) A new, tenth subunit of TFIIH is responsible for the DNA repair syndrome trichothiodystrophy group A. *Nature Genetics*, **36**, 714–19.

57 Lehmann, A.R. (2001) The xeroderma pigmentosum group D (*XPD*) gene: one gene, two functions, three diseases. *Genes & Development*, **15**, 15–23.

58 Taylor, E.M., Broughton, B.C., Botta, E., Stefanini, M., Sarasin, A., Jaspers, N.G., Fawcett, H., Harcourt, S.A., Arlett, C.F. and Lehmann, A.R. (1997) Xeroderma pigmentosum and trichothiodystrophy are associated with different mutations in the *XPD* (ERCC2) repair/transcription gene. *Proceedings of the National Academy of Sciences of the United States of America*, **94**, 8658–63.

59 Bootsma, D. and Hoeijmakers, J.H. (1993) DNA repair. Engagement with transcription. *Nature*, **363**, 114–15.

60 Broughton, B.C., Steingrimsdottir, H., Weber, C.A. and Lehmann, A.R. (1994) Mutations in the xeroderma pigmentosum group D DNA repair/transcription gene in patients with trichothiodystrophy. *Nature Genetics*, **7**, 189–94.

61 Vermeulen, W., van Vuuren, A.J., Chipoulet, M., Schaeffer, L., Appeldoorn, E., Weeda, G., Jaspers, N.G., Priestley, A., Arlett, C.F. and Lehmann, A.R. (1994) Three unusual repair deficiencies associated with transcription factor BTF2(TFIIH): evidence for the existence of a transcription syndrome. *Cold Spring Harbor Symposia on Quantitative Biology*, **59**, 317–29.

62 Broughton, B.C., Berneburg, M., Fawcett, H., Taylor, E.M., Arlett, C.F., Nardo, T., Stefanini, M., Menefee, E., Price, V.H., Queille, S., Sarasin, A., Bohnert, E., Krutmann, J., Davidson, R., Kraemer, K.H. and Lehmann, A.R. (2001) Two individuals with features of both xeroderma pigmentosum and trichothiodystrophy highlight the complexity of the clinical outcomes of mutations in the *XPD* gene. *Human Molecular Genetics*, **10**, 2539–47.

63 Graham, J.M. Jr , Hennekam, R., Dobyns, W.B., Roeder, E. and Busch, D. (2004) MICRO syndrome: an entity distinct from COFS syndrome. *American Journal of Medical Genetics Part A*, **128**, 235–45.

64 Graham, J.M. Jr , Anyane-Yeboa, K., Raams, A., Appeldoorn, E., Kleijer, W.J., Garritsen, V.H., Busch, D., Edersheim, T.G. and Jaspers, N.G. (2001) Cerebro-oculo-facio-skeletal syndrome with a nucleotide excision-repair defect and a mutated *XPD* gene, with prenatal diagnosis in a triplet pregnancy. *American Journal of Human Genetics*, **69**, 291–300.

65 Meira, L.B., Graham, J.M. Jr , Greenberg, C.R., Busch, D.B., Doughty, A.T., Ziffer, D.W., Coleman, D.M., Savre-Train, I. and Friedberg, E.C. (2000) Manitoba aboriginal kindred with original cerebro-oculo- facio-skeletal syndrome has a

mutation in the Cockayne syndrome group B (*CSB*) gene. *American Journal of Human Genetics*, **66**, 1221–8.

66 Johnson, R.E., Kondratick, C.M., Prakash, S. and Prakash, L. (1999) *hRAD30* mutations in the variant form of xeroderma pigmentosum. *Science*, **285**, 263–5.

67 Broughton, B.C., Cordonnier, A., Kleijer, W.J., Jaspers, N.G., Fawcett, H., Raams, A., Garritsen, V.H., Stary, A., Avril, M.F., Boudsocq, F., Masutani, C., Hanaoka, F., Fuchs, R.P., Sarasin, A. and Lehmann, A. R. (2002) Molecular analysis of mutations in DNA polymerase eta in xeroderma pigmentosum-variant patients. *Proceedings of the National Academy of Sciences of the United States of America*, **99**, 815–20.

68 Masutani, C., Kusumoto, R., Yamada, A., Dohmae, N., Yokoi, M., Yuasa, M., Araki, M., Iwai, S., Takio, K. and Hanaoka, F. (1999) The XP-V (xeroderma pigmentosum variant) gene encodes human DNA polymerase eta. *Nature*, **399**, 700–4.

69 Masutani, C., Araki, M., Yamada, A., Kusumoto, R., Nogimori, T., Maekawa, T., Iwai, S. and Hanaoka, F. (1999) Xeroderma pigmentosum variant (XP-V) correcting protein from HeLa cells has a thymine dimer bypass DNA polymerase activity. *EMBO Journal*, **18**, 3491–501.

70 Gratchev, A., Strein, P., Utikal, J. and Goerdt, S. (2003) Molecular genetics of Xeroderma pigmentosum variant. *Experimental Dermatology*, **12**, 529–36.

71 van Steeg, H. and Kraemer, K.H. (1999) Xeroderma pigmentosum and the role of UV-induced DNA damage in skin cancer. *Molecular Medicine Today*, **5**, 86–94.

72 Emmert, S., Kobayashi, N., Khan, S.G. and Kraemer, K.H. (2000) The xeroderma pigmentosum group C gene leads to selective repair of cyclobutane pyrimidine dimers rather than 6-4 photoproducts. *Proceedings of the National Academy of Sciences of the United States of America*, **97**, 2151–6.

73 Khan, S.G., Muniz-Medina, V., Shahlavi, T., Baker, C.C., Inui, H., Ueda, T., Emmert, S., Schneider, T.D. and Kraemer, K.H. (2002) The human *XPC* DNA repair gene: arrangement, splice site information

content and influence of a single
nucleotide polymorphism in a splice
acceptor site on alternative splicing and
function. *Nucleic Acids Research*, **30**,
3624–31.

74 Khan, S.G., Oh, K.S., Shahlavi, T., Ueda,
T., Busch, D.B., Inui, H., Emmert, S.,
Imoto, K., Muniz-Medina, V., Baker, C.
C., DiGiovanna, J.J., Schmidt, D.,
Khadavi, A., Metin, A., Gozukara, E.,
Slor, H., Sarasin, A. and Kraemer, K.H.
(2006) Reduced *XPC* DNA repair gene
mRNA levels in clinically normal parents
of xeroderma pigmentosum patients.
Carcinogenesis, **27**, 84–94.

75 Keeney, S., Chang, G.J. and Linn, S.
(1993) Characterization of a human
DNA damage binding protein implicated
in xeroderma pigmentosum E. *Journal
of Biological Chemistry*, **268**, 21293–300.

76 Wang, Q.E., Zhu, Q., Wani, G., Chen, J.
and Wani, A.A. (2004) UV radiation-
induced *XPC* translocation within
chromatin is mediated by damaged-DNA
binding protein, DDBIX2. *Carcinogenesis*,
25, 1033–43.

77 Fitch, M.E., Nakajima, S., Yasui, A. and
Ford, J.M. (2003) In vivo recruitment of
XPC to UV-induced cyclobutane
pyrimidine dimers by the DDBIX2 gene
product. *Journal of Biological Chemistry*,
278, 46906–10.

78 El-Mahdy, M.A., Zhu, Q., Wang, Q.E.,
Wani, G., Praetorius-Ibba, M. and Wani,
A.A. (2006) Cullin 4A-mediated
proteolysis of DDBIX2 protein at DNA
damage sites regulates *in vivo* lesion
recognition by *XPC*. *Journal of Biological
Chemistry*, **281**, 13404–11.

79 Sugasawa, K., Okuda, Y., Saijo, M.,
Nishi, R., Matsuda, N., Chu, G., Mori, T.,
Iwai, S., Tanaka, K., Tanaka, K. and
Hanaoka, F. (2005) UV-induced
ubiquitylation of XPC protein mediated
by UV-DDB-ubiquitin ligase complex.
Cell, **121**, 387–400.

80 Mu, D. and Sancar, A. (1997) Model for
XPC-independent transcription-coupled
repair of pyrimidine dimers in humans.
Journal of Biological Chemistry, **272**,
7570–3.

81 Selby, C.P., Drapkin, R., Reinberg, D.
and Sancar, A. (1997) RNA polymerase II
stalled at a thymine dimer: footprint and

effect on excision repair. *Nucleic Acids
Research*, **25**, 787–93.

82 Svejstrup, J.Q. (2002) Mechanisms of
transcription-coupled DNA repair. *Nature
Reviews Molecular Cell Biology*, **3**, 21–9.

83 Venema, J., van Hoffen, A., Karcagi, V.,
Natarajan, A.T., van Zeeland, A.A. and
Mullenders, L.H. (1991) Xeroderma
pigmentosum complementation group C
cells remove pyrimidine dimers selectively
from the transcribed strand of active
genes. *Molecular and Cellular Biology*, **11**,
4128–34.

84 van Hoffen, A., Natarajan, A.T., Mayne,
L.V., van Zeeland, A.A., Mullenders, L.H.
and Venema, J. (1993) Deficient repair of
the transcribed strand of active genes in
Cockayne's syndrome cells. *Nucleic Acids
Research*, **21**, 5890–5.

85 Holstege, F.C., van der Vliet, P.C. and
Timmers, H.T. (1996) Opening of an RNA
polymerase II promoter occurs in two
distinct steps and requires the basal
transcription factors IIE and IIH. *EMBO
Journal*, **15**, 1666–77.

86 Riedl, T., Hanaoka, F. and Egly, J.M.
(2003) The comings and goings of
nucleotide excision repair factors on
damaged DNA. *EMBO Journal*, **22**,
5293–303.

87 Missura, M., Buterin, T., Hindges, R.,
Hubscher, U., Kasparkova, J., Brabec, V.
and Naegeli, H. (2001) Double-check
probing of DNA bending and unwinding
by *XPA-RPA*: an architectural function in
DNA repair. *EMBO Journal*, **20**, 3554–64.

88 Matsunaga, T., Mu, D., Park, C.H.,
Reardon, J.T. and Sancar, A. (1995)
Human DNA repair excision nuclease.
Analysis of the roles of the subunits
involved in dual incisions by using anti-
XPG and anti-ERCC1 antibodies. *Journal of
Biological Chemistry*, **270**, 20862–9.

89 Emmert, S., Schneider, T.D., Khan, S.G.
and Kraemer, K.H. (2001) The human
XPG gene: gene architecture, alternative
splicing and single nucleotide polymorphisms. *Nucleic Acids Research*, **29**,
1443–52.

90 Moggs, J.G., Yarema, K.J., Essigmann,
J.M. and Wood, R.D. (1996) Analysis of
incision sites produced by human cell
extracts and purified proteins during
nucleotide excision repair of a 1,3-

intrastrand d(GpTpG)-cisplatin adduct. *Journal of Biological Chemistry*, **271**, 7177–86.

91 Goukassian, D.A., Helms, E., van Steeg, H., van Oostrom, C., Bhawan, J. and Gilchrest, B.A. (2004) Topical DNA oligonucleotide therapy reduces UV-induced mutations and photocarcino-genesis in hairless mice. *Proceedings of the National Academy of Sciences of the United States of America*, **101**, 3933–8.

92 Shivji, M.K., Podust, V.N., Hubscher, U. and Wood, R.D. (1995) Nucleotide

excision repair DNA synthesis by DNA polymerase epsilon in the presence of *PCNA, RFC*, and *RPA. Biochemistry*, **34**, 5011–17.

93 Araujo, S.J., Tirode, F., Coin, F., Pospiech, H., Syvaoja, J.E., Stucki, M., Hubscher, U., Egly, J.M. and Wood, R.D. (2000) Nucleotide excision repair of DNA with recombinant human proteins: definition of the minimal set of factors, active forms of TFIIH, and modulation by CAK. *Genes and Development*, **14**, 349–59.

26
Hereditary Tumors in Children

Simone Fulda

Summary

Cancer predisposition syndromes during infancy are rare and only 1–10% of child-hood malignancies are caused by hereditary factors. A variety of familial and genetic syndromes is associated with an increased risk of cancer during childhood. Known hereditary syndromes account for almost all the excess risk of cancer among first-degree relatives of children with cancer. The genetic basis of cancer predisposition provides many opportunities for the management of patients and their families.

26.1
Introduction

Cancer is a very rare disease among children throughout the world [1, 2]. Child-hood malignancies comprise histologically very diverse entities, while the majority of adult cancers are carcinomas. Therefore, pediatric tumors are usually classified according to histology rather than primary site. The standard scheme is the International Classification of Childhood Cancer [3]. There, diagnostic groups are defined according to codes for morphology as well as topography in the second edition of the International Classification of Diseases for Oncology (ICD-O). The major groups are leukemias and lymphomas, brain and spinal tumors, sympathetic nervous system tumors, retinoblastoma, kidney tumors, liver tumors, bone tumors, soft-tissue sarcomas, gonadal and germ-cell tumors, epithelial tumors, and other and unspecified malignant neoplasms. This review provides an overview of hereditary cancers in childhood.

Hereditary Tumors: From Genes to Clinical Consequences
Edited by Heike Allgayer, Helga Rehder and Simone Fulda
Copyright © 2009 WILEY-VCH Verlag GmbH & Co. KGaA, Weinheim
ISBN: 978-3-527-32028-8

26.2
Familial Neoplastic Syndromes Associated with Childhood Cancer

Among other factors, genetic alterations contribute to carcinogenesis. As far as many childhood cancers are concerned, the age-incidence patterns and cell types of origin point to an origin at latest in utero. For example, studies of monozygotic twins concordant for leukemia and studies performed on neonatal blood spots that analyzed chromosome translocations involved in many childhood leukaemias argue an origin during fetal hematopoiesis [4, 5]. To this end, studies on familial aggregations have provided important insights into the genetic etiology of cancers in children. Pairs of siblings with cancer certainly occur more often than would be expected by chance [6]. Also, the risk of childhood cancer in a sibling of an affected child in the absence of a known family history is approximately twice as high [6]. When cancer does occur in a second sibling, however, this will often be the defining event for the existence of a known syndrome in the respective family. Vice versa, large population-based studies in the Nordic countries revealed that there is virtually no excess risk of cancer in the siblings, parents, or offspring of children with cancer that cannot be accounted for by known hereditary syndromes [7–9]. Therefore, the likelihood of the contribution of any as yet undefined familial syndromes can be considered as very small.

Table 26.1 gives an overview on the most common familial neoplastic syndromes that give rise to an increased risk of childhood cancer. Among these, *retinoblastoma* is the classic example of a malignancy arising in childhood that results from an inherited genetic abnormality. Retinoblastoma is a malignant tumor of the eye that originates from the developing cells of the retina [10]. There are numerous families with more than one generation affected and with more than one member in one generation. In the majority of familial cases, both eyes are affected. By definition, heritable retinoblastoma is any case with bilateral tumors or a family history. Retinoblastoma is the typical example of the two-hit hypothesis of human cancers, as it results from two mutations in the *RBIX1* tumor suppressor gene [11]. In heritable cases, the first of these two mutations is prezygotic and is either inherited or alternatively, a rare germ-cell mutation. By comparison, both mutations are postzygotic in nonheritable cases. The retinoblastoma gene (*RBIX1*) located on chromosome 13 (13q14) was cloned as the first tumor suppressor gene in 1986 [12]. The pattern of inheritance of familial retinoblastoma is autosomal dominant. The penetrance is very high with about 90% where an affected parent has bilateral tumors. Somewhat lower is the penetrance in the rare cases of unilateral heritable retinoblastoma. Since the survival rate from retinoblastoma has been very high for many decades in sharp contrast to other pediatric malignancies, several families affected with retinoblastoma in multiple generations had already been reported half a century ago. It is interesting to note that survivors have a remarkably high risk of developing further primary tumors, many of which cannot be directly linked to treatment received for retinoblastoma. For example, the incidence of osteosarcoma is markedly elevated compared to the general population and occurs mainly in the first three decades [13, 14]. The

Table 26.1 Familial neoplastic syndromes associated with childhood cancer.

Syndrome	Inheritance	Locus	Gene	Childhood cancers
Familial retinoblastoma	AD	13q14	*RB1*	Retinoblastoma, osteosarcoma
Familial Wilms' tumor	AD	17q1221	*FWT1*	Wilms' tumor
Familial Wilms' tumor 2	AD	19q13	*FWT2*	Wilms' tumor
Li–Fraumeni syndrome	AD	17p13	*TP53*	Adrenocortical carcinoma,
	AD	22q12	*CHK2*	Soft-tissue sarcoma,
	AD	22q11	*SNF5*	Osteosarcoma, CNS tumors
Multiple endocrine neoplasia type 2B	AD	10q11	*RET 1*	Medullary thyroid carcinoma
Neurofibromatosis type 1	AD	17q11	*NF*	Astrocytoma, JMML, ALL, rhabdomyosarcoma, MPNST
Neurofibromatosis type 2	AD	22q12	*NF2*	Meningioma
	AD	3p21	*MLH1*	
	AD	7p22	*PMS2*	
Hereditary nonpolyposis colon cancer	AD	2p22-21	*MSH2*	Glioma
Familial adenomatous polyposis	AD	5q21	*APC*	Medulloblastoma, hepatoblastoma
Gorlin syndrome	AD	9q31	*PTCH*	Medulloblastoma, basal cell carcinoma

increased risk of developing subsequent unrelated malignancies continues also later in life, although the specific types of cancer change with advancing age. In adulthood, the excess risk is especially high for malignant melanoma and for lung and bladder carcinoma [15, 16].

Compared to retinoblastoma, familial aggregations of other characteristic embryonal tumors of childhood are relatively rare. To give an example, only 1.5% of 6209 children with *Wilms' tumor*, a malignant tumor of the kidney, in the National Wilms' Tumor Study (NWTS) in the US had a family history of the disease [17]. In Wilms' tumors, bilateral disease represents a much smaller proportion of total cases than in retinoblastoma [17]. In addition, family history of the same tumor is also much rarer in Wilms' tumors compared to retinoblastoma [17]. Although the proportion of familial cases is anticipated to rise because of increased survival, it will always be small compared to familial retinoblastoma [18]. There are at least three familial Wilms' tumor susceptibility genes, the best known being *WT1* [19].

Familial aggregations of *neuroblastoma* are even less frequent than in retinoblastoma or Wilms' tumor. Neuroblastoma is the most common extracranial solid cancer in infancy arising from the sympathetic nervous system [20]. While several chromosomal regions have been investigated, no candidate region or gene has yet been linked to familial neuroblastoma [21].

The *Li–Fraumeni* cancer family syndrome (LFS) was first identified in children with the diagnosis of rhabdomyosarcoma. By definition, LFS is a patient with sarcoma diagnosed before the age of 45 years, a first-degree relative with any cancer also before the age of 45 years, and another first or second-degree relative with sarcoma at any age or any cancer before the age of 45 years [22]. Malignancies that are characteristic of LFS comprise soft-tissue sarcomas, adrenocortical carcinoma, central nervous system tumors, premenopausal breast carcinoma, and osteosarcoma. The relative risk of childhood cancer is about 20. By comparison, Li–Fraumeni-like syndrome (LFL) is defined as a patient with any tumor before the age of 45 years, or a sarcoma, brain tumor or adrenocortical tumor before the age of 45 years, together with a first-or second-degree relative with a typical LFS tumor at any age, and another first-or second-degree relative with any cancer before the age of 60 years [23]. Germline mutations of the tumor suppressor gene *p53* have been detected in 77% of LFS and 40% of LFL families in the largest single study [24]. In cases of LFS in which no *p53* mutation were found, it has been argued that this could be due to failure of detection. However, some LFS or LFL families have been found to have germline mutations of other genes, including *CHK2* and *SNF5* [25, 26]. Interestingly, mutations of *SNF5* have been particularly associated with choroid plexus tumors and atypical teratoid rhabdoid tumors of the brain [27, 28].

Medullary thyroid carcinoma is another malignancy that may arise during childhood in families with multiple endocrine neoplasia type 2 (*MEN2*) [29]. This particular type of thyroid carcinoma has been linked to a mutation in the proto-oncogene *RET* [30].

Children with *neurofibromatosis type 1* (NF1) have an increased risk of several types of childhood cancer. CNS tumors, especially astrocytoma, are the most frequent among them. For example, the risk of optic nerve glioma (astrocytoma) by age 15 years among children with NF1 is markedly increased up to 4–5% [31]. Besides CNS tumors, there is a similar relative risk for soft-tissue sarcomas, with the excess accounted for by malignant peripheral nerve sheath tumors and rhabdomyosarcoma [29]. *Neurofibromatosis type 2* (NF2) accounts for a much lower proportion of childhood cancer than NF1. The most commonly associated CNS tumors are meningiomas.

Turcot's syndrome includes two distinct groups of patients with brain tumors and colorectal polyposis or cancer [32]. The first encompasses children with gliomas, usually high-grade astrocytomas, and colorectal adenomas without polyposis, and their siblings with glioma and/or colorectal adenoma. The risk of a brain tumor in members of families with hereditary nonpolyposis colorectal cancer is about five times that in the general population [33]. The second group encompasses children with brain tumors that are usually medulloblastomas and occur in members of familial adenomatous polyposis (FAP) families. Hepatoblastoma is about 100 times commoner in FAP families than in the general population [34].

The proportion of childhood medulloblastoma due to *Gorlin syndrome* is 2–3% [35]. A characteristic feature of these medulloblastoma is their desmoplastic subtype [35, 36].

26.3
Non-Neoplastic Genetic Syndromes Associated with Childhood Cancer

Besides these familial neoplastic syndromes that are associated with childhood cancers, there are also some non-neoplastic genetic syndromes that harbor an increased risk of cancer occurrence during childhood (Table 26.2).

Among these, two syndromes that involve the Wilms' tumor suppressor gene *WT1* are probably the best known ones. Over one third of children with *Wilms' tumor, Aniridia, Genitourinary Anomalies and Mental Retardation (WAGR) syndrome* develop Wilms' tumor [37]. Patients with WAGR syndrome develop Wilms' tumor in addition to aniridia, genitourinary abnormalities, and mental retardation. A much higher risk of Wilms' tumor is also found in patients with *Denys–Drash syndrome* [37]. Both syndromes usually occur sporadically. Also associated with Wilms' tumor are the *Simpson–Golabi–Behmel syndrome* and the *Perlman syndrome* [38, 39].

Beckwith–Wiedemann syndrome is the most common overgrowth syndrome that is linked to childhood cancer [40]. The most frequent type of cancer for children with Beckwith–Wiedemann syndrome is Wilms' tumor [40, 41]. In addition, the risk of developing hepatoblastoma, neuroblastoma, and pancreatoblastoma is increased in these patients [40, 41]. The cumulative cancer risk for one of these cancers is elevated up to 10% by age 4 years [40]. Moreover, hemihypertrophy, as part of the Beckwith–Wiedemann syndrome or alone, is associated with Wilms' tumor, adrenocortical carcinoma, and hepatoblastoma [42]. Rhabdomyosarcoma and bladder carcinoma are the typical types of cancers that may arise in children with *Costello syndrome* [43]. Patients with *tuberous sclerosis* typically develop brain tumors in childhood [44, 45]. Hepatocellular carcinoma is characteristically seen in children with *tyrosinaemia* [46]. For *Sotos syndrome*, no uniform pattern of malignancies can be listed, since a wide variety of childhood cancers has been associated with this syndrome [47, 48].

Table 26.2 Non-neoplastic genetic syndromes associated with childhood cancers.

Syndrome	Inheritance	Locus	Gene	Childhood cancers
WAGR syndrome	Sporadic	11p13	*WT1*	Wilms' tumor
Denys–Drash syndrome	Sporadic	11p13	*WT1*	Wilms' tumor
Simpson–Golabi–Behmel syndrome	X-linked	Xq26	*GPC3*	Wilms' tumor
Perlman syndrome	?	11p	?	Wilms' tumor
Beckwith–Wiedemann syndrome	Sporadic/AD	11p15	Complex	Wilms' tumor, hepatoblastoma, neuroblastoma, pancreatoblastoma
Costello syndrome	AD	11p15?a	?	Rhabdomyosarcoma, bladder carcinoma
Tuberous sclerosis	AD	9q34	*TSC1*	Subependymal giant cell astrocytoma
		16p13	*TSC2*	
Tyrosinaemia	AR	15q23-25	*FAH*	Hepatocellular carcinoma
Sotos syndrome	Sporadic	5q35	*NSD1*	Various

Table 26.3 Numerical chromosome abnormalities associated with childhood cancers.

Syndrome	Childhood cancers
Down syndrome (Trisomy 21)	Leukaemia, germ-cell tumors
Trisomy 18	Wilms' tumor
Turner syndrome (45,X)	Neuroblastoma, Wilms' tumor
Klinefelter syndrome (47,XXY)	Germ-cell tumors

26.4
Numerical Chromosome Abnormalities Associated with Childhood Cancer

There are several numerical chromosome abnormalities that harbor an increased risk of childhood cancer (Table 26.3). *Down syndrome* is not only the best known of these, but also accounts for the largest number of cases. To this end, markedly elevated relative risks of leukemia have been reported with an up to 50-fold rise in the first 5 years of life and a 10-fold increase in the next 10 years [49, 50]. The most common form of leukemia in children with Down syndrome is ALL followed by AML. What is less well known is that there is also an increased risk of germ-cell tumors in these patients [49, 51, 52]. *Trisomy 18* is characterized by a higher risk of Wilms' tumor than expected [53]. Neuroblastoma and Wilms' tumor may arise more frequently in patients with *Turner syndrome* [54, 55], however, the evidence for this association needs to be confirmed by large studies. Germ-cell tumors, especially those localized in the mediastinum, may point to *Klinefelter syndrome* [56].

26.5
Inherited Immune Deficiency Syndromes Associated with Childhood Cancer

It is also known that the risk of childhood cancer is elevated in several inherited immune deficiency syndromes (Table 26.4). In particular, such patients carry an increased risk of developing lymphomas and leukemias. However, since inherited immune deficiency syndromes are rare, these malignancies account only for a very small proportion of all childhood cancers. The most frequent type of inherited immune deficiency syndrome that is associated with childhood cancer is *Ataxia*

Table 26.4 Inherited immunodeficiency syndromes associated with childhood cancer.

Syndrome	Inheritance	Locus	Gene	Childhood cancers
Ataxia telangiectasia	AR	11q22	*ATM*	Lymphoma, leukaemia
Wiskott–Aldrich syndrome	X-linked	Xp11	*WAS*	NHL
Bloom syndrome	AR	15q26	*BLM*	NHL, Wilms' tumor, osteosarcoma
Common variable immunodeficiency	Various	Various	Various	Lymphoma
X-linked agammaglobulinaemia	X-linked	Xq21-22	*BTK*	Lymphoma
IgA deficiency	AD	6p21	*IGAD1*	Lymphoma
Severe combined immunodeficiency	X-linked	Xq13	*IL2RG*	Lymphoma
Duncan disease	X-linked	Xq25	Various	Lymphoma
Nijmegen breakage syndrome	AR	8q21	*NBS1*	NHL

telangiectasia. In this disease, more than 10% of affected children develop leukemia or lymphoma before 15 years [57]. *Wiskott–Aldrich syndrome* is known for a higher risk of Non-Hodgkin Lymphoma (NHL) [58]. The relative risk of leukemia and NHL is also increased in a number of rare syndromes, including *Bloom syndrome, common variable immunodeficiency syndrome, X-linked agammaglobulinaemia, IgA deficiency, severe combined immunodeficiency* (SCID), *Duncan's disease,* and *Nijmegen breakage syndrome* [59–61]. In patients with Bloom syndrome, Wilms' tumor and osteosarcoma are unusual tumors that may occasionally occur [60]. In a gene therapy trial for children with SCID, 20% developed T-cell ALL, possibly due to insertional oncogenesis [62].

26.6
Inherited Bone Marrow Failure Syndromes Associated with Childhood Cancer

There are also several inherited bone marrow failure syndromes that have been linked to an increased risk of childhood cancer (Table 26.5), for example, *Fanconi anemia, Diamond–Blackfan anemia* and *Shwachman–Diamond syndrome.* Patients with Fanconi anemia harbor an increased risk of AML or myelodysplasia [63, 64]. There are some indications that children with Diamond–Blackfan anemia have an elevated risk of AML and osteosarcoma [65]. Shwachman-Diamond syndrome has been reported to show an increased risk of AML [66].

Table 26.5 Inherited bone marrow failure syndromes associated with childhood cancer.

Syndrome	Inheritance	Locus	Gene	Childhood cancers
Fanconi anemia	AR	16q24	*FANCA*	AML
Diamond–Blackfan anemia	Various	Various	Various	AML
Shwachman–Diamond syndrome	AR	7q11	*SBDS*	Myelodysplasia

26.7
Conclusions

Overall, childhood cancer is rare everywhere in the world and even less frequent are cases that can be accounted for by known hereditary syndromes. Over recent decades, there have been rapid advances in our understanding of the molecular basis of inherited cancer susceptibility syndromes in childhood. Genetic testing is available for many conditions and is an important aspect in the care of patients and their families. In many cases, this will improve the management of relatives that are at risk or provide information about the possible course of the disease. These advancements are likely to provide long-term benefits for families affected by hereditary cancer syndromes.

References

1 McGregor, L.M., Metzger, M.L., Sanders, R. and Santana, V.M. (2007) Pediatric cancers in the new millennium: dramatic progress, new challenges. *Oncology (Williston)*, **21**, 809–20.

2 Parkin, D.M., KramaÂrovaÂ, E., Draper, G.J., Masuyer, E., Michaelis, J. and Neglia, J. (1998) *International Incidence of Childhood Cancer, Vol. II. IARC Scientific Publication no. 144*, Vol. **246**, IARC, Lyon.

3 Kramarova, E. and Stiller, C.A. (1996) The international classification of childhood cancer. *International Journal of Cancer*, **68**, 759–65.

4 Greaves, M.F., Maia, A.T., Wiemels, J.L. and Ford, A.M. (2003) Leukemia in twins: lessons in natural history. *Blood*, **102**, 2321–33.

5 Greaves, M.F. and Wiemels, J. (2003) Origins of chromosome translocations in childhood leukaemia. *Nature Reviews Cancer*, **3**, 639–49.

6 Draper, G.J., Heaf, M.M. and Kinnier Wilson, L.M. (1977) Occurrence of childhood cancers among sibs and estimation of familial risks. *Journal of Medical Genetics*, **14**, 81–90.

7 Olsen, J.H., Boice, J.D. Jr, Seersholm, N., Bautz, A. and Fraumeni, J.F. Jr (1995) Cancer in the parents of children with cancer. *New England Journal of Medicine*, **333**, 1594–9.

8 Sankila, R., Olsen, J.H., Anderson, H., Garwicz, S., Glattre, E., Hertz, H., Langmark, F., Lanning, M., Moller, T. and Tulinius, H. (1998) Risk of cancer among offspring of childhood-cancer survivors. Association of the Nordic Cancer Registries and the Nordic Society of Paediatric Haematology and Oncology. *New England Journal of Medicine*, **338**, 1339–44.

9 Winther, J.F., Sankila, R., Boice, J.D., Tulinius, H., Bautz, A., Barlow, L., Glattre, E., Langmark, F., Moller, T.R., Mulvihill, J.J., Olafsdottir, G.H., Ritvanen, A. and Olsen, J.H. (2001) Cancer in siblings of children with cancer in the Nordic countries: a population-based cohort study. *Lancet*, **358**, 711–17.

10 Lohmann, D.R. and Gallie, B.L. (2004) Retinoblastoma: revisiting the model prototype of inherited cancer. *American Journal of Medical Genetics Part C, Seminars in Medical Genetics*, **129**, 23–8.

11 Knudson, A.G. Jr (1971) Mutation and cancer: statistical study of retinoblastoma. *Proceedings of the National Academy of Sciences of the United States of America*, **68**, 820–3.

12 Friend, S.H., Bernards, R., Rogelj, S., Weinberg, R.A., Rapaport, J.M., Albert, D. M. and Dryja, T.P. (1986) A human DNA segment with properties of the gene that predisposes to retinoblastoma and osteosarcoma. *Nature*, **323**, 643–6.

13 Draper, G.J., Sanders, B.M. and Kingston, J.E. (1986) Second primary neoplasms in patients with retinoblastoma. *British Journal of Cancer*, **53**, 661–71.

14 Wong, F.L., Boice, J.D. Jr, Abramson, D.H., Tarone, R.E., Kleinerman, R.A., Stovall, M., Goldman, M.B., Seddon, J.M., Tarbell, N., Fraumeni, J.F. Jr and Li, F.P. (1997) Cancer incidence after retino-blastoma. Radiation dose and sarcoma risk. *The Journal of the American Medical Association*, **278**, 1262–7.

15 Sanders, B.M., Jay, M., Draper, G.J. and Roberts, E.M. (1989) Non-ocular cancer in relatives of retinoblastoma patients. *British Journal of Cancer*, **60**, 358–65.

16 Kleinerman, R.A., Tarone, R.E., Abramson, D.H., Seddon, J.M., Li, F.P. and Tucker, M.A. (2000) Hereditary retinoblastoma and risk of lung cancer. *Journal of the National Cancer Institute*, **92**, 2037–9.

17 Breslow, N.E., Olson, J., Moksness, J., Beckwith, J.B. and Grundy, P. (1996) Familial Wilms' tumor: a descriptive study. *Medical and Pediatric Oncology*, **27**, 398–403.

18 Li, F.P., Williams, W.R., Gimbrere, K., Flamant, F., Green, D.M. and Meadows, A.T. (1988) Heritable fraction of unilateral Wilms tumor. *Pediatrics*, **81**, 147–9.

19 Rapley, E.A., Barfoot, R., Bonaiti-Pellie, C., Chompret, A., Foulkes, W., Perusinghe, N., Reeve, A., Royer-Pokora, B., Schumacher, V., Shelling, A., Skeen, J.,

de Tourreil, S., Weirich, A., Pritchard-Jones, K., Stratton, M.R. and Rahman, N. (2000) Evidence for susceptibility genes to familial Wilms tumour in addition to WT1, FWT1 and FWT2. *British Journal of Cancer*, **83**, 177–83.

20 Brodeur, G.M. (2003) Neuroblastoma: biological insights into a clinical enigma. *Nature Reviews Cancer*, **3**, 203–16.

21 Perri, P., Longo, L., McConville, C., Cusano, R., Rees, S.A., Seri, M., Conte, M., Romeo, G., Devoto, M. and Tonini, G.P. (2002) Linkage analysis in families with recurrent neuroblastoma. *Annals of the New York Academy of Sciences*, **963**, 74–84.

22 Li, F.P., Fraumeni, J.F. Jr, Mulvihill, J.J., Blattner, W.A., Dreyfus, M.G., Tucker, M.A. and Miller, R.W. (1988) A cancer family syndrome in twenty-four kindreds. *Cancer Research*, **48**, 5358–62.

23 Birch, J.M., Hartley, A.L., Tricker, K.J., Prosser, J., Condie, A., Kelsey, A.M., Harris, M., Jones, P.H., Binchy, A., Crowther, D. *et al.* (1994) Prevalence and diversity of constitutional mutations in the *p53* gene among 21 Li–Fraumeni families. *Cancer Research*, **54**, 1298–304.

24 Varley, J.M. (2003) Germline *TP53* mutations and Li–Fraumeni. Syndrome. *Human Mutation*, **21**, 313–20.

25 Bell, D.W., Varley, J.M., Szydlo, T.E., Kang, D.H., Wahrer, D.C., Shannon, K.E., Lubratovich, M., Verselis, S.J., Isselbacher, K.J., Fraumeni, J.F., Birch, J.M., Li, F.P., Garber, J.E. and Haber, D.A. (1999) Heterozygous germ line *hCHK2* mutations in Li- Fraumeni syndrome. *Science*, **286**, 2528–31.

26 Sevenet, N., Sheridan, E., Amram, D., Schneider, P., Handgretinger, R. and Delattre, O. (1999) Constitutional mutations of the *hSNF5/INI1* gene predispose to a variety of cancers. *American Journal of Human Genetics*, **65**, 1342–8.

27 Biegel, J.A., Zhou, J.Y., Rorke, L.B., Stenstrom, C., Wainwright, L.M. and Fogelgren, B. (1999) Germ-line and acquired mutations of *INI1* in atypical teratoid and rhabdoid tumors. *Cancer Research*, **59**, 74–9.

28 Taylor, M.D., Gokgoz, N., Andrulis, I.L., Mainprize, T.G., Drake, J.M. and Rutka, J.T. (2000) Familial posterior fossa brain tumors of infancy secondary to germline mutation of the *hSNF5* gene. *American Journal of Human Genetics*, **66**, 1403–6.

29 Narod, S.A., Stiller, C. and Lenoir, G.M. (1991) An estimate of the heritable fraction of childhood cancer. *British Journal of Cancer*, **63**, 993–9.

30 Marsh, D.J., Mulligan, L.M. and Eng, C. (1997) RET proto-oncogene mutations in multiple endocrine neoplasia type 2 and medullary thyroid carcinoma. *Hormone Research*, **47**, 168–78.

31 McGaughran, J.M., Harris, D.I., Donnai, D., Teare, D., MacLeod, R., Westerbeek, R., Kingston, H., Super, M., Harris, R. and Evans, D.G. (1999) A clinical study of type 1 neurofibromatosis in north west England. *Journal of Medical Genetics*, **36**, 197–203.

32 Paraf, F., Jothy, S. and Van Meir, E.G. (1997) Brain tumor-polyposis syndrome: two genetic diseases? *Journal of Clinical Oncology*, **15**, 2744–58.

33 Vasen, H.F., Sanders, E.A., Taal, B.G., Nagengast, F.M., Griffioen, G., Menko, F.H., Kleibeuker, J.H., Houwing-Duistermaat, J.J. and Meera Khan, P. (1996) The risk of brain tumours in hereditary non-polyposis colorectal cancer (HNPCC). *International Journal of Cancer*, **65**, 422–5.

34 Garber, J.E., Li, F.P., Kingston, J.E., Krush, A.J., Strong, L.C., Finegold, M.J., Bertario, L., Bulow, S., Filippone, A. Jr, Gedde-Dahl, T. Jr, *et al.* (1988) Hepatoblastoma and familial adenomatous polyposis. *Journal of the National Cancer Institute*, **80**, 1626–8.

35 Cowan, R., Hoban, P., Kelsey, A., Birch, J.M., Gattamaneni, R. and Evans, D.G. (1997) The gene for the naevoid basal cell carcinoma syndrome acts as a tumour-suppressor gene in medulloblastoma. *British Journal of Cancer*, **76**, 141–5.

36 Amlashi, S.F.A., Riffaud, L., Brassier, G. and Morandi, X. (2003) Nevoid basal cell carcinoma syndrome: relation with desmoplastic medulloblastoma in infancy. A population-based study and review of the literature. *Cancer*, **98**, 618–24.

37 Coppes, M.J., Haber, D.A. and Grundy, P.E. (1994) Genetic events in the development of Wilms' tumor. *New England Journal of Medicine*, **331**, 586–90.

38 Lindsay, S., Ireland, M., O'Brien, O., Clayton-Smith, J., Hurst, J.A., Mann, J., Cole, T., Sampson, J., Slaney, S., Schlessinger, D., Burn, J. and Pilia, G. (1997) Large scale deletions in the *GPC3* gene may account for a minority of cases of Simpson–Golabi–Behmel syndrome. *Journal of Medical Genetics*, **34**, 480–3.

39 Henneveld, H.T., van Lingen, R.A., Hamel, B.C., Stolte-Dijkstra, I. and van Essen, A.J. (1999) Perlman syndrome: four additional cases and review. *American Journal of Medical Genetics*, **86**, 439–46.

40 DeBaun, M.R. and Tucker, M.A. (1998) Risk of cancer during the first four years of life in children from The Beckwith–Wiedemann Syndrome Registry. *Journal of Pediatrics*, **132**, 398–400.

41 Drut, R. and Jones, M.C. (1988) Congenital pancreatoblastoma in Beckwith–Wiedemann syndrome: an emerging association. *Pediatric Pathology*, **8**, 331–9.

42 Sotelo-Avila, C., Gonzalez-Crussi, F. and Fowler, J.W. (1980) Complete and incomplete forms of Beckwith–Wiedemann syndrome: their oncogenic potential. *Journal of Pediatrics*, **96**, 47–50.

43 Gripp, K.W., Scott, C.I. Jr, Nicholson, L., McDonald-McGinn, D.M., Ozeran, J.D., Jones, M.C., Lin, A.E. and Zackai, E.H. (2002) Five additional Costello syndrome patients with rhabdomyosarcoma: proposal for a tumor screening protocol. *American Journal of Medical Genetics*, **108**, 80–7.

44 Webb, D.W., Fryer, A.E. and Osborne, J.P. (1996) Morbidity associated with tuberous sclerosis: a population study. *Developmental Medicine and Child Neurology*, **38**, 146–55.

45 Lindor, N.M. and Greene, M.H. (1998) The concise handbook of family cancer syndromes. Mayo Familial Cancer Program. *Journal of the National Cancer Institute*, **90**, 1039–71.

46 Weinberg, A.G., Mize, C.E. and Worthen, H.G. (1976) The occurrence of hepatoma in the chronic form of hereditary tyrosinemia. *Journal of Pediatrics*, **88**, 434–8.

47 Hersh, J.H., Cole, T.R., Bloom, A.S., Bertolone, S.J. and Hughes, H.E. (1992) Risk of malignancy in Sotos syndrome. *Journal of Pediatrics*, **120**, 572–4.

48 Opitz, J.M., Weaver, D.W. and Reynolds, J.F. Jr (1998) The syndromes of Sotos and Weaver: reports and review. *American Journal of Medical Genetics*, **79**, 294–304.

49 Hasle, H., Clemmensen, I.H. and Mikkelsen, M. (2000) Risks of leukaemia and solid tumours in individuals with Down's syndrome. *Lancet*, **355**, 165–9.

50 Hermon, C., Alberman, E., Beral, V. and Swerdlow, A.J. (2001) Mortality and cancer incidence in persons with Down's syndrome, their parents and siblings. *Annals of Human Genetics*, **65**, 167–76.

51 Hasle, H. (2001) Pattern of malignant disorders in individuals with Down's syndrome. *The Lancet Oncology*, **2**, 429–36.

52 Satge, D., Sasco, A.J., Carlsen, N.L., Stiller, C.A., Rubie, H., Hero, B., de Bernardi, B., de Kraker, J., Coze, C., Kogner, P., Langmark, F., Hakvoort-Cammel, F.G., Beck, D., von der Weid, N., Parkes, S., Hartmann, O., Lippens, R.J., Kamps, W.A. and Sommelet, D. (1998) A lack of neuroblastoma in Down syndrome: a study from 11 European countries. *Cancer Research*, **58**, 448–52.

53 Olson, J.M., Hamilton, A. and Breslow, N.E. (1995) Non-11p constitutional chromosome abnormalities in Wilms' tumor patients. *Medical and Pediatric Oncology*, **24**, 305–9.

54 Blatt, J., Olshan, A.F., Lee, P.A. and Ross, J.L. (1997) Neuroblastoma and related tumors in Turner's syndrome. *Journal of Pediatrics*, **131**, 666–670.

55 Swerdlow, A.J., Hermon, C., Jacobs, P.A., Alberman, E., Beral, V., Daker, M., Fordyce, A. and Youings, S. (2001) Mortality and cancer incidence in persons with numerical sex chromosome abnormalities: a cohort study. *Annals of Human Genetics*, **65**, 177–88.

56 Hasle, H., Mellemgaard, A., Nielsen, J. and Hansen, J. (1995) Cancer incidence in men with Klinefelter syndrome. *British Journal of Cancer*, **71**, 416–20.

57 Morrell, D., Cromartie, E. and Swift, M. (1986) Mortality and cancer incidence in 263 patients with ataxia-telangiectasia. *Journal of the National Cancer Institute*, **77**, 89–92.

58 Sullivan, K.E., Mullen, C.A., Blaese, R.M. and Winkelstein, J.A. (1994) A multiinstitutional survey of the Wiskott–Aldrich syndrome. *Journal of Pediatrics*, **125**, 876–85.

59 Mueller, B.U. and Pizzo, P.A. (1995) Cancer in children with primary or secondary immunodeficiencies. *Journal of Pediatrics*, **126**, 1–10.

60 German, J. (1997) Bloom's syndrome. XX. The first 100 cancers. *Cancer Genetics and Cytogenetics*, **93**, 100–6.

61 The International Nijmegen Breakage Syndrome Study Group (2000) Nijmegen breakage syndrome. *Archives of Disease in Childhood*, **82**, 400–6.

62 Kohn, D.B., Sadelain, M. and Glorioso, J.C. (2003) Occurrence of leukaemia following gene therapy of X-linked SCID. *Nature Reviews Cancer*, **3**, 477–88.

63 Kutler, D.I., Singh, B., Satagopan, J., Batish, S.D., Berwick, M., Giampietro, P.F., Hanenberg, H. and Auerbach, A.D. (2003) A 20-year perspective on the International Fanconi Anemia Registry (IFAR). *Blood*, **101**, 1249–56.

64 Rosenberg, N.A., Pritchard, J.K., Weber, J.L., Cann, H.M., Kidd, K.K., Zhivotovsky, L.A. and Feldman, M.W. (2002) Genetic structure of human populations. *Science*, **298**, 2381–5.

65 Lipton, J.M., Federman, N., Khabbaze, Y., Schwartz, C.L., Hilliard, L.M., Clark, J.I., Vlachos, A. (2001) Osteogenic sarcoma associated with Diamond-Blackfan anemia: a report from the Diamond-Blackfan Anemia Registry. *Journal of Pediatric Hematology/Oncology*, **23**, 39–44.

66 Dror, Y. and Freedman, M.H. (2002) Shwachman–Diamond syndrome. *British Journal of Haematology*, **118**, 701–13.

27
Sarcomas and Bone Tumors in Adulthood

Eva Wardelmann

Summary

As for sporadic tumors, recent studies have improved our understanding of the genetic background of hereditary tumors of soft tissue and bone. A large number of syndromes associated with neoplasms is well-known and is becoming more precisely characterized. The knowledge of the Mendelian inheritance of different diseases is the prerequisite for counseling of patients and relatives to prevent life-threatening stages of disease by early recognition and appropriate treatment. Furthermore, the knowledge of which pathways might be involved in the development of specific soft tissue and bone tumors will probably help to also better understand sporadic tumors.

The minority of bone and soft tissue tumors is due to inherited susceptibility, often associated with syndromes. In the following chapter, several syndromes with known or highly suspected underlying genetic causes are described, whereas rare groups with a very low incidence are not. As such, the list is not complete and preferentially comprises the most common syndromes. The overlap with other chapters concerning familial syndromes is not avoidable, but this chapter focuses on the tumor manifestations in soft tissue and bone.

27.1
Epidemiology

27.1.1
Incidence of Soft Tissue and Bone Sarcomas in General

Soft tissue tumors amount to less than 1% of all malignant tumors, with an annual incidence of up to 30 per million. The frequency of bone tumors, with 0.2% of all neoplasms, is even lower [1] (http://seer.cancer.gov/csr/1975_2004/, based on the November 2006 SEER data submission, posted to the SEER web site, 2007). Comparing the subgroup of bone sarcomas (BS) with soft tissue sarcomas (STS),

Hereditary Tumors: From Genes to Clinical Consequences
Edited by Heike Allgayer, Helga Rehder and Simone Fulda
Copyright © 2009 WILEY-VCH Verlag GmbH & Co. KGaA, Weinheim
ISBN: 978-3-527-32028-8

the first may occur at a rate of approximately one-tenth of the latter. In both groups, benign tumors of soft tissue and bone by far outnumber malignant lesions.

27.1.2
Mortality

The mortality in STS and BS highly depends on the histomorphological subtype and, as in other malignancies, on the stage at primary diagnosis. More details are given with the different tumor entities.

27.1.3
Proportion of Hereditary Tumors

The number of cases with STS or BS, occurring on a familial or inherited basis, is low. However, the intensive study of underlying genetic predispositions may highlight the pathogenesis of sporadic tumors also, which seems worthwhile, especially considering there is little knowledge about the nature of both tumor groups. Furthermore, bone tumors occurring in a syndromal or familial setting during childhood may be precursors of BS in adults, the risk depending on the underlying syndrome. For example, whereas enchondromatosis and the familial retinoblastoma syndrome are associated with a high risk, other lesions such as polyostotic Paget disease or multiple osteochondromas are thought to be correlated with a moderate, and fibrous dysplasia with a low risk of malignant transformation.

27.2
Syndromes

Familial adenomatous polyposis (FAP, Gardner's syndrome) is described in detail elsewhere in this book (see also Chapter 16 on gastrintestinal polyposis syndromes). Its estimated frequency is between 1 : 7000 and 1 : 30 000. Besides the occurrence of multiple colorectal polyps with an increasing risk to progress to colorectal cancer, polyps may also develop in the upper gastrointestinal tract and malignancies may occur at other sites such as brain or thyroid. Furthermore, more than 50% of patients develop abnormalities in the facial bones (such as dental abnormalities and osteomas) and, in a much lower percentage, fibromatoses from the desmoid type (Figure 27.1). Furthermore, since the first description of Gardner's syndrome in the 1950s, there have been numerous descriptions of other associated soft tissue or bone tumors such as lipomas [2], fibrous dysplastic lesions [3], familial infiltrative fibromatosis [4], fibromatous mesenteric plaques similar to Gardner's fibroma [5, 6], juvenile nasopharyngeal angiofibroma [7], and rhabdomyosarcoma [8].

The frequency of **desmoid fibromatosis** associated with FAP is estimated to be around 10%. Numerous studies have recognized this association [9–12]. Distinct

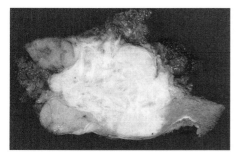

Figure 27.1 Macroscopic aspect of a desmoid tumor: whorled fibrous cut surface at cut margins and poorly defined margins to the surrounding skeletal muscle.

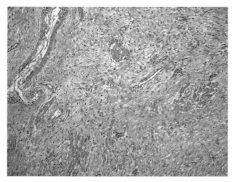

Figure 27.2 Microscopic findings in an abdominal fibromatosis: spindled or stellated cells with bland nuclei (HE, 20 × obj.).

mutational subtypes in the APC gene are associated with a higher frequency of desmoids whereas mutations in the β-Catenin gene are frequently found in sporadic forms of fibromatosis [13]. The nuclear expression of β-Catenin as detectable by immunohistochemistry is one major diagnostic parameter to divide fibromatosis from other spindle cell tumors (Figures 27.2 and 27.3). Gardner's fibroma is now recognized as an initial event often preceding the development of adenomatous polyps and sometimes coincides with fibromatosis. A subgroup of patients presenting with familial infiltrative fibromatosis also carry germline mutations in the APC gene but lack colonic polyps. For lesions such as nasopharyngeal angiofibroma and rhabdomyosarcoma [14], it is still not clear whether these tumors occur as part of the syndrome or if they are sporadic.

Bone tumors occurring in association with FAP are benign and thought to be dysplasias rather than true neoplasms, since they never evolve into other bone tumors such as osteoblastomas or BS. Osteomas consist of mature lamellar bone developing in the flat bones of the head, and again are often associated with

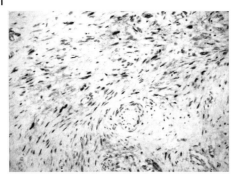

Figure 27.3 Strong nuclear immunohistochemical expression of β-Catenin in fibromatosis (Transduction Laboratories, Lexington, KY, USA; 20 × obj.).

particular APC mutational subtypes [15]. APC gene mutations in FAP are inherited autosomally dominant with an almost complete penetrance. About 20% of patients are thought to carry *de novo* mutations because of no family history [16]. More details about function and mutations of the *APC* gene can be found in Chapter 16 of this book.

The **Beckwith–Wiedemann syndrome** (BWS) is also termed EMG (exomphalus-macroglossa-gigantism syndrome) syndrome. Elliot and DeBaun [17, 18] have proposed clinical criteria for the BWS diagnosis, with Elliot being more strict than DeBaun. For the first, major features are abdominal wall defects, macroglossia, increased pre- and/or postnatal growth, and minor features are ear creases or pits, naevus flammeus, hypoglycaemia, nephromegaly, and hemihypertrophy. Patients with three major features or two major and at least three minor features are thought to be BWS patients. For the latter, two of the most common five parameters are enough. Patients with BWS have an increased risk to mostly develop intra-abdominal tumors such as Wilms tumor (see also Chapter 14 on Wilms and rhabdoid tumors of the kidney), adrenocortical carcinoma, rhabdomyosarcoma, and hepatoblastoma. Furthermore, myxomas, fibromas, and hamartomas have been described. The majority of tumors develop during childhood.

BWS is characterized by a number of involved genes that are subject to genomic imprinting [19]. A maternal transmission is predominant and the genetic changes map to chromosome 11q15. In this region, translocations, LOI, and gene mutations may occur, leading to imprinting of the encoded genes. As three different regions within 11p13.5pter could be identified, BWS can be subgrouped into BWSCR1, 2, and 3, depending on the involved genomic region. Phenotypic differences between the different types have been already identified. One gene known to be involved at least indirectly is *KCNQ1*, which encodes a potassium channel. The closely related *KCNQ1OT1*, which is transcribed from this region in an antisense orientation shows a high degree of methylation in a high percentage of BWS cases. In other cases, heterozygous mutations of the *CDKN1C* gene, encoding an inhibitor of cyclin-dependent kinases, have been found which may be associated with specific phenotypes. Finally, there are reports about an involvement of insulin growth factor 2 (IGF2) and its downstream interactor H19, since mouse models overexpressing IGF2 show a phenotype overlapping with BWS. It is important to know that BWS exists also in a mosaic form in the case of uniparental disomy, leading to aberrant methylation of *KCNQ1OT1* with or without aberrant methylation of H19/IGF2. H19 methylation defects seem to be associated with an increased risk of tumor development. Regional differences concerning epigenetic and genetic alterations are described [20]. For BWS, see also other chapters of this book, especially Chapter 14 on Wilms and rhabdoid tumors of the kidney).

Enchondromatosis can occur with two different phenotypes. **Ollier's disease** is characterized by the development of multiple cartilaginous lesions, preferentially involving the short and long tubular bones of the limbs. If these bone lesions are found in combination with haemangiomas in the cutis, soft tissue, or viscera, it is called **Mafucci syndrome**. The majority of cases occur sporadically, but families with multiple affected members have also been described, suggesting an autosomal dominant inheritance with variable penetrance [21]. Both subtypes of enchondromatosis usually present in childhood and stop growing at puberty. However, for patients with Malfucci syndrome, the risk to develop a chondrosarcoma during adulthood is higher than for those with Ollier's disease. Renewed enlargement of the tumors in adults is highly suspect for malignant transformation. Altogether, the estimated risk to develop a chondrosarcoma is 15 to 30%. Some patients may develop angiosarcomas, brain tumors, and tumors of the hepatobiliary system [22].

Molecular genetic analysis in patients with Ollier's disease revealed mutations of the *PTHR1* gene encoding a receptor for parathyroid hormone and parathyroid hormone-related protein. The result may be an increased cAMP signaling and a constitutively activated hedgehog signaling leading to a decreased differentiation of proliferating chondrocytes. Models with transgenic mice substantiate this hypothesis [23].

Another group of genes involved in the development of normal cartilage are the *EXT* genes. The syndrome of multiple osteochondromas (MO) is genetically heterogeneous, with different mutations in the *EXT* genes. The incidence is about 1 : 50 000 persons. More than half of the patients with multiple osteochondromas report a positive family history. The diagnosis can be made with at least two lesions in the long bones in the juxta-epiphyseal region. Osteochondromas develop during the first decade of life, and grow until puberty. The long bones of the extremities are predisposed, especially around the knees. Furthermore, patients may develop complex deformities and abnormalities in other long bones, often leading to short stature [24–26]. In 0.5 to 3% of patients, osteochondromas may transform to secondary chondrosarcoma, which has to be suspected in cases with growing lesions after puberty, pain, or increasing thickness of cartilaginous caps in adults. If an osteochondroma transforms, it results in chondrosarcoma in the vast majority of cases, while secondary osteosarcoma and spindle cell sarcomas are very rare. The latter develop in the stalk of the osteochondroma, while chondrosarcomas develop in the cap. A dedifferentiation of these chondrosarcomas into high grade lesions such as fibrosarcoma, malignant fibrous histiocytoma/pleomorphic high grade sarcoma, or osteosarcoma, occurs very rarely.

The gene products of EXT 1 and 2, exostosin 1 and 2, are type II transmembrane glycoproteins, which form an oligomeric complex involved in heparan sulfate polymerization. Heparan sulfate proteoglycans are required for fibroblastic growth factor interaction with its receptor. Furthermore, it is suspected that exostosin-1 and 2 influence the Indian hedgehog pathway, which is important for segment polarity in the growth plate. Germline mutations in one of both genes are most often located in the first 5 to 6 exons of the genes, without mutational hotspots. The genes are located on chromosome 8q24 (EXT 1) and chromosome 11p11–12 (EXT 2). All known mutational subtypes such as missense, splice-site, non-sense, or frameshift mutations may be found, leading to defects of the EXT function [27]. Other studies found evidence of a tumor suppressor gene function, since losses of the remaining wildtype allele have been identified in a subgroup of patients [28].

Paget's disease of bone (PDB) is a disorder with a predilection for older individuals. Over the age of 50 years, 2 to 3%, and over the age of 80 years, 10% of the population are affected by PDB, respectively. The symptoms are variable, varying from asymptomatic cases to significant morbidity. The most severe complication is the sarcomatous transformation of affected bone. Familial clustering has been observed in a subgroup of cases. Several reports in the literature describe pagetoid osteosarcomas with an autosomal dominant trait. The identification of the exact gene locus is still missing; however, several regions are highly suspected to be involved as indicated by linkage analyses and the detection of losses of heterozygosity: these are chromosome 18q21, involving a gene named *TNFRSF11A*, encoding the receptor activator of factor NF kappa B (RANK), and the chromosomal regions 5q31 and 5q35 [29]. Several mutations affecting different RANK-NF-kappa B signaling components have been identified, probably involving aberrant RANK-mediated osteoclast signaling. Other potential contributors, such as viruses and environmental factors, still have to be identified [30]. The region 18q21 has first been identified as involved in the pathogenesis of familial expansile osteolysis, which is a very rare disease with similiarities to PDB, in which osteosarcomas may develop. Further studies are needed to identify further candidate genes potentially functioning as tumor suppressor genes.

The **Retinoblastoma syndrome** (see also Chapter 7 on retinoblastoma), besides the most common intraocular tumor of children, is associated with the frequent occurrence of secondary site primary tumors including osteosarcomas, fibrosarcomas, chondrosarcomas, Ewing sarcomas, and several non-sarcomatous neoplasms. Osteogenic sarcomas are the most frequent second site neoplasms. More recent studies found that the occurrence of such secondary neoplasms is similar in groups receiving radiation, and those without previous radiation [31, 32].

The **Carney triad** (CT) consists of gastrointestinal stromal tumors (GISTs), multiple pulmonary chondromas, and functionally active extra-adrenal paragangliomas. CT is an extremely rare syndrome, with fewer than 30 cases reported with all three tumors present, and fewer than 100 incomplete cases presenting with

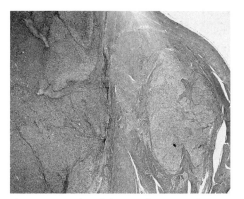

Figure 27.4 Multinodular growth pattern of a gastrointestinal stromal tumor in Carney triad (HE, 1 × obj). (Courtesy of H. U. Schildhaus, Department of Pathology, University of Bonn, Medical School, Germany).

two of the three tumor types (usually GISTs and chondromas). The syndrome predominately affects females (>80% of cases), with the first tumor often appearing between 10 and 20 years of age in the stomach. Paragangliomas are rare tumors arising from neural-crest-derived chromaffin cells. These cells are located in certain areas of the head, neck, and torso. Paragangliomas may raise blood pressure by producing adrenalin. Pulmonary chondromas are benign cartilaginous lung tumors, also known as chondromatous hamartomas. The GISTs in CT are usually located in the stomach [33, 34]. Because GISTs often precede the occurrence of other tumors types of this syndrome, all pediatric GIST cases should be considered as potential CT cases. These GISTs are typically multifocal (displaying more than one tumor nodule, Figure 27.4), and show an epithelioid phenotype. The prognosis is better than in adult GIST, with a slow course of progression even after metastasis has occurred. However, repeated surgeries may be required due to recurring tumors.

Recently Carney [33] described two other conditions (adrenocortical adenoma and esophageal leiomyoma) as additional components occurring in some triad patients. Furthermore, in 2002 he described another hereditary syndrome with paragangliomas and multifocal GIST, but without pulmonary chondromas in 5 distinct families with an average onset age of 23. He concluded that this syndrome is different from the classical CT [35]. This dyad of paraganglioma and GIST was later called **Carney–Stratakis syndrome** (see also Chapter 18 on gastrointestinal stromal tumors (GISTs)). GIST samples from two Carney triad patients have been tested for mutations in the *KIT* and *PDGFRα* gene, which are known to be responsible for the vast majority of sporadic GISTs [36–38], but none were found. Glivec (Novartis, Basel, Switzerland) had no apparent effect on liver metastases in the patient described by Diment *et al.* [36]. However, Delemarre *et al.* [39] did report a case for whom Imatinib (Glivec) was effective. Very recently, it could be shown that germline mutations of the genes encoding the succinate dehydrogenase subunits B, C, and D (SDHB, SDHC, and SDHD) were found in five different kindreds with this dyad, obviously implicating an autosomal dominant inheritance [40]. These mutations had been already described by Bayley *et al.* in familial paraganglioma and/or pheochromocytoma [41] and seem to play a pathogenetic role in these diseases, needing further clarification.

The **Rothmund–Thomson syndrome** (RTS), at least in a subset of cases, is associated with inherited mutations in the *RECQL4* helicase gene, and has an autosomal recessive trait. More than 250 cases have been described until now. The central feature is a sunset-dependent rash occurring during the first 6 months after birth. It is located on the face, the buttocks, and extremities. With time, patients develop hyper- and hypo-pigmentations, skin atrophy, and teleangiektasias. Besides abnormalities of the skin, hair, eyes, nails, and skeleton, up to one-third of patients develop osteosarcomas, the majority during childhood. Furthermore, cutaneous malignancies are observed (see also Chapter 4 on genetic dysmorphic syndromes leading to tumorigenesis).

Genetically, a subgroup of RTS patients carry different types of mutations in the *RECQL4* helicase gene on chromosome 8q24.3. Its gene product is highly expressed in the thymus and testis and, to a lower level, in multiple other tissues. There is an overlap with Bloom and Werner syndromes due to homology of the genes.

The **Werner syndrome** (WS) is a rare autosomal recessive genetic instability syndrome, which is caused by mutations in the *WRN* gene [42]. Its frequency is estimated to be between 1:22 000 and 1:1 000 000 per population, varying with the founder mutations and consanguinity. It is characterized by a progeria in the second and third decade of life, associated with an increased risk to develop neoplastic and non-neoplastic diseases. Patients develop STSs and thyroid cancer of different histological subtypes, melanomas, meningiomas, haematological diseases, and osteosarcomas. It is estimated that the risk to develop such neoplasms is elevated 30-fold as compared to the normal population. To identify patients with WS, a scoring system has been developed that can be found on the International Registry of Werner Syndrome Web site: (www.pathology.washington.edu/research/werner/registry/diagnostic.html).

As previously mentioned, there is an overlap with Bloom syndrome and Rothmund–Thomson syndrome, since all syndromes are associated with a loss of function of a human RecQ helicase protein. This protein encodes for both DNA helicase and exonuclease activities [43], and is likely to play an important physiological role in homologous recombinational repair in human somatic cells [44, 45].

The **Li–Fraumeni syndrome** (LFS) is characterized by an increased risk for many cancers, including sarcomas, leukemia, breast cancer, ovarian cancer, and others (see also Chapter 5 on hereditary brain tumors). The patients develop multiple primary neoplasms, already in childhood and as young adults. There is a predominance of STS, osteosarcomas, breast cancer, brain tumors, leukemia, and adrenocortical carcinomas [46]. In 2007, more than 380 families with proven LFS were registered in the IARC database (http://www_p53.iarc.fr/Germline.html).

The diagnostic criteria for LFS are the occurrence of sarcomas before the age of 45, at least one first-degree relative with any tumor before the age of 45, and a second- or first-degree relative with cancer before age 45 or a sarcoma at any age [47]. Patients with LFS often develop breast cancer at an earlier age than the normal population, probably with a worse prognosis. The next most frequent cancers are brain tumors and sarcoma of soft tissue or bone.

The majority of LFS cases are caused by a *TP53* germline mutation located on chromosome 17p13.1. Its gene product p53 belongs to the family of tumor suppressors. The gene is composed of 11 exons. Its gene product is expressed in most cell types, but does not accumulate due to rapid turnover. Under stress, p53 is released from negative control of MDM2, which regulates its degradation by post-translational modifications. It may then accumulate in the nucleus where it may act as a transcription factor for several gene types: these are cell-cycle regulatory, pro-apoptotic, and DNA-repairing genes. As a consequence, two different mechanisms of cellular responses may be modulated. First, cell-cycle arrest leads to DNA repair after different forms of cellular stress. Second, apoptosis is induced in damaged cells which cannot be repaired efficiently. If the mutation leads to an inactivation of these mechanisms, the number of damaged cells increases continuously. Mutations of the *TP53* gene are also frequently found in sporadic cancers, the majority clustering between exons 5 and 8 encoding the DNA binding domain. There are several mutational hotspots (codons 175, 245, 248, 273, and 282), which carry missense or non-sense mutations due to single base substitutions. In families with germline mutations, a subgroup fulfils the strict criteria of LFS, but others do not fall into the strict criteria and thus are called Li–Fraumeni-like syndrome. The mutational hotspots are identical to the sporadic cases. [48].

Another gene which might be involved in the pathogenesis of LFS is *CHEK2* located on chromosome 22q12.1. It has 14 exons, with exon 10 to 14 also often found in other regions of the whole genome due to duplication. To avoid errors when looking for germline mutations, it is important to run long-range PCRs, with primers located outside of this duplicated region. As *p53*, *CHEK2* is involved in the control of cell/DNA damage by causing cell-cycle arrest, DNA repair, or apoptosis. There are several downstream substrates such as *p53*, *BRCA1*, *Cdc25A*, and *Cdc25C*. Further studies are needed to rule out the possibility of polymorphisms or mutations in this gene. Until now, no germline mutations have been found in other possible candidates in patients without *p53* mutations such as *PTEN* or *p16*.

Neurofibromatosis (NF) (see also Chapter 6 on neurofibromatosis) results in developmental changes in the nervous system, causing nerve sheath tumors. Other abnormalities associated with neurofibromatosis include skin changes, bone deformities, GISTs, and somatostatin-producing tumors in the gastrointestinal tract. The latter tumors may be associated with phaeochromocytomas, involving one or both of the adrenal glands [49]. Neurofibromatosis type 1 (NF1) is an autosomal dominant disease characterized by multiple neurofibromas, malignant peripheral nerve sheath tumors (MPNST), optic nerve gliomas and other astrocytomas, multiple café-au-lait spots, freckling in the axilla and groin,

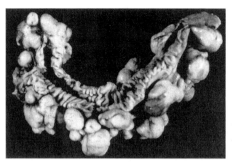

Figure 27.5 Multiple synchronous GIST of the small bowel. (Courtesy of R. Stiens, Institute of Pathology, Gummersbach, Germany).

iris hamartomas, and different lesions of the bone. With two or more of these symptoms, an NF1 patient can be diagnosed. The prevalence is estimated at about 1 : 4000, with 50% of cases resulting from new germline mutations.

Neurofibromas may occur in the dermis as well circumscript tumors, but may also be plexiform, growing over years and deforming the body. About 5% of plexiform tumors transform to MPNST, whereas this transformation is very rare in other types of neurofibromas. Besides MPNST, tumors may include heterologous differentiations, then being called Triton tumors, which are highly characteristic for NF1 [50]. The risk for the development of rhabdomyosarcoma is increased. Furthermore, patients with NF1 may develop multiple GISTs and may present with up to 100 nodules in the gastrointestinal wall, preferentially in the small bowel (Figure 27.5). The prevalence of GISTs is about 5 to 25% in the NF1 population [51, 52]. GISTs in NF1 usually do not show mutations in the *c-KIT* gene or the *PDGFRα* gene, and have normal or wildtype *KIT* and *PDGFRA* [53]. One exception involving a patient with an exon 11 mutation in *c-KIT* was described by Yantiss *et al.* [54]. Cheng [55] also reported one mutant case. Takazawa *et al.* [56] reported mutations in at least one tumor from 3 of 9 NF1 patients investigated. Both *KIT* and *PDGFRA* mutations were identified. Different tumors from a single patient showed different mutations, and it was observed that the same patient could have both, GISTs with mutations and other tumors that were wildtype. When *KIT* or *PDGFRA* mutations are found, they apparently are a late, but not necessary pathogenetic event. Andersson *et al.* [57] discussed the possibility that NF1 inactivation could lead to constitutive activation of RAS and increased MAP kinase signaling. Maertens *et al.* [58] also demonstrated that inactivation of neurofibromin was sufficient to hyperactivate the MAPK pathway, which is more important in NF1 GISTs than in sporadic GISTs. A subgroup of patients with multiple GISTs in the small bowel, lacking neurofibromas in other locations or other typical NF1, signs are thought to carry mutations in the *NF1* gene in a mosaic pattern, because of morphologic similarities with typical NF1 cases. However, this has not been proven until now. More details regarding other tumor manifestations and the genomic findings are found in the Chapter 6 on neurofibromatosis.

Neurofibromatosis type 2 (NF2) is not further mentioned, since besides benign neural tumors, soft tissue or bone sarcoma are not typical for this syndrome.

27.2.1
Prevention/Prediction

To date, one of the most important prerequisites to lower the mortality of hereditary sarcoma is early detection. Especially for the group of sarcomas which are rare, the recognition of an inherited trait is of central relevance. The physician has to know the syndromes of concern, and has to be aware of the possibility that an aggregation of sarcomas in one family is highly suggestive for inheritance. As a result, referral to a hereditary cancer consultation center with genetic counseling and DNA testing might be helpful to identify family members at risk [59]. These will need a special survey depending on the results of the genetic testing and on the underlying syndrome to achieve the diagnosis of a tumor as early as possible.

References

1 Ries, L.A.G., Melbert, D., Krapcho, M., Mariotto, A., Miller, B.A., Feuer, E.J., Clegg, L., Horner, M.J., Howlader, N., Eisner, M.P., Reichman, M. and Edwards, B.K. (1975–2004) *SEER Cancer Statistics Review*, National Cancer Institute, Bethesda, MD.

2 Pierce, E.R. (1970) Gardner's syndrome: formal genetics and statistical analysis of a large canadien kindred. *Clinical Genetics*, **1**, 65–80.

3 Naylor, E.W., Gardner, E.J. and Richards, R.C. (1979) Desmoid tumors and mesenteric fibromatosis in Gardner's syndrome: report of kindred 109. *Archives of Surgery*, **114**, 1181–5.

4 Scott, R.J., Frogggattt, N.J., Trembath, R.C., Evans, D.G., Hodgen, S.V. and Maher, E.R. (1996) Familial infiltrative fibromatosis (demoid tumours) (MIM135290) caused by a recurrent 3'APC gene mutation. *Human Molecular Genetics*, **5**, 1921–4.

5 Clark, S.K., Smith, T.G., Katz, D.E., Reznek, R.H. and Phillips, R.K. (1998) Identification and progression of a desmoid precursor lesion in patients with familial adenomatous polyposis. *The British Journal of Surgery*, **85**, 970–3.

6 Wehrli, B.M., Weiss, S.W., Yandow, S. and Coffin, C.M. (2001) Gardner-associated fibromas (GAF) in young patients: a distinct fibrous lesin that identifies unsuspected Gardner's syndrome and risk for fibromatosis. *The American Journal of Surgical Pathology*, **25**, 645–51.

7 Giardiello, F.M., Hamilton, S.R., Krush, A.J., Offerhaus, J.A., Booker, S.V. and Peterson, G.M. (1993) Nasopharyngeal angiofibroma in patients with familial adenomatous polyposis. *Gastroenterology*, **105**, 1550–2.

8 Armstrong, S.J., Duncan, A.W. and Mott, M.G. (1991) Rhabdomyosarcoma associated with familial adenomatous polyposis. *Pediatric Radiology*, **21**, 445–6.

9 Bertario, E., Russo, A., Sala, P., Eboli, M., Giarola, M., D'amico, F., Giismondi, V., Varesco, L., Pierotti, M.A. and Radice, P. (2001) Genotype and phenotype factors as determinants of desmoid tumors in patients with familial adenomatous polyposis. *International Journal of Cancer*, **95**, 102–7.

10 Heiskanen, I. and Jarvinen, H.J. (1996) Occurance of desmoiid tumours in familial adenomatous polyposis and results of treatment. *International Journal of Colorectal Disease*, **11**, 157–62.

11 Hizawa, K., Iida, M., Mibu, R., Aoyagi, K., Yao, T. and Fujishima, M. (1997) Desmoid tumors in familial adenomatous polyposis/Gardner's syndrome. *Journal of Clinical Gastroenterology*, **25**, 334–7.

12 Sarovia, C., Berk, T., McLeod, R.S. and Cohan, Z. (2000) Desmoid disease in patients with familial adenomatous polyposis. *Diseases of the Colon and Rectum*, **43**, 363–9.

13 Heinrich, M.C., McArthur, G.A., Demetri, G.D., Joenssuu, H., Bono, P., Herrmann, R., Hirte, H., Cresta, S., Koslin, D.B., Corless, C.L., Dirnhofer, S., van Oosterom, A.T., Nikolova, Z., Dimitriijevic, S. and Fletcher, J.A. (2006) Clinical and molecular studies of the effect of Imatinib on advanced aggressive fibromatosis (desmoid tumor). *Journal of Clinical Oncology*, **24**, 1195–203.

14 Lynch, H.T., Ruma, T.A., Albano, W.A., Lynch, J.F. and Lynch, P.M. (1982) Phenotypic variation in hereditary adenomatosis: unusual tumor spectrum. *Diseases of the Colon and Rectum*, **25**, 235–8.

15 Takeuchi, T., Takenoshita, Y., Kubo, K. and Iida, M. (1993) Natural course of jaw lesions in patients with familial adenomatosis coli (Gardner's syndrome). *International Journal of Oral and Maxillofacial Surgery*, **22**, 226–30.

16 Bisgaard, M.L., Fenger, K., Bulow, S., Niebuhr, E. and Mohr, J. (1994) Familial adenomatous polyposis (FAP): frequency, penetrance, and mutation rate. *Human Mutation*, **3**, 121–5.

17 DeBaun, M.R. and Tucker, M.A. (1998) Risk of cancer during in first four years of life in children from The Beckwith–Wiedemann Syndrome Registry. *Journal of Pediatrics*, **132**, 398–400.

18 Elliott, M., Bayly, R., Cole, T., Temple, I.K. and Maher, E.R. (1994) Clinical features and natural history of Beckwith-Wiedemann syndrome: presentation of 74 new cases. *Clinical Genetics*, **46**, 168–74.

19 Temple, I.K. (2007) Imprinting in human disease with special reference to transient neonatal diabetes and Beckwith–Wiedemann syndrome. *Endocrine Development*, **12**, 113–23.

20 Sasaki, K., Soejima, H., Higashimoto, K., Yatsuki, H., Ohashi, H., Yabakke, S., Joh, K., Niikawa, N. and Mukai, T. (2007) Japanese and North American/European patients with Beckwith–Wiedemann syndrome have different frequencies of some epigenetic and genetic alterations. *European Journal of Human Genetics*, **15** (12), 1205–10.

21 McKusick, V.A. (1998) *Mendelian Inheritance in Man, Catalogs of Human Genes and Genetic Disorders*, 12th edn, Johns Hopkins University Press, Baltimore.

22 Schwarz, H.S., Zimmermann, N.B., Simon, M.A., Wroble, R.R., Millar, E.A. and Bonfiglio, M. (1987) The malignant potential of enchondromatosis. *The Journal of Bone and Joint Surgery. American Volume*, **69**, 269–74.

23 Hopyan, S., Gokgoz, N., Poon, R., Gensure, R.C., Yu, C., Cole, W.G., Bell, R.S., Juppner, H., andrulis, I.L., Wunder, J.S. and Alman, B.A. (2002) A mutant PTH/PTHrP type I receptor in enchondromatosis. *Nature Genetics*, **30**, 306–10.

24 Legeai-Mallet, L., Munnich, A., Maroteaux, P. and Le Merrer, M. (1997) Incomplete penetrance and expressivity skewing in hereditary multiple exostoses. *Clinical Genetics*, **52**, 12–16.

25 Francannet, C., Cohen-Tanugi, A., Le Merrer, M., Munnich, A., Bonaventure, J. and Legeai-Mallet, L. (2001) Genotype-phenotype correlation in hereditary multiple exostoses. *Journal of Medical Genetics*, **38**, 430–4.

26 Wicklund, C.L., Pauli, R.M., Johnston, D. and Hecht, J.T. (1995) Natural history study of hereditary multiple exostoses. *American Journal of Medical Genetics*, **55**, 43–6.

27 Cheung, P.K., McCormick, C., Crawford, B.E., Esko, J.D., Tufaro, F. and Duncan, G. (2001) Etiological point mutations in the hereditary multiple exostoses gene EXT1: a functional analysis of heparin sulphate polymerase activity. *American Journal of Human Genetics*, **69**, 55–66.

28 Signori, E., Massi, E., Matera, M.G., Poscente, M., Gravina, C., Falcone, G., Rosa, M.A., Rinaldi, M., Wuyts, W., Deripa, D., Dallapiccola, B. and Fazio,

V.M. (2007) A combined analytical approach reveals novel *EXT1/2* gene mutations in a large cohort of Italian multiple osteochondromas patients. *Genes, Chromosomes and Cancer*, **46** (5), 470–7.

29 McNairn, J.D.K., Damron, T.A., St. Landas, K., Ambrose, J.L. and Shrimpton, A.E. (2001) Inheritance of osteosarcoma and Paget's disease of bone. *The Journal of Molecular Diagnostics*, **3**, 171–7.

30 Layfield, R. (2007) The molecular pathogenesis of Paget's disease of bone. *Expert Reviews in Molecular Medicine*, **99** (27), 1–13.

31 Kleinerman, R.A., Tucker, M.A., Abramson, D.H., Seddon, J.M., Tarone, R.E. and Fraumeni, J.F. Jr (2007) Risk of soft tissue sarcomas by individual subtype in survivors of hereditary retinoblastoma. *Journal of the National Cancer Institute*, **99**, 24–31.

32 Meadows, A. (ed.) (2007) Retinoblastoma survivors: sarcomas and surveillance. *Journal of the National Cancer Institute*, **99**, 3–5.

33 Carney, J.A. (1999) Gastric stromal sarcoma, pulmonary chondroma, and extra-adrenal paraganglioma (Carney Triad): natural history, adrenocortical component, and possible familial occurrence. *Mayo Clinic Proceedings*, **74** (6), 543–52.

34 Appleman, H.D. (1999) The Carney Triad: a lesson in observation, creativity, and perseverance. *Mayo Clinic Proceedings*, **74** (6), 638–40.

35 Carney, J.A. and Stratakis, C.A. (2002) Familial paraganglioma and gastric stromal sarcoma: a new syndrome distinct from the Carney triad. *American Journal of Medical Genetics*, **108**, 132–9.

36 Diment, J., Tamborini, E., Casali, P., Gronchi, A., Carney, J.A. and Colecchia, M. (2005) Carney triad: case report and molecular analysis of gastric tumor. *Human Pathology*, **36**, 112–16.

37 Knop, S., Schupp, M., Wardelmann, E., Stueker, D., Horger, M.S., Kanz, L., Einsele, H. and Kroeber, S.M. (2006) A new case of Carney triad: gastrointestinal stromal tumours and leiomyoma of the oesophagus do not show activating

mutations of *KIT* and platelet-derived growth factor receptor alpha. *Journal of Clinical Pathology*, **59**, 1097–9.

38 Agaimy, A., Pelz, A.F., Corless, C.L., Wünsch, P.H., Heinrich, M.C., Hofstaedter, F., Dietmaier, W., Blanke, C.D., Wieacker, P., Roessner, A., Hartmann, A. and Schneider-Stock, R. (2007) Epithelioid gastric stromal tumours of the antrum in young females with the Carney triad: a report of three new cases with mutational analysis and comparative genomic hybridization. *Oncology Reports*, **18**, 9–15.

39 Delemarre, L., Aronson, D., van Rijn, R., Bras, H., Arets, B. and Verschuur, A. (2008) Respiratory symptoms in a boy revealing Carney triad. *Pediatric Blood & Cancer*, **50** (2), 399–401, Oct 12.

40 McWhinney, S.B., Pasini, B. and Stratakis, C.A. (2007) International carney triad and Carney–Stratakis syndrome consortium, familial gastrointestinal stromal tumors and germline mutations. *New England Journal of Medicine*, **357**, 1054–6.

41 Bayley, J.P., van Minderhout, I., Weiss, M.M., Jansen, J.C., Oomen, P.H.N., Menko, F.H., Pasini, B., Ferrando, B., Wong, N., Alpert, L.C., Williams, R., Blair, E., Devilee, P. and Taschner, P.E.M. (2006) Mutation analysis of SDHB and SDHC: novel germline mutations in sporadic head and neck paraganglioma and familial paraganglioma and/or pheochromocytoma. *BMC Medical Genetics*, **7**, 1–10, DOI:10.1186/1471-2350-7-1.

42 Kudlow, B.A., Kennedy, B.K. and Monnat, R.J. Jr (2007) Werner and Hutchinson–Gilford progeria syndromes: mechanistic basis of human progeroid diseases. *Nature Reviews Molecular Cell Biology*, **88** (5), 394–404.

43 Moynahan, M.E., Chiu, J.W., Koller, B.H. and Jasin, M. (1999) *BRCA1* controls homology-directed DNA repair. *Molecular Cell*, **4**, 511–18.

44 Hicks, M.J., Roth, J.R., Kozinetz, C.A. and Wang, L.L. (2007) Clinicopathologic of osteosarcoma in patients with Rothmund–Thomson syndrome. *Journal of Clinical Oncology*, **25** (4), 370–5.

45 Dietschy, T., Shevelev, I. and Stagljar, I. (2007) The molecular role of the Rothmund–Thomson-, RAPADILINO- and

Baller–Gerold–gene product, RECQL4: recent progress. *Cellular and Molecular Life Sciences*, **64** (7-88), 796–802.

46 Li, F.P. and Fraumeni, J.F. Jr (1969) Soft tissue syndroms, breast cancer, and other neoplasms. A familial syndrome? *Annals of Internal Medicine*, **71**, 747–52.

47 Li, F.P., Fraumeni, J.F. Jr, Mulvihill, J.J., Blattner, W.A., Dreyfus, M.G., Tucker, M.A. and Miller, R.W. (1988) A cancer family syndrome in twenty-four kindreds. *Cancer Research*, **48**, 5358–6362.

48 Kleihues, P., Cavenee, W.K., zur Hausen, A., Esteve, J. and Ohgaki, H. (1997) Tumors associated with *p53* germline mutations: a syndrome of 91 families. *American Journal of Pathology*, **150**, 1–13.

49 Burke, A.P., Sobin, L.H., Shekitka, K.M., Federspiel, B.H. and Helwig, E.B. (1990) Somatostatin-producing duodenal carcinoids in patients with von Recklinghausen's neurofibromatosis. A predilection for black patients. *Cancer*, **65**, 1591–5.

50 Woodruff, J.M. (1996) Pathology of malignant peripheral nerve sheat tumors, in *Soft Tissue Tumors (International Academy of Pathology Monograph)* (eds S.W. Weiss and J.S J. Brooks), Williams and Wilkens, Baltimore, pp. 129–61.

51 Guily, J.A., Picand, R., Giuly, D., Monges, B. and Ngyuen-Cat, R. (2003) von Recklinghausen disease and gastrointestinal stromal tumors. *Am J Serg*, **185**, 86–7.

52 Zöller, M.E., Rembeck, B., Odén, A., Samuelsson, M. and Angervall, L. (1997) Malignant and benign tumors in patients with neurofibromatosis type 1 in a defined Swedish population, *Cancer*, **79**, 2125–31.

53 Kinoshita, K., Hirota, S., Isozaki, K., Ohashi, A., Nishida, T., Kitamura, Y.,

Shinomura, Y. and Matsuzawa, Y. (2004) Absence of *c-kit* gene mutations in gastrointestinal stromal tumors from neurofibromatosis type I patients. *The Journal of Pathology*, **202**, 80–5.

54 Yantiss, R.K., Rosenberg, A.E., Sarraan, L., Besmer, P. and Antonescu, C.R. (2005) Multiple gastrointestinal stromal tumors in type I neurofibromatosis: a pathologic and molecular study. *Modern Pathology*, **18** (4), 475–84.

55 Cheng, S.P., Huang, M.J., Yang, T.L., Tzen, C.Y., Liu, C.L., Liu, T.P. and Hsiao, S.C. (2004) Neurofibromatosis with gastrointestinal stromal tumors: insights into the association. *Digestive Diseases and Sciences*, **49** (7–8), 1165–9.

56 Takazawa, Y., Sakurai, S., Sakuma, Y., Ikeda, T., Yamaguchi, J., Hashizume, Y., Yokoyama, S., Motegi, A. and Fukayama, M. (2005) Gastrointestinal stromal tumors from neurofibromatosis type I (von Recklingshausen disease). *The American Journal of Surgical Pathology*, **29**, 755–63.

57 Andersson, J., Sihto, H., Meis-Kindblom, J.M., Joensuu, H., Nupponen, N. and Kindblom, L.G. (2005) NNF1-associated gastrointestinal stromal tumors have unique clinical, phenotypic, and genotypic characteristics. *The American Journal of Surgical Pathology*, **29** (9), 1170–6.

58 Maertens, O., Prenen, H., Debiec-Rychter, M., Wozniak, A., Sciot, R., Pauwels, P., De Wever, I., Vermeesch, J.R., de Raedt, T., De Paepe, A., Speleman, F., van Osterom, A., Messiaen, L. and Legius, E. (2006) Molecular pathogenesis of multiple gastrointestinal stromal tumors in NF1 patients. *Human Molecular Genetics*, **15** (6), 1015–23.

59 Lynch, H.T., Deters, C.A., Hogg, D., Lynch, J.F., Kinarsky, Y. and Gatalica, Z. (2003) Familial sarcoma, challenging pedigrees. *Cancer*, **98**, 1947–57.

Part IV
Genetic Counseling, Psycho-Oncology, and
General Perspectives for Therapeutic Strategies

28
Genetic Counseling for Hereditary Tumors

Dorothea Gadzicki and Brigitte Schlegelberger

Summary

The goal of cancer genetic counseling is to educate counselees about their risk of developing cancer, help them to derive the personal significance from cancer genetic information, to empower them to make educated, informed decisions ("informed consent") about genetic testing, cancer screening, and cancer prevention, and to support them in coping with the situation. Thus, genetic counseling is an integral part of the cancer risk assessment process and should be offered before and after genetic testing. In this chapter, different aspects of cancer genetic counseling, for example, documentation of the pedigree and the medical history of the family, tailored information giving, shared decision-making regarding genetic testing, risk assessment tools, interaction with other specialists, and transmission of the information within the family, are discussed.

28.1
Introduction

Cancer is a genetic disease caused by mutations in genes that are involved in the regulation of cell growth, differentiation, and survival. Mutations in so-called tumor suppressor genes and oncogenes are implicated in carcinogenesis. In most cases the disease-causing mutations are induced by age-related factors, as the result of life-long environmental exposures, or acquired by chance because of DNA replication errors during continuous cell division. Mutations acquired in somatic cells (somatic mutations) lead to sporadic cancer. On the other hand, there are families with an accumulation of specific types of malignancies in the absence of an identifiable carcinogenic exposure. These cancers are classified as familial cancers and are caused by germline mutations in so-called cancer genes. Familial cancer may be due to a combination of genetic variants and transmitted according to a polygenic trait. In this case, close relatives of an affected individual are at a moderately increased cancer risk, for example, first-

Hereditary Tumors: From Genes to Clinical Consequences
Edited by Heike Allgayer, Helga Rehder and Simone Fulda
Copyright © 2009 WILEY-VCH Verlag GmbH & Co. KGaA, Weinheim
ISBN: 978-3-527-32028-8

degree relatives of an affected person usually have double the risk of the general population.

In contrast, about 5% of cancers are monogenic disorders caused by alterations of a single gene. These diseases are classified as hereditary cancer syndromes. In these cancer families, in which the predisposition to a specific group of cancers is the result of an inherited germline mutation in a cancer-related gene, at-risk individuals tend to develop the tumors at an earlier age than individuals with sporadic or familial cancer, and they are prone to develop more than one primary tumor. Usually, the disease is transmitted from one generation to the other, according to the autosomal-dominant pattern of inheritance. That means that siblings and offspring of an affected person have a 50% risk of inheriting the cancer-predisposing mutation – or vice versa a 50% chance to inherit the normal allele. Those that have inherited the mutation are at a highly increased risk to develop cancer that can approach 90% over a lifetime. Recently, hereditary cancer syndromes transmitted according to the autosomal-recessive pattern of inheritance have been identified, for example, *MYH*-associated colon cancer (see Chapter 17 on Lynch syndrome (HNPCC)).

If the responsible cancer-related gene is known, genetic testing can be offered. Identification of the at-risk individuals opens up the chance to improve clinical management, that is, to implement screening programs for the early detection of cancer prior to the time at which general population screening would be initiated. Moreover, preventive measures, like removal of organs such as the bowels in the case of FAP, can be discussed.

Genetic counseling is an integral part of the cancer risk assessment process [1–3]. According to the recommendations of the National Society of Genetic Counselors [4], a referral for genetic counseling should be considered for individuals with personal or family history features suggestive of familial or hereditary cancer and should not be limited to just those individuals who are potential candidates for genetic testing. Usage of the pedigree analysis combined with available risk assessment models enables the identification of at-risk individuals and facilitates the familial cancer syndrome classification. The purpose of cancer genetic counseling is to educate clients about their risk of developing cancer, help them derive the personal significance from cancer genetic information, and empower them to make educated, informed decisions ("informed consent") about genetic testing, cancer screening, and cancer prevention.

The over 30 years old and still valid definition of genetic counseling published by the (American and Canadian) Ad Hoc Committee on Genetic Counseling, describes it as "a communication process which deals with the human problems associated with the occurrence, or risk of occurrence, of a genetic disorder in a family." This process involves "an attempt to help the individual or family (1) comprehend the medical fact and the available management; (2) appreciate the way heredity contributes to the disorder; (3) understand the options for dealing with the risk of recurrence; (4) choose the course of action which seems appropriate; and (5) make the best possible adjustment to the disorder" [5]. This definition also applies to cancer genetic counseling.

Because individuals presenting for tumor genetic counseling can be healthy and not affected by cancer, they should not be called patients, but be more appropriately called counselees.

The aim of cancer genetic counseling is to support the counselee in assessing her/his personal risk of developing cancer and to educate her/him about medical and potential behavioral options to decrease their risk. It also includes obtaining an informed consent about genetic testing, to provide psychological support, guidance about medical options, and referral to clinical specialists as a means of early detection or prevention of cancer.

Initially, genetic counseling has been developed as a nondirective approach. The reason of this approach is, especially in a situation when no useful medical options are available, to avoid the counselee being manipulated by the counselors' personal preferences. However, in the context of cancer genetic counseling, bearing in mind the medical options to improve survival because of the possibility of early detection and treatment or even prevention of cancer, a more direct approach may be appropriate. Kenneth Offit, a leading expert in the field of clinical cancer genetics, states "For a number of reasons, including the strong presumption of benefit of some cancer screening and early detection options, cancer genetic counseling may be more directive than reproductive counseling" [6].

In general, counseling should be offered to individuals from families that fulfill the following criteria:

- Clustering of the same cancer within the family,
- Clustering of cancer typically associated with cancer syndromes,
- Occurrence of cancer in several generations,
- Early age of onset of cancer,
- Multiple primary cancer in one individual,
- Bilateral cancer.

Not only the occurrence of the identical cancer, but also the occurrence of cancer typically associated with defined hereditary cancer syndromes, for example, pancreas cancer and melanoma, colon and endometrial cancer, or breast and ovarian cancer should be considered. This is a major task of cancer genetic expertise, because investigating the family history for cancer occurring in "other" fields is often not daily practice for clinical specialists. Cancer developing at least 10 years earlier than the average age, and multiple or bilateral cancer in the same individual, are also indicators of possible hereditary origin.

Because different issues and aspects play a role in comprehensive cancer genetic counseling, a multidisciplinary approach is recommended. In addition to the medical geneticist, a clinical specialist from the respective field should be integrated into the counseling process [7]. Since a severely elevated cancer risk can be associated with psychosocial problems, support from a psychologist familiar with oncology should be available (for further details see Chapter 29 on psycho-oncologic and aspects of hereditary tumors and predictive testing).

Up to now there have been no data available as to whether a simultaneous (a counseling session with both the geneticist and the clinician) or sequential counseling approach, that is, meeting the geneticist and the clinician in separate sessions, is more appropriate for the counselee. A simultaneous counseling session enables questions from the counselee concerning different fields to be answered at the same time, and prevents different messages from different experts, but harbors the risk of overloading the counselee with too much new information and makes it more difficult to build up a personal relationship. On the other hand, the sequential counseling session allows a more personal and confidential atmosphere to be created, but harbors the risk of non-uniform and therefore confusing information.

28.2
Counseling Process

The structure of the cancer genetic counseling process is shown in the flow diagram (Figure 28.1).

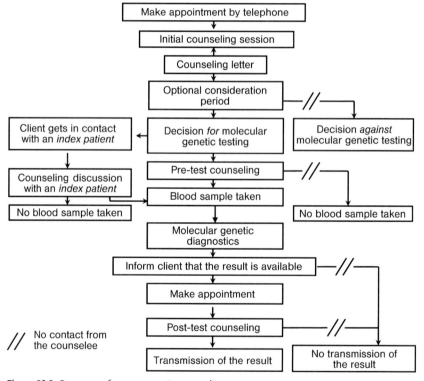

Figure 28.1 Structure of cancer genetic counseling.

28.2.1
First Contact and Counseling Session

To initiate the counseling process, the counselee arranges an appointment for the first counseling session, usually by telephone. It may be helpful to explain the counseling process to the counselees in advance. In particular, they should be prepared at an early stage for the fact that uncertainties will often remain. Moreover, in the first counseling session, the motivation for seeking cancer genetic counseling should be determined [8]. Reasons for undergoing genetic counseling could be to assess the personal risk or the risk for the children. It should be clarified what the counselees' goals for the consultation are and what information she/he hopes to obtain. These questions are essential to guarantee a tailored information strategy. The aim of tailored counseling is to give all the information that best fits the relevant needs and characteristics of the individual without overloading her/him [9].

The counselor's role is to educate and inform about genetic and clinical options, answer questions about what is known, and suggest appropriate referrals to help reach difficult decisions. The counselee should be in a situation after the counseling to undertake shared decision-making (informed consent), that is, for genetic testing.

The content of a cancer genetic counseling session is (modified according to [10]):

- Documentation of the family history/drawing a pedigree,
- Taking the medical history of the counselee,
- Classification of medical records,
- If necessary, physical examination of the counselee, or arranging further medical examinations,
- Determining an as precise as possible genetic diagnosis,
- Transmission of information to the counselee about:
  - Clinical presentation of the disease,
  - Clinical outcome, if possible,
  - Inheritance,
  - Genetic risk for relatives,
  - Possible impact of molecular genetic findings for life and family planning,
  - Risk-reducing strategies and advice about preventive medical check-ups,
- Support in decision-making "informed consent",
- Offer of further assistance (self-help groups, psychologists, clinical specialists),
- Offer of molecular genetic diagnostics, if available,
- Writing a summarizing report of the counseling session.

After clarifying the motives for genetic counseling, the collection of the individuals' personal and the family medical history is the essential first step for cancer risk assessment counseling.

28.2.2
Documentation of the Pedigree and the Medical History

Pedigree documentation is a critical adjunct to taking the family history. The full family structure, including all relatives over at least three generations from the maternal as well as the paternal line, should be recorded. Absolutely essential information for pedigree documentation are:

- At least three generations,
- Gender and age of all relatives (current age or age of death),
- Paternal and maternal line,
- Cancer history of all affected relatives (type(s) of cancer, age at diagnosis, names of affected relatives),
- Hospital/pathology records for all relevant cancers,
- Other medical conditions.

In practice, it may be advantageous to send the counselee a family history questionnaire, which can be assembled into a pedigree working draft to be checked and updated during the interview. To ensure the greatest extent possible, the data collection should include the hospital records of the affected individuals, pathology records and, in special circumstances, histological sections or paraffin blocks to confirm diagnoses. If the counselee is not able to acquire these documents, the counselor should help to obtain them after receiving the signed release forms from the relatives.

It should be stated during the counseling session that the interpretation of a pedigree may change dramatically after the change in health status of even one family member.

28.2.3
Risk Calculation

Family history as evidenced in the pedigree provides the most important information to assess the individual cancer risk. For some cancer syndromes, criteria defined by international expert committees, for example, the Amsterdam and Bethesda criteria in the case of hereditary non-polyposis colorectal cancer (see Chapter 17 on Lynch syndrome (HNPCC)), or the LFS criteria originated from Li and Fraumeni's published work in the case of Li–Fraumeni syndrome [11], are available to facilitate the diagnosis of a hereditary cancer syndrome. These criteria are based on the occurrence of defined malignancies in first-degree relatives, and on age of onset. Families that fulfill these criteria are generally accepted to have hereditary cancer. However, the opposite is not true, thus making it very difficult in some family constellations to decide whether a repeated occurrence of cancer in a family is due to a random accumulation of sporadic cancer, due to a polygenic background leading to a moderately increased risk, or whether cancer has indeed developed due to a monogenic hereditary cancer syndrome.

In the case of hereditary breast and ovarian cancer, different risk calculation models have been developed to improve individual cancer risk assessment, for example, the individual's risk of being a mutation carrier, or the risk of developing breast cancer within the next 10 years or during her lifetime, and/or to better assess the risk of an individual to carry a pathogenic BRCA1/2 mutation. The risk calculation models are helpful tools to evaluate which women will most likely benefit from genetic testing, but usually defined family constellations are taken as a basis for the decision as to which women qualify for mutation analysis [3, 12]. Currently, no international guidelines recommend usage of a certain risk calculation model, since all available models have considerable weaknesses. Instead, a careful qualified genetic analysis of the family history is essential to determine the real individual risk [3, 13].

There are empirical, genetic, and mixed models [13, 14], see Table 28.1 for more details [15–22]. Empirical models consider the family history, for example, the degree of relationship of the counselee to affected women in the family and the age of diagnosis, or additional risk factors, for example, reproductive history, and include them in a logistic regression model. Genetic models are based on the assumption that one autosomal dominant gene (1-gene model) or two autosomal dominant genes (2-gene models) with age-dependent penetrance are responsible for hereditary breast cancer. Newer mixed models include a polygenetic component or empirical risk factors, for example, reproductive history, histopathology or body-mass index, in addition to the 2-gene models.

Only a few studies have compared the accuracy of the different models. According to Euhus et al. [23], genetic counselors and the risk calculation model BRCAPRO had a comparable sensitivity, but BRCAPRO had a significantly higher specificity. Evaluating 272 pedigrees, genetic counselors determined a heterozygous risk of less than 10%, in which no mutation analysis is offered usually, in 8 to 29% and BRCAPRO in 16%. The positive predictive value (PPV) for BRCAPRO was 74%, given a probability to carry a mutation of over 95%, whilst the genetic counselors achieved a PPV of 65 to 100% (median 75%). However, in 2 out of 5 families with a BRCA1/2 mutation, for whom BRCAPRO had determined a heterozygous risk of less than 10%, 7 out of 8 genetic counselors correctly determined a heterozygous risk of more than 10%. This may be explained by the fact that BRCAPRO significantly underestimates the risk of families with ovarian cancer. In three recent studies, only a few of the available models were compared. In an Italian study, BRCAPRO, and in a study in the United States, BOADICEA turned out to be the best model to predict the real mutation frequency [24, 25]. In a British study considering 3150 women, the calculation models were compared in a prospective manner. The newly introduced IBIS model turned out to be the best model, probably because further risk factors are taken into account in addition to the genetic components [26]. All the other prediction models clearly tend to underestimate the risk for developing breast cancer. An alternative, fast and easy-to-use approach to select families most suitable for genetic testing was suggested by Evans et al. [27]. The Manchester scoring system includes a cut-off at 10 points for each gene. This scoring system is shown to be far superior to BRCAPRO regarding the

Table 28.1 Risk prediction models for hereditary breast and ovarian cancer (no guarantee of completeness, modified according to [13]).

Risk prediction model	Model type	Information included	Reference
Gail model (prediction of cancer risk)	Empirical	Number and age of first-degree relatives with breast cancer, age at menarche, reproduction history, biopsies, atypical hyperplasia	Gail, M.H. *et al.* (1989) *Journal of the National Cancer Institute 81*, 1879–86 [15]
Couch model (prediction of *BRCA1/2* carrier probability)	Empirical	Ashkenazi Jewish origin, personal and familial history of breast and ovarian cancer, average age at diagnosis of breast cancer in the family	Couch, F.J. *et al.* (1997) *New England Journal of Medicine 336*, 1409–17 [16]
Myriad tables (prediction of *BRCA1/2* carrier probability)	Empirical	Ashkenazi Jewish origin, personal and familial history of breast and ovarian cancer, age at diagnosis, number of breast cancers diagnosed before 50 years	Frank, T.S. *et al.* (2002) *Journal of Clinical Oncology. 20*, 1480–90 [17]
Claus model (prediction of *BRCA1/2* carrier probability) (incorporated in Cyrillic)	Genetic	Family history, age at diagnosis of breast cancer, age at last follow-up	Claus, E.B. *et al.* (1994) *Cancer 73*, 643–51 [18] adapted for the German population: Chang-Claude, J. *et al.* (1995) *Zentralblatt für Gynäkologie 117*, 423–34 [19]
BRCAPRO (prediction of *BRCA1/2* carrier probability)	Genetic	Family history, age at diagnosis of breast cancer and ovarian cancer, bilateral breast cancer, age at last follow-up, bilateral breast cancer, male breast cancer	Parmigiani, G. *et al.* (1998) *American Journal of Human Genetics. 62*, 145–58 [20]
IBIS (prediction of *BRCA1/2* carrier probability)	Genetic	Family history, age at diagnosis of breast and ovarian cancer, bilateral breast cancer, age at last follow-up, age at menarche, reproduction history, biopsies, atypical hyperplasia, height, body mass index	Tyrer, J. *et al.* (2004) *Statistics in Medicine 23*, 1111–30 [21]
BOADICEA (prediction of *BRCA1/2* carrier probability)	Genetic	Family history, age at diagnosis of breast cancer and ovarian cancer, bilateral breast cancer, age at last follow-up, bilateral breast cancer, male breast cancer	Antoniou, A.C. *et al.* (2004) *British Journal of Cancer 91*, 1580–90 [22]

sensitivity and specificity at 10% prediction for the presence of mutations. Details regarding all prediction models can be found in the excellent review of Antoniou and Easton about the Gail model, BOADICEA, BRCAPRO, Couch model, IBIS, Claus tables, and Myriad tables [13]. After reviewing and comparing these risk prediction models, Antoniou and Easton stated that "some risk models are highly predictive, (but) they cannot determine the mutation status of an individual nor their future disease outcome, with certainty. Thus, they can aid management but cannot substitute for genetic testing. Furthermore, any risk assessment can only be as accurate as the available data, and the accuracy of medical and family history data will continue to be paramount".

28.2.4
Risk Communication Strategies

The goal of cancer genetic counseling is to assess as precisely as possible the individual's risk to develop a primary or secondary cancer. It is not an easy task communicating the determined risk to the counselee. There are different strategies to communicate risks. Risks can be presented in a probability-based fashion, focusing on numerical information, or in a contextualized approach informing a person about the antecedents and consequences of a health problem. These two approaches should be considered as complementary [9]. Because many people have difficulties in understanding quantitative information such as numerical probabilities, communication strategies based on broader information using several presentation formats should be preferred. For a better understanding, the individual risk should be compared with that of the general population. Furthermore, the risk should be given as a percentage, that is, 20%, rather than as a lifetime risk, for example, 0.2. In addition, the percentage should be explained in words, for example, 20% means that 20 out of 100 women in the same situation will develop cancer. To give a better idea, the inverted information should also be provided, for example, 80 of these 100 women will not develop cancer. It can be helpful to illustrate the risk estimation as pie charts or bar graphs. Moreover, the risk should be presented for different time lines, for example, for the next 5 or 10 years and for lifetime.

28.2.5
Pre-Test Counseling

If the family could be classified as having a known hereditary cancer syndrome and the responsible gene is known, a genetic test for the cancer-causing gene can be offered. To obtain the best information, a DNA sample from an affected person from the family, a so-called index patient, should be analyzed first. If she/he is carrying a disease-related mutation, further healthy relatives can undergo genetic testing to find out whether they are also mutation carriers and have an increased risk for developing cancer or whether they did not inherit the mutation and thus have the average cancer risk of the general population. If the counselee decides to undergo genetic testing, informed consent has to be obtained. Many counselees need more than one counseling session to fully understand the facts related to hereditary cancer and to "translate" this information for their individual situation. This is of the utmost importance to develop a mature decision for or against undergoing genetic testing.

Since the results from genetic testing are often relevant for the diseased index patient her/himself, for example, for determining the risk to develop a second cancer, she/he should have received all necessary information to be aware of possible consequences before initiating the genetic testing. Therefore, it should be ensured that genetic counseling has been offered.

It is very helpful to allow to the person undergoing genetic testing time to think over the consequences of genetic testing for her/his life [7]. This has to be considered, particularly in the case of predictive genetic testing.

Before offering genetic testing, the counselee should be prepared to deal with all the medical, psychological, and social consequences of a positive, a negative, or an ambiguous result. Furthermore, she/he should be prepared for the different outcomes of the genetic test result. Besides clear disease-causing mutations, polymorphisms without obvious clinical relevance and/or sequence variants with unknown clinical significance (so-called unclassified variants) may be found.

In addition, the limited sensitivity and specificity of the genetic tests employed should be explained and documented. It should also be ensured that the counselee has understood that the recommended measures for cancer screening do not necessarily guarantee that cancers will not occur.

The education about the basic genetics, like the manner of inheritance, and also the medical information, for example, about the clinical presentation of the disease, should be transmitted in understandable terms. This educational presentation can vary according to the background and characteristics of the counselee. To be most effective, the counselor should come prepared with illustrative charts and tables.

A challenging aspect of cancer risk counseling is the discussion of the medical options to decrease the risk of cancer or to diagnose it at an early stage. It may be that within the counseling session counselees are confronted for the first time with drastic surgical procedures, like the removal of healthy organs, an established management for some syndromes (FAP, MEN 2a). In this counseling situation, it is wise to integrate a clinician, for example a surgeon, into the counseling to clarify the clinical impact and to select the appropriate screening program.

Counselees should be advised from the beginning of the counseling process, before performing genetic testing, that a test result can reveal genetic information about family members not directly involved in the counseling process. The counselee should be prepared for this situation and the possible ways of how to cope with this situation should be discussed.

The decision of the individual to proceed with genetic testing must follow a careful process of pre-test counseling regarding the medical, psychological risks, and benefits of testing. The relevance of genetic test results for insurance and employment issues should also be discussed.

28.2.6
Physical Examination

In special situations, a targeted physical examination should be performed. Some rare hereditary cancer syndromes are associated with physical stigmata, for example, of the head, neck, and skin. Therefore, the observation of alterations (sebaceous cysts, epidermoid cysts, skin lesions like café-au-lait spots or melanin spots) can be essential for the diagnosis and for risk assessment.

28.2.7
Written Report

After every counseling session, a personalized letter summarizing the consultation contents in easily understandable words is sent to the counselee.

To ensure confidentiality it should also be discussed with the counselee beforehand, to whom a copy of the written summary should be additionally sent. The report is addressed in first priority to the counselee her/himself. It may also be useful for the preventive medical recommendation that the individual's physician and/or another healthcare professional are informed.

28.2.8
Post-Test Counseling

When the result of the genetic testing is available, the counselee is informed of this fact. To obtain the test result at a suitable time, the counselee should contact the counseling team to arrange an appointment for test result transmission (see Figure 28.1).

The explanation of the potential impact of the test result requires profound knowledge about the technical details, potential, and limitations of the molecular methods and about the correct interpretation of the genetic test result. Therefore, test result interpretation should be transmitted by geneticists, because the test result is only of clinical value if the interpretation is correct [28].

Genetic test results have to be treated with the utmost confidentiality to prevent misuse. Communicating this information to others is only allowed after the express consent of the counselee.

28.2.9
Psychosocial Aspects

Cancer genetic risk assessment can raise a number of psychosocial issues. Individuals with a familial risk continue to deal with considerable uncertainty, concerning the risk of developing cancer and the associated possibility of death. They are confronted with potentially difficult decisions for managing their future health and worry about potential risks for their children and other family members. An accurate evaluation of the motives and concerns during the first counseling session is essential for a better understanding of how the genetic information will impact this individual's life. Anticipating the psychological and social consequences of a positive, a negative, or an ambiguous result during genetic counseling prior to initiating genetic testing can help to avoid problems. Multiple studies referring to hereditary breast and ovarian cancer show that risk communication and predictive genetic testing can be undertaken without causing significant psychological distress [29]. Immediately after receiving the information of carrying a mutation, depression and anxiety are only minimally increased and adjust back to an almost normal level within a short time after test result disclosure [30, 31]. A systematic review and a meta-analysis found no evidence for adverse psychological effects of informing women about an increased risk of cancer [32, 33].

28.2.10
Communication of Genetic Test Results within the Family

The communication process within the family about the genetic risk is necessary to alert those who may benefit from identification of a hereditary risk. Family communication is a complex and dynamic issue and only a limited number of surveys have been carried out so far about counselees' attitudes towards the disclosure of genetic risk information and the problems that might arise during the dissemination of the genetic test results within the family. Most studies focus on the disclosure of genetic test results in families with hereditary breast and ovarian cancer.

All the studies demonstrate that a relevant proportion of women undergoing genetic testing as the first member of a family have severe problems communicating their genetic risk to relatives. Thus, subsequent diffusion of genetic risk information and interfamily communication may cause difficulties for high-risk individuals [29, 34]. There is research emphasis on the short-term psychological effects of predictive mutation testing with largely reassuring results, but very little is known about the long-term outcome. The first long-term surveys revealed that difficulties can occur, in particular from divulging the test result to family members, and that emotional response within the family differs according to the mutation status [35, 36]. A recent study has shown that mutation carriers are more likely to experience difficulties and distress during the communication of their test result and have less positive feedback from family members [37].

This indicates that there are potential difficulties experienced by mutation carriers during the communication of genetic test results. Thus, it is a major challenge to develop strategies to facilitate dissemination of information within hereditary breast and ovarian cancer families without "overstraining the messenger patient".

Informed counselees are the key players for disclosing genetic risk information to the family. One goal of an effective genetic counseling process is to motivate the counselee to share the risk information with other at-risk relatives. Therefore, the counselor should remind the counselee of the importance the information obtained may have for other family members, at best both prior to genetic testing and on receipt of results. The American Society of Clinical Oncology states in its Policy Statement Update: Genetic Testing for Cancer Susceptibility [38]: "ASCO believes that the cancer care provider's obligations (if any) to at-risk relatives are best fulfilled by communication of familial risk to the person undergoing testing, emphasizing the importance of sharing this information with family members so that they may also benefit".

28.2.11
Problems Due to Failed Communication

Nevertheless, providers of genetic services are likely to deal with counselees who are not willing to disclose the genetic risk information to relatives who may benefit from this knowledge, even though the counselor has stressed the importance of sharing such information [39, 40]. Different international stances exist addressing the question of how to act in this situation. What should have priority? The privacy and confidentiality of the counselee? Or the duty to warn at-risk relatives? In the United States, in exceptional circumstances, the patient's desire for confidentiality may be overridden. This situation is given if the harm is serious, imminent, and likely, and if prevention and treatment are available. According to the statement of the American Society of Human Genetics [41], the healthcare professional has the permission to warn the at-risk family members when attempts to encourage a patient to inform his or her family about the existence of a hereditary risk have failed, if the genetic information reveals that family members are at a substantially higher risk of suffering from a serious and otherwise undetected genetic disorder, and if prevention or treatment is available. In contrast, the national law in Denmark does not authorize physicians to directly transmit genetic information to relatives but accepts such a physician's disclosure at the patient's request [42]. In Germany, in accordance with the Guidelines for Genetic Counseling published by the Berufs-verband Medizinische Genetik e.V. in 1996 [43], it is not permitted to actively contact family members not directly involved in the counseling process, without their consent.

The question of ethical responsibilities of healthcare professionals to warn at-risk relatives will remain a topic of future debate.

28.2.12
Testing Children for Cancer Susceptibility

All existing guidelines strongly oppose the performance of genetic testing for cancer susceptibility in children. Genetic testing should be delayed, even against a strong demand by the parents, until a child is old enough to make its own informed decision regarding genetic testing. Exceptions are hereditary cancer syndromes with a high probability of developing a malignancy during childhood, and the availability of risk-reducing strategies (e.g. FAP, MEN2) [38, 43].

28.3
Outlook

Our knowledge about the molecular basis of hereditary cancer syndromes has dramatically increased during the last decade. With the identification of the genes involved, genetic testing has become available and has been incorporated into modern medical practice. An important component of responsible medical care is the identification of the at-risk individuals to enable the initiation of strategies for prevention or early detection of cancer. Currently, targeted therapeutic drugs, that is, treatment with PARP (poly(ADP-ribose)polymerase) inhibitors for *BRCA1/2*-associated breast cancer, are being developed. Thus, knowledge about the individual mutation status will be even more important in future, since this information will have direct consequences for the individual care, for example, the selection of adjuvant chemotherapy and surgical strategy [44, 45]. However, this knowledge is of lifelong relevance, also for further family members, and may cause psychosocial problems. Therefore, a purely "clinically orientated" pragmatism has to be avoided. The individual's right of "not to know" should be respected [7]. According to all valid guidelines and recommendations, genetic testing should only be offered embedded in a counseling setting including pre- and post-test counseling. Genetic counseling is a multi-step process with the aim of educating the counselee about her/his genetic risk, to enable the individual to make "informed consent" decisions, and to support her/him to cope with the situation. This will become more and more important in the future.

References

1 American Society of Clinical Oncology (ASCO) (1996) Statement of the American Society of Clinical Oncology: genetic testing for cancer susceptibility. *Journal of Clinical Oncology*, **14**, 1730–6.

2 Eisinger, F., Alby, N., Bremond, A., Dauplat, J., Espie, M., Janiaud, P., Kuttenn, F., Lebrun, J.P. *et al.* (1998) Recommendations for management of hereditary breast and ovarian cancer. The French National Ad Hoc Committee. *Annals of Oncology*, **9**, 939–50.

3 NICE (National Institute for Clinical Excellence) (2004) *NICE Clinical Guideline 14: Familial Breast Cancer. The Classification and Care of Women at Risk of Familial Breast Cancer in Primary, Secondary and Tertiary Care*, National Institute for Clinical Excellence, London.

4 Trepanier, A., Ahrens, M., McKinnon, W., Peters, J., Stopfer, J., Grumet, S.C.,

Manley, S., Culver, J.O. *et al.* (2004) Genetic cancer risk assessment and counseling: recommendations of the National Society of Genetic Counselors. *Journal of Genetic Counseling*, **13**, 83–114.

5 Ad Hoc Committee on Genetic Counseling (1975) Report to the American Society of Human Genetics. *American Journal of Human Genetics*, **27**, 240–2.

6 Offit, K. (1998) Clinical cancer genetics and risk counseling, in *Clinical Cancer Genetics* (ed. K. Offit), Wiley-Liss, New York, pp. 1–20.

7 Bundesärztekammer (1998) Richtlinien zur Diagnostik der genetischen Disposition für Krebserkrankungen. *Deutsches Ärzteblatt*, **95**, A1396–1403.

8 Schlegelberger, B. and Hoffrage, U. (2005) Implikationen der genetischen Beratung bei Hochrisiko-Familien für erblichen Brust- und eierstockkrebs, in *BRCA-*

Erblicher Brust- und Eierstockkrebs, (eds A. Gerhardus, H. Schleberger, B. Schlegelberger and F.W. Schwartz), Springer Medizin Verlag, Heidelberg, pp. 33–58.

9 Julian-Reynier, C., Welkenhuysen, M., Hagoel, L., Decruyenaere, M., Hopwood, P. and CRISCOM Working Group (2003) Risk communication strategies: state-of-the-art and effectiveness in the context of cancer genetic services. *European Journal of Human Genetics*, **11**, 725–36.

10 Jungck, M. and Propping, P. (2001) Humangenetische Beratung bei erblichen Tumordispositionserkrankungen, in *Molekularmedizinische Grundlagen von hereditären Tumorerkrankungen* (eds D. Ganten and K. Ruckpaul), Springer-Verlag, Berlin, Heidelberg, pp. 13–21.

11 Li, F.P., Fraumeni, J.E., Mulvihill, J.J., Blattner, W.A., Dreyfus, M.G., Tucker, M.A. and Miller, R.W. (1988) A cancer family syndrome in twenty-four kindreds. *Cancer Research*, **48**, 5358–62.

12 Schmutzler, R., Schlegelberger, B., Meindl, A., Gerber, W.D. and Kiechle, M. (2003) Beratung, genetische Testung und Prävention von Frauen mit einer familiären Belastung für das Mamma- und Ovarialkarzinom. Interdisziplinäre Empfehlungen des Verbundprojektes "Familiärer Brust- und Eierstockkrebs" der Deutschen Krebshilfe. *Medgen*, **15**, 385–95.

13 Antoniou, A.C. and Easton, D.F. (2006) Risk prediction models for familial breast cancer. *Future Oncology*, **2**, 257–74.

14 Fischer, C. and Bickeböller, H. (2007) Risikokalkulationen bei erblichen Krebserkrankungen. *Medgen*, **2**, 245–9.

15 Gail, M.H., Brinton, L.A., Byar, D.P., Corle, D.K., Gree, S.B., Schairer, C. and Mulvihill, J.J. (1989) Projecting individualized probabilities of developing breast cancer for white females who are being examined annually. *The Journal of the National Cancer Institute*, **81**, 1879–86.

16 Couch, F.J., DeShano, M.L., Blackwood, M.A., Calzone, K., Stopfer, J., Campeau, L., Ganguly, A., Rebbeck, T. and Weber, B.L. (1997) *BRCA1* mutation in women

attending clinics that evaluate the risk of breast cancer. *New England Journal of Medicine*, **336**, 1409–15.

17 Frank, T.S., Deffenbaugh, A.M., Reid, J.E., Hulick, M., Ward, B.E., Lingenfelter, B., Gumpper, K.L., Scholl, T. *et al.* (2002) Clinical characteristics of individuals with germline mutations in *BRCA1* and *BRCA2*: analysis of 10 000 individuals. *Journal of Clinical Oncology*, **20**, 1480–90.

18 Claus, E.B., Risch, N. and Thompson, W.D. (1994) Autosomal dominant inheritance of early-onset breast cancer. Implications for risk prediction. *Cancer*, **73**, 643–51.

19 Chang-Claude, J., Becher, H., Hamann, U. and Schroeder-Kurth, T. (1995) Risikoabschätzung für das familiäre Auftreten von Brustkrebs. *Zentralblatt für Gynäkologie*, **117**, 423–34.

20 Parmigiani, G., Berry, D. and Aguilar, O. (1998) Determining carrier probabilities for breast cancer-susceptibility genes *BRCA1* and *BRCA2*. *American Journal of Human Genetics*, **62**, 145–58.

21 Tyrer, J., Duffy, S.W. and Cuzick, J. (2004) A breast cancer prediction model incorporating familial and personal risk factors. *Statistics in Medicine*, **23**, 1111–30.

22 Antoniou, A.C., Pharoah, P.P., Smith, P. and Easton, D.F. (2004) The BOADICEA model of genetic susceptibility to breast and ovarian cancer. *British Journal of Cancer*, **91**, 1580–90.

23 Euhus, D.M., Smith, K.C., Robinson, L., Stucky, A., Olopade, O.I., Cummings, S., Garber, J.E., Chittenden, A. *et al.* (2002) Pretest prediction of *BRCA1* or *BRCA2* mutation by risk counselors and the computer model BRCAPRO. *The Journal of the National Cancer Institute*, **94**, 844–51.

24 Marroni, F., Aretini, P., D'Andrea, E., Caligo, M.A., Cortesi, L., Viel, A., Ricevuto, E., Montagna, M. *et al.* (2004) Evaluation of widely used models for predicting *BRCA1* and *BRCA2* mutations. *Journal of Medical Genetics*, **41**, 278–85.

25 Barcenas, C.H., Hosain, G.M., Arun, B., Zong, J., Zhou, X., Chen, J., Cortada, J.M., Mills, G.B. *et al.* (2006) Assessing *BRCA* carrier probabilities in extended families. *Journal of Clinical Oncology*, **24**, 354–60.

26 Amir, E., Evans, D.G., Shenton, A., Lalloo, F., Moran, A., Boggis, C., Wilson, M. and Howell, A. (2003) Evaluation of breast cancer risk assessment packages in the family history evaluation and screening programme. *Journal of Medical Genetics*, **40**, 807–14.

27 Evans, D.G.R., Eccles, D.M., Rahman, N., Young, K., Bulman, M., Amir, E., Shenton, A., Howell, A. and Lalloo, F. (2004) A new scoring system for the chances of identifying a *BRCA1/2* mutation outperforms existing models including BRCAPRO. *Journal of Medical Genetics*, **41**, 474–80.

28 Giardiello, F.M., Brensinger, J.D., Petersen, G.M., Luce, M.C., Hylind, L. M., Bacon, J.A., Booker, S.V., Parker, R.D. and Hamilton, S.R. (1997) The use and interpretation of commercial *APC* gene testing for familial adenomatous polyposis. *New England Journal of Medicine*, **336**, 823–7.

29 Hopwood, P. (2005) Psychological aspects of risk communication and mutation testing in familial breast-ovarian cancer. *Current Opinion in Oncology*, **17**, 340–4.

30 Reichelt, J.G., Heimdal, K., Moller, P. and Dahl, A.A. (2004) *BRCA1* testing with definitive results: a prospective study of psychological distress in a large clinic-based sample. *Familial Cancer*, **3**, 21–8.

31 Watson, M., Foster, C., Eeles, R., Eccles, D., Ashley, S., Davidson, R., Mackay, J., Morrison, P.J., Hopwood, P., Evans, D.R.G. and Psychosocial Study Collaborators (2004) Psychosocial impact of breast/ovarian (*BRCA1/2*) cancer-predictive genetic testing in a UK multi-centre clinical cohort. *British Journal of Cancer*, **91**, 1787–94.

32 Meiser, B. and Halliday, J.L. (2002) What is the impact of genetic counselling in women at risk of developing hereditary breast cancer? A meta-analytic review. *Social Science & Medicine*, **54**, 1463–70.

33 Butow, P.N., Lobb, E.A., Meiser, B., Barratt, A. and Tucker, K.M. (2003) Psychological outcomes and risk perception after genetic testing and counselling in breast cancer: a systematic

review. *The Medical Journal of Australia*, **178**, 77–81.

34 Patenaude, A.F., Dorval, M., DiGianni, L.S., Schneider, K.A., Chittenden, A. and Garber, J.E. (2006) Sharing *BRCA1/2* test results with first-degree relatives: factors predicting who women tell. *Journal of Clinical Oncology*, **24**, 700–6.

35 Nippert, I. and Schlegelberger, B. and the members of The Consortium "Hereditary Breast and Ovarian Cancer of the Deutsche Krebshilfe" (2003) Women's experiences of undergoing *BRCA1* and *BRCA2* testing: organisation of the German Hereditary Breast and Ovarian Cancer Consortium survey and preliminary data from Münster. *Community Genetics*, **6**, 249–58.

36 Lim, J., Macluran, M., Price, M., Bennett, B., Butow, P. and the kConFab Psychosocial Group (2004) Short- and long-term impact of receiving genetic mutation results in women at increased risk for hereditary breast cancer. *Journal of Genetic Counseling*, **13**, 115–33.

37 Gadzicki, D., Wingen, L.U., Teige, B., Horn, D., Bosse, K., Kreuz, F., Goecke, T., Schäfer, D. *et al.* and German Cancer Aid Consortium on Hereditary Breast and Ovarian Cancer (2006) Communicating *BRCA1* and *BRCA2* genetic test results. *Journal of Clinical Oncology*, **24**, 2969–70.

38 American Society of Clinical Oncology (2003) American Society of Clinical Oncology policy statement update: genetic testing for cancer susceptibility. *Journal of Clinical Oncology*, **21**, 2397–406.

39 Julian-Reynier, C., Eisinger, F., Chabal, F., Lasset, C., Nogues, C., Stoppa-Lyonnet, D., Vennin, P. and Sobol, H. (2000) Disclosure to the family of breast/ovarian cancer genetic test results: patient's willingness and associated factors. *American Journal of Medical Genetics*, **94**, 13–8.

40 Narod, S.A. and Offit, K. (2005) Prevention and management of hereditary breast cancer. *Journal of Clinical Oncology*, **23**, 1656–63.

41 The American Society of Human Genetics Social Issues Subcommittee on Familial Disclosure (1998) ASHG statement professional disclosure of familial genetic information. *American Journal of Human Genetics*, **62**, 474–83.

42 Wilcke, J.T., Seersholm, N., Kok-Jensen, A. and Dirksen, A. (1999) Transmitting genetic risk information in families: attitudes about disclosing the identity of relatives. *American Journal of Human Genetics*, **65**, 902–9.

43 Berufsverband Medizinische Genetik e.V. Deutsche Gesellschaft für Humangenetik (1996) Leitlinien zur Erbringung humangenetischer Leistungen: 1. Leitlinien zur genetischen Beratung. *Medgen*, **8**, Heft 3, Sonderbeilage 1–2.

44 Farmer, H., McCabe, N., Lord, C., Tutt, A., Johnson, D., Richardson, T., Santarosa, M., Dillon, K. *et al.* (2005) Targeting the DNA repair defect in *BRCA* mutant cells as a therapeutic strategy. *Nature*, **434**, 917–21.

45 Bryant, H., Schultz, N., Thomas, H., Parker, K., Flower, D., Lopez, E., Kyle, S., Meuth, M. *et al.* (2005) Specific killing of *BRCA2*-deficient tumours with inhibitors of poly(ADP-ribose) polymerase. *Nature*, **434**, 913–17.

29
Psycho-Oncologic Aspects of Hereditary Tumors and Predictive Testing

Mechthild Neises

Summary

Genetic counseling is a highly specialized service in medical care. The service is expensive and its task is comprehensive, including the family perspective. It often starts a communication process which deals with human problems associated with the risk of occurrence of a genetic disorder in a family. For a breast cancer service, which is the most explored cancer, this process is an attempt to assist the counselee in understanding the medical facts, the mode of inheritance, the risk of getting breast and/or ovarian cancer (again), and the implications and consequences for daily life, the family, and partnership. This includes decision-making regarding surgical options and notification to offspring and family, along with a sense of isolation, which may lead to psychological and emotional distress.

Genetic analyzes in general and preventive options depend on the individual situation and can only be recommended in an interdisciplinary setting. Guidelines including standards for genetic analyzes and comprehensive counseling have been established aiming at the prevention of negative consequences for persons at risk. During the pretest-phase, counseling aims at supporting the process of decision-making, in individuals and their families. After disclosure of test results, psychosocial support aims to enhance adjustment and communication within families. A small subgroup at risk for increased psychosocial distress needs additional support, for example, psychotherapy.

29.1
Introduction

Extensive progress has been made in scientific research in medicine over the past few decades, particularly in the field of genetics. For example, the gynecologists made a radical discovery that breast cancer could well have a genetic disposition (see also Chapter 11 on hereditary breast cancer). The genes responsible, *BRCA1*

Hereditary Tumors: From Genes to Clinical Consequences
Edited by Heike Allgayer, Helga Rehder and Simone Fulda

and *BRCA2* (breast cancer genes), were observed and localized in the years 1994 and 1995. A mutation in one of these genes presents one of the most significant risk factors for the formation of such a carcinoma. After several years of uncertain prognoses, finally a plausible clarification was ascertained for the increase of breast cancer in family members. It has been estimated that 5 to 10% of all breast and ovarian carcinomas has a genetic disposition. In cases of carcinoma of the breast commencing before the age of 35, around 25 to 40% are the cause of a genetic disposition [1]. The hereditary tendency of this affliction is most likely to be passed on to 50% of the offspring. The genes *BRCA1* and *BRCA2* have been shown in around 50% of the severe cases of mutation and could be identified with molecular genetic methods [2]. The remaining 50% of the severe cases revealed changes due to other breast cancer genes, yet to be identified. Women presenting with a disease-associated mutation in the *BRCA1* or *BRCA2* genes suffer a life-long risk of being afflicted with carcinoma of the breast (up to 85%) and ovarian carcinoma (20–60%) [3]. Compared to the state of health of the general population, the life-long risk of carcinoma of the breast is increased to around 10-fold, and for ovarian cancer around 50-fold. It is not a rare occurrence to experience these familiar forms of cancer before the age of 50, as well as a heightened risk of other forms of cancer, for example, cancer of the bowels, uterine cancer, and cancer of the pancreas [4].

Diagnostics for hereditary tumors may indicate the genetic disposition; however, the question still remains if the disease will occur at all, and if so, when. The determination of a genetic tendency results in long-range consequences for the afflicted patient. On the one hand, there is the possibility to detect the disease in the early stages by means of timely diagnosis, and such cases may well be effectively treated by curative measures. The predictive genetic diagnostics of cancer may indeed reduce the feelings of concern and anxiety initially; however, the underlying fear with regard to future health and well-being is awakened, and intensified within the social environment of the afflicted patients. Furthermore, information on the genetic disposition does not only influence the private spheres, but also other areas of life, for example, profession and matters pertaining to insurance.

As is often the case in medicine, progress in scientific research introduces new but not necessarily positive results, particularly for the psychic state of the patients. For example, due to the discovery of the breast cancer genes it may be possible to assess the degree of risk involved for those afflicted with this genetic hereditary tendency. Furthermore, the discovery also enables those women without cancer of the breast to be made aware of their personal genetic disposition, and therefore their chances of being affected at some stage in life with this disease. The problems concerning the psychosomatic – more aptly, somato-psychic field – present a considerable emotional strain both in the knowledge of a breast cancer tendency, or in the difficulties connected with the progress of breast cancer.

With this in mind, the Federal Board of Physicians in 1998 (Bundesärztekammer 1998) laid down in the "Guidelines for the diagnostics of genetic disposition for cancerous diseases". These guidelines were revised in 2003 (Bundesärztekammer

2003) to include an introduction pertaining to human-genetic diagnostics, and the associated consultation with patients with genetic disposition.

Seen from the perspective of the patients, this prospect introduced hope to many, and the awareness of the risk of being afflicted with cancer. Besides, for those risk patients, a certain degree of hope was imparted that the affliction would be discovered in its early stages, by means of special early detection methods, some of which are not presented in the routine services provided by the Health Services. It is common that the actual medical possibilities stand in contradiction to the high expectations of those seeking advice, and also their families. Often, the genetic testing of those seeking advice does not provide the assurance they anticipated. The uncertainty lies in both directions. Twenty to thirty percent of those with genetic disposition showed no tendency towards cancer during the course of their lives. The reasons for this remain, for the main part, unclear. On the other hand, even if the investigation revealed no evidence of a genetic disposition, this does not indicate any general exclusion of risk.

29.2
The Psychosomatics Concerning the Discrepancies Between Physician, Patient, and Diagnosis

The genetic investigation of healthy individuals from families with increased risk of cancer is known as predictive diagnostics. These diagnostics predict a genetic hereditary tendency towards cancer diagnosed previously in a member of the family already afflicted with cancer. This predictive genetic investigation may be performed, given that the family member suffering from cancer consents to such an examination. Specifically, the introduction of predicting the risk of cancer of the breast in healthy women brings about new medical-psychological problems that were not evident prior to the discovery of the breast cancer genes. This leads to the question as to whether or not healthy women or men wish to be informed about their disposition, and their risk of getting cancer, respectively. Would they prefer not to know? In the case that cancer of the breast is a hereditary factor in the female line of the family, particularly if more than one member has suffered, the question of a genetic investigation is considered essential, and not only should be discussed with those women seeking counseling, but also actively approached by the treating physician. However, some patients with a hereditary history of cancer will develop a certain adverse reaction to such an investigation, to avoid any confrontation with the disease.

To be informed about a genetic affliction if cancer has already been diagnosed, appears to affect the patient to a lesser extent. In most cases, clinical treatment has already commenced using surgical and possibly chemotherapeutic and/or radio-therapeutic, as well as antihormonal measures. The therapy offered is based on the primary diagnosis, and continued for the course of the illness. It may occur that the patient is so preoccupied with his illness that he does not wish to be burdened with the additional knowledge of a positive genetic investigation. It is of greater importance that he is prepared to accept his prognosis of cancer, and to concentrate on the therapeutic responses, positively or negatively. For those women or men already afflicted with cancer, it is imperative that they seek counseling so that they are aware of the risk that cancer might be passed on to their children. According to the autosomal-dominant hereditary pattern, there is a 1:1 risk that the children of afflicted mothers will also inherit the mutation. It is not so much the knowledge of the risk involved, rather than the ability to learn how to accept this knowledge, both on the part of the mothers as well as of the daughters. Adolescents of families with a genetic tendency generally take their state of health most seriously, especially the risk of being afflicted with cancer. These anxieties and fears result in considerable psychic stress in three-quarters of all adolescents [5].

29.3
Expectations Concerning the Diagnostics

The above-mentioned aspects make clear that clarification and consultation, regarding the genetic tendency, are of great personal significance. It is highly important to inform the families during the first consultation of all the possibilities, already including the restrictions and consequences of molecular-genetic diagnostics. In this way, any false expectations may be avoided concerning the course of diagnostics and consultations. One must consider – as is the case with each physician-patient encounter – to not only impart professional knowledge to the patient, but to do this in a way that the highly complex medical and genetic jargon is made perfectly clear since, in general, most patients are not conversant with the technicalities of medical language. More often than not, the patients form their own ideas on the subjective theory of the illness, based on what they have seen and heard; notions which may be totally irrational and vague. In each case, inadequate expectations or ideas must be explained in detail and put into perspective. A number of patients seeking counseling may show a very vague or even a very insistent motivation – this is often the result of an ambivalent reaction towards the investigation. It may be necessary to conduct several consultations to decide for or against predictive diagnostics. The reason behind such an attitude may reveal a high degree of psychic stress, requiring, in some cases, therapy. This may include an addictive illness, severe psychic disorders, for instance, specific personality disorders, or even severe depression. Should these illnesses be diagnosed, an appropriate therapy is called for before the genetic diagnostics are undertaken.

The initial consultation may reveal that a clarification of the actual position in life is of primary importance, for instance, existing deep-lying conflicts in a relationship, or separation from a partner. In several cases, the motivation leading to an investigation is often the outcome of an illness, or loss of a relative due to cancer. Should the loss of a family member be a recent event, the patient must be allowed first to undertake a period of mourning. In such a situation, the decision on the part of the physician to postpone a gene test may be a wise move, since it would involve a number of consultations for the patient, a situation she or he may not be ready for.

29.4
Function of Psychosomatics in the Interdisciplinary Consultation Setting

The primary role of predictive diagnostics is to provide information also for healthy individuals who, until now, have suffered no adverse symptoms. By means of these diagnostics, they are taught how to cope with an increased risk of illness, that is, to accept the knowledge of a genetic tendency towards breast cancer. This knowledge often has a profound effect on the private and professional lifestyle of the individual, and indeed affects the personal rights of those seeking counseling. In order to protect these rights, the Federal Board of Physicians set up certain guidelines in 1998, summarized in Table 29.1.

The essential points concerning the guidelines for consultation are that the individual is of age, that sufficient time is allowed between the consultation and the decision, that the decision is based on a specific concept pertaining to consultation, and that the decision lies exclusively with the individual seeking counseling. It is essential that during the first consultation, all details referring to the possibilities, restrictions, and the consequences of molecular-genetic diagnostics are clarified. First, the afflicted member of the family, the so-called index patient, should be examined. Should the causative mutation be identified, then the next step should involve investigation of all the healthy female members in the family (in case of hereditary breast/ovarian cancer) in order to assess whether the mutation, and thus the increased risk of illness, has been inherited or not. It is

Table 29.1 Counseling for those individuals with genetic cancer disposition corresponding to the publication of the Federal Board of Physicians, pertaining to the "Guidelines to the diagnostics of genetic disposition for cancer patients" of 1998.

Intelligible documentation of each counseling session
Written substantiation of indication according to type of illness and/or family case history
Predictive genetic investigation, in general, for those individuals of age
Sufficient time for decision for diagnostics
Decision concerning the course of events lies alone with the individual seeking counseling. Written consent is required.
Inclusion of predictive genetic diagnostics in a counseling concept: counseling/diagnostics/counseling
Further specific synopses of genetic counseling by a qualified physician for human genetics

an unavoidable fact that all members of the family are involved in the decision and diagnostic processes, and the specific family dynamics, that is, "who should speak with whom", "who should receive certain information", and so on, may often result in tension among the family members. For those patients already afflicted with the mutation, the result of the molecular-diagnostic diagnosis is of direct relevance since this indicates a markedly increased risk for recurrence, as well as a secondary renewed illness [6]. Significant grounds for extensive diagnostics in family members enable the afflicted women, as well as the healthy individuals, to gain some knowledge as to the risk involved for their own children. It must be considered that the Federal Board of Physicians pays special attention to the case of children since, according to the aforementioned guidelines; they should not be subjected to genetic investigation.

The patients seeking counseling are informed in detail during the consultation as to the appropriate early detection, follow-up care program, and additionally the possible prophylactic operative measures to combat any further risk of illness. The most important features of the consultation are summarized in a detailed and intelligible letter, which is then forwarded to the patient. Then, should the patient wish for molecular-genetic diagnostics, a second appointment is made for the index patient. This consultation is carried out within an interdisciplinary setting to include professionals in the fields of, for example, breast/ovarian cancer, human genetics, gynecology, and psychosomatics. Again, all the possibilities are discussed concerning the consequences of the diagnostics, and the reasons for the decision. Only then, a blood sample is taken for further laboratory diagnostics. Once the results have been processed, the patient is then contacted again with a written letter, and invited for a third consultation. This consultation is also carried out within an interdisciplinary setting, and all consequences of the findings discussed again in detail, including the further course of treatment. It goes without saying that the patient seeking advice has the right to discontinue the consultation and diagnostic sessions at any time – without stating reasons (Figure 29.1). Always, a psychological/psychotherapeutic attendance is present within the interdisciplinary setting. This may be a psychologist with the knowledge of somatics, a physician of psychosomatic medicine and psychotherapy, or of a somatic field such as gynecology with corresponding additional psychotherapeutic qualifications.

The presence of a qualified psychotherapist or psychologist in the session enables the parallel undertaking of psycho-diagnostics. Several important aspects are usually revealed, such as the motivation of the patient regarding molecular-genetic diagnostics, the patient's psycho-social position, present psychic state of health, and the resources and relevant strategies for coping with the illness. Should it be necessary that extensive psychotherapeutic-oriented counseling during the first consultation is required, this should be introduced subtly to cover all the significant aspects. It is of importance to find out the source of the motivation leading to consultation and diagnostics, and what expectations are awaited by whom, be it a member of the family, a relative, or acquaintance. It is of primary importance to discover how those individuals with a close relationship to the

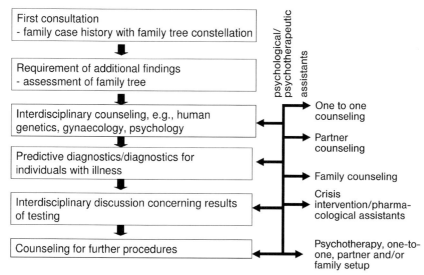

Figure 29.1 Psychological support during interdisciplinary counseling.

afflicted patient perceive this illness, also those distantly acquainted. Based on the biographical case history, vulnerability factors are to be perceived, such as stressful experiences and how these were overcome. This can be done by self-assessment of the patient seeking advice, as well as an assessment of the inter-viewer with a view to both the individual resources and the resources, within the social environment. On clarification of the actual state of health, it is essential to consider experiences of anxiety, and the methods used to cope with anxiety, be it fear of life in general, a specific fear of getting cancer, or of the progress of already detected cancer (Damocles syndrome). In conjunction with psychothera-peutic competence, the first consultation enables the early detection of any psychic risk factors, and ensues in the support and development of a motivation to include an extensive consultation and possibly psychotherapy, should this be necessary [7]. Relevant aspects of psychotherapeutic primary consultation for tumor-genetic diagnostics include:

- Motivation for diagnostics by individual seeking counseling, within the family and in personal environment;

- Personal view, information status, expectation of discussion, subjective theory of illness, experience of counseling, course of counseling, and diagnostics;

- Observation of family system and its members, specific clarification of relations towards family members already suffering from cancer;

- Biographical case history;

- Present biopsychosocial state of health, individual and familial psychiatric and psychosomatic illnesses;

- Conclusive clarification of further course of events, e.g., further counseling sessions, clarification of indication and motivation for psychotherapeutic treatment.

29.5
Psychosomatic Aspects of the Patient

It is basically the decision of the patient whether or not to undergo genetic testing. More often than not, the patient will seek advice in order to help make the final decision, be it from a close contact or a physician, even from a competent psychotherapist. The decision usually depends on how the patient copes with mental stress in general. Variables determining this aspect have much to do with the personality structure. It must be emphasized that it is usually the compulsive type who tends to demand detailed information on the whole situation, also the genetic disposition. It is often the more phobic individuals who wish to avoid any detailed knowledge. Those with a histrionic personality may play down the severity of the illness at first; however, once the facts are put before them, then the actual situation is recognized as apparent and real.

A particular variable is how much risk the patient is prepare to take. Past history can serve to determine this factor, especially if the patient has previously found herself in an ambivalent stress situation requiring her to make a decision. It is usually the case that those patients who are willing to undertake a higher risk are more likely to agree to a genetic testing than those with a lower risk-taking capacity. The reasons leading to the motivation for genetic testing tend to vary among the women who have personally experienced breast cancer, or those who have a member of the family with evidence of BRCA 1 or BRCA2. For persons who are already afflicted with cancer, the main motive for a genetic investigation is to gain more information with a view that their own children may also be one day afflicted. Another motive is the fear of a recurrent episode of cancer and finally, a number of patients wish to be of help for the purpose of scientific research. For example women stemming from a family with evidence of BRCA1 or BRCA2 state that this was their motive to go ahead with genetic testing. It has been shown that women with a lower degree of education are usually those who wish for genetic testing, so that they are aware of the risk involved for their own offspring, and also to support scientific research. Also, they have a higher interest in a prophylactic mastectomy. While younger women are more inclined to be motivated by their own personal risk of getting cancer, combined with the interest to gain more information on prophylactic mastectomy, the older generation is more motivated by the wish to support scientific progress, and to be informed of the risk involved for their children [8].

Frequent motives for genetic testing for breast cancer are:

1. For women with a medical history of breast cancer:
   - risk for their children,
   - worry about getting cancer again,
   - helping scientific research.

2. With evidence of *BRCA1* and *BRCA2* in the family:
   - because a family member asked for appointment for genetic counseling,
   - risk for their children,
   - interest in prophylactic mastectomy.

An important factor is the familial situation of the patient with known genetic disposition, since an arrangement of further investigations and the course of events is a matter also concerning the family, in particular the partner. A sound and supportive relationship is of paramount importance for the mental ability of the patient to come to terms with the genetic disposition. The partner should, if possible, be included in the decision for genetic testing, since it is often the partner's wish to be informed in detail of the situation, thus so providing the necessary support for the partner, especially if evidence of a *BRCA1* or *BRCA2* gene is detected [9]. Unrestrained communication between all family members reduces considerably the intensive mental strain on the part of the patient. It must be said that openness within a relationship may lead to an increased psychological stress, although this usually happens when information is withheld concerning the possible consequences [10].

The general early case history of the patient presents an idea of how the patient was able to cope with her previous somatic illnesses, and also the experiences she has made with other psychological and possibly psychiatric illness. In general, it may be expected that she will react in a similar way towards her actual genetic situation as she did towards her previous illnesses. Other areas in her past history will also indicate how she dealt with stress, for example, in the case of fleeing from a situation, a person can experience of physical abuse, or even loss of a partner. All these factors reveal the possible reactions to expect when informing of a genetic disposition.

29.6
Variables on Notification of Diagnosis

A decisive factor is the stability of the physician-patient relationship, in particular, concerning the following aspects:

One of the essential questions is whether the actual physician-patient relationship was formed as a result of previous medical care, or if the relationship was formed when a genetic disposition had been diagnosed. The patient may already have gained confidence in the physician, but should the patient have been introduced to the physician only recently, it is important for the physician to realize how the patient is coping with coming to terms with the diagnosis. Attention should be paid to the psychosomatic care administered, and previous variables offer an insight into the degree of support required. The perspectives in life of the patient, in view of the previous lifestyle, as well as in view of the basic perspectives in life for the future, should be taken into account. Such a situation depends on the acceptance and tolerance in the knowledge of the genetic affliction. This experience can influence the reflection and meaning of aims and values in one's life. Even without the aid of psychotherapy, it is highly important for the physician to identify with the patient, and to recognize and treat the somato-psychic condition with utmost sensitivity and care. A corresponding stable and compatible physician-patient relationship may take some time to form. This is essential in the case of a psychotherapeutic intervention.

The theory of consultation as compiled by the Federal Board of Physicians may be of help as a guideline for the orientation and general direction for the physician. On the one hand, the motivation of the patient is a most important factor together with clear indications for a psychotherapeutic intervention. In some cases, the motivation must be first developed, in order to assure an optimal outcome for coming to terms with the illness and planning for the future.

29.7
Psychosomatic–Psychotherapeutic Procedures

From a psychosomatic view, questions raised are indication of a genetic testing, the notification and coming to terms with a possibly stressful outcome, how this will affect the actual lifestyle, the family and other contact persons, the basic attitude towards life, that is, the sense and values of ones' own future life, and, in particular, the self-perception of the patient. Crucial is the resource-mobilization, that is, reflexion on the particular spheres of life that would enable the stability of self-esteem, security in life, and fulfilment of life. It must be heeded, however, that stress factors might be problems caused by the partner, illness, financial matters, or the family. From a psychosomatic point of view, attention must be paid to the internal and external resources, the latter stemming from the social environment. All these factors may influence the patient coming to terms with her/his illness.

Within the consultation setting, special attention should be paid as to whether a family member has already suffered from cancer. This is of particular significance when a sister of the patient seeking counseling is afflicted with cancer [11]. Apart from routine consultation, a one-to-one discussion should take place, this if possible, in the company of another person. Intensive support and care should be made available to those patients who were closely involved with members of the family in need of care and have died of cancer. Taking care of those gravely ill leads to an enormous strain, and makes one acutely aware of the increased risk of oneself being afflicted with the same illness. Generally speaking, those women or men with a minimum of education and training require a higher degree of attention, since such individuals with socio-demographic attributes are more prone towards anxiety and depression.

Those individuals who refuse to undergo diagnostics should also receive special attention as they constitute the type of women with a high psychological morbidity rate, which is not recognized when a hasty decision is made. The decision for or against a gene test often presents with repercussions on the other family members, so that the refusal to undergo such a test may result in the family forming a stronger bond and expressing emotions more freely. Mutation patients already tested tend to be less emboldened, do not show emotions as openly, or exchange information as easily, with other persons [12]. Also women or men who generally are less compliant in their perception of preventive measures often show signs of a higher psychological morbidity. These aspects emphasize not only the necessity of a number of successive consultations in the course of the diagnostic process, but also the necessity of psychological and psychotherapeutic competence in the form of an interdisciplinary consultation. Furthermore, there is always the possibility that a crisis intervention will be called for, or an admission to outpatient psychotherapy.

Finally, it is of great importance to point out that many of those seeking advice are able to come to terms with the result of their diagnostics [13], that is, around 80% of women with hereditary breast or ovarian cancer are able to overcome the process of making a decision, and the result of the diagnostics, using their own resources. Around half of those women seeking advice and diagnostics put priority on gynecological and genetic topics, not on psycho-oncological aspects. However, it is assumed that every fifth woman seeking counseling had the need to undergo psycho-oncological care.

29.8
Conclusion

The molecular and gene-diagnostic progress over the past few years has served to increase the interest in predictive diagnostics, especially, for example, for hereditary breast and ovarian cancer. Although women with a minimal risk may not profit from such a test, studies have shown an increase in the interest of women in the general public [14]. Information and communication strategies should be developed for the purpose of consultation, and these should focus on balancing unrealistic expectations concerning genetic testing, as well as reducing the known risk of cancer and the raised level of anxiety and fear. During a consultation, it should be taken into account that the genetic risk and the result of molecular-genetic diagnostics usually affect the family entirely. Interdisciplinary cooperation is the best prerequisite available for both the patient seeking counseling and the family, to correctly interpret an increased risk of cancer, the optimal measures for treatment and, in particular, to undergo extensive counseling and psychotherapy. Supportive group psychotherapy for patients suffering *BRCA1* and *BRCA2* mutations showed that those participating in the session had a high level of knowledge prior to the intervention, and that this showed no change during the course of intervention. Significant improvements were achieved in the psychological condition of the patients as to their anxiety and depressive state. A large number of women considered company to be beneficial for making the decision as to a prophylactic operation (ovarectomy or mastectomy) [15]. However, it is too early to determine the long-term effects resulting from the knowledge of genetic cancer predispositions. There is the probability that a specific group of persons will react with increased feelings of anxiety or raised tendencies towards physical complaints and for these individuals, the knowledge on their personal risk of cancer will rather be a stress factor than a positive declaration [16]. The ability to identify the risk persons early enough, and to develop the appropriate supportive measures, will prove to be a significant task in the future.

References

1 Lux, M.P., Fasching, P.A., Barny, M. and Beckmann, MW. (2004) Heriditäres Mamma- und Ovarialkarzinom – ein update. *Geburtsh Frauenheilk*, **64**, 1037–51.

2 Miki, Y., Swensen, J., Shattuck-Eidens, D., Futreal, P.A., Harshman, K., Tavtigian, S., Liu, Q., Cochran, C., Bennett, L.M. and Ding, W. (1994) A strong candidate for the breast and ovarian cancer susceptibility gene *BRCA1*. *Science*, **166**, 66–71.

3 King, M.C., Marks, J.H. and Mandell, J.B. for the New York Breast Cancer Study Group (2003) Breast and ovarian cancer risks due to inherited mutations in *BRCA1* and *BRCA2*. *Science*, **302**, 643–46.

4 Thompson, D. and Easton, D.F. (2002) The Breast Cancer linkage Consortium: cancer incidence in *BRCA1* mutation carriers. *Journal of the National Cancer Institute*, **94**, 1358–65.

5 Capelli, M., Verma, S., Korneluk, Y., Hunter, A., Tomiak, E., De Allanson, J.G., Grasse, C., Corsini, L. and Humphreys, L. (2005) Psychological and genetic counseling implications for adolescent daughters of mothers with breast cancer. *Clinical Genetics*, **67**, 481–91.

6 Haffty, B.G., Harrold, E., Khan, A.J., Pathare, P., Smith, T.E., Turner, B.C., Glazer, P.M., Ward, B., Carter, D., Matloff, E., Bale, A.E. and Alvarez-Franco, M. (2002) Outcome of conservatively managed early-onset breast cancer by *BRCA1/2* status. *Lancet*, **359**, 1471–7.

7 Bodden-Heidrich, R. (2001) Psychosomatische Aspekte der prädiktiven Diagnostik in der Frauenheilkunde. *Gynäkologie*, **34**, 189–93.

8 Van Asperen, C.J., Van Dijk, S., Zoeteweij, M.W., Timmermans, D.R., De Bock, G.H., Meijers-Heijboer, E.J., Niermeijer, M.F., Breuning, M.H., Kievit, J. and Otten, W.J. (2002) *Medical Genetics*, **39**, 410–14.

9 Bluman, L.G., Rimer, B.K., Regan Sterba, K., Lancaster, J., Clark, S., Borstelmann, N., Iglehart, J.D. and Winer, E.P. (2003) Attitudes, knowledge, risk perceptions and decision-making among women with breast and/or ovarian cancer considering testing for *BRCA1* and *BRCA2* and their spouses. *Psychooncology*, **12**, 410–27.

10 Manne, S., Audrain, J., Schwartz, M., Main, D., Finch, C. and Lerman, C. (2004) Associations between ralationship support and psychological reactions of participants and partners to *BRCA1* and *BRCA2* testing in a clinic-based sample. *Annals of Behavioral Medicine*, **28**, 211–25.

11 van Dooren, S., Seynaeve, C., Rijnsburger, A.J., Duivenvoorden, H.J., Essink-Bot, M.L., Bartels, C.C.M., Klijn, J.G.M., de Koning, H.J. and Tibben, A. (2005) The impact of having relatives affected with breast cancer on psychological distress in

women at increased risk for hereditary breast cancer. *Breast Cancer Research and Treatment*, **89**, 75–80.

12 McInerney-Leo, A., Biesecker, B.B., Hadley, D.W., Kase, R.G., Giambarresi, T.R., Johnson, E., Lerman, C. and Struewing, J.P. (2005) BRCA1/2 testing in hereditary breast and ovarian cancer families II. Impact on relationships. *American Journal of Medical Genetics. Part A*, **133**, 165–9.

13 Schwartz, M.D., Peshkin, B.N., Hughes, C., Main, D., Isaacs, C. and Lerman, C. (2002) Impact of *BRCA1/BRCA2* mutation testing on psychologic distress in a clinic-based sample. *Journal of Clinical Oncology*, **20**, 514–20.

14 Reitz, F., Barth, J. and Bengel, J. (2004) Predictive value of breast cancer cognitions and attitudes toward genetic testing on women's interest in genetic testing for breast cancer risk. Psycho-Social-Medicine : 1: Doc03, www.egms.de/en/journals/psm/ 2004-1/psm000003.shtml (accessed 15.10.2007).

15 Esplen, M.J., Hunter, J., Leszcz, M., Warner, E., Narod, S., Metcalfe, K., Glendon, G., Butler, K., Liede, A., Young, M.A., Kieffer, S., DiProspero, L., Irwin, E. and Wong, J. (2004) A multicenter study of supportive-expressive group therapy for women with *BRCA1/BRCA2* mutations. *Cancer*, **15**, 2327–40.

16 Keller, M. (2000) Psychosocial issues in cancer genetics: State of the art. *Zeitschrift für Psychosomatische Medizin und Psychotherapie*, **46**, 80–97.

17 Bundesärztekammer (1998) Richtlinien zur Diagnostik der genetischen Disposition für Krebserkrankungen. *Dt Ärztebl*, **95**, B1120–7.

18 Bundesärztekammer (2003) Richtlinien zur prädiktiven genetischen Diagnostik (verabschiedet vom Vorstand der Bundesärztekammer am 14.02.2003. *Dt Ärztebl*, **100**, B1085–93.

30
Molecular Targeted Therapy

Heike Allgayer and Simone Fulda

Summary

Progress in the elucidation of molecular targets in human cancers in the last decades has provided the basis for the development of novel therapeutics. A huge variety of potential target structures have been identified, many of which are already exploited for therapeutic purposes. To conclude this book on hereditary tumors, with an outlook on general diagnostic and therapeutic challenges and chances, this review introduces the reader into the concept of molecular targeted therapies, and provides some prototypic examples.

30.1
Introduction

During recent years, there has been a rapid development of molecular markers as targets for innovative therapeutic concepts ("Targeted Therapy"). A high number of molecules have already become therapeutic targets, especially growth factors and growth factor receptors, molecules of signal transduction, tumor-associated antigens, molecules of intracellular protein metabolism (proteasome inhibitors), factors regulating cell survival, cell cycle and cell death, and molecules associated with invasion, metastasis, and angiogenesis. An overview on major examples for targets that already entered first clinical trials is given in Figure 30.1. Some of these molecular targeted compounds are not only efficient as tumor therapeutics, but also improve quality of life by, for example, reducing pain associated with the reduction of bone metastasis [1–6].

30.2
Example for Success: Targeting Tyrosine Kinase Receptors, for Example, EGF-R

There has been an especially impressive development of compounds targeted against tyrosine kinase receptors [7]. Here, targeting concepts directed against

Hereditary Tumors: From Genes to Clinical Consequences
Edited by Heike Allgayer, Helga Rehder and Simone Fulda
Copyright © 2009 WILEY-VCH Verlag GmbH & Co. KGaA, Weinheim
ISBN: 978-3-527-32028-8

Tumor cell

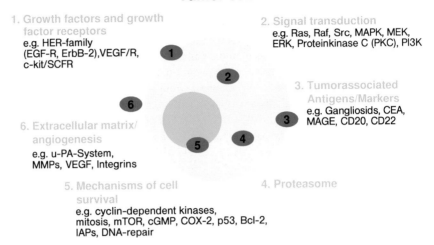

1. Growth factors and growth factor receptors
e.g. HER-family (EGF-R, ErbB-2),VEGF/R, c-kit/SCFR

2. Signal transduction
e.g. Ras, Raf, Src, MAPK, MEK, ERK, Proteinkinase C (PKC), PI3K

3. Tumorassociated Antigens/Markers
e.g. Gangliosids, CEA, MAGE, CD20, CD22

6. Extracellular matrix/ angiogenesis
e.g. u-PA-System, MMPs, VEGF, Integrins

5. Mechanisms of cell survival
e.g. cyclin-dependent kinases, mitosis, mTOR, cGMP, COX-2, p53, Bcl-2, IAPs, DNA-repair

4. Proteasome

Figure 30.1 Overview on major examples of molecules that have become therapeutic targets, for compounds that already have entered early clinical trials.

c-erb-B2 (HER2), such as Herceptin, especially in breast cancers, c-Kit-targeted therapy (Gleevec) in Bcr/Abl-positive leukemias and GIST-tumors, VEGF/VEGF-R-targeted compounds [8, 9], and a number of therapeutic concepts targeting EGF-receptors, are standing out as major examples that have led, or will almost certainly lead, to paradigm shifts in the treatment of major tumor diseases. With increasing numbers of clinical studies, a part of them accompanied by molecular translational studies, it becomes clear that the therapeutic response towards such-like compounds to a considerable extent will be defined by the individual molecular conditions of the individual patient, the genetic- or population-based background of a patient, and either acquired or inherited peculiar characteristics and changes within the gene encoding the target, such as amplifications, mutations, or polymorphisms.

This can be illustrated by first experiences from clinical studies on compounds targeting, e.g. the EGF-receptor. The EGF-receptor is overexpressed in a number of solid carcinomas, such as colorectal or certain types of lung cancers [10], and its prognostic impact has already been shown for these tumor entities for certain patient subgroups [10–12]. Binding of the ligand EGF leads to dimerization, either with another EGF-R-molecule or with a molecule from the Erb-B-receptor tyrosine-kinase family. This is followed by the phosphorylation of the intracellular domain, activating a number of, for example, Ras-associated signaling cascades that can initiate phenomena such as tumor cell proliferation, invasion, metastasis, or anti-apoptosis [5, 6]. During recent years, diverse therapeutic strategies targeting EGF-R have been developed. Small molecular compounds targeting EGF-R are directed against the tyrosine kinase domain of EGF-R and inhibit its activation, thereby inhibiting EGF-R initiated signaling [13–15]. Other EGF-R-targeted strategies are based on antibodies [16–24]. A number of studies have already been conducted, especially concerning the tyrosine-kinase inhibitors in colorectal [10] and lung cancer [25–28]. Large studies of non-small cell lung cancer, such as the ISEL- or BR21-study on 1692 or 731 patients, have shown that the best response to therapy and best survival was observed in patient subgroups with an Asian population background, female gender, adenocarcinoma, and no history of smoking.

Furthermore, in various studies, the level of EGF-R protein expression or amplification of the EGF-R gene was associated with response to EGF-R-based tyrosine-kinase inhibitor therapy [29–35]. Certain studies show an association of certain mutations within the EGF-R gene with the clinical response towards small molecular EGF-R targeted compounds [31]. Most of these mutations have been found within exons 18 to 21 within the *EGF-R* gene [30]. In addition, it has been shown that certain mutations within the *EGF-R* gene can be associated with the development of a secondary resistance to therapy [30, 31]. On the other hand, initial results on antibody-based therapy suggest an independence of EGFR-antibody-based therapy of EGFR-expression or -mutations, but rather on molecules such as E-cadherin (see Chapter 1), suggesting considerations of differential, or combined, strategies depending on the individual situation ([16–24, 71] and own unpublished observations). Patients harboring activating *k-ras*-mutations in non-small cell lung cancers most often show resistance towards EGF-R-based tyrosine kinase inhibitors most likely also antibodies [30]. In such cases, a combination with, for example, Ras-targeted compounds may be necessary for an individual patient. An excellent introduction to Ras-targeted therapy (e.g. farnesyltransferase inhibitors) is given for the particular example of neurofibromatosis-related tumors (see Chapter 6 on neurofibromatosis). Taken together, the initial results of the particular EGF-R-targeted therapy illustrate that especially molecular, and also potentially genetic, conditions can modify and affect the response to targeted therapy concepts. This emphasizes the notion that detailed molecular analysis of the individual tumor in the individual patient needs to accompany further studies on molecular targeted compounds, to precisely classify the subgroups of patients that best respond to novel targeted compounds (see below).

30.3
Example: Targeting Apoptosis Pathways for Cancer Therapy

Moreover, a number of strategies have been developed that target the apoptotic machinery in cancer cells, and therefore, this should serve as a second example. Apoptosis or programmed cell death is the cell's intrinsic death program that plays an important role in various physiological and pathological situations and is highly conserved throughout evolution [36]. Tissue homeostasis is maintained by a subtle balance between proliferation on one side and cell death on the other [37]. As a consequence, too little apoptosis can contribute to tumor formation, progression, and resistance to treatment [38]. Moreover, one of the most important advances in cancer research in recent years is the recognition that killing of tumor cells by anticancer therapies commonly used in the treatment of human cancer, for example, chemotherapy, γ-irradiation, immunotherapy, or suicide gene therapy, is predominantly mediated by initiating programmed cell death, that is, apoptosis in cancer cells [39, 40]. The elucidation of signaling pathways involved in the regulation of apoptosis in cancer cells over the last decade has led to the identification of key apoptosis regulatory molecules that may serve as molecular targets for cancer therapy. In principle, apoptosis-based cancer therapeutics may aim at directly activating apoptosis pathways in cancer cells, at restoring defects in the apoptotic machinery, or at disabling the antiapoptotic function of molecules involved in treatment resistance. Such strategies may open up new perspectives to overcome apoptosis resistance in a variety of human cancers. Some examples of how apoptosis pathways could be targeted for cancer therapy will be discussed in the following sections.

30.3.1
Apoptosis Signaling Pathways

There are two principle pathways of apoptosis, the receptor or extrinsic and the mitochondrial or intrinsic pathway (Figure 30.2) [40]. Stimulation of either pathway eventually activates caspases, a family of cysteine proteases that act as common effector molecules in various forms of cell death [41]. Caspases are synthesized as inactive proenzymes. Once activated, they cleave various substrates in the cytoplasm or nucleus, causing characteristic morphological features of apoptotic cell death [41]. In the extrinsic apoptosis pathway, stimulation of death receptors (DR) of the tumor necrosis factor (TNF) receptor superfamily, for example, CD95 (APO-1/Fas) or TRAIL receptors, results in activation of the initiator caspase-8, which in turn can directly cleave downstream effector caspases, such as caspase-3 [42]. Also, activation of caspase-8 may link the receptor to the mitochondrial pathway by cleaving Bid, a Bcl-2 family protein with a BH3 domain that only translocates to mitochondria upon cleavage to initiate a mitochondrial amplification loop [43]. In the mitochondrial pathway, the release of apoptogenic factors such as cytochrome c, apoptosis-inducing factor (AIF), second mitochondria-derived activator of caspase (Smac)/direct IAP Binding protein with Low PI (DIABLO) or Omi/high temperature requirement protein A (HtrA2) from the mitochondrial intermembrane space into the cytosol initiates caspase-3 activation [44]. Cytochrome c promotes caspase-3 activation through formation of the cytochrome c/Apaf-1/caspase-9-containing apoptosome complex, while Smac/DIABLO promotes caspase activation through neutralizing the inhibitory effects of IAPs [44]. Because of the potential detrimental effects on cell survival in cases of inappropriate caspase activation, activation of caspases has to be tightly controlled. The anti-apoptotic mechanisms regulating cell death have also been implicated in conferring drug resistance to tumor cells.

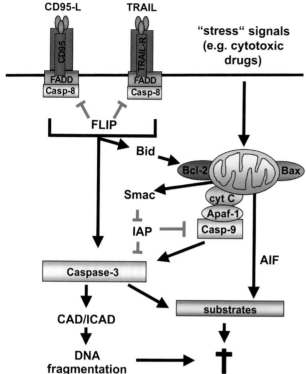

CD95-L   **TRAIL**

**"stress" signals
(e.g. cytotoxic
drugs)**

Figure 30.2 Apoptosis pathways. Apoptosis pathways can be initiated by ligation of death receptors (DR) such as CD95 or TRAIL receptors (TRAIL-Rs) by their respective ligands, for example, CD95 ligand (CD95L) or TRAIL, followed by receptor trimerization, recruitment of adaptor molecules (FADD) and activation of caspase-8 (receptor pathway). The mitochondrial pathway is initiated by the release of apoptogenic factors such as cytochrome c, Smac, or AIF from mitochondria in the cytosol. Apoptosis can be inhibited by Bcl-2 or by "Inhibitor of Apoptosis Proteins" (IAPs). Smac promotes apoptosis by neutralizing IAP-mediated inhibition of caspase-3 and -9. See text for more details.

30.3.2
Exploiting the Apoptotic Machinery for Cancer Therapy

Based on the concept that resistance to apoptosis is a characteristic feature of human cancers that contributes to tumor formation and progression, strategies designed to restore defective apoptosis programs in cancer cells may overcome intrinsic or acquired resistance of tumor cells to current regimens [45]. Also, apoptosis targeted therapies may enhance the responsiveness of human cancers towards conventional treatments that are currently used in clinics, for example, chemo- or radiotherapy, since these therapies primarily exert their anti-tumor activity by triggering apoptosis in cancer cells [40].

30.3.2.1 Targeting Death Receptors for Cancer Therapy

The idea to trigger death receptors in order to induce apoptosis in cancer cells is attractive for cancer therapy, since death receptors are directly linked to the cell's intrinsic death machinery [46]. Death receptors are members of the TNF receptor gene superfamily, which exhibit a broad range of biological functions besides triggering cell death, including regulation of survival, differentiation, or immune responses [42, 46, 47]. Death receptors share an intracellular domain called "death domain", which transmits the death signal from the cell's surface to intracellular signaling pathways. The best-characterized death receptors include CD95 (APO-1/Fas), TNF receptor 1 (TNFRI), TNF-related apoptosis-inducing ligand (TRAIL) receptor 1 (TRAIL-R1), and TRAIL-R2. The corresponding ligands of the TNF superfamily comprise CD95 ligand, TNFα or TRAIL. Death receptors are activated upon oligomerization in response to bind their cognate ligand or by agonistic antibodies.

Among the death receptor ligands, TRAIL is the most promising candidate for clinical development, since it predominantly kills cancer cells, while sparing normal cells [48]. Recombinant soluble TRAIL or monoclonal antibodies targeting TRAIL receptors TRAIL-R1 or TRAIL-R2 were reported to induce apoptosis in a wide range of cancer cell lines and also *in vivo* in several xenograft models of human cancers [48–50]. Interestingly, TRAIL-R2 antibody-based therapy was recently reported as an efficient strategy not only to eliminate TRAIL-sensitive tumor cells, but also to induce tumor-specific T cell memory that afforded long-term protection from tumor recurrence [51].

Moreover, TRAIL-based combination therapies were developed, since a large proportion of human cancer turned out to be partially or completely resistant towards monotherapy with TRAIL, despite the expression of both agonist TRAIL receptors. For example, synergistic interaction between TRAIL and chemotherapy or γ-irradiation was found in various cancers [52, 53].

30.3.2.2 Targeting the Mitochondrial Pathway for Cancer Therapy

Another approach to target apoptosis pathways for cancer therapy is to antagonize antiapoptotic Bcl-2 family members. The Bcl-2 family of proteins consists of both antiapoptotic members, for example, Bcl-2, Bcl-X_L, Mcl-1, as well as proapoptotic molecules [43]. The latter comprise, on the one hand, multidomain proteins such as Bax, Bak, and Bad and, on the other hand, BH3-domain-only molecules, for example, Bim, Bid, Bmf, Noxa, or Puma [43]. Bcl-2 family proteins play an important role in the regulation of the mitochondrial pathway of apoptosis, since they are involved in the control of mitochondrial outer membrane permeabilization [43]. There are currently two models of how BH3-only proteins activate Bax and Bak during the course of apoptosis. According to the direct activation model [54], putative activators such as Bim and cleaved Bid (tBid) bind directly to Bax and Bak to trigger their activation, while BH3-only proteins that act as sensitizers, for example, Bad, bind to the pro-survival Bcl-2 proteins. By comparison, the indirect activation model holds that BH3-only proteins activate Bax and Bak by binding and thus inactivating the various antiapoptotic Bcl-2 proteins that in turn inhibit Bax and Bak [55]. Imbalances in the ratio of anti- versus pro-apoptotic Bcl-2 proteins may tip the balance towards tumor cell survival and thus may contribute to tumor formation and progression. Since high expression of anti-apoptotic Bcl-2 family proteins may confer resistance to chemo- or radiotherapy by blocking the mitochondrial pathway of apoptosis, there has been much interest in developing strategies to overcome the cytoprotective effect of Bcl-2 and related molecules. A prominent example of these efforts is the development of the small molecule antagonist ABT-737, which binds to the surface groove of Bcl-2, Bcl-X_L, and Bcl-w that normally interacts with the BH3 domain of Bax or Bak [56]. By preventing the binding of antiapoptotic Bcl-2 proteins to Bax or Bak, ABT-737 frees Bax and Bak to oligomerize and form pores in the outer mitochondrial membrane, promoting the release of cytochrome c from mitochondria into the cytosol. Studies in cancer cell lines and preclinical models demonstrate that ABT-737 as a single agent can trigger apoptosis in some susceptible cancer types, for example, those that critically depend on Bcl-2 for survival [56]. In addition, ABT-737 sensitize cancer cells for apoptosis when combined with conventional chemotherapeutics [57]. Since ABT-737 targets Bcl-2/Bcl-xL but not Mcl-1, high expression of Mcl-1 may confer resistance to this novel agent. Indeed, several recent reports indicate that Mcl-1 represents a key determinant of ABT-737 sensitivity and resistance in cancer cells [58, 59]. Collectively, these findings suggest that small molecule inhibitors of antiapoptotic Bcl-2 family proteins may open new perspectives to reactivate the mitochondrial pathway of apoptosis in cancer cells.

30.3.2.3 Targeting "Inhibitor of Apoptosis Proteins" (IAPs) for Cancer Therapy

Another promising therapeutic strategy directed at apoptosis regulators is the neutralization of "Inhibitor of Apoptosis Proteins" (IAPs). The family of endogenous caspase inhibitors, IAPs, comprise eight human analogues, XIAP, c-IAP1, c-IAP2, survivin, apollon, livin/melanoma-IAP (ML-IAP), NAIP, and ILP-2 [60]. IAPs have been reported to directly inhibit active caspase-3 and -7 and to block caspase-9 activation [60]. The role of survivin in the regulation of apoptosis and proliferation is more complex compared to other IAP family proteins, since in addition to regulation of apoptosis, survivin is involved in regulation of mitosis [61]. There is mounting evidence that cancer cells have an intrinsic drive to apoptosis that is held in check by IAPs. To this end, high basal levels of caspase-3 and caspase-8 activities and active caspase-3 fragments in the absence of apoptosis were detected in various tumor cell lines and cancer tissues, but not in normal cells [62]. Tumor cells in contrast to normal cells also expressed high levels of IAPs, suggesting that upregulated IAP expression counteracts the high basal caspase activity selectively in tumor cells [62].

Since IAPs are expressed at high levels in the majority of human cancers, they present an attractive molecular target. Consequently, several strategies have been developed to target enhanced expression of IAPs in human malignancies. For the design of therapeutic small molecules directed against XIAP, the binding groove of the BIR3 domain of XIAP, to which Smac binds after its release from the mitochondria, has attracted most attention [63]. Smac peptides that neutralize XIAP through binding to its BIR2 and BIR3 domains were able to promote caspase activation and enhanced TRAIL- or chemotherapy-induced apoptosis. In addition, Smac peptides even substantially increased the antitumor activity of TRAIL *in vivo* in an intracranial malignant glioma xenograft model, resulting in complete eradication of established tumors [64]. Also, XIAP antisense oligonucleotides exhibited potent antitumor activity as a single agent and in combination with clinically relevant chemotherapeutic drugs [65, 66]. Currently, XIAP antisense oligonucleotides are evaluated in phase I/II clinical trials, either as single agents or in combination with chemotherapy in advanced tumors. Thus, Smac agonists, low molecular weight XIAP antagonists, or XIAP antisense oligonucleotides are promising new approaches to either directly engage apoptosis or to lower the threshold for apoptosis induction in cancer cells.

30.4
The Challenge of Today: Defining the Right Patients for the Right Therapeutic Concept

The examples given above illustrate the promising potential of molecular targeted therapy. However, they also illustrate the increasing importance of including molecular diagnosis to achieve an appropriate patient selection for therapy. Increasing attention is being given to the field of pharmacogenomics, which investigates the genetic conditions of patients defining a particular type of response to certain therapeutics [67]. For example, there is increasing evidence that genetic polymorphisms which, under normal conditions, are not relevant for a disease or a phenotype, can significantly modify the response to certain types of therapies, for example, cytochrome p450-dependent substances [67]. Such polymorphisms can also influence the response not only to novel molecular targeted therapies, but also classical chemo- or radiation therapy. Prominent examples for this notion are certain enzymes involved in DNA-repair mechanisms. For example, certain polymorphisms within the XRCC3 gene (X-ray repair cross complementing group 3) have are associated with a significantly longer survival following Cisplatinum/Gemcitabine-based therapy in non-small cell lung cancer, as compared to Cisplatinum/Docetaxel-based therapy. The survival benefit resulting from these polymorphisms was observed especially in young patients with non-small cell lung cancer [68]. The consequence of such a study would be that younger patients with non-small cell lung cancer harboring particular polymorphisms of the *XRCC3* gene would be treated with Cisplatinum/Gemcitabine rather than Cisplatinum/Docetaxel. In another study [69] it was shown that a particular polymorphism of the *ERCC1* gene (excision repair cross complementing group 1), ERCC1-8092A/A, defines particularly poor survival following treatment with Cisplatinum/Docetaxel. ERCC1 is an important enzyme conducting nucleotide-excision DNA repair that is known to remove DNA adducts following Cisplatinum-based therapy. Certain ERCC1 polymorphisms affect ERCC1 expression, and it has been shown that NSCLC patients with low ERCC1 expression respond better to Cisplatinum-based therapy than patients with high ERCC1 expression [70]. For information on DNA-repair diagnostics in lung cancer, see also the Chapter 10 on lung tumors in this book.

These are only two of many recent examples illustrating that genetic polymorphisms within DNA repair relevant for metabolizing DNA changes following particular types of chemotherapy can significantly modify the therapeutic response of tumor patients towards classical therapy concepts. They illustrate that pharmacogenomics will be of increasing importance for optimizing therapeutic compounds towards the individual genetic and molecular conditions of an individual tumor patient in the future. Certainly, novel generations of targeted therapy strategies will also increasingly have to consider particular molecular or genetic variations and changes within patients for further significant improvement of therapy response and survival of cancer patients. Therefore, individual genetic or inherited conditions, which by themselves might not cause disease, will become increasingly important, even for sporadic types of cancers, and for the therapy of tumors with a non-familiar background.

30.5
Conclusion

Over the last two decades the elucidation of molecular conditions, among them signal transduction pathways involved in regulation of tumor growth, cell death in human cancers, or molecular markers of cancer progression, have provided the fundamental basis for the development of molecular targeted therapies. Since such strategies are specifically directed against key components that are crucial for the cancer cell's survival and function, they may be more selective and effective in killing malignant rather than non-malignant cells. While several approaches have already been translated into medical application, many concepts have still to be evaluated in (pre)clinical trials. Another main goal with molecular targeted therapies will be considering appropriate patient selection to enrich for a more responsive population. This will certainly include sporadic as well as inherited molecular conditions that become increasingly elucidated. Eventually, these efforts are expected to yield more effective yet less toxic treatment options for patients suffering from cancer.

Acknowledgments

Work in the authors' laboratory is supported by the Deutsche Forschungsgemeinschaft, the Deutsche Krebshilfe, the Bundesministerium für Forschung und Technologie, Wilhelm-Sander-Stiftung, Else-Kröner-Fresenius Stiftung, the European Community, Inter University Attraction Pole and the Landesstiftung Baden-

Württemberg, the Alfred Krupp von Bohlen und Halbach Stiftung, B. Braun Stiftung, Merck, Darmstadt, Dr Hella Bühler Stiftung, and Dr Ingrid zu Solms Stiftung, Frankfurt.

References

1 Green, J.R. (2004) Bisphosphonates: preclinical review. *Oncologist*, **9** (Suppl 4), 3–13.

2 Green, J.R. (2003) Antitumor effects of bisphosphonates. *Cancer*, **97**, 840–7.

3 Jonathan, R. and Green, M.J.R. (2002) Pharmacologic profile of zoledronic acid: a highly potent inhibitor of bone resorption. *Drug Development Research*, **55**, 210–24.

4 Rogers, M.J., Gordon, S., Benford, H.L., Coxon, F.P., Luckman, S.P., Monkkonen, J. and Frith, J.C. (2000) Cellular and molecular mechanisms of action of bisphosphonates. *Cancer*, **88**, 2961–78.

5 Liu, D., Aguirre Ghiso, J., Estrada, Y. and Ossowski, L. (2002) EGFR is a transducer of the urokinase receptor initiated signal that is required for *in vivo* growth of a human carcinoma. *Cancer Cell*, **1**, 445–57.

6 Festuccia, C., Angelucci, A., Gravina, G.L., Biordi, L., Millimaggi, D., Muzi, P., Vicentini, C. and Bologna, M. (2005) Epidermal growth factor modulates prostate cancer cell invasiveness regulating urokinase-type plasminogen activator activity. EGF-receptor inhibition may prevent tumor cell dissemination. *Journal of Thrombosis and Haemostasis*, **93**, 964–75.

7 Jain, R.K., Duda, D.G., Clark, J.W. and Loeffler, J.S. (2006) Lessons from phase III clinical trials on anti-VEGF therapy for cancer. *Nature Clinical Practice Oncology*, **3**, 24–40.

8 Ranieri, G., Patruno, R., Ruggieri, E., Montemurro, S., Valerio, P. and Ribatti, D. (2006) Vascular endothelial growth factor (VEGF) as a target of bevacizumab in cancer: from the biology to the clinic. *Current Medicinal Chemistry*, **13**, 1845–57.

9 Hurwitz, H., Fehrenbacher, L., Novotny, W., Cartwright, T., Hainsworth, J., Heim, W., Berlin, J., Baron, A., Griffing, S., Holmgren, E., Ferrara, N., Fyfe, G., Rogers, B., Ross, R. and Kabbinavar, F. (2004) Bevacizumab plus irinotecan, fluorouracil, and leucovorin for metastatic colorectal cancer. *New England Journal of Medicine*, **350**, 2335–42.

10 Lund, L.R., Romer, J., Ronne, E., Ellis, V., Blasi, F. and Dano, K. (1991) Urokinase-receptor biosynthesis, mRNA level and gene transcription are increased by transforming growth factor beta 1 in human A549 lung carcinoma cells. *Embo Journal*, **10**, 3399–407.

11 Dumler, I., Petri, T. and Schleuning, W.D. (1994) Induction of *c-fos* gene expression by urokinase-type plasminogen activator in human ovarian cancer cells. *FEBS Letters*, **343**, 103–6.

12 Wang, Y., Kristensen, G.B., Helland, A., Nesland, J.M., Borresen-Dale, A.-L. and Holm, R. (2005) Protein expression and prognostic value of genes in the erb-b signaling pathway in advanced ovarian carcinomas. *American Journal of Clinical Pathology*, **124**, 392–401.

13 Pollack, V.A., Savage, D.M., Baker, D.A., Tsaparikos, K.E., Sloan, D.E., Moyer, J.D., Barbacci, E.G., Pustilnik, L.R., Smolarek, T.A., Davis, J.A., Vaidya, M.P., Arnold, L.D., Doty, J.L., Iwata, K.K. and Morin, M.J. (1999) Inhibition of epidermal growth factor receptor-associated tyrosine phosphorylation in human carcinomas with CP-358,774: dynamics of receptor inhibition *in situ* and antitumor effects in athymic mice. *The Journal of Pharmacology and Experimental Therapeutics*, **291**, 739–48.

14 Akita, R.W. and Sliwkowski, M.X. (2003) Preclinical studies with Erlotinib (Tarceva). *Seminars in Oncology*, **30**, 15–24.

15 Moyer, J.D., Barbacci, E.G., Iwata, K.K., Arnold, L., Boman, B., Cunningham, A., DiOrio, C., Doty, J., Morin, M.J., Moyer, M.P., Neveu, M., Pollack, V.A.,

Pustilnik, L.R., Reynolds, M.M., Sloan, D., Theleman, A. and Miller, P. (1997) Induction of apoptosis and cell cycle arrest by CP-358,774, an inhibitor of epidermal growth factor receptor tyrosine kinase. *Cancer Research*, **57**, 4838–48.

16 Mendelsohn, J. (2006) Targeting the EGF receptor: experience and lessons. *European Journal of Cancer Supplements*, **4**, 25–6.

17 Schlessinger, J. (2006) Cell signaling by receptor tyrosine kinases: From basic concepts to clinical applications. *European Journal of Cancer Supplements*, **4**, 3.

18 Schlessinger, J. (2004) Common and distinct elements in cellular signaling via EGF and FGF receptors. *Science*, **306**, 1506–7.

19 Fleishman, S.J., Schlessinger, J. and Ben-Tal, N. (2002) A putative molecular-activation switch in the transmembrane domain of erbBIX2. *Proceedings of the National Academy of Sciences of the United States of America*, **99**, 15937–40.

20 Schlessinger, J. (2003) Signal trans-duction. Autoinhibition control. *Science*, **300**, 750–2.

21 Klein, P., Mattoon, D., Lemmon, M.A. and Schlessinger, J. (2004) A structure-based model for ligand binding and dimerization of EGF receptors. *Proceedings of the National Academy of Sciences of the United States of America*, **101**, 929–34.

22 Schlessinger, J. (2002) Ligand-induced, receptor-mediated dimerization and activation of EGF receptor. *Cell*, **110**, 669–72.

23 Lax, I., Wong, A., Lamothe, B., Lee, A., Frost, A., Hawes, J. and Schlessinger, J. (2002) The docking protein FRS2alpha controls a MAP kinase-mediated negative feedback mechanism for signaling by FGF receptors. *Molecular Cell*, **10**, 709–19.

24 Reinmuth, N., Meister, M., Muley, T., Steins, M., Kreuter, M., Herth, F.J.F., Hoffmann, H., Dienemann, H. and Thomas, M. (2006) Molecular deter-minants of response to RTK-targeting agents in nonsmall cell lung cancer. *International Journal of Cancer*, **119**, 727–34.

25 Thatcher, N. (2006) The ISEL and BR21 trials – outcomes similar or different? *European Journal of Cancer Supplements*, **4**, 23–4.

26 Thatcher, N., Chang, A., Parikh, P., Rodrigues Pereira, J., Ciuleanu, T., von Pawel, J., Thongprasert, S., Tan, E.H., Pemberton, K., Archer, V. and Carroll, K. (2005) Gefitinib plus best supportive care in previously treated patients with refractory advanced non-small-cell lung cancer: results from a randomised, placebo-controlled, multicentre study (Iressa Survival Evaluation in Lung Cancer). *Lancet*, **366**, 1527–37.

27 Shepherd, F.A., Rodrigues Pereira, J., Ciuleanu, T., Tan, E.H., Hirsh, V., Thongprasert, S., Campos, D., Maoleekoonpiroj, S., Smylie, M., Martins, R., van Kooten, M., Dediu, M., Findlay, B., Tu, D., Johnston, D., Bezjak, A., Clark, G., Santabarbara, P., Seymour, L. and National Cancer Institute of Canada Clinical Trials (2005) Erlotinib in previously treated non-small-cell lung cancer. *New England Journal of Medicine*, **353**, 123–32.

28 Blackhall, F., Ranson, M. and Thatcher, N. (2006) Where next for gefitinib in patients with lung cancer? *The Lancet Oncology*, **7**, 499–507.

29 Hirsch, F.R. (2006) The role of EGFR family in preneoplasia and lung cancer. Perspectives for targeted therapies and selection of patients. *European Journal of Cancer Supplements*, **4**, 13–14.

30 Van Zandwijk, N., Mathy, A., De Jong, D., Baas, P., Burgers, S. and Nederlof, P. (2006) Impact of epidermal growth factor receptor (EGFR) mutations on responsiveness of non-small cell lung cancer (NSCLC) to tyrosine kinase inhibitors (TKIs): Prospective observations. *European Journal of Cancer Supplements*, **4**, 14–15.

31 Pao, W., Miller, V., Zakowski, M., Doherty, J., Politi, K., Sarkaria, I., Singh, B., Heelan, R., Rusch, V., Fulton, L., Mardis, E., Kupfer, D., Wilson, R., Kris, M. and Varmus, H. (2004) EGF receptor gene mutations are common in lung cancers from "never smokers" and are associated with sensitivity of tumors to gefitinib and erlotinib. *Proceedings of the National*

Academy of Sciences of the United States of America, **101**, 13306–11.

32 Cappuzzo, F., Hirsch, F.R., Rossi, E., Bartolini, S., Ceresoli, G.L., Bemis, L., Haney, J., Witta, S., Danenberg, K., Domenichini, I., Ludovini, V., Magrini, E., Gregorc, V., Doglioni, C., Sidoni, A., Tonato, M., Franklin, W.A., Crino, L., Bunn, P.A. Jr and Varella-Garcia, M. (2005) Epidermal growth factor receptor gene and protein and gefitinib sensitivity in non-small-cell lung cancer. *Journal of the National Cancer Institute*, **97**, 643–55.

33 Hirsch, F.R., Varella-Garcia, M., McCoy, J., West, H., Xavier, A.C., Gumerlock, P., Bunn, P.A. Jr, Franklin, W.A., Crowley, J., Gandara, D.R. (2005) Increased epidermal growth factor receptor gene copy number detected by fluorescence in situ hybridization associates with increased sensitivity to gefitinib in patients with bronchioloalveolar carcinoma subtypes: a Southwest Oncology Group Study. *Journal of Clinical Oncology*, **23**, 6838–45.

34 Tsao, M.-S., Sakurada, A., Cutz, J.-C., Zhu, C.-Q., Kamel-Reid, S., Squire, J., Lorimer, I., Zhang, T., Liu, N., Daneshmand, M., Marrano, P., Santos, G., Lagarde, A., Richardson, F., Seymour, L., Whitehead, M., Ding, K., Pater, J. and Shepherd, F.A. (2005) Erlotinib in lung cancer–molecular and clinical predictors of outcome. *New England Journal of Medicine*, **353**, 133–44.

35 Hirsch, F.R., Varella-Garcia, M., Bunn, P.A. Jr, Franklin, W.A., Dziadziuszko, R., Thatcher, N., Chang, A., Parikh, P., Pereira, J.R., Ciuleanu, T., von Pawel, J., Watkins, C., Flannery, A., Ellison, G., Donald, E., Knight, L., Parums, D., Botwood, N. and Holloway, B. (2006) Molecular predictors of outcome with gefitinib in a phase III placebo-controlled study in advanced non-small-cell lung cancer. *Journal of Clinical Oncology*, **24**, 5034–42.

36 Hengartner, M.O. (2000) The biochemistry of apoptosis. *Nature*, **407**, 770–6.

37 Evan, G.I. and Vousden, K.H. (2001) Proliferation, cell cycle and apoptosis in cancer. *Nature*, **411**, 342–8.

38 Lowe, S.W. and Lin, A.W. (2000) Apoptosis in cancer. *Carcinogenesis*, **21**, 485–95.

39 Makin, G. and Dive, C. (2001) Apoptosis and cancer chemotherapy. *Trends in Cell Biology*, **11**, S22–26.

40 Fulda, S. and Debatin, K.M. (2006) Extrinsic versus intrinsic apoptosis pathways in anticancer chemotherapy. *Oncogene*, **25**, 4798–811.

41 Degterev, A., Boyce, M. and Yuan, J. (2003) A decade of caspases. *Oncogene*, **22**, 8543–67.

42 Walczak, H. and Krammer, P.H. (2000) The CD95 (APO-1/Fas) and the TRAIL (APO-2L) apoptosis systems. *Experimental Cell Research*, **256**, 58–66.

43 Adams, J.M. and Cory, S. (2007) The Bcl-2 apoptotic switch in cancer development and therapy. *Oncogene*, **26**, 1324–37.

44 Saelens, X., Festjens, N., Van de Walle, L., van Gurp, M., van Loo, G. and Vandenabeele, P. (2004) Toxic proteins released from mitochondria in cell death. *Oncogene*, **23**, 2861–74.

45 Johnstone, R.W., Ruefli, A.A. and Lowe, S.W. (2002) Apoptosis: a link between cancer genetics and chemotherapy. *Cell*, **108**, 153–64.

46 Ashkenazi, A. (2002) Targeting death and decoy receptors of the tumour-necrosis factor superfamily. *Nature Reviews Cancer*, **2**, 420–30.

47 Krammer, P.H. (2000) CD95's deadly mission in the immune system. *Nature*, **407**, 789–95.

48 LeBlanc, H.N. and Ashkenazi, A. (2003) Apo2L/TRAIL and its death and decoy receptors. *Cell Death and Differentiation*, **10**, 66–75.

49 Chuntharapai, A., Dodge, K., Grimmer, K., Schroeder, K., Marsters, S.A., Koeppen, H., Ashkenazi, A. and Kim, K.J. (2001) Isotype-dependent inhibition of tumor growth *in vivo* by monoclonal antibodies to death receptor 4. *Journal of Immunology*, **166**, 4891–8.

50 Ichikawa, K., Liu, W., Zhao, L., Wang, Z., Liu, D., Ohtsuka, T., Zhang, H., Mountz, J.D., Koopman, W.J., Kimberly, R.P. and Zhou, T. (2001) Tumoricidal activity of a novel anti-human DR5 monoclonal antibody without hepatocyte cytotoxicity. *Nature Medicine*, **7**, 954–60.

51 Takeda, K., Yamaguchi, N., Akiba, H., Kojima, Y., Hayakawa, Y., Tanner, J.E., Sayers, T.J., Seki, N., Okumura, K., Yagita, H. and Smyth, M.J. (2004) Induction of tumor-specific T cell immunity by anti-DR5 antibody therapy. *The Journal of Experimental Medicine*, **199**, 437–48.

52 Gliniak, B. and Le, T. (1999) Tumor necrosis factor-related apoptosis-inducing ligand's antitumor activity *in vivo* is enhanced by the chemotherapeutic agent CPT-11. *Cancer Research*, **59**, 6153–8.

53 Chinnaiyan, A.M., Prasad, U., Shankar, S., Hamstra, D.A., Shanaiah, M., Chenevert, T.L., Ross, B.D. and Rehemtulla, A. (2000) Combined effect of tumor necrosis factor-related apoptosis-inducing ligand and ionizing radiation in breast cancer therapy. *Proceedings of the National Academy of Sciences of the United States of America*, **97**, 1754–9.

54 Letai, A., Bassik, M.C., Walensky, L.D., Sorcinelli, M.D., Weiler, S. and Korsmeyer, S.J. (2002) Distinct BH3 domains either sensitize or activate mitochondrial apoptosis, serving as prototype cancer therapeutics. *Cancer Cell*, **2**, 183–92.

55 Willis, S.N., Fletcher, J.I., Kaufmann, T., van Delft, M.F., Chen, L., Czabotar, P.E., Ierino, H., Lee, E.F., Fairlie, W.D., Bouillet, P., Strasser, A., Kluck, R.M., Adams, J.M. and Huang, D.C. (2007) Apoptosis initiated when BH3 ligands engage multiple Bcl-2 homologs, not Bax or Bak. *Science*, **315**, 856–9.

56 Oltersdorf, T., Elmore, S.W., Shoemaker, A.R., Armstrong, R.C., Augeri, D.J., Belli, B.A., Bruncko, M., Deckwerth, T.L., Dinges, J., Hajduk, P.J., Joseph, M.K., Kitada, S., Korsmeyer, S.J., Kunzer, A.R., Letai, A., Li, C., Mitten, M.J., Nettesheim, D.G., Ng, S., Nimmer, P.M., O'Connor, J.M., Oleksijew, A., Petros, A. M., Reed, J.C., Shen, W., Tahir, S.K., Thompson, C.B., Tomaselli, K.J., Wang, B., Wendt, M.D., Zhang, H., Fesik, S.W. and Rosenberg, S.H. (2005) An inhibitor of Bcl-2 family proteins induces regression of solid tumours. *Nature*, **435**, 677–81.

57 Shoemaker, A.R., Oleksijew, A., Bauch, J., Belli, B.A., Borre, T., Bruncko, M., Deckwirth, T., Frost, D.J., Jarvis, K., Joseph, M.K., Marsh, K., McClellan, W., Nellans, H., Ng, S., Nimmer, P., O'Connor, J.M., Oltersdorf, T., Qing, W., Shen, W., Stavropoulos, J., Tahir, S.K., Wang, B., Warner, R., Zhang, H., Fesik, S.W., Rosenberg, S.H. and Elmore, S.W. (2006) A small-molecule inhibitor of Bcl-XL potentiates the activity of cytotoxic drugs *in vitro* and *in vivo*. *Cancer Research*, **66**, 8731–9.

58 Konopleva, M., Contractor, R., Tsao, T., Samudio, I., Ruvolo, P.P., Kitada, S., Deng, X., Zhai, D., Shi, Y.-X., Sneed, T., Verhaegen, M., Soengas, M., Ruvolo, V.R., McQueen, T., Schober, W.D., Watt, J.C., Jiffar, T., Ling, X., Marini, F.C., Harris, D., Dietrich, M., Estrov, Z., McCubrey, J., May, W.S., Reed, J.C. and Andreeff, M. (2006) Mechanisms of apoptosis sensitivity and resistance to the BH3 mimetic ABT-737 in acute myeloid leukemia. *Cancer Cell*, **10**, 375–88.

59 Van Delft, M.F., Wei, A.H., Mason, K.D., Vandenberg, C.J., Chen, L., Czabotar, P.E., Willis, S.N., Scott, C.L., Day, C.L., Cory, S., Adams, J.M., Roberts, A.W. and Huang, D.C.S. (2006) The BH3 mimetic ABT-737 targets selective Bcl-2 proteins and efficiently induces apoptosis via Bak/Bax if Mcl-1 is neutralized. *Cancer Cell*, **10**, 389–99.

60 Salvesen, G.S. and Duckett, C.S. (2002) IAP proteins: blocking the road to death's door. *Nature Reviews Molecular Cell Biology*, **3**, 401–10.

61 Altieri, D.C. (2003) Validating survivin as a cancer therapeutic target. *Nature Reviews Cancer*, **3**, 46–54.

62 Yang, L., Cao, Z., Yan, H. and Wood, W.C. (2003) Coexistence of high levels of apoptotic signaling and inhibitor of apoptosis proteins in human tumor cells: implication for cancer specific therapy. *Cancer Research*, **63**, 6815–24.

63 Shiozaki, E.N. and Shi, Y. (2004) Caspases, IAPs and Smac/DIABLO: mechanisms from structural biology. *Trends in Biochemical Sciences*, **29**, 486–94.

64 Fulda, S., Wick, W., Weller, M. and Debatin, K.M. (2002) Smac agonists sensitize for Apo2L/TRAIL- or anticancer drug-induced apoptosis and induce regression of malignant glioma *in vivo*. *Nature Medicine*, **8**, 808–15.

65 LaCasse, E.C., Kandimalla, E.R., Winocour, P., Sullivan, T., Agrawal, S., Gillard, J.W. and Durkin, J. (2005) Application of XIAP antisense to cancer and other proliferative disorders: development of AEG35156/ GEM640. *Annals of the New York Academy of Sciences*, **1058**, 215–34.

66 LaCasse, E.C., Cherton-Horvat, G.G., Hewitt, K.E., Jerome, L.J., Morris, S.J., Kandimalla, E.R., Yu, D., Wang, H., Wang, W., Zhang, R., Agrawal, S., Gillard, J.W. and Durkin, J.P. (2006) Preclinical characterization of AEG35156/GEM 640, a second-generation antisense oligonucleotide targeting X-linked inhibitor of apoptosis. *Clinical Cancer Research*, **12**, 5231–41.

67 Tribut, O., Lessard, Y., Reymann, J.-M., Allain, H. and Bentue-Ferrer, D. (2002) Pharmacogenomics. *Medical Science Monitor*, **8**, RA152–63.

68 Rosell-Costa, R., Alberola, V., Camps, C., Lopez-Vivanco, G., Moran, T., Etxaniz, O., De Las Peñas, R., Gupta, J., Taron, M. and Sanchez, J. (2006) Clinical outcome of gemcitabine (gem)/cisplatin (cis)-vs docetaxel (doc)/cis-treated stage IV non-small cell lung cancer (NSCLC) patients (p) according to X-ray repair cross-complementing group 3 (XRCC3)

polymorphism and age. *Journal of Clinical Oncology*, **24**, 7055.

69 Taron, M., Alberola, V., Lopez Vivanco, G., Camps, C., De Las Penas, R., Alonso, G., Provencio, M., Salvatierra, A., Sanchez, J. and Rosell, R. (2006) Excision cross-complementing group 1 (ERCC1) single nucleotide polymorphisms (SNPs) and survival in cisplatin (cis)/docetaxel (doc)-treated stage IV non-small cell lung cancer (NSCLC) patients (p): A Spanish Lung Cancer Group study. *Journal of Clinical Oncology*, **24**, 7053.

70 Olaussen, K.A., Dunant, A., Fouret, P., Brambilla, E., Andre, F., Haddad, V., Taranchon, E., Filipits, M., Pirker, R., Popper, H.H., Stahel, R., Sabatier, L., Pignon, J.-P., Tursz, T., Le Chevalier, T., Soria, J.-C. and Investigators, I.B. (2006) DNA repair by ERCC1 in non-small-cell lung cancer and cisplatin-based adjuvant chemotherapy. *New England Journal of Medicine*, **355**, 983–91.

71 Sobrero, A.F., Maurel, J., Fehrenbacher, L., Scheithauer, W., Abubakr, Y.A., Lutz, M.P., Vega-Villegas, M.E., Eng, C., Steinhauer, E.U., Prausova, J., Lenz, H.-J., Borg, C., Middleton, G., Kröning, H.K., Luppi, G., Kisker, O., Zubel, A., Langer, C., Kopit, J. and Burris, III H.A. (2008) EPIC:Phase-III trial of cetuximab plus irinotecan after fluoropyrimidine and oxaliplatin failure in patients with metastatic colorectal cancer. *J Clin Oncol*, **26** (*14*), 2311–19.

Index

Hereditary Tumors: From Genes to Clinical Consequences
Edited by Heike Allgayer, Helga Rehder and Simone Fulda
Copyright © 2009 WILEY-VCH Verlag GmbH & Co. KGaA, Weinheim
ISBN: 978-3-527-32028-8